Fundamental Principles of Veterinary Anesthesia

Fundamental Principles of Veterinary Anesthesia

Edited by

Gareth E. Zeiler
Valley Farm Animal Hospital, Pretoria
and
University of Pretoria
South Africa

Daniel S.J. Pang
University of Calgary
Canada

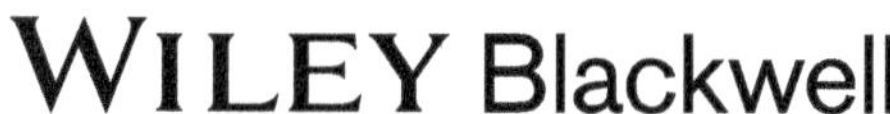

This edition first published 2024

Registered Office
John Wiley & Sons, Inc., 111 River Street, Hoboken, NJ 07030, USA

For details of our global editorial offices, customer services, and more information about Wiley products visit us at www.wiley.com.

Wiley also publishes its books in a variety of electronic formats and by print-on-demand. Some content that appears in standard print versions of this book may not be available in other formats.

A catalogue record for this book is available from the Library of Congress

Paperback ISBN: 9781119791249; ePub ISBN: 9781119791270; ePDF ISBN: 9781119791300

Cover Images: © Vlad Klok/Shutterstock Gareth E. Zeiler -
Author Provided Image © Igor Djurovic/iStock/Getty Images
Cover Design: Wiley

Set in 9.5/12.5pt STIXTwoText by Integra Software Services Pvt. Ltd, Pondicherry, India

SKY10065181_011724

To BJZ and SJZ for their patience, understanding, and encouragement during the creation of this textbook, and to all my colleagues (especially LB, GFS, BTD, LCRM, and ERG) who taught me anesthesia and scientific writing, completed research projects together, and helped train the next generation in anesthesia. What a ride!

Gareth Zeiler

To J, for her support, kindness, and patience, and to all the clinicians, researchers, technicians, and residents who have taught me the art and science of anesthesia (DF, SC, ET, YR, NF, JL, CB, JK, GD, FRB, and MR).

Daniel Pang

Contents

Contributors

This textbook was written by 27 authors from nine countries with a range of different specializations and working at university hospitals or in private practice.

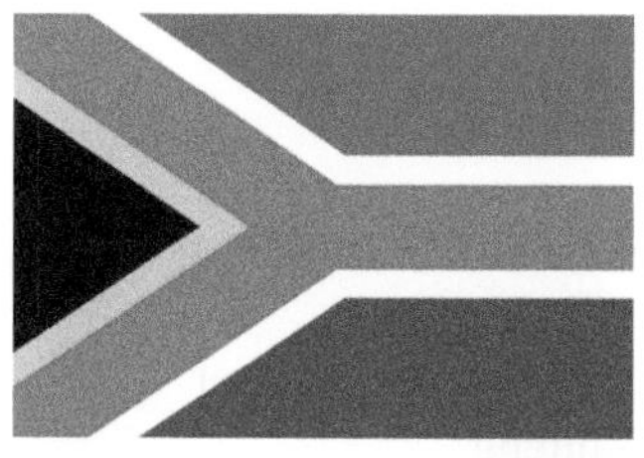

Abdur R. Kadwa
BSc (Vet Bio), BVSc, MMedVet (Anaesthesiology), Diplomate ECVAA
Senior Lecturer
Affiliation 1: Department of Companion Animal Clinical Studies, Faculty of Veterinary Science, University of Pretoria

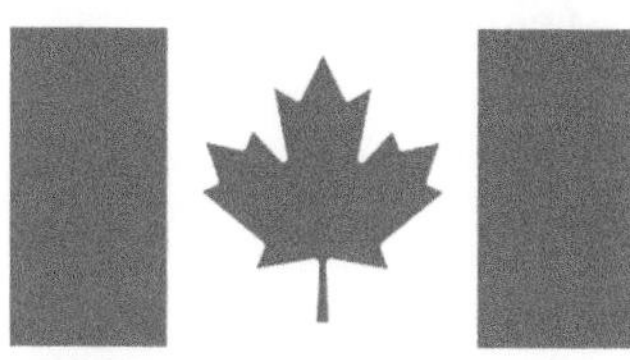

Alicia M. Skelding
BScAgr, DVM, MSc, DVSc, Diplomate ACVAA
Assistant Professor, Veterinary Anesthesia
Affiliation 1: Michigan State University College of Veterinary Medicine

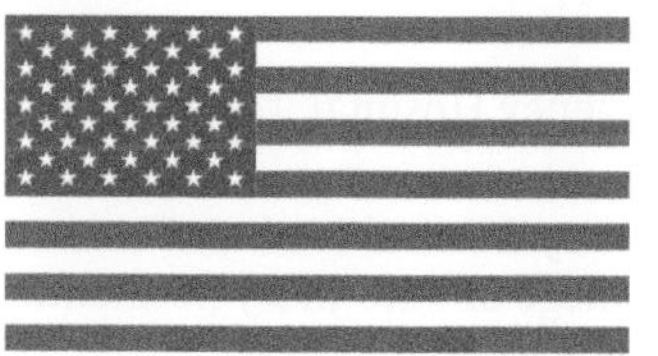

Benjamin M. Brainard
VMD, Diplomate ACVAA, Diplomate ACVECC
Edward H Gunst Professor of Small Animal Critical Care and Director of Clinical Research
Affiliation 1: College of Veterinary Medicine, University of Georgia

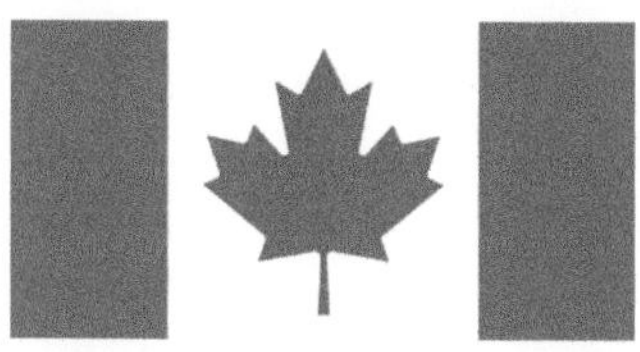

Carolyn Kerr
DVM, DVSc, PhD, Diplomate ACVAA
Professor
Affiliation 1: Department of Clinical Studies, Ontario Veterinary College, University of Guelph

Chantal McMillan
DVM, MVSc, Diplomate ACVIM
Senior Instructor
Affiliation 1: Faculty of Veterinary Medicine, University of Calgary

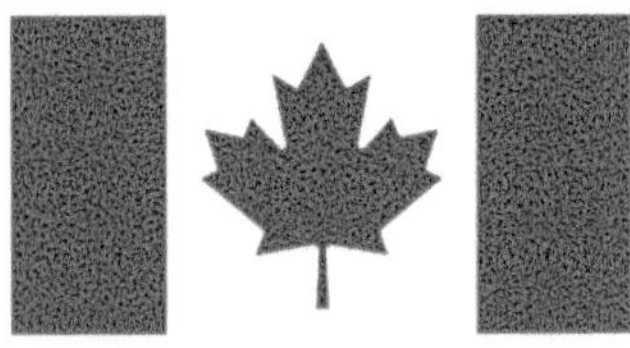

Daniel S. J. Pang
BVSc, PhD, Diplomate ACVAA, Diplomate ECVAA FRCVS
Professor
Affiliation 1: Faculty of Veterinary Medicine, University of Calgary
Affiliation 2: Department of Clinical Sciences, Faculty of Veterinary Medicine, Université de Montréal

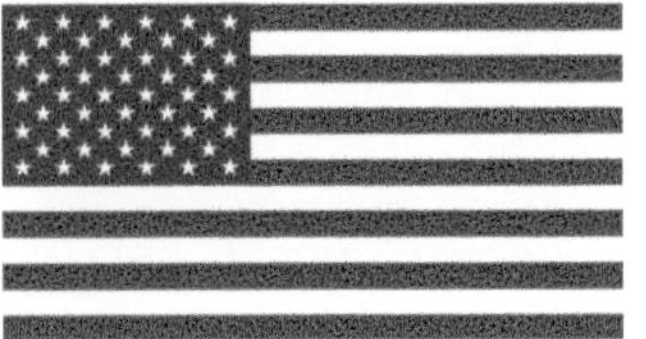

Eugene P. Steffey
VMD, PhD, Diplomate ACVAA, Diplomate ECVAA (retired)
Emeritus Professor (University of California, Davis)
Affiliation 1: Department of Surgical and Radiological Sciences, University of California, Davis
Affiliation 2: Department of Clinical Sciences, College of Veterinary Medicine and Biomedical Sciences, Colorado State University

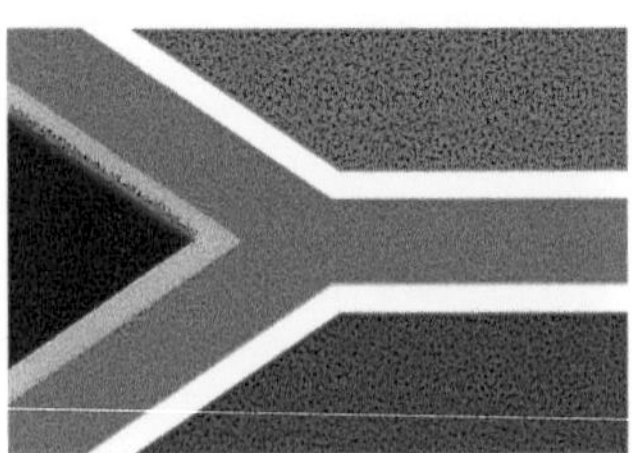

Gareth E. Zeiler
BVSc (Hons), MMedVet (Anaesthesiology), PhD (UP), PhD (WITS), Diplomate ECVAA, Diplomate ACVAA, Diplomate ECVECC
Head of Anaesthesia and Critical Care Services and Extraordinary Lecturer
Affiliation 1: Valley Farm Animal Hospital, Pretoria, Gauteng
Affiliation 2: Department of Companion Animal Clinical Studies, Faculty of Veterinary Science, University of Pretoria

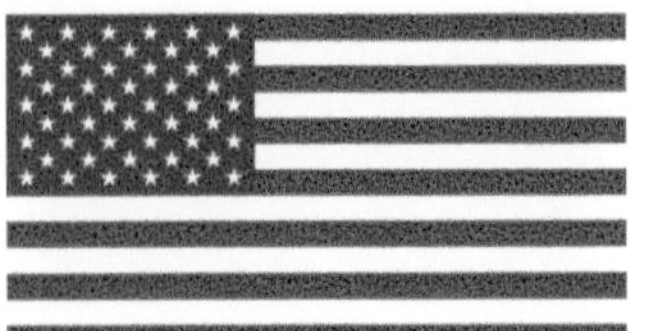

H. Nicole Trenholme
DVM, MS, Diplomate ACVECC, Diplomate ACVAA
Medical director, Head of services for emergency and critical care as well as anesthesia
Affiliation 1: Evolution Veterinary Specialty and Emergency Hospital, Lakewood, CO, United States
Affiliation 2: Adjunct Professor, Department of Veterinary Clinical Medicine and Veterinary Teaching Hospital, University of Illinois College of Veterinary Medicine

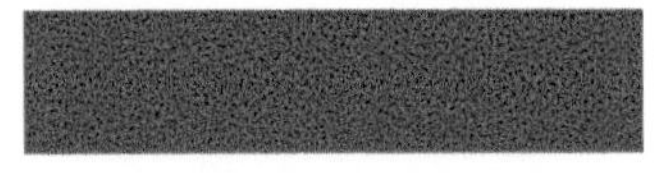

Hugo van Oostrom
DVM, PhD, Diplomate ECVAA
Head of Anaesthesia Services
Affiliation 1: IVC Evidensia The Netherlands

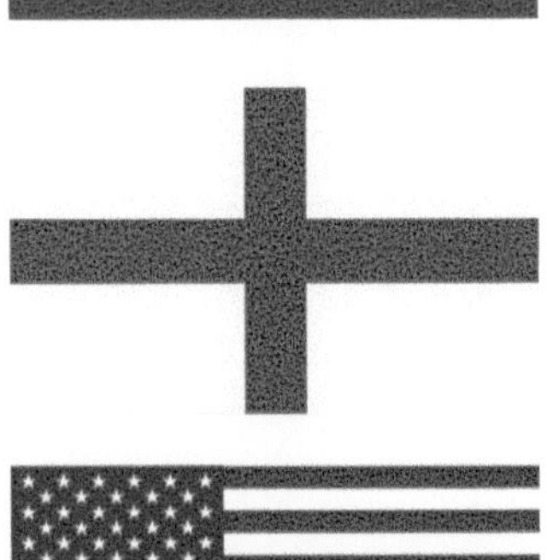

Jo Murrell
BVSc (hons), PhD, Diplomate ECVAA, MRCVS
Clinical Anesthesiologist
Affiliation 1: Highcroft Veterinary Referrals

John A.E. Hubbell
DVM, MSc, Diplomate ACVAA
Chief of Anesthesia Service and Emeritus Professor
Affiliation 1: Rood and Riddle Equine Hospital
Affiliation 2: Department of Veterinary Clinical Sciences, College of Veterinary Medicine, The Ohio State University

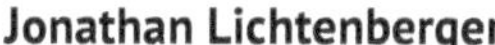

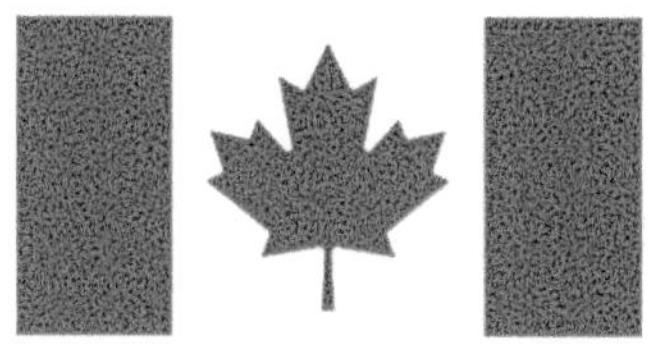

Jonathan Lichtenberger
DVM, MSc, Diplomate ACVIM (Cardiology)
Board-certified Veterinary Cardiologist and Founder of Pacific Coast Veterinary Cardiology
Affiliation 1: Pacific Coast Veterinary Cardiology

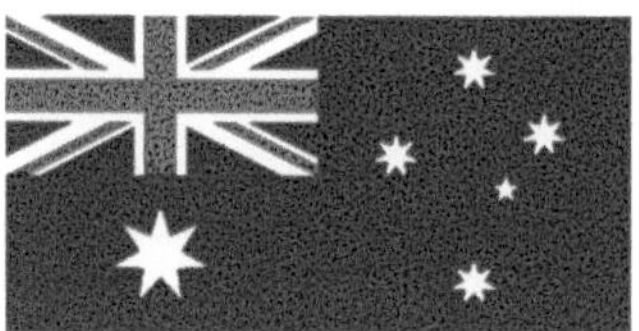

Justin F. Grace
BVSc, MMedVet (Anaesthesiology), MRCVS
Senior Lecturer
Affiliation 1: Sydney School of Veterinary Science, University of Sydney 2006, Australia
Affiliation 2: Department of Companion Animal Clinical Studies, Faculty of Veterinary Science, University of Pretoria

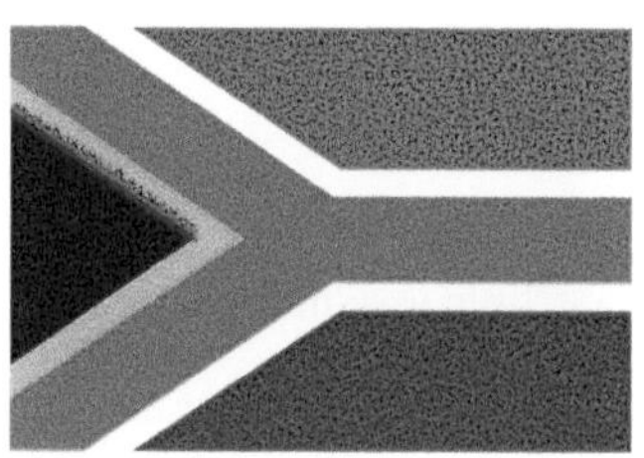

Keagan J. Boustead
BVSc, MSc, Diplomate ECVAA
Clinical Anesthesiologist
Affiliation 1: Westville Veterinary Hospital, Durban, KwaZulu Natal
Affiliation 2: Department of Companion Animal Clinical Studies, Faculty of Veterinary Science, University of Pretoria

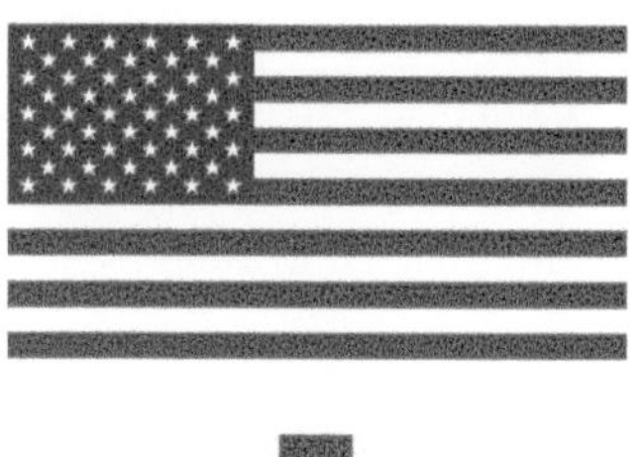

Khursheed Mama
DVM, Diplomate ACVAA
Professor
Affiliation 1: Department of Clinical Sciences, College of Veterinary Medicine and Biomedical Sciences, Colorado State University

Matthew Gurney
BVSc, CertVA, PgCertVBM, Diplomate ECVAA, FRCVS
Anesthesiologist
Affiliation 1: Anderson Moores Veterinary Specialists
Affiliation 2: The Zero Pain Philosophy

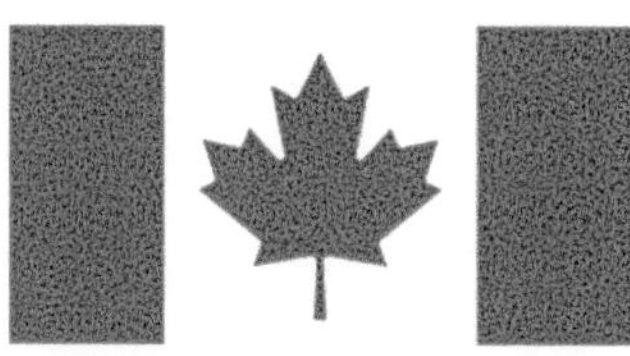

Nigel Caulkett
DVM, MVetSci, Diplomate ACVAA
Professor
Affiliation 1: Faculty of Veterinary Medicine, University of Calgary

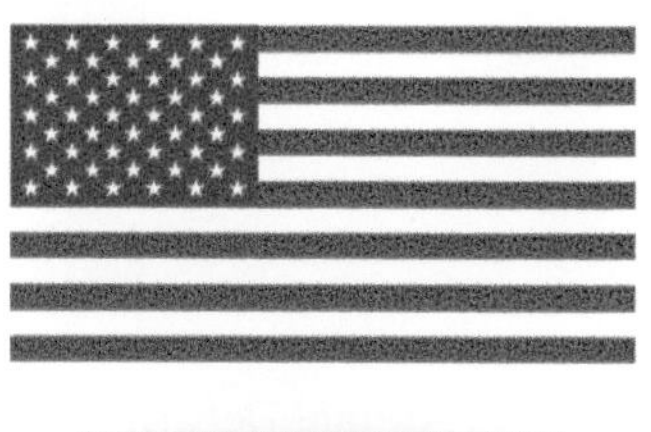

Nora Matthews
DVM, Diplomate ACVAA
Emeritus Professor
Affiliation 1: Department of Small Animal Clinical Sciences, College of Veterinary Medicine and Biomedical Sciences, Texas A&M University

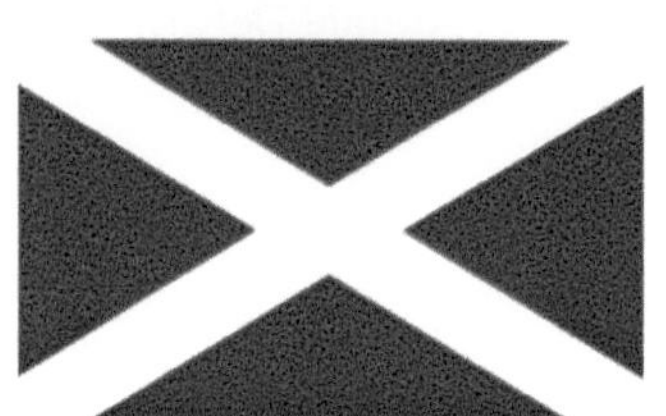

Pamela J. Murison
BVMs, PhD, Diplomate ECVAA, DVA, FHEA, MRCVS
Professor
Affiliation 1: School of Biodiversity, One Health and Veterinary Medicine, University of Glasgow

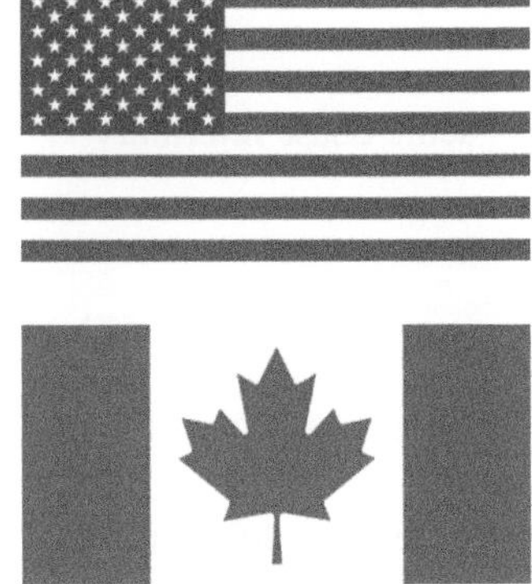

Robert E. Meyer
DVM, Diplomate ACVAA (Emeritus)
Emeritus Professor
Affiliation 1: Department of Clinical Sciences, College of Veterinary Medicine, Mississippi State University

Roxanne K. Buck
BVSc, MSc, MMedVet (Anaesthesiology), PhD, Diplomate ECVAA
Clinical Anesthesiologist
Affiliation 1: Department of Clinical Studies, Ontario Veterinary College, University of Guelph
Affiliation 2: Department of Companion Animal Clinical Studies, Faculty of Veterinary Science, University of Pretoria

Sabine B.R. Kästner
Prof. Dr. Med. Vet., MVetSci, Diplomate ECVAA
Professor
Affiliation 1: Department of Anaesthesia and Analgesia, Clinic for Small Animals, University of Veterinary Medicine Hannover

Samantha Swisher
DVM, MPH, DABVP (Exotic Companion Mammal), DACVPM
Exotic companion mammal specialist and resident in veterinary public health
Affiliation 1: Department of Veterinary Preventive Medicine, The Ohio State University College of Veterinary Medicine

Stijn Schauvliege
DVM, PhD, Diplomate ECVAA
Associate Professor
Affiliation 1: Department of Large Animal Surgery, Anaesthesia and Orthopaedics, Faculty of Veterinary Medicine, Ghent University

Tamara Grubb
DVM, PhD, Diplomate ACVAA
Anesthesiologist
Affiliation 1: International Veterinary Academy of Pain Management (President-Elect)
Affiliation 2: Veterinary Anesthesia, Analgesia and Continuing Education Services

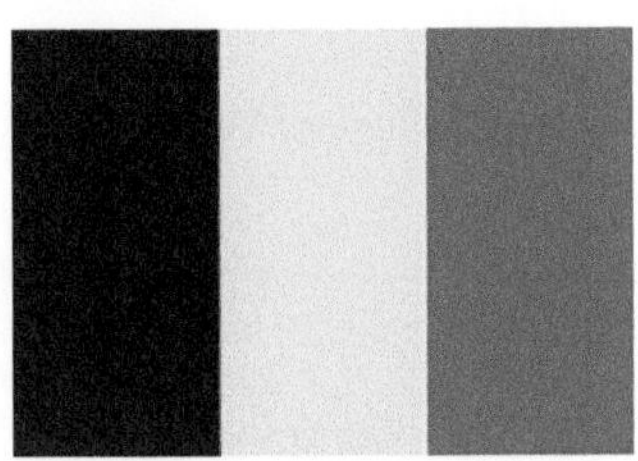

Tim Bosmans
DVM, PhD
Anesthesiologist
Affiliation 1: Section of Anaesthesiology and Analgesia, Small Animal Department, Faculty of Veterinary Medicine, Ghent University

Preface

Providing anesthesia with appropriate patient care, including pre-anesthetic assessment, stabilization (as necessary), monitoring and management of physiologic variables, and a smooth recovery, is a fundamental skill, essential to facilitate a wide range of procedures. Nonetheless, we are aware that anesthesia can be daunting when faced with the many options available for drugs and equipment, and specific patient and procedure considerations.

Our goal in this book is to provide practical, accessible guidance on how to anesthetize frequently encountered companion, farm, and exotic species. We hope that it proves useful to veterinarians in general practice, those in their final years of veterinary study, and veterinary technicians (nurses). The material presented is intended to support and complement content covered in veterinary anesthesia courses and veterinary technician training. We are particularly pleased with the large number of figures presented in support of the text and complementary online resources.

Chapters are organized to cover general considerations applicable to all patients, with species-specific chapters describing anesthetic approaches in healthy and sick animals. Each chapter ends with questions to test the reader's knowledge and understanding, with more questions available online.

As this is not intended to be an exhaustive reference textbook, we have intentionally limited lists of references to key articles for interested readers or to highlight more controversial areas.

We are indebted to the many co-authors who made this book possible. They have been generous in sharing their knowledge, experience and expertise, and have been patient with our many questions and numerous revisions as we strove to create the book we envisioned.

Every effort has been made to confirm accuracy of the text.

Gareth Zeiler and Daniel Pang

Glossary

Analgesia is defined as the inability to feel pain (https://www.iasp-pain.org/resources/terminology).

Anesthesia (as in general anesthesia) is defined as a state of drug-induced, controlled, and temporary loss of awareness that is induced for medical purposes.

Anesthetist is the person managing the anesthetic. This includes one or more of the following: administering the anesthetic, monitoring the patient, recording monitored variables, and providing analgesia. An anesthetist could be a veterinarian or a veterinary technician in the context of veterinary anesthesia. Note: The role of technicians will vary according to local regulations.

Anesthesiologist, though not strictly defined, it is generally accepted that the term is restricted to a veterinarian, and it is often, though not always, assumed that they have achieved specialist status, as recognized by their country's veterinary professional body or by a specialty college.

Anxiolysis is defined as the reduction of anxiety.

Induction of general anesthesia describes the transition from a conscious state to an unconsciousness state (general anesthesia, as defined earlier).

Local anesthesia is defined as administering a local anesthetic drug, using various techniques, to induce the absence of sensation in a specific part of the animal's body. Generally, the aim of inducing local anesthesia is to provide a local insensitivity to pain but often other local senses (feeling of sensations such as touch, heat, pressure, etc.) may also be lost.

Maintenance of general anesthesia is the phase of the anesthetic during which a stable plane of anesthesia and analgesia is maintained, and physiologic variables are ideally maintained within species-specific reference intervals to preserve optimal respiratory and hemodynamic stability.

Nociception is defined as the neural process of encoding noxious stimuli. The encoding may be autonomic (e.g., elevated blood pressure) or behavioral (e.g., motor withdrawal reflex). A sensation of pain is not necessarily implied (https://www.iasp-pain.org/resources/terminology).

Pain is an unpleasant sensory and emotional experience associated with, or resembling that associated with, actual or potential tissue damage. An inability to communicate does not negate the possibility that an animal is experiencing pain (https://www.iasp-pain.org/resources/terminology).

Premedication is when drugs are administered alone, or in combination, to the patient before induction of general anesthesia. A sufficient time is necessary for these drugs to take effect before induction. This time period is typically around 15–20 min following intramuscular administration.

Recovery comprises the period from the end of anesthesia (stopping delivery of anesthetic drugs) to the return of consciousness and recovery of physiologic function.

Sedation describes a drug-induced decreased level of consciousness, from an awake state to a sleepy, but rousable, state.

About the Companion Website

This book is accompanied by a companion website which includes a number of resources created by author for students and instructors that you will find helpful.

www.wiley.com/go/VeterinaryAnesthesiaZeiler

The Instructor website includes the following resources for each chapter:

- Extra questions and answers
- PowerPoint presentation templates
- Figures of the textbook

Section 1

Foundational Knowledge

1

Veterinary Anesthesia

Gareth Zeiler and Daniel Pang

Introduction to Veterinary Anesthesia

Veterinary anesthesia is a fundamental discipline within the broad field of veterinary medicine that deals with anesthesia (local and general) and analgesia of all animals. Many aspects of veterinary anesthesia directly relate to the aims of an oath of ethics (oaths or credos are country dependent) that a veterinarian or veterinary technician (nurse) must take before being allowed to practice veterinary medicine. An example of such an oath is the American Veterinary Medical Association Veterinarian's Oath:

> "Being admitted to the profession of veterinary medicine, I solemnly swear to use my scientific knowledge and skills for the benefit of society through the protection of animal health and welfare, the prevention and relief of animal suffering, the conservation of animal resources, the promotion of public health, and the advancement of medical knowledge.
>
> I will practice my profession conscientiously, with dignity, and in keeping with the principles of veterinary medical ethics.
>
> I accept as a lifelong obligation the continual improvement of my professional knowledge and competence."

Furthermore, many of these oaths address the five freedoms of animal welfare, which are as follows: the freedom (1) from hunger and thirst, (2) from discomfort, (3) from pain, injury and disease, (4) to express normal behavior, and (5) from fear and distress. Specifically, practicing anesthesia and providing analgesia in animals facilitates a wide range of procedures (e.g., surgery and many diagnostic imaging procedures) and prevents discomfort and pain. Furthermore, for example, treating painful age-related disease processes, such as providing analgesia to an old dog suffering debilitating osteoarthritis, addresses the freedom to express normal behavior. Pain-free animals are also more likely to eat and drink which addresses the freedom from thirst and hunger. Thus, the practice of veterinary anesthesia can address all freedoms, enabling veterinarians and technicians to meet their ethical obligation to uphold their oath.

Anesthesia (as in general anesthesia) is defined as a state of controlled, temporary loss of sensation or awareness that is induced for medical purposes.

Local anesthesia is defined as administering a local anesthetic drug, using various techniques, to induce the absence of sensation in a specific part of the animal's body. Generally, the aim of inducing local anesthesia is to provide a local insensitivity to pain but often other local senses (feeling of sensations such as touch, heat, pressure, etc.) may also be lost.

Analgesia is defined as the inability to feel pain. However, many drugs that are used to treat pain (opioids, nonsteroidal anti-inflammatory drugs, etc.) are more accurately described as "hypoalgesics," as they decrease the sensation of pain rather than abolishing it completely. Local anesthetic drugs provide loss of sensation and are thus considered true analgesics.

The anesthetist is the person administering the anesthetic and providing analgesia. An anesthetist could be a veterinarian or a veterinary technician. *Note*: The role of technicians will vary according to local regulations.

Though not strictly defined, it is generally accepted that the term "anesthesiologist" is restricted to a veterinarian, and it is often, though not always, assumed that they have completed postgraduate, discipline-specific clinical training and are registered by their country's veterinary professional body, or board-certified by a college, conferring specialist status as a veterinary anesthesiologist.

Fundamental Principles of Veterinary Anesthesia, First Edition. Edited by Gareth E. Zeiler and Daniel S. J. Pang.

Companion Website: www.wiley.com/go/VeterinaryAnesthesiaZeiler

The Stages of Learning and Developing Skills in Veterinary Anesthesia

There are three major areas that require development to become proficient at practicing anesthesia and analgesia (Figure 1.1). These are focused on (1) your development (knowledge and practice of anesthesia, to achieve proficiency as a new graduate through practice and situational awareness), (2) understanding your patient, and (3) understanding the drugs.

Your development begins with building your knowledge and understanding. This involves enrolling into a veterinary degree course where fundamental aspects of veterinary anesthesia are taught in a classroom environment.

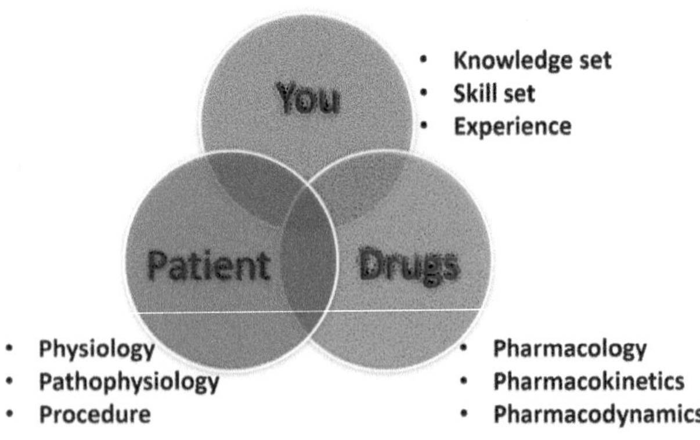

Figure 1.1 The three major fields that require development to become proficient at practicing anesthesia and analgesia. These fields are focused on your development, your understanding of the patient, and an understanding of the drugs used during the peri-anesthetic period.

At this early stage of development, you are classified as a *novice* on the learning and development staircase framework (Figure 1.2). Many of the aspects of veterinary anesthesia will be foreign to you because you have not necessarily been exposed to clinical practice. This makes the initial learning of this subject a challenge. As you progress through classroom learning, some faculties have a skills laboratory where you will be exposed to the practical aspects of performing certain procedures on purpose-built training models (simulators). Once that phase of learning is completed you are considered an *apprentice* and you will be ready for clinical training with live patients (academic hospitals or at private practice rotation programs, depending on your school). During this period of training, you will gain practical experience and begin to develop your skill set while applying the theory from the classroom. Upon graduation from the veterinary program, you are considered *proficient* at veterinary anesthesia.

Over and above learning the fundamental principles of veterinary anesthesia is the need to incorporate knowledge gained from other courses, such as physiology (species-specific and disease pathophysiology). Understanding and integrating this knowledge is essential to practicing anesthesia at an acceptable level. In most anesthesia courses, there is not enough time to review physiology and pathophysiology so it is therefore expected that a student recalls and integrates this knowledge during the course. This also applies to the core concepts of pharmacology (such as receptor function and location, and principles of pharmacokinetics and pharmacodynamics).

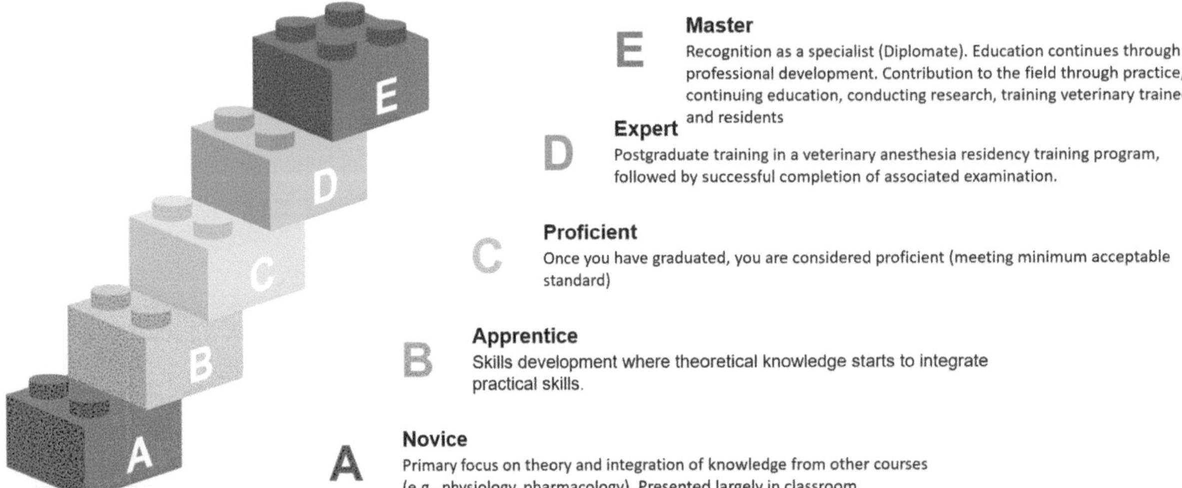

Figure 1.2 The hypothetical learning and development staircase that starts in the lecture halls (A), graduating from a degree in veterinary science (C), and then specializing in veterinary anesthesia (D and E).

Colleges and Associations

There are a number of colleges and academies where a veterinarian or veterinary technician can enroll for postgraduate training with the goal of becoming a specialist. Acquiring this status will classify you as an *expert* (specialist) in veterinary anesthesiology. The differentiation between expert and *master* is not formally structured, but Diplomates would be expected to achieve master status with experience. However, veterinarians or veterinary technicians who have a keen interest in anesthesiology but do not want to pursue a specialist degree can join an association to keep up to date with developments in the field or gain additional knowledge at their own pace and level of interest. Table 1.1 lists a few internationally recognized organizations that offer specialist training or information to interested persons. Your country may offer some regional organizations where advanced training or information can be found; it is best to consult your local associations or schools for information.

Referral and Advice Considerations

There are specialists in veterinary anesthesiology all over the world who will accept a case referral or be prepared to consult on a case if physical referral is not an option. The ACVAA and ECVAA websites have directories listing board-certified veterinary anesthesiologists. If that approach is unsuccessful, then phoning your local region's registering body or association could be helpful.

Table 1.1 A list of some internationally recognized organizations that offer specialist training in veterinary anesthesia or provide a source of information to an interested person.

Entity	Criteria for membership	Description	Website
ACVAA	Membership requires diplomate status. Diplomate status is achieved by completing a residency and passing the board-certifying examination.	The American College of Veterinary Anesthesia and Analgesia. The ACVAA exists to promote the highest standards of clinical practice of veterinary anesthesia and analgesia and defines criteria for designating veterinarians with advanced training as specialists in the clinical practice of veterinary anesthesiology. The ACVAA issues certificates to those meeting these criteria, maintains a list of such veterinarians, and advances scientific research and education in veterinary anesthesiology and analgesia.	www.acvaa.org
ECVAA	Membership requires diplomate status. Diplomate status is achieved by completing a residency and passing the board-certifying examination.	The European College of Veterinary Anaesthesia and Analgesia. The mission of the ECVAA is to contribute significantly to the maintenance and enhancement of the quality of European Veterinary Specialists in Anaesthesia and Analgesia across all European countries at the highest possible level so as to ensure that improved veterinary medical services will be provided to the public.	www.ecvaa.org
AVTAA	Veterinary technician specialist (anesthesia and analgesia) status is achieved by completing credentials and passing a certifying examination.	The Academy of Veterinary Technicians in Anesthesia and Analgesia. The AVTAA exists to promote interest in the discipline of veterinary anesthesia. The Academy provides a process by which a veterinary technician may become credentialed as a Veterinary Technician Specialist (Anesthesia and Analgesia). The Academy provides the opportunity for members to enhance their knowledge and skills in the field of veterinary anesthesia.	www.avtaa-vts.org
AVA	All professions and animal caregivers with an interest in veterinary anesthesia, analgesia, and associated animal welfare can join the association.	The Association of Veterinary Anaesthetists. The AVA is an active, enthusiastic group of veterinary surgeons and others (e.g., researchers, technicians, and pharmacologists) who share an interest in animal anesthesia, analgesia, and animal welfare. The AVA promotes the study of, and research into, the subject of anesthesia and analgesia in animals; and to promote collaboration between anesthetists in all places, and actively encourage the establishment and taking of diplomas and degrees in veterinary anesthesia.	www.ava.eu.com
NAVAS	All professions and animal caregivers with an interest in veterinary anesthesia, analgesia, and associated animal welfare can join the society.	The North American Veterinary Anesthesia Society. The NAVAS helps veterinary professionals and caregivers advance and improve the safe administration of anesthesia and analgesia to all animals through development of standards consistent with recent findings documented in high-quality basic and clinical scientific publications and texts. The NAVAS encourages discussion and disseminates information to all those interested in veterinary anesthesia and analgesia, including the general public. The NAVAS strives to be a community of, and an accessible resource for, all veterinary caregivers and interested individuals within the general public on matters relevant to veterinary anesthesia, analgesia, and related animal welfare.	www.mynavas.org

When to Consider Referral

A good rule of thumb is to consider the predicted risk of peri-anesthetic mortality for the patient's physical status classification (see Chapter 2 for a description of the American Society of Anesthesiologists physical status classification). As physical status classification increases, the risk of mortality increases. A further consideration is veterinarian familiarity with the species to be anesthetized. For example, it is not unreasonable to consider that a veterinarian who primarily works with cats and dogs will be less proficient anesthetizing a pet reptile. This lack of familiarity will increase the anesthetic risk as it is likely to impact the quality of anesthetic management. Another consideration for referral is access to a specialist. Some anesthesiologists are prepared to travel and assist with a case at your practice.

Asking for Advice when Referral Is Not an Option

While referral may not always be an option, with potential financial and geographic limitations, modern communications increase the options available for specialist consultation, such as teleconsulting/telemedicine. Other sources of free advice can be found on professional networks (often hosted by associations and controlling bodies), invited email lists (ACVA-L), social media groups (e.g., interest groups on Facebook), and in some cases anesthesiologists employed at local veterinary specialty/academic hospitals. Information provided by those without recognized advanced training is not subject to any form of quality control and practitioners should be aware of the associated risks.

Interpreting the Science

How to Find Quality Information in a Hurry

When looking for information quickly most of us turn to an internet search engine; however, information available on websites is often inaccurate and incomplete. This explains the commonly held misconception that there are a large number of dog and cat breeds that are especially "sensitive" to anesthetic drugs (see Further Reading). Unfortunately, distinguishing between reliable and unreliable sources may not be obvious. A helpful approach is to examine the credentials of the person/group providing information. At an individual level, only Diplomates of the American College of Veterinary Anesthesia and Analgesia or European College of Veterinary Anaesthesia and Analgesia are entitled to use the post-nominal "DACVAA" or "DECVAA," respectively. The terms "specialist," "anesthetist," and "anesthesiologist" can be misleading as these are not necessarily defined or protected terms in all countries. Any association or group producing anesthesia resources should include Diplomates within its membership. Such groups include the ACVAA, ECVAA, and the Association of Veterinary Anaesthetists and Continental/National Anesthesia Associations (e.g., NAVAS, North American Veterinary Anesthesia Society).

Evaluating Scientific Articles

A detailed description of interpreting scientific articles is beyond the scope of this chapter. Interested readers are referred to the Further Reading section. Research quality can be viewed as a hierarchy, ranging from personal opinion and case reports to systematic reviews and meta-analysis (Figure 1.3). Based on this, some of the more popular means for veterinarians to gain new information, such as through conference (congress) presentations, should be assessed based on the credentials (qualifications and relevant experience) of the speaker and quality of evidence (including a description of strengths/weaknesses) presented.

In general, much of the reporting of research in veterinary medicine falls below well-established guidelines. This reflects a risk of bias and weak study design in published articles, highlighting that publication is not a guarantee of the quality of work. For example, in a study to compare treatment A versus treatment B, if the treatment an animal receives is not randomly assigned it is possible that some other factors biased the allocation of treatments. Similarly, if the outcome of treatment depends on a researcher evaluation (e.g., pain assessment), researcher awareness of the treatment given to an animal could affect subsequent evaluation. A particularly common limitation in veterinary clinical research is insufficient sample size, i.e., too few animals were studied to identify an important difference between treatments on an outcome of interest (e.g., pain relief). Therefore, when assessing the results and conclusions from an article it is helpful to confirm if comparable articles reported similar findings, whether research findings have been successfully applied, and the interpretation of research results by independent experts.

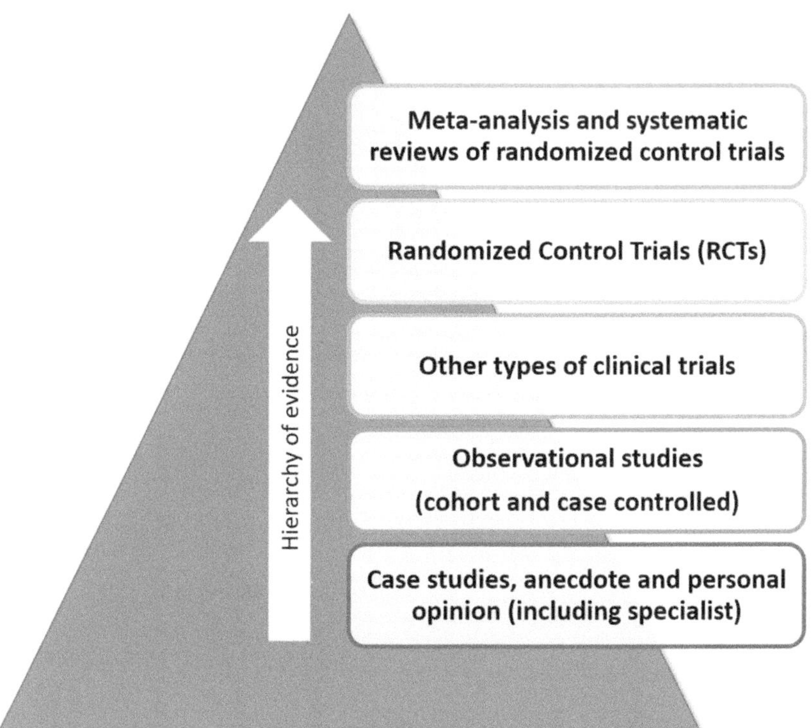

Figure 1.3 Hierarchy of evidence, ranging from low quality (bottom layer of pyramid) to high quality (top layer of pyramid). *Note*: Quality varies within individual layers, such as may occur with strengths/weaknesses in the design and reporting of clinical trials. *Source:* Figure adapted from Greenhalgh (2019).

Further Reading

Cockcroft, P. and Holmes, M. (2003). *Handbook of Evidence-based Veterinary Medicine*, 1e. Wiley-Blackwell. ISBN: 1405108908.

Greenhalgh, T. (2019). *How to Read a Paper: The Basics of Evidence-based Medicine*, 6e.Wiley-Blackwell. ISBN-10: 1119484745.

Hofmeister, E.H., Watson, V., Snyder, L.B.C., and Love, E.J. (2008). Validity and client use of information from the World Wide Web regarding veterinary anesthesia in dogs. *J Am Vet Med Assoc* 233: 1860–1864.

Rufiange, M., Rousseau-Blass, F., and Pang, D.S.J. (2019). Incomplete reporting of experimental studies and items associated with risk of bias in veterinary research. *Vet Rec Open* 6: e000322. https://doi.org/10.1136/vetreco-2018-000322.

2

Patient Assessment, Planning, and Preparation

Tim Bosmans, Roxanne Buck, and Gareth Zeiler

Sedation Compared to General Anesthesia

Sedation is the depression of awareness, whereby the patient's response to external stimuli is reduced, but consciousness is maintained. Depending on the patient's level of alertness before sedation and on the combination and dose of sedatives used, the effect of sedation can be described as mild, moderate, or deep. The aim of mild sedation is to provide anxiolysis with minimal suppression of consciousness. Moderate sedation depresses consciousness, but the patient will still respond to external tactile and auditory stimuli. With deep sedation, the patient will only respond to noxious stimuli. It is a common misconception that sedation is safer than general anesthesia. Although patients usually maintain their physiological reflexes and breathe spontaneously, deep sedation can result in levels of cardiovascular, respiratory, and thermoregulatory depression, and it should not be assumed that reflexes are always maintained. These effects might even be exacerbated when different classes of drugs are used in combination. For example, the combination of alpha-2 adrenergic receptor agonists and opioids results in a synergistic effect and might lead to depression of airway reflexes which can cause upper airway obstruction that leads to asphyxia (e.g., in brachycephalic dogs). Also, sedated patients are generally not monitored as closely as anesthetized patients and, if sedated for procedures like radiographs, their body position is often changed regularly which can increase the risk of regurgitation and aspiration. Thus, monitoring of the sedated animal should always be performed.

General anesthesia, on the other hand, is an induced, reversible, loss of consciousness, whereby the animal is thought to have no recognition of all types of stimuli that occur. Three criteria should ideally be met under general anesthesia and this "triad of anesthesia" includes, unconsciousness, muscle relaxation, and analgesia. Specific drugs that act on one or more components of the triad are used in combination to reduce the side effects of each individual drug. This concept is termed "balanced anesthesia."

Defining the Purpose of Performing Anesthesia

Before anesthetizing any patient, it is vital that the veterinarian appreciates why this particular patient requires anesthesia. As anesthesia may be required for a variety of procedures, understanding the purpose of anesthesia enables the veterinarian to better plan and prepare for the procedure. For example, a patient having orthopedic surgery will likely require more potent analgesics than one having a small cutaneous mass removed. Likewise, the condition of the patient, the nature, and anticipated duration of the procedure will influence the choice of drugs and method of delivery. Additionally, by understanding why the patient is being anesthetized, the veterinarian can make informed choices about fluid management, the extent of monitoring required, and better appreciate any potential risks to the patient.

Safe and efficient anesthesia requires an optimized patient because inadequate pre-operative preparation is generally accepted as a major contributory factor to pre-anesthetic mortality. A thorough pre-anesthetic assessment allows the veterinarian to develop a pre-anesthetic plan with the goal of reducing patient morbidity and mortality and improving patient and owner experience. The pre-anesthetic plan encompasses the following processes:

1) Documentation of the condition(s) for which the anesthesia is required.
2) Assessment of the patient's overall health status and identification of any hidden conditions that could cause problems during the procedure.
3) Peri-anesthetic risk determination.

Fundamental Principles of Veterinary Anesthesia, First Edition. Edited by Gareth E. Zeiler and Daniel S. J. Pang.

Companion Website: www.wiley.com/go/VeterinaryAnesthesiaZeiler

4) Education of the owner about the procedure and post-procedure care to reduce anxiety and facilitate recovery.
5) Optimization of the patient's medical condition before anesthesia.
6) Development of an appropriate peri-anesthetic care plan.

Patient Assessment

Anesthesia is accompanied by depression of normal physiologic function, most often manifested as hypoventilation, hypotension, and hypothermia due to depression of respiratory, cardiovascular, and neurological functions. Healthy patients are often, though not always, able to compensate enough for these changes to maintain adequate system function. Stressors, such as hypovolemia, hypothermia, pain, or coexisting diseases, can leave animals physiologically compromised, thereby increasing the risk of peri-anesthetic morbidity and mortality.

Before anesthesia, the veterinarian should endeavor to learn as much about the patient as possible to identify individual risk factors that could impact anesthesia. A thorough history and physical examination, in combination with appropriately directed laboratory and other diagnostic procedures, can help identify underlying physiologic and pathologic changes that could impact the anesthetic plan. Thereafter, medical treatment of coexisting diseases and stabilization of the patient before anesthesia play an important role in reducing peri-anesthetic morbidity and mortality.

History Taking

A history should be collected before anesthesia. The history should begin with the signalment of the patient, as species, breed, sex, and age can all alter the patient's response to anesthesia. Thereafter, the history should focus on the main reason for presentation and the details of current illness (as applicable). History of previous illnesses and medical care, including any previous reactions to anesthetic or other drugs (such as antibiotics), should also be discussed. The history should include a complete review of systems to identify undiagnosed disease or inadequately controlled chronic diseases, with particular focus on the cardiopulmonary and nervous systems (for example exercise intolerance or a history of seizures), which are the most relevant systems in respect of fitness for anesthesia. Confirmation of any current medication, in particular any behavior modifying drugs, cardiac drugs, chronically administered analgesics (e.g., nonsteroidal anti-inflammatory drugs), herbal medicines, and their dosing schedules, is also essential. During this time, it is also important that the veterinarian verifies the client's contact details, outlines potential risks of the anesthetic and procedure, and obtains consent before proceeding with drafting an anesthetic plan.

There can be some important breed-specific considerations in anesthesia though these are less common than often perceived. For example, greyhounds can have prolonged recovery after receiving some drugs (barbiturates), and other breeds affected by the multiple drug resistance mutation 1 (MDR1; now known as "ABCB1") gene should initially receive reduced dosages of some drugs (e.g., opioids) and should be reassessed. Some breed-associated conditions can also influence anesthesia. Brachycephalic dogs, for example, are predisposed to upper airway obstruction, miniature schnauzers may have sick sinus syndrome, and Cavalier King Charles Spaniels are predisposed to mitral valve disease. These are examples of common breed-specific considerations and other examples are described in species-specific chapters.

Patient age is also an important consideration. Pediatric and geriatric patients may require dose adjustments. Older patients tend to have more comorbidities than younger patients and more pre-operative diagnostic tests may be warranted (Chapter 15).

Patient sex should also be considered. Pregnancy alters physiology and can affect drug pharmacokinetics. In some species, such as horses, intact males can be more difficult to handle because of their temperament, and they often have higher drug requirements.

Physical Clinical Examination

A physical examination should be completed to build on the information gathered during the history. Documenting physical examination findings forms an important part of the clinical record, and it has been shown that failure to record a physical exam increases the odds for anesthetic-related death in dogs.

For elective cases, it is recommended to perform a clinical examination within 12–24 h before anesthesia. At a minimum, the focused pre-anesthesia examination should encompass assessment of the airway, lungs and heart, with documentation of vital signs. Any abnormal findings on the physical examination should be investigated before proceeding.

Assessment of the cardiovascular system should focus on hydration status and determining the adequacy of tissue perfusion. Heart rate and rhythm, as well as pulse quality and regularity, should be assessed (Table 2.1). Additionally, capillary refill time and mucous membrane color should be noted. Thoracic auscultation should be performed to detect any cardiac murmurs.

Table 2.1 Normal reference intervals of heart rate and mean arterial pressure ranges for common veterinary species during general anesthesia.

Animal	Heart rate (beats/min)	Mean arterial blood pressure (mmHg)
Dog	70–100	70–100
Cat	100–200	80–120
Horse (adult)	35–45	70–90
Horse (foal)	50–80	60–80
Cow	60–80	90–140
Sheep and goat	60–90	80–110
Pig	60–90	80–110

The pulmonary system is assessed through respiratory rate, volume, and effort in combination with auscultation of the lungs. Respiratory rates are usually between 12 and 25 breaths/min for small animals and 8 and 20 breaths/min for large animals. Tidal volumes are usually 8–14 mL/kg at rest. Additionally, the veterinarian should assess for potential upper airway obstruction or difficult intubation.

Evaluation of the nervous system should focus particularly on demeanor, mentation, level of pain, and the presence of any paralysis or weakness. Temperament can impact the ability to perform a physical examination and also affect the response of the patient to drugs. Anxious and highly stressed patients may require higher doses of sedatives, or more potent sedatives, which can predispose to respiratory or cardiovascular depression.

The renal and hepatic systems are also of importance given their role in drug metabolism and excretion. Therefore, if signs of renal (e.g., polyuria/polydipsia) or hepatic disease (e.g., icterus) are identified during the physical examination then they should be investigated further.

Hematology and Biochemical Investigation

Generally, a good clinical history combined with physical examination represents the best method of screening for the presence of disease. Hematologic and biochemical investigation should be performed if a disease is detected or suspected based on clinical examination.

Pre-anesthetic laboratory screening generally includes complete blood cell (CBC) count, serum biochemistry, and urinalysis. Hypoproteinemia and anemia are two of the more common abnormalities that may affect how the patient responds to anesthesia, and urinalysis can be useful in early detection of renal disease (Table 2.2).

However, the costs of tests, patient stress associated with blood sampling, and questionable significance of abnormal values in changing the anesthetic drug protocol have called into question whether pre-anesthetic screening is necessary in healthy veterinary patients. In human anesthesia, pre-anesthetic screening in healthy patients is not recommended and does not change patient management, predict peri-operative complications, or affect outcomes. In veterinary anesthesia, there is no consensus on the usefulness or necessity of blood tests, and the Association of Veterinary Anesthetists (AVA) voted in 1998 that routine pre-anesthetic screening is unnecessary if the patient is healthy based on physical examination and history, and the clinical use of pre-anesthetic blood tests remains at the discretion of the veterinarian. However, in geriatric animals, evidence suggests that there is value in documenting pre-anesthetic blood tests to appreciate possible progression of undiagnosed or chronic diseases after an anesthetic.

Table 2.2 Normal reference intervals for total plasma protein and packed cell volume (PCV) in veterinary species that are commonly anesthetized.

Parameter	Dog	Cat	Horse	Cow	Sheep	Pig
Total plasma protein (g/dL)	5.7–7.2	5.6–7.4	6.5–7.8	7.0–9.0	6.3–7.1	6.0–7.5
PCV (%)	36–54	25–46	27–44	23–35	30–50	30–48

The timing of performing pre-anesthetic blood work is also controversial. It has been suggested that blood tests obtained within 3–6 months before an anesthetic that were within normal reference intervals for the patient are reasonable in clinically healthy animals with no change in history. However, pre-anesthetic laboratory screening has been recommended within two weeks of anesthesia in all otherwise healthy geriatric dogs and cats. Where laboratory values or the patient's health are abnormal, blood work should be repeated immediately before anesthesia.

Additional biochemical testing in individual patients should be considered when indicated by abnormalities found during the physical examination or in the history. Serum biochemical profiles should be tailored according to the patient, for example, serum glucose and liver function should be investigated in diabetic patients and clotting function tests should be performed where prolonged hemostasis is suspected. The clinician should consider the risk–benefit ratio of any ordered laboratory test, as guided by the age of the patient, complexity of the surgical procedure, and completeness of the history and physical examination.

Other Pre-anesthetic Assessments

The need for any additional pre-anesthetic assessments is usually dictated by historical and clinical findings. For example, blood pressure should be measured in patients with known renal, cardiovascular, or endocrine disease. An electrocardiogram should be performed where arrhythmias are detected on auscultation. Additionally, an echocardiogram may provide detailed information on the structure and function of the heart. Thoracic radiographs should be performed where lower airway disease or cardiac disease is suspected.

The veterinarian should practice good judgment when ordering pre-anesthetic tests, balancing the need for information with test cost and the likelihood of useful information being received.

Risk Assessment and Patient Stratification

Anesthesia is not without risk of morbidity and mortality. Numerous studies have attempted to estimate mortality ranging in commonly anesthetized species, with reported mortality figures across all cases of 0.17–1.5% in dogs, 0.24–2.2% in cats, and 0.9–1.9% in horses, based on large-scale multicenter studies (see Further Reading).

Although anesthetic mortality risk cannot be simply predicted before anesthesia, the American Society of Anesthetists (ASA) formalized a classification system that summarizes patient assessment to a numerical value, thereby helping to identify those patients who warrant special attention. The five category ASA physical status classification system has been used in human anesthesia since 1963, and in veterinary anesthesia, as in humans, mortality is associated with increased ASA class. Each risk category has been defined to provide guidelines to the clinician, and approved examples have been established for human anesthesia. The definitions commonly used in veterinary patients are derived from these examples although the veterinarian should remember that the ASA status classification is a clinical judgment based on multiple factors, with inherent subjectivity (Table 2.3). To improve communication and assessments at a specific institution, institutional-specific examples can be developed.

It is important to understand the purpose of the system is to assess and communicate pre-anesthetic comorbidities. While the system alone does not predict peri-operative risks, when used alongside other factors, it can be useful in predicting peri-operative risks. Dogs and cats with ASA status ≥ III have an increased risk of anesthesia-related death and severe complications (hypotension and hypothermia) compared to those with ASA status < III (see Further Reading).

As highlighted in the preceding text, patient status is not the only factor contributing to anesthetic risk. Other factors include the type of surgical intervention (duration and invasiveness of surgery), the experience of both the anesthetist and surgeon, and the anesthetic techniques used. Additionally, the urgency of the procedure is important, with emergency anesthesia usually carrying greater risk than elective anesthesia because less time is available to perform diagnostics, prepare the patient for anesthesia, and often performed outside regular working hours. The facilities available and the availability of personnel also influence procedure success. Duration of both anesthesia and surgery also affect outcome, with longer procedures (generally > 2 h) being associated with greater risk.

Table 2.3 American Society of Anesthesiologists (ASA) physical status classification system.

ASA classification	Definition	Patient examples
ASA I	A normal healthy patient	Healthy patient with a normal body condition score
ASA II	A patient with mild systemic disease	Mild diseases without any substantiative functional limitations, e.g., well-controlled epilepsy, pregnancy, obesity, and fractures without shock
ASA III	A patient with severe systemic disease	Substantive functional limitations with one or more moderate-to-severe diseases, e.g., poorly controlled diabetes mellitus and mitral valve disease with moderate reduction of ejection fraction
ASA IV	A patient with severe systemic disease that is a constant threat to life	Cardiac valve dysfunction with severe reduction of ejection fraction or congestive heart failure, shock, sepsis, disseminated intravascular coagulation, and severe trauma
ASA V	A moribund patient that is not expected to survive without the procedure	Severe hemorrhage, multiple organ dysfunction syndrome, and decompensated congestive heart failure

The addition of "E" denotes an emergency procedure. With *emergency* defined as existing when delay in treatment of the patient would lead to a significant increase in the threat to life or body part.

Overview of an Anesthetic Plan

When drafting an anesthetic plan, the anesthetist should take into consideration the entire peri-anesthetic period. This starts with a thorough understanding of the patient's pre-anesthetic status and the assessment of the risks related to the specific anesthesia (see in the preceding text). When necessary, pre-anesthetic stabilization should be performed to return physiology toward normal function. Stabilization can involve fluid therapy, diuresis, analgesia, anxiolysis and sedation, pre-oxygenation, normalization of body temperature, and medical and interventional support. The anesthetist should be familiar with and have a full understanding of the type of surgery that will be performed and be aware of the level of nociception that is to be expected during and following the intervention. Both the results of patient physical status classification, pre-anesthetic risk assessment and knowledge of the type of surgery to be performed, serve as a guide for the choice of anesthetic and analgesic drugs. Additionally, the most efficient approach (e.g., standing sedation versus inhalant anesthesia) and analgesic technique (e.g., locoregional analgesia versus intravenous infusion of analgesic drugs such as an opioid) can be selected and the full anesthetic protocol can be developed.

The anesthetic plan takes into account the four phases of the anesthetic period: premedication, induction, maintenance, and recovery. The plan describes the drugs used during each phase to provide anesthesia and analgesia, patient monitoring, and fluid therapy. Before the start of anesthesia, it is necessary to ensure that all equipment for anesthesia is present and operational. Here, equipment checklists can be a very useful aid (see Chapter 20). Additionally, the anesthetist must ensure that adequate monitoring of the patient is planned (see Chapter 4). Emergency drugs should be readily available, doses calculated, and preferably drawn up in high-risk patients, to prevent delay in treating life-threatening events (see Chapter 20). Last but not least, it is the task of the anesthetist to communicate early with hospital or intensive care staff and to optimize patient handover and post-operative support.

The Phases of the Peri-anesthetic Period

Premedication Phase

Drugs are administered alone or in combination to the patient before induction of anesthesia, with, in general, a minimum lag time of 15–20 min between premedication and induction. They are either administered orally (including at-home treatment in very anxious patients), subcutaneously (rarely recommended), intramuscularly, or intravenously. When patients are severely debilitated, the premedication phase is sometimes omitted and induction of anesthesia is subsequently the first step of the anesthetic protocol.

The aims of premedication are as follows:

- Providing anxiolysis with or without causing sedation, which facilitates animal handling (e.g., placement of an intravenous catheter) and reduction of stress, which is beneficial for the patient, the anesthetist, and support staff.
- Providing analgesia, which is mandatory if surgery is performed, and during short procedures these analgesic drugs may contribute to post-operative analgesia.
- To provide a smooth transition from an awake, conscious state to an unconscious state during the induction of anesthesia.
- Dose reduction of induction and maintenance anesthetic drugs, by which premedication contributes to a balanced anesthetic technique.
- Protection against adverse effects from anesthetic induction and maintenance drugs (e.g., to decrease the sympathetic nervous system response and associated risk of arrhythmias).
- To provide some degree of muscle relaxation, which could be beneficial in some patients (e.g., dogs and cats), but it is not beneficial in all patients (e.g., ataxia in horses).
- To contribute to a calm recovery and to prevent emergence delirium (depending on the duration of the surgery and the duration of effect of the premedication drug(s)).
- Prevention of pre- and post-anesthetic nausea and vomiting.

Not all aims of premedication can always be met, but all should be considered when drafting an anesthetic plan.

Induction Phase

By definition, it is the transition from a conscious state to a drug-induced, unconscious, anesthetized state. Induction drugs can be administered intramuscularly (ketamine, tiletamine, and alfaxalone), intravenously (ketamine, tiletamine, propofol, barbiturates, alfaxalone, and etomidate), or by inhalation (inhalational anesthetics). During the administration of the induction drug(s), the animal passes through different states. Typically, intravenous injection of the induction drug is started by giving a bolus as a fraction of the total calculated dose (depending on the type of drug and the level of sedation following premedication). The rest of the induction drug is then given "to effect," usually over a period of 30–60 seconds, targeted to an endpoint, which is usually endotracheal intubation. Induction dose titration is thus given to achieve loss of consciousness, loss of righting reflexes (in small exotic species), decrease of jaw tone, and loss of swallowing reflexes, so the airway can be secured by inserting an endotracheal tube into the trachea. Additionally, dose titration serves to prevent an overdose of anesthesia ("too deep"), with risks of induction apnea and cardiovascular depression. By contrast, if induction dose titration is performed too slowly, a state of excitement may occur, which is recognized by signs of involuntary movement, vocalization, uncontrolled head movements, repetitive movements of the limbs, tachycardia, and tachypnea. This state should not be confused with a "hypersensitivity reaction" to the induction drug, or convulsions, and progression through the induction phase should not be stopped. Hypersensitivity reactions are rare, usually presenting with cutaneous wheals (hives and urticaria), swelling of the lips and eyelids, which can occur within 10 min of drug administration. When early signs of excitement are observed, it is important to continue induction drug administration, so the animal becomes unconsciousness as soon as possible. In some species, there is a risk of developing of laryngospasm (e.g., cats, pigs, and rabbits) during this light state of anesthesia, particularly if endotracheal intubation is attempted when the depth of anesthesia is too superficial ("light"), such as when an animal is coughing and swallowing during intubation. In large animals (horses and cattle), induction drugs are not titrated to effect but rather a precalculated dose is rapidly injected to minimize any risk of excitement.

Maintenance Phase

This is the phase of the anesthetic during which a stable plane of surgical anesthesia and analgesia is maintained and physiological variables are maintained within species-specific reference intervals to preserve optimal respiratory and hemodynamic stability. Techniques for maintenance of anesthesia are total intravenous anesthesia (TIVA; e.g., intermittent boluses or infusions of induction drugs), inhalant anesthesia, and partial intravenous anesthesia (PIVA; administration of a combination of injectable and inhalational anesthetic drugs). Fluid therapy during an operation often begins shortly after induction and is continued during the maintenance phase of anesthesia (see later). Fluid therapy could be continued in the recovery phase but may require revision on administration rate and fluid type.

During maintenance of anesthesia, the animal can be in different states of anesthetic depth and it is important for the anesthetist to differentiate between light, surgical, and deep states ("planes") of anesthesia. To do this properly, an integrated assessment of the animal (e.g., position of the eyes, presence/absence of palpebral reflexes, jaw tone, muscle movement, and response to surgical stimulus) and information from monitoring physiological variables (e.g., heart and respiratory rate, tidal volume, and blood pressure) should be made (Table 2.4 and Figure 2.1). Additionally, communication between the anesthetist and the surgery team is important to ensure awareness of the situation at all times.

Table 2.4 Physiological variables and their relation to assessment of depth of anesthesia in common veterinary species during inhalant anesthesia.

Variable	Species	Light plane of anesthesia	Surgical plane of anesthesia	Deep plane of anesthesia
Eye position	Small animals	Central	Ventromedially rotated	Central with dilated pupils
	Horses	Rapid nystagmus	Variable position	Central with dilated pupils
	Ruminants	Central	Ventrally rotated	Central with dilated pupils
Palpebral reflex	All species	Present	Absent	Absent
Jaw tone	All species	Present	Relaxed	Relaxed (to absent)
Tear production	All species	Moist cornea	Moist cornea	Dry cornea
Heart rate	Small animals	Generally increased	Normal	Decreased
	Horses	Usually normal	Normal	Decreased
	Ruminants	Generally increased	Normal	Decreased
Blood pressure in hemodynamically stable animals	All species	Generally increased	Normal	Decreased
Respiratory rate	All species	Generally increased	Normal	Decreased
Tidal volume	All species	Generally decreased, shallow breathing	Normal	Decreased
Muscle movement and response to surgical stimulation	All species	Possible	Absent	Absent

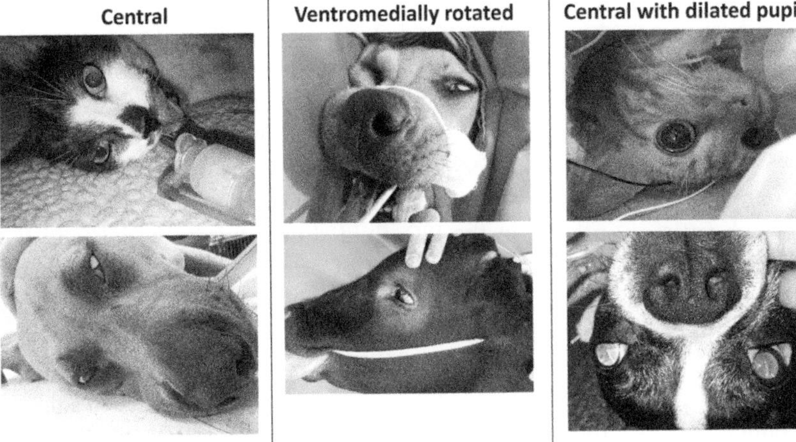

Figure 2.1 Examples of different eye positions under general anesthesia. Eye position (orientation of ocular globe) varies with depth of anesthesia in some species and is one of several variables used to determine the depth of anesthesia (see text for detailed description). Ocular changes can also be induced by other factors. For example, some drugs may promote a more central position (e.g., ketamine), and opioids (in cats) and anticholinergics (in all animals) cause pupil dilation (mydriasis). Note that the example of the dog in the central column has the nondependent eye ventromedially rotated and the dependent eye is central. The different eye positions in the same animal can be a common observation.

Recovery Phase

The recovery phase comprises the period between the end of anesthesia (stopping delivery of anesthetic drugs), the return of consciousness, and the recovery of cardiopulmonary and thermoregulatory function. The importance of the recovery phase is often overlooked. However, it is critically important: approximately half to two-thirds of peri-anesthetic deaths (47% of dogs, 61% of cats, and 64% of rabbits) occur within the first four hours of the recovery phase (see Further Reading). Likely contributing factors for this are the transition from a highly controlled setting of surgical anesthesia to a much less controlled recovery environment (e.g., absence of a secured airway, reduced monitoring or lack of monitoring, monitoring by less experienced personnel, and loss of direct continuous observation). Residual sedation and hypothermia, for example, can be "silent killers" if the animal is insufficiently monitored in the post-operative period. It is important to monitor the patient until return of near normal baseline values of vital signs. Additionally, one must not forget to assess and treat post-operative pain.

Peri-anesthetic Fluid Therapy

Fluid therapy is frequently applied in the peri-anesthetic period. It must be stressed that fluids should be considered drugs, with the following considerations: correct type (solution content) and volume, appropriate route, and recommended rate. With appropriate use, fluid administration can be lifesaving. When used inappropriately (incorrect plan or by accident), fluids can cause patient morbidity and mortality. Appropriate fluid therapy is key to treating dehydration, hypovolemia, and electrolyte imbalances, but excessive fluid administration can lead to hypervolemia and overhydration with serious complications (e.g., pulmonary edema, electrolyte disturbances, edema of the gastrointestinal tract, edema of tissue injury sites, hemodilution, and coagulopathies).

Pre-operatively, fluids might be administered to stabilize sick patients in order to restore volume status (e.g., dehydration and blood loss), treat electrolyte imbalances (e.g., hyperkalemia), and to correct acid–base balance. During the maintenance phase of anesthesia while surgery is occurring, fluids are administered to correct and maintain circulating volume (correct normal ongoing and extra fluid losses) and to maintain adequate cardiac output and tissue perfusion in the face of anesthetic-induced cardiovascular depression. Ultimately, the primary goal of peri-anesthetic fluid administration is to support hemodynamic stability and adequate blood oxygen content. This will result in a clinical situation where tissue perfusion and oxygen delivery are maintained. Traditional methods for monitoring the need for fluid therapy are by evaluating clinical variables that indirectly reflect perfusion (e.g., arterial blood pressure, heart rate, urine output, capillary refill time, and mucous membrane color). However, these variables do not always ensure adequate hemodynamic status in all patients (see Further Reading). Guidance is provided on fluid support during anesthesia (see later). If cardiovascular variables are lower than a lower acceptable threshold, then other therapies should be considered. These commonly include reducing the depth of anesthesia or administering drugs that act directly on the cardiovascular system (e.g., catecholamines) or both. In the post-operative period, fluids can be administered to restore fluid and electrolyte balance, as needed. Typically, maintenance fluid therapy is indicated for patients who have adequate fluid status but are not yet drinking or eating.

Basic Concepts of Water Balance

Water accounts for approximately two-thirds (60%) of the total body weight (TBW) in adult mammals, with variations according to age (e.g., 80% of TBW in neonatal animals), species, and body fat percentage. Body water is distributed among the different body compartments as shown in Figure 2.2.

The main compartments are the intracellular (ICC) and extracellular (ECC) compartments, which account for 40% and 20% of the TBW, respectively. The ECC is further subdivided into the interstitial compartment (ISC), which represents fluid between the cells (15% of TBW), and the intravascular compartment (IVC), which accounts for the plasma in the blood vessels (5% of TBW). The total blood volume is dependent on both the plasma volume and the hematocrit (approximately 4% of TBW). Total blood volume therefore accounts for approximately 9% of TBW, but this can vary with age and between species. Transcellular fluid (fluids within the respiratory, gastrointestinal and urogenital tracts, synovial fluid, cerebrospinal fluid, lymph, and intraocular fluid) makes up a fourth compartment that accounts for approximately 1% of the TBW in humans, but it can vary greatly among species and is usually not considered during fluid therapy calculations.

The volume of each of the four compartments is not fixed and fluid (i.e., water) moves between the compartments by means of hydrostatic pressure, osmosis, and lymph circulation. Fluid shift between the IVC and the ISC is mainly driven by *hydrostatic pressure*. Intravascular colloid oncotic pressure (COP) was thought to be partly responsible for the maintenance of intravascular volume, but its role in fluid shifts is being revised and is considered less important (see Further Reading). In the tissues, intravascular capillary hydrostatic pressure is higher compared to the ISC hydrostatic pressure, promoting fluid transfer into the ISC over the entire length of the capillary in a gradually decreasing manner. Once fluid is present in the ISC, fluid shift between the ISC and the ICC occurs by means of *osmosis*. With osmosis, water moves across the semipermeable cell membrane, from the ISC to the ICC and vice versa, in response to the difference in concentration of solutes, also referred to as "osmotically active particles" (osmoles), on both sides of the cell membrane. The solute concentrations between the ISC and ICC vary. This is because some of the solutes (e.g., blood urea nitrogen) can pass freely through the semipermeable membrane while others have their movement modulated by membrane transport systems (e.g., Na^+ and glucose). A change in the concentrations of osmoles within a compartment, without a change in the volume of water, will lead to a change in equilibrium between the compartments, and water will be redistributed until the tonicity between the compartments reaches equilibrium again. The main osmoles are Na^+, Cl^- and some proteins (primarily albumin) in the ISC, and K^+ and proteins in the ICC. Plasma in the IVC exerts an osmolarity that is chiefly determined by the concentration of Na^+ ions. Doubling the measured [Na^+] gives a good approximation of plasma osmolarity (normal value of 280–320 mOsm/L). Effective osmolarity is expressed by the term "tonicity." Tonicity only takes into account the osmoles that do not freely move across a semipermeable membrane and exert a pull (osmotic effect) on water over the semipermeable membrane. In the IVC, proteins, such as globulins and especially albumin, exert intravascular

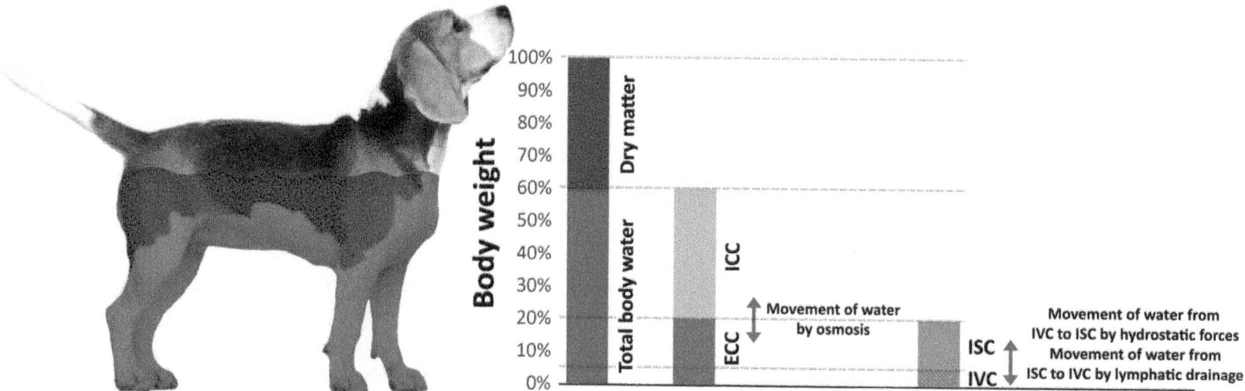

Figure 2.2 The total body water in adult animals is distributed between the intracellular compartment (ICC) and extracellular compartment (ECC). Water in the ECC compartment is distributed into the interstitial compartment (ISC) and intravenous compartment (IVC). Various factors influence the movement of water into and out of these compartments (see text for details and Chapter 16).

tonicity since they cannot freely move across a semipermeable membrane (e.g., the vascular endothelium) in a healthy animal. They contribute little to the plasma osmolarity but exert COP or oncotic pressure (18–25 mmHg in plasma) that is important for the maintenance of volume in the IVC. Reuptake of fluid from the ISC into the IVC is regulated by *lymphatic circulation* and does not occur at the venous end of the capillary, as was considered by the original Starling equation (see Further Reading).

In summary, the main mechanism for water movement from the IVC to the ISC is hydrostatic pressure, whereas osmosis is the determinant of water shifts between the ISC and the ICC. Water returns from the ISC to the IVC by the lymphatic circulation and is maintained in the IVC by the plasma COP.

Fluid Types

A description of the characteristics and indications of the commonly used peri-anesthetic fluid types (crystalloids and colloids) is given in the following text and displayed in Tables 2.5 and 2.6, respectively. A brief summary of the indications and characteristics of natural colloids, blood, and blood products used in veterinary medicine is presented in Table 2.7. An in-depth discussion of the latter fluid types is beyond the scope of this chapter and the reader is directed to other references (see Further Reading).

Crystalloids

A crystalloid fluid is an aqueous solution containing mineral salts (electrolytes) and water-soluble molecules (sugars). These solutions may be buffered with lactate, acetate, or gluconate to approach plasma pH. Crystalloids can be classified according to their tonicity, application (maintenance fluids or replacement fluids), and electrolyte composition.

Classification of Crystalloid Fluids based on their Tonicity

Isotonic crystalloid solutions have a sodium concentration that is similar to that of plasma (close to 140 mmol/L) and therefore exert a similar tonicity as plasma (280–320 mOsm/L). Isotonicity of the fluids prevents osmotic damage to the blood cells, especially erythrocytes. Some "isotonic" solutions, such as dextrose containing solutions (e.g., dextrose 5% in water D5W) and, to a milder extent, lactate-containing solution (lactated Ringer's solution and Hartmann's solution), become hypotonic once dextrose and lactate, respectively, are metabolized *in vivo*. Isotonic crystalloids are frequently used for intra-operative fluid therapy and are used to replace fluid deficits in case of hypovolemia (intravascular fluid deficit) and dehydration (interstitial fluid deficit). Approximately one-third of administered isotonic replacement fluid remains in the IVC 40 min after administration, with two-thirds entering the ISC. Isotonic fluids can be further classified into balanced (polyionic solutions where the electrolytes are similar to those found in plasma) and nonbalanced fluids (0.9% NaCl). The risk of large volume infusions (>30 mL/kg) of a nonbalanced isotonic solution is the development of a hyperchloremic acidosis.

Hypertonic crystalloid solutions (e.g., 7.2% and 7.5% NaCl) have a high sodium concentration and are specifically administered to rapidly expand the IVC, by pulling fluid from the ISC. The volume expansion is short-lived (approximately 45 min) because the sodium quickly redistributes throughout the extracellular compartment. They should be used with caution and for hypovolemic patients who are not dehydrated. Hypertonic saline should not be administered at a rate faster than 1 mL/kg/min since vagally mediated bradycardia and cardiopulmonary arrest may occur at high infusion rates (see Further Reading).

Hypotonic fluids (e.g., 0.45% NaCl, Normosol-M) have a low sodium concentration and are mainly used as maintenance fluids of total body water and are frequently supplemented with dextrose. Hypotonic fluids are more likely to be used in animals that are hospitalized and being kept on fluid therapy for longer than 2–3 days. They are not recommended for use during the peri-anesthetic period and should never be used for rapid volume resuscitation.

Classification of Crystalloid Fluids based on their Mode of Application

Replacement fluids are designed to replace losses of electrolytes, mainly sodium and body water in the ECC. The composition of these fluids in terms of electrolytes is therefore very close to that of the extracellular fluids (high in sodium and chloride and low in potassium, calcium, and magnesium). Commercially available replacement fluids are Hartmann's solution, 0.9% NaCl, lactated Ringer's solution, Normosol-R, and Plasma-Lyte A. Hypertonic crystalloids are also classified as replacement fluids for resuscitation purposes in very hypovolemic, but not dehydrated patients, but should be used together with isotonic crystalloids.

Maintenance fluids are designed to maintain body fluid homeostasis by correcting for expected sensible (urine and feces) and insensible (sweating and respiration) losses, while also providing requirements for maintenance needs. These fluids are typically low in sodium (close to total body sodium concentration of 70 mmol/L) and chloride, while containing sufficient potassium and dextrose. Hence, they are appropriate for long-term administration. Normosol-M and Plasma-Lyte 56 are typical maintenance fluids. Note, however, that both are not licensed for veterinary use in most countries. Other maintenance fluid options are 0.45%

Table 2.5 Characteristics and composition of some commonly used commercial fluid types in veterinary medicine.

Fluid type	Osmolarity (mOsm/L)	COP (mmHg)	Volume expansion (%)	MS	MW (kDa)	C2/C6 ratio	$[Na^+]$ (mmol/L)	$[Cl^-]$ (mmol/L)	$[K^+]$ (mmol/L)	$[Ca^{2+}]$ (mmol/L)	$[Mg^{2+}]$ (mmol/L)	Buffer (mmol/L)	pH
Isotonic crystalloids													
Lactated Ringer's solution	272	0	NA	NA	NA	NA	130	109	4	3	0	Lactate 28	6.5
Hartmann's solution	273	0	NA	NA	NA	NA	131	111	5	2	0	Lactate 29	6.7
0.9% NaCl	308	0	NA	NA	NA	NA	154	154	0	0	0	NA	5.0
Plasma-Lyte A	295	0	NA	NA	NA	NA	140	98	5	0	1.5	NA	7.4
Normosol-R	295	0	NA	NA	NA	NA	140	98	5	0	1.5	Acetate 27 and Gluconate23	6.6
Hypotonic crystalloids			-										
0.45% NaCl	154	0	NA	NA	NA	NA	77	77	0	0	0	NA	5.0
Normosol-M	110	0	NA	NA	NA	NA	40	40	16	0	1.5	Acetate 16	5.0
Plasma-Lyte 56	110	0	NA	NA	NA	NA	40	40	13	0	1.5	Acetate 16	5.5
Hypertonic crystalloids													
7.2% NaCl	2464	0	4:1 ratio compared to 0.9% NaCl short-lived because of rapid redistribution	NA	NA	NA	1232	1232	0	0	0	NA	5.2
7.5% NaCl	2566	0	4:1 ratio compared to 0.9% NaCl short-lived because of rapid redistribution	NA	NA	NA	1283	1283	0	0	0	NA	5.0
Gelatins													
Geloplasma	274	34	70	NA	30	NA	150	100–125	5	0	1.5	NA	
HES solutions													
6% 450/0.7 0.9% NaCl (Hespan)	310	32	100	0.7	450	5:1	154	154	0	0	0	NA	5.5
10% 200/0.5 (Hemohes 10%)	326	72	145–150	0.5	200	5:1	154	154	0	0	0	NA	5.0
6% 130/0.4 (Voluven)	308	36–38	100–130	0.4	130	9:1	154	154	0	0	0	NA	4–5.5

COP: colloid osmotic pressure; MS: molar substitution ratio; MW: average molecular weight; HES: hydroxyethyl starches; NA: not applicable.

Table 2.6 Fluid therapy guidelines and recommendations for specific peri-anesthetic indications in different species.

Species	Fluid indication	Fluid type	Bolus (mL/kg)	Recommended infusion rate (mL/kg/h)	Important considerations
Dog	Daily maintenance	Maintenance crystalloids		2–6 or 132 x body weight $(kg)^{0.75}$	
	Anesthetic maintenance	Replacement isotonic crystalloids		5	If patient remains hemodynamically stable reduce rate by 25% every hour until minimum maintenance rate is reached
	Hypotension due to relative hypovolemia during anesthesia	Replacement isotonic crystalloids	3–10 (over 5 min); repeat once if needed		1) Before bolus, first check anesthetic depth and decrease when necessary 2) If inadequate, consider administration of a colloid bolus (5–10 mL/kg over 15 min; max dose: 20 mL/kg/day) 3) If still inadequate, patient might not be hypovolemic and vasopressor/inotropic therapy might be necessary
	Volume resuscitation	Replacement isotonic crystalloids	Up to 80–90		1) Administer 25% of the calculated shock dose over 5–15 min (≈20 mL/kg) 2) Reassess patient cardiovascular parameters for the need to continue with an additional 25% dose administered over 15 min 3) If steps 1 and 2 are insufficient, consider adding colloid administration (5–10 mL/kg over 15 min), maximum dose 20 mL/kg/day
		7.2% or 7.5% hypertonic saline	4–5 over 5–10 min		1) Administration must be followed by replacement isotonic crystalloids 2) Beware of hypernatremia 3) Maximum rate of 1 mL/kg/min
		Hydroxyethyl starches	4–5 over 10 min	1 (for treatment of hypo-oncotic states)	Maximum 20 mL/kg/day
Cat	Daily maintenance	Maintenance crystalloids		2–3 or 80 x body weight $(kg)^{0.75}$	
	Anesthetic maintenance	Replacement isotonic crystalloids		3	If patient remains hemodynamically stable, reduce rate by 25% every hour until minimum maintenance rate is reached
	Hypotension due to relative vasodilation during anesthesia	Replacement isotonic crystalloids	3–10 over 5 min; repeat once if needed		1) Before bolus, first check anesthetic depth and decrease when necessary 2) If inadequate, consider administration of a colloid bolus (1–5 mL/kg over 15 min) 3) If still inadequate, patient might not be hypovolemic and vasopressor/inotropic therapy might be necessary

(Continued)

Table 2.6 (Continued)

Species	Fluid indication	Fluid type	Bolus (mL/kg)	Recommended infusion rate (mL/kg/h)	Important considerations
	Volume resuscitation	Replacement isotonic crystalloids	Up to 50–55		1) Administer 25% of the calculated shock dose over 5–15 min (≈10 mL/kg) 2) Reassess patient cardiovascular parameters for the need for an additional 25% dose administered over 15 min 3) If steps 1 and 2 are insufficient, consider adding colloid administration (2.5–5 mL/kg slowly)
		7.2% or 7.5% hypertonic saline	2–2.5 over 5–10 min		1) Administration must be followed by replacement isotonic crystalloids 2) Beware of hypernatremia 3) Maximum rate of 1 mL/kg/min
		Hydroxyethyl starches	4–5 over 10 min	1 (for treatment of hypo-oncotic states)	Maximum 20 mL/kg/day
Horse	Daily maintenance	Maintenance isotonic crystalloids		1.6–2.5 (adults) 3.5–5 (neonatal foals)	
	Anesthetic maintenance	Replacement isotonic crystalloids		2–5	
	Resuscitation	Replacement isotonic crystalloids	Up to 80–90		1) Administer 20–25% of the calculated shock dose rapidly 2) Reassess patient cardiovascular parameters for the need for an additional dose (repeat up to 4–5 times)
		7.2% or 7.5% hypertonic saline	4–5 over 10 min		1) Administration must be followed by replacement isotonic crystalloids 2) Beware of hypernatremia
		Hydroxyethyl starches	4–5 over 10 min		Maximum 10 mL/kg/day since higher rates are associated with higher risk of coagulation derangements
Cattle	Daily maintenance	Maintenance isotonic crystalloids		3–5	be aware of extensive amounts of fluid lost through salivation and regurgitation during anesthesia
	Resuscitation	Replacement isotonic crystalloids	20–40 L/adult cow	40 (adult cattle); max 80 (calves)	In adult cattle flow rate is determined by gravity through a 14 gauge catheter

Table 2.7 Indications and characteristics of natural colloids, blood, and blood products used in veterinary medicine.

Fluid type	Indications	Characteristics and useful information
Natural colloids		
Canine serum albumin (CSA)	Acute intravascular volume expansion of patients with hypoalbuminemia	Commercially available as a lyophilized preparation that has to be reconstituted with sodium chloride to obtain an iso-osmotic 5% or hyperosmotic 16% solution
Human serum albumin (HSA)	1) PLE and PLN with an [albumin] < 15 g/L 2) Sepsis	1) Commercially available as 5% (iso-osmotic), 20% and 25% (hyperoncotic) monodisperse solutions 2) Risk of immunologic reactions in dogs is high, especially after repeated infusion. Although HSA was used in the past, its administration is now strongly discouraged
Blood and blood products		
Fresh whole blood	1) Massive hemorrhage 2) Coagulopathy with active bleeding 3) Anemia + liver disease (pre-operative stabilization)	1) Contains erythrocytes, WBC, plasma, clotting factors, platelets, proteins, and anticoagulant 2) Infuse within 4–6 h following collection, using a filtered giving set
Stored whole blood	Increase of oxygen-carrying capacity in hypoproteinemic patients	Fresh whole blood can be stored in a refrigerator for up to four weeks at 1–6 °C, but platelets become nonfunctional after 1–5 days; indication for administration: increase of oxygen-carrying capacity in hypoproteinemic patients
Packed red blood cells (PRBC)	1) Chronic anemia in normovolemic patients 2) Correction of anemia before surgery	1) Contains erythrocytes (hematocrit = 60–70%), resuspended in saline solution 2) Use a filtered giving set for administration 3) Can be stored in a refrigerator for 28–42 days at 1–6 °C
Fresh frozen plasma (FFP)	1) Coagulopathies: vWd, warfarin toxicity 2) SIRS 3) DIC 4) Acute hemorrhage replaced by PRBC 5) Colostrum replacement in neonates	1) Contains plasma that is separated from whole blood; contains labile and nonlabile clotting factors 2) Frozen at −20 °C within 6 h following collection; can be used for up to 12 months after freezing 3) Infuse within 6 h following thawing
Frozen plasma	1) Vitamin K-dependent coagulopathies 2) Hypoproteinemia	1) Contains nonlabile clotting factors II, VII, IX, and X; albumin and immunoglobulins 2) Obtained from plasma frozen later than 6 h following collection; refrozen FFP; derived from FFP that was frozen for more than 1 year 3) Can be stored for 4 years at −20 °C 4) If used for treatment of hypoproteinemia, high volumes are required and is generally not recommended
Cryoprecipitate	Congenital factor deficiencies (vWd, hemophilia A, and hypofibrogenemia)	1) Contains clotting factors (high concentrations of vWf, fibrinogen, and clotting factors VIII and XIII) 2) Precipitate is obtained through thawing and centrifugation of FFP 3) Can be stored frozen at −20 °C for 1 year
Cryo-poor plasma or cryo-supernatant	Plasma exchanges	1) Contains nonlabile clotting factors, albumin, and immunoglobin 2) What remains from the FFP after removal of the cryoprecipitate
Platelet-rich plasma (PRP)	Thrombocytopenia	1) Supernatant from centrifugated fresh whole blood 2) Contains platelets 3) Difficult to obtain and store (at >18 °C and slowly agitated) 4) Can be stored for 1–5 days

Note: Blood typing is necessary in all cats to avoid transfusion reactions. For dogs, the first transfusion with blood or blood products is usually without an immunologic or nonimmunologic response, but blood typing should be performed before a second transfusion is given 24–48 h after the first.

COP: colloid oncotic pressure; DIC: disseminated intravascular coagulopathy; PLE: protein-losing enteropathy; PLN: protein-losing nephropathy; SIRS: systemic inflammatory response syndrome; vWd: von Willebrand disease; vWf: von Willebrand factor; WBCs: white blood cells.

NaCl + 5% glucose or 5% glucose in water. Maintenance fluids are generally administered to hospitalized patients with no ongoing fluid losses, who are not yet drinking or eating. Maintenance fluids do not remain in the IVC and do not expand intravascular volume.

Colloids

Colloids are large molecules with a molecular weight (MW >30–1000+ kDa) and are either naturally occurring (e.g., albumin, plasma, blood, and blood products) or synthetic (e.g., gelatins and hydroxyethyl starches [HES] are commonly used in veterinary medicine). In the case of an intact endothelium, colloids remain in the intravascular space for a longer period of time than crystalloid solutions. They are osmotically active molecules that increase the plasma COP, attract fluid from the ISC, and expand intravascular volume. Compared with crystalloids, smaller volumes of colloids achieve a similar or greater volume expansion effect. The number of colloid molecules, rather than their size, is responsible for the magnitude of the osmotic effect. This is similar to plasma, where albumin, albeit much smaller than globulin, is primarily responsible for the plasma oncotic pressure since it is more abundant. The primary indications for colloids are rapid intravascular volume expansion, particularly when a low fluid volume is desirable, and/or in patients with hypoproteinemia. Synthetic colloids are designed to provide rapid and sustained volume expansion and not as a replacement or maintenance of intravascular water or total body water. The administration of synthetic colloids has been associated with several complications, mainly in humans. Reported adverse effects are hypersensitivity reactions, accumulation of colloids in the tissues, pruritus, coagulopathies (due to a dilutional effect and interference with platelet function, clotting factors, and the fibrinolysis system), acute kidney injury (AKI) (especially in patients with sepsis and burns), and mortality following administration of HES solutions. In human medicine, this has led to a general avoidance of the use of HES solutions in the peri-operative period (see Further Reading). In veterinary medicine, the adverse effects of colloid administration are less studied and reported. To the authors' knowledge, there are no clinical reports on hypersensitivity reactions and tissue accumulation of synthetic colloids. Interference of HES solutions with coagulation have been documented *in vitro* in cats and dogs (see Further Reading) and *in vivo* in healthy horses (see Further Reading). The effects of HES solutions on the occurrence of AKI have been studied in dogs and cats, with varied results in dogs and no evidence of AKI in cats (see Further Reading).

Types of Synthetic Colloids used in Veterinary Anesthesia

Gelatins

Gelatins are small size polypeptide colloids (MW 30–35 kDa) derived from bovine collagen (bovine skin and bone). Volume expansion lasts around 2–3 h and elimination by the kidneys is rapid. The colloid-associated adverse effects described in the preceding text are all reported for gelatins. In particular, the incidence of hypersensitivity reactions in humans is higher for gelatins (especially succinylated gelatins compared to urea-linked gelatins) than with other colloids.

Hydroxyethyl starches

HES solutions are branched chains of chemically modified waxy maize or potato starches, which are typically characterized by their concentration, mean MW, molar substitution (MS), substitution ratio (C2/C6 ratio), and their carrier solution. As such, a HES solution is identified by four numbers reporting each of these items (e.g., 10% HES 250/0.5/5:1) and a designation of the carrier solution.

Concentration

HES solutions are available in 4%, 6%, and 10% concentrations. The concentration determines the initial intravascular volume expanding effect.

Mean MW

Each HES solution is polydisperse and thus contains molecules with a large range of molecular weights. The displayed MW is the mean MW, which determines the size of the COP effect and the longevity of it. Larger molecules remain longer in circulation since the degradation of the molecules by plasma alpha-amylase takes longer. Eventually, degraded smaller molecules are eliminated through the kidneys. Molecules that are not eliminated by the kidneys are taken up by the reticuloendothelial system in the tissues. Based on their mean MW, HES are classified as low-MW HES (≤70 kDa), medium-MW (130–200 kDa), and high-MW HES (450–670 kDa).

Molar Substitution (MS), Degree of Substitution (DS) and Substitution Ratio (C2/C6 Ratio)

To slow degradation of the starch molecule and to prolong the intravascular expansion effect, hydroxyethyl groups ($-CH_2CH_2OH$) can be added to some of the side chains of the glucose molecule as substitutes for hydroxyl groups. The typical sites for substitution are the carbon 2 and 6 (C2 and C6) positions, with some substitution at the C3 position. Substitution at the C2 position slows degradation of the molecule more than substitution at the C6 position; therefore a higher C2/C6 ratio prolongs the duration of effect of the HES solution. The MS represents the number of hydroxyethyl groups per glucose subunit and is used to classify the starches as tetrastarches (MS = 0.4), pentastarches (MS = 0.5), hexastarches (MS = 0.6), and hetastarches (MS = 0.7). The DS represents the number of substituted glucose units as a proportion of the total number of possible substitution sites.

In conclusion, a more concentrated HES solution, with a higher MW, a greater percentage of overall substitution, and a higher C2/C6 ratio all prolong the intravascular volume expansion effects of the HES solution. As such, the effects of a high-MW, high-substitution HES solution may last up to 24–48 h in comparison to 4–6 h with the low-MW solutions.

Fluid Selection and Rates of Administration

Fluid selection should be based on whether the goal of fluid therapy is meeting daily requirements, replacement of deficits or urgent resuscitation. A fluid protocol should always include considerations of volume, rate, required fluid composition, and the location where the fluid is needed (intravascular versus interstitial). Additionally, context consideration (e.g., fluid loss due to hemorrhage, hypotension, trauma, or sepsis) is important for the choice of fluids.

The majority of the veterinary literature on the subject of IV fluid therapy in dogs, cats, horses, and cattle is descriptive and does not comply with evidence-based research standards (major areas of noncompliance include identification of predefined outcome variables, sample size determination, randomization, and blinding) and as such it does not adequately translate to veterinary clinical practice (see Further Reading). Moreover, standardized IV fluid protocols are increasingly replaced by patient-specific fluid administration, guided by published guidelines, which emphasize that fluid therapy should always be tailored to individual needs and re-evaluated according to changes in status (see Further Reading). Tables 2.6 and 2.7 provide some fluid therapy guidelines and recommendations for common indications in different species in clinical practice using synthetic fluids and blood products, respectively.

Patient Preparation

Principles of Obtaining Intravenous Access

It is always recommended to secure intravenous access in any patient being anesthetized regardless of whether injectable or inhalation drugs will be used for the procedure. Furthermore, intravenous access should be considered during sedation, particularly for long duration or profound sedation, in unstable patients or those with elevated ASA status.

Obtaining intravenous access is achieved by aseptically placing a catheter or cannula into a peripheral (e.g., cephalic vein and saphenous vein) or major vein (e.g., jugular vein or vena cava). *Note*: In this textbook, the terms "catheter" and "cannula" are used interchangeably at the discretion of the main author of the chapter. However, the original uses of these terms differ. A "catheter" refers to a long flexible tube passed into a blood vessel (e.g., central intravenous catheter), body cavity (e.g., thoracic drain and peritoneal drain), or urinary bladder (e.g., urinary catheter). It is usually inserted using an over-the-wire technique and kept in place for a longer period of time than a cannula (i.e., a few days). A "cannula" refers to a more rigid, shorter tube, usually inserted with an over-the-needle technique and kept in place for a shorter period of time. While cannulas can be used to drain body cavities (e.g., thoracocentesis, abdominocentesis, etc.), they are not usually kept in place for this purpose. Their design is for obtaining intravenous access. The term "catheter" is more frequently used in North America, while "cannula" is more often used in Europe, particularly the United Kingdom.

An intravenous catheter enables quick and efficient delivery of sedative, anesthetic, analgesic and emergency drugs, allows for the provision of intravenous fluids or infusions of drugs, and lowers the risk of inadvertent extravascular injection.

A variety of sterilized polythene, nylon, or Teflon intravenous catheters are available in various diameters and lengths, with the most appropriate size being dictated by the vessel to be catheterized. Fluid flow through the catheter is directly related to the radius of the catheter and inversely affected by the length. Radius has the greatest effect, with flow being related to the radius to the fourth power, as described by the Hagen–Poiseuille equation:

$$Q = \frac{(P_2 - P_1)\pi r^4}{8\eta l}$$

where Q represents flow, P is pressure, r is the tube radius, η is fluid viscosity, and l is length of the catheter.

The Birmingham gauge wire system is used to describe catheter diameter. The system works on a descending scale, with higher gauge (G) values indicating smaller diameter (e.g., 18 G is 0.8 mm internal diameter and 24 G is 0.3 mm). Catheter length also impacts flow rate, with shorter catheters allowing a faster rate of flow. The influence of catheter length is not as great as the radius and catheter length is generally chosen based on patient size.

Infections associated with IV catheters are reported to be one of the most frequent causes of nosocomial infection in hospitalized patients (see Further Reading); therefore, particular attention should be placed on aseptic technique during placement. While gloves are not necessary when placing catheters (except in immunocompromised or leukopenia patients), the World Health Organization recommends hands are washed before catheter placement and alcohol solution is applied to the hands of the person placing the catheter. Patient hair/fur is usually removed to assist visualizing the vein, promote asepsis, and facilitate securing the catheter. Clippers are considered superior to razor blades for hair removal to reduce the risk of skin damage (which increases infection risk) (see Further Reading). Preparation of the skin with a 1:1 solution of 4% chlorhexidine gluconate (for a final concentration of 2%) in combination with 70% isopropyl alcohol has been shown in people and animals to cause less infection than povidone–iodine or 70% alcohol alone.

The site of catheter placement will be influenced by the patient, procedure, and veterinarian preference. In dogs and cats, the cephalic vein, which is relatively large and easy to visualize and locate, is most frequently used. The lateral (dogs) or medial (cat) saphenous vein can also be used, but these sites are more prone to contamination from urine and fecal matter, which can increase the risk of infection. In horses, the jugular vein is most commonly catheterized; the lateral thoracic vein represents an alternative when no jugular vein is suitable. In adult cattle, the jugular veins or an auricular vein are usually catheterized. In small ruminants and calves, the jugular, cephalic, or auricular veins can be used. Pigs are notoriously difficult to catheterize, with the auricular vein, and occasionally the cephalic or dorsal metatarsal veins (piglets and young pigs) being the most accessible.

Application of a dressing over the catheter can help to prevent contamination and secure the catheter in place. Care should be taken to check dressing and tape tension. Tissue swelling can arise if the placement is too tight while loose taping can result in catheter dislodgement.

Catheters should be monitored frequently. The insertion site and blood vessel should be checked for inflammation and infection at least daily. Additionally, the catheter should be checked for leaks or perivascular displacement regularly. The securing dressing and tape should also be monitored. It is recommended to flush catheters every two to four hours with physiologic saline to ensure catheter patency and prevent the development of clots (heparinized solutions are commonly recommended for flushing catheters, but heparin can interact with drugs and this should be taken into consideration) (see Further Reading).

It has been suggested that keeping a "short-stay" catheter (those described in this section and commonly used when performing anesthesia) in place for longer than 72–96 h increases the risk of infection. It is recommended to replace an intravenous catheter every 72 h to reduce this risk (see Further Reading). In patients requiring long-term intravenous access, placement of a long-stay catheter (i.e., central line; usually a single or multi-lumen catheter placed via a jugular vein and the tip advanced past the thoracic inlet) while the patient is anesthetized is recommended, if feasible.

Other reported complications associated with intravenous catheters include mechanical irritation caused by the catheter, air embolism, and excessive bleeding at the site of placement which can lead to hematoma formation.

Pre-anesthetic Withholding of Food and Water

Pre-anesthetic fasting (withholding of food) is performed to protect the patient from the risks associated with the presence of a full gastrointestinal system. The risks of not withholding food before anesthesia are species dependent. In dogs and cats, pre-anesthetic fasting serves to reduce nausea, vomiting, and, in dogs, gastroesophageal regurgitation (GER). The latter can lead to peri-anesthetic complications such as esophageal and choanal stricture (narrowing of the nasal airway at the caudal parts of the choanae) and aspiration pneumonia. Regarding fasting times, the traditional practice of withholding food for periods of 12 h or longer to ensure an empty stomach in healthy adult dogs and cats before the anesthetic procedure is outdated since compelling evidence (canine studies) links prolonged fasting to reduced gastric pH (increases gastric acidity) and increased sequestration of fluids increasing gastric volume, which can increase the risk of GER and associated complications (see Further Reading). Since horses are unable to vomit, although reflux and regurgitation can occur when intestinal obstruction is present, the goal of pre-anesthetic fasting in horses is to reduce pressure of the gastrointestinal system on the diaphragm in a recumbent horse. Pressure reduction is an attempt to preserve functional residual capacity of the lungs, and thus maintain alveolar ventilation and minimize hypoxemia. Furthermore, fasting could also reduce compression of the caudal vena cava, which may help maintain venous return to the heart and cardiac output. In ruminants, the fasting aims to reduce the rate of fermentation in the gastrointestinal system and to minimize the development of bloat and increased salivation during anesthesia. In pigs, gastric emptying is generally rapid and pre-anesthetic withholding of food is less important but may be required for gastrointestinal surgery. In rabbits, food is allowed up to the time of premedication since fasting may result in hypoglycemia and contributes to gastrointestinal stasis, which results in gastrointestinal tympany and ileus in the peri-anesthetic period.

Regarding the pre-anesthetic withholding of water, current opinions are that it is better to refrain from prolonged water withholding in most species and to provide water up to two hours before or until the time of premedication. The continuation of water uptake up to a shorter period before the onset of anesthesia has the main benefit of reducing the potential for hypovolemia during anesthesia. Since all ruminants are a high risk for anesthesia and recumbency-related tympany, gastric regurgitation and aspiration pneumonia, prolonged water withholding is generally performed to decrease the volume of fermentable ingesta, to reduce salivation and the amount of gastric regurgitation.

When considering a pre-anesthetic fasting protocol, it is not only the duration of food and water restriction prior to anesthesia that is of concern, but, in many species, the type of food (dry, wet, liquid, and concentrate), the composition of food (protein, carbon, fat, and fiber content), and meal size also influence the gastrointestinal emptying time (see Further Reading). Individual factors, such as breed (brachycephalic dog breeds show prolonged gastric emptying and are more prone to regurgitation), age (juvenile animals are predisposed to hypoglycemia), body conformation, health status, and medication also influence the decision of what is an appropriate fasting protocol for an individual patient. Furthermore, in many species there is lack of evidence and subsequently no consensus for when and how long water and food should be withheld before anesthesia. Therefore, pre-anesthetic fasting should be carefully considered and tailored to an individual patient. Current recommendations for pre-anesthetic fasting and water withholding times in different species are displayed in Table 2.8 and can serve as a guideline.

Table 2.8 Current guidelines and recommendations for pre-operative fasting times in common veterinary species.

Species	Patient status	Withhold water (h)	Recommended type of food	Withhold food (h)
Dogs and cats	<8 weeks or < 2 kg	0		1–2
	Healthy adult	0–2*	Half daily rate of "wet" canned food of low fat and low fibre content	(4)–6
	Healthy adult	0–2*	Half daily rate of dry, fat, or high in protein content food	10+
Horses	Foals	0		0
	Healthy adult	0		8–12
	Healthy adult	0	Concentrates and large meals of forages	4–6
	Healthy adult	0	Grazing or *ad lib* access to conserved or ensiled forages (preserved forages)	1–2
Ruminants	Nonruminating calves, lambs, and kids	0	Milk	0
	Nonruminating calves, lambs, and kids	0	Creep feeds	1–2
	Healthy large species adult	12		24–36
	Healthy small species adult	12		12–16
Pigs	Pre-weaning piglets	0	Milk and creep feeds	0
	Micropigs/minipigs	0		0
	Other pigs	0		0–1 6–12
	Abdominal surgery	0	Liquid food	4–6
	Gastrointestinal surgery	12	Carbohydrate-dense drink	12
Rabbits		0		0

Information in this table is a summary of the expert opinions from an open discussion between European College of Veterinary Anaesthesia (ECVAA) Diplomates on the subject of food and water withholding before anesthesia, held at the 2019 Spring meeting of the Association of Veterinary Anaesthetists (AVA).

*For the recommended short periods of water withholding, water is usually removed at the time of premedication.

Questions and Answers

There are more practice questions and answers available for this chapter on the website. Please visit http://www.wiley.com/go/VeterinaryAnesthesiaZeiler.

Questions

1) A dog presents with a femur fracture and is tachycardic with weak pulses and depressed. The other clinical, hematological, and biochemical variables are within normal reference intervals. Describe your fluid plan, in brief notes, that you will use during the peri-anesthetic period. Provide fluid examples and volumes of administration.
2) What is the purpose of the ASA classification?
   a) Pre-operative score denoting anesthetic risk based on physical status
   b) Post-operative score assigned based on surgical outcome
   c) Post-operative score assigned based on occurrence of anesthetic complications
   d) Pre-operative score denoting surgical risk
   e) Pre-operative score denoting anesthetic risk based on risk of surgery
3) A dog presents for emergency surgery due to a ruptured duodenal ulcer, how long should it be fasted prior to surgery?
   a) Remove food and water immediately to starve the patient for 4–6 h before surgery
   b) Remove food only for 4–6 h before surgery
   c) Withhold food and water during the stabilization and preparation period
   d) Remove water only for 4–6 h before surgery because it is unlikely to eat

Answers

1) The dog is presumed to be in shock and requires volume resuscitation. Any of the isotonic crystalloids or synthetic colloids could be used for the initial volume replacement to stabilize the cardiovascular system function before anesthesia. For the isotonic crystalloids, an initial bolus of 20 mL/kg can be given over 5–15 min and then heart rate, pulse quality, and demeanor can be re-evaluated. For synthetic colloids, a bolus of 5–10 mL/kg can be given over 5–15 min and then re-evaluation of cardiovascular function is required. Once stabilized, general anesthesia can be induced for surgical repair of the femur. During the operation, an isotonic crystalloid can be administered at 5 mL/kg/h during the anesthesia.
2) a
3) c

Further Reading

Albrecht, N.A., Howard, J., Kovacevic, A. et al. (2016). In Vitro effects of 6% hydroxyethyl starch 130/0.42 solution on feline whole blood coagulation measured by rotational thromboelastometry. *BMC Vet Res* 12: 1–8.

Bednarski, R. (2011). AAHA anesthesia guidelines for dogs and cats. *J Am Anim Hosp Assoc* 47: 377–385.

Benzimra, C., Cerasoli, I., Rault, D. et al. (2020). Computed tomographic features of gastric and esophageal content in dogs undergoing CT myelography and factors influencing the presence of esophageal fluid. *J Vet Sci* 21: e84.

Berry, A., Watt, B., Goldacre, M. et al. (1982). A comparison of the use of povidone–iodine and chlorhexidine in the prophylaxis. *J Hosp Infect* 3: 55–63.

Bradbury, G.A. and Clutton, E.R. (2016). Review of practices reported for preoperative food and water restriction of laboratory pigs (Sus Scrofa). *J Am Assoc Lab Anim Sci* 55: 35–40.

Brodbelt, D.C., Blissit, K.J., Hammond, R.A. et al. (2008). The risk of death: the confidential enquiry into perioperative small animal fatalities. *Vet Anaesth Analg* 35: 365–373.

Chandra, A. (2014). The role of pre-operative investigations in relatively healthy general surgical patients – a retrospective study. *Anaes Pain Intens Care* 18: 241–244.

Crabtree, N.E. and Epstein, K.L. (2021). Current concepts in fluid therapy in horses. *Front Vet Sci* 8: 1–16.

Davidbow, B. (2013). Transfusion medicine in small animals. *Vet Clinic N Am: Sm Anim Prac* 43: 735–756.

Davis, H. (2015). Nursing care. *V Clinic N Am: Sm Anim Prac* 45: 1029–1048.

Davis, H., Jensen, T., Knowles, P. et al. (2013). AAHA/AAFP fluid therapy guidelines for dogs and cats. *J Am Anim Hospl Assoc* 49: 149–159.

Epstein, K., Bergren, A., Giguere, S. et al. (2014). Cardiovascular, colloid osmotic pressure, and hemostatic effects of 2 formulations of hydroxyethyl starch in healthy horses. *J Vet Intern Med* 28: 223–233.

Fielding, C.L. (2018). Practical fluid therapy and treatment modalities for field conditions for horses and foals with gastrointestinal problems. *Vet Clinic: Equi Prac* 34: 155–168.

Galatos, A.D. and Raptopoulos, D. (1995). Gastro-esophageal reflux during anesthesia in the dog: the effect of preoperative fasting and premedication. *Vet Rec* 137: 479–483.

Hayes, G., Benedicenti, L., and Mathews, K. (2016). Retrospective cohort study on the incidence of acute kidney injury and death following hydroxyethyl starch (HES 10% 250/0.5/5:1) administration in dogs (2007 – 2010). *J Vet Emerg Crit Care* 26: 35–40.

Iannucci, C., Dirkman, D., Howard, J. et al. (2020). A prospective randomized open-label trial on the comparative effects of 6% hydroxyethyl starch 130/0.4 versus polyionic isotonic crystalloids on coagulation parameters in dogs with spontaneous hemoperitoneum. *J Vet Emerg Crit Care* 31: 32–42.

Johnston, G.M., Eastment, J.K., Wood, J., and Taylor, P.M. (2002). The confidential enquiry into perioperative equine fatalities (CEPEF): mortality results of Phases 1 and 2. *Vet Anaesth Analg* 29: 159–170.

Jones, I.D., Case, A.M., Stevens, K.B. et al. (2009). Factors contributing to the contamination of peripheral intravenous catheters in dogs and cats. *Vet Rec* 164: 616–618.

Mathews, K.A., Brooks, M.J., and Valliant, A.E. (1996). A prospective study of intravenous catheter contamination. *J Vet Emerg Crit Care* 6: 33–43.

McCluskey, S.A. and Karkouti, K. (2013). Starches for fluid therapy: is it time for a re-appraisal or has the horse left the barn? *Can J Anesth* 60: 630–633.

Muir, W.W., Ueyama, Y., Noel-Morgan, J. et al. (2017). A systematic review of the quality of IV fluid therapy in veterinary medicine. *Front Vet Sci* 4: 127.

Osuna, D.J., Deyoung, D.J., and Walker, R.L. (1990). Comparison of three skin preparation techniques Part 1: clinical trial in 100 dogs. *Vet Surg* 19: 14–19.

Portier, K. and Ida, K.K. (2018). The ASA physical status classification: what is the evidence for recommending its use in veterinary anesthesia? A systematic review. *Front Vet Sci* 5: 204.

Robertson, S.A., Gogolski, S.M., Pascoe, P. et al. (2018). AAFP feline anesthesia guidelines. *J Fel Med Surg* 20: 602–634.

Roussel, A.J. (2014). Fluid therapy in mature cattle. *Vet Clin: Food Anim Prac* 30: 429–439.

Savvas, I., Rallis, T., and Raptopoulos, D. (2009). The effect of pre-anesthetic fasting time and type of food on gastric content volume and acidity in dogs. *Vet Anaesth Analg* 36: 539–546.

Savvas, I. and Raptopoulos, D. (2000). Incidence of gastro-esophageal reflux during anesthesia, following two different fasting times in dogs. *Vet Anaesth Analg* 27: 59–60.

Senior Care Guidelines Task Force: AAHA, Epstein, M., Kuehn, N.F., Landsberg, G. et al. (2005). AAHA senior care guidelines for dogs and cats. *J Am Anim Hosp Assoc* 41: 81–91.

Sigrist, N.E., Kalin, N., and Dreyfus, A. (2017a). Effects of hydroxyethyl starch 130/0.4 on serum creatinine concentration and development of acute kidney injury in nonazotemic cats. *J Vet Intern Med* 31: 1749–1756.

Sigrist, N., Kalin, N., and Dreyfus, A. (2017b). Changes in serum creatinine concentration and acute kidney injury (AKI) grade in dogs treated with hydroxyethyl starch 130/0.4 from 2013 to 2015. *J Vet Intern Med* 31: 434–441.

Tanner, J., Norrie, P., and Melen, K. (2011). Preoperative hair removal to reduce surgical site infection. *Cochrane Data Syst Rev* 9 (11): CD004122.

Viskjer, S. and Sjöström, L. (2017). Effect of the duration of food withholding prior to anesthesia on gastroesophageal reflux and regurgitation in healthy dogs undergoing elective orthopedic surgery. *Am J Vet Res* 78: 144–150.

Woodcock, T.E. and Michel, C.C. (2021). Advances in the Starling principle and microvascular fluid exchange: consequences and implications for fluid therapy. *Front Vet Sci* 8: 623–671.

Woodcock, T.E. and Woodcock, T.M. (2012). Revised Starling equation and the glycocalyx model of transvascular fluid exchange: an improved paradigm for prescribing intravenous fluid therapy. *Br J Anaesth* 108: 384–394.

3

Pain Physiology, Assessment, and Principles of Treatment

Jo Murrell and Daniel Pang

The Definition of *Pain*

The International Association for the Study of Pain (IASP) define *pain* in humans and animals as "An unpleasant sensory and emotional experience associated with, or resembling that associated with, actual or potential tissue damage." Importantly, this definition is supported by a number of key notes, one of which is that "Verbal description is only one of several behaviors to express pain; inability to communicate does not negate the possibility that a human or a nonhuman animal experiences pain." This note is particularly pertinent to the definition of pain in animals, highlighting the fact that animals process pain as a sensory and emotional experience despite the lack of their ability to verbally communicate. Other notes that accompany this definition of pain are as follows:

- Pain is always a personal experience that is influenced to varying degrees by biological, psychological, and social factors.
- Pain and nociception are different phenomena. Pain cannot be inferred solely from activity in sensory neurons.
- Through their life experiences, individuals learn the concept of pain.
- A person's report of an experience as pain should be respected.
- Although pain usually serves an adaptive role, it may have adverse effects on function and social and psychological well-being.

These notes highlight the global effect that pain has on every aspect of an individual's life, a phenomenon that, although more difficult to detect in animals, is likely also to be the case.

Nociception is defined differently to pain as the neural process of encoding noxious stimuli. Although nociception may lead to pain sensation, it is not necessarily implied. For example, in an anesthetized animal undergoing surgery, nociception will be present but if the animal is adequately anesthetized pain will not be experienced. This is because the cerebral cortex is effectively "knocked out" of the pain pathway in an adequately anesthetized animal and a functioning cerebral cortex is essential for pain perception. However, providing analgesia during anesthesia is still important because otherwise activation of nociceptive pathways caused by tissue injury and surgery will lead to upregulation of the pain pathways and enhanced, uncontrolled, pain in the recovery period.

An Overview of the Somatic Nociceptive Pathway

The somatic pain pathway begins with nociceptors that are located in peripheral soft and hard tissues (the skin, muscles, bone, joint, and joint capsules) and detect noxious stimuli in the environment and ends in pain perception due to processes occurring in the cerebral cortex. Information related to noxious environmental stimuli is transduced by nociceptors and transmitted via afferent primary order neurons to the dorsal horn of the spinal cord. The signal is then relayed via secondary order neurons in the spinal cord to the brain stem and thalamus and finally the cerebral cortex (Figure 3.1).

Nociceptors

Nociceptors are the free nerve endings of sensory fibers that are activated when subjected to stimuli that are of sufficient magnitude to be damaging to tissue. Different nociceptors that respond to different types of noxious stimuli have been characterized using electrophysiological

Fundamental Principles of Veterinary Anesthesia, First Edition. Edited by Gareth E. Zeiler and Daniel S. J. Pang.

Companion Website: www.wiley.com/go/VeterinaryAnesthesiaZeiler

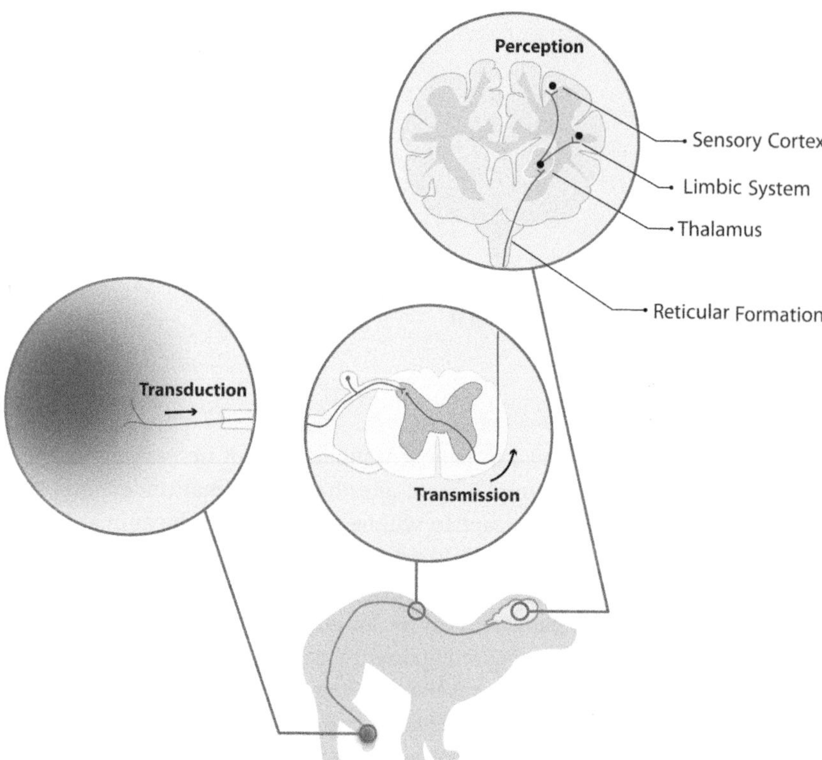

Figure 3.1 Overview of the somatic pain pathway, showing transduction of noxious stimuli into a nerve signal (by nociceptors) that is transmitted from the periphery to the central nervous system (via the dorsal horn of the spinal cord), where perception of pain occurs as the signal terminates in the cerebral cortex.

techniques. It is important to note that nociceptors are extremely heterogenous, with a variety of different receptors being expressed and neurotransmitters released.

Nociceptors that are associated with myelinated Aδ (A-delta) fibers mediate acute, well-localized, fast pain, in effect the onset of pain perception associated with a particular stimulus, whereas unmyelinated C fiber nociceptors mediate slow, poorly localized, "second pain." Aδ nociceptors are divided into two types: Type I and Type II. Type I Aδ nociceptors are described as high threshold mechanical receptors that respond primarily to mechanical and chemical stimuli, although they are also activated by heat at high temperatures (>50 °C). Type I receptors become sensitized following tissue damage so that thresholds for stimulation by both heat and mechanical stimuli decrease. This means that low levels of heat and mechanical stimuli, normally insufficient to trigger activation, are capable of eliciting a response leading to allodynia (see the following section on sensitization for more detail). Type II Aδ nociceptors have lower heat thresholds and higher mechanical thresholds than type I receptors and are primarily responsible for the first acute pain response to noxious heat. C fiber nociceptors are polymodal, responding to heat, mechanical, and chemical stimuli, with some C fibers responding to innocuous stimuli such as cooling.

How Does Activation of the Nociceptor by a Noxious Stimulus Result in Generation of an Action Potential in the Afferent Fiber?

The nervous system encodes and transmits information electrically in the form of action potentials. Activation of the nociceptors described in the preceding text by different noxious stimuli, if of sufficient magnitude, will cause a depolarization of the receptor membrane, termed a "receptor potential." Receptor potentials have the capacity to generate an action potential in the sensory afferent fiber, allowing onward transmission of the signal to the spinal cord. Voltage-gated sodium, calcium, and potassium channels expressed on C and Aδ fibers are recognized to be important in the translation of receptor potentials to generate an action potential and so they are important potential targets for novel analgesics.

Spinal Cord

Primary afferent sensory fibers synapse in the gray matter of the dorsal horn of the spinal cord, which is organized into 10 anatomical and functionally distinct layers or laminae. Different primary afferent fibers synapse in distinct lamina, depending on whether the sensory fiber is transmitting noxious or non-noxious (innocuous) information. The more superficial laminae (I and II) are associated with the processing of noxious stimuli, although laminae I to V all receive sensory input (Figure 3.2). Aδ and C fibers synapse primarily in laminae I and II. Aβ (A-beta) fibers primarily relay non-nociceptive input related to mechanosensation and touch synapse in laminae III and IV. Lamina V is unusual compared to others because the primary afferent terminals of sensory fibers conveying both noxious and non-noxious information can synapse here. Aβ, Aδ, and, indirectly, C fibers, all terminate in this layer. Cells of the dorsal horn can be subdivided into nociceptive-specific cells, which predominate in laminae I and II, non-nociceptive (predominantly in laminae III and IV), and wide dynamic range neurons that respond to a range of stimuli from non-noxious to noxious. Wide dynamic range neurons predominate in lamina V. A number of different neurotransmitters are released at the primary afferent terminal, described in more detail in the section on central sensitization (see the following text). The precise structural organization is likely to facilitate differentiation between noxious stimuli of different intensities and qualities, for example heat or mechanostimulation.

Ascending Projection Neurons

Projection neurons are predominantly located in laminae I, III, and IV and send axons in the white spinal matter to the brain. Afferent, primary order neurons, arising from nociceptors, may directly synapse with projection neurons (secondary order neurons) or via interneurons. Projection neurons ascend in specific fiber tracts relating to transmission of different types of noxious stimuli so that the precise structural organization of the dorsal horn of the spinal cord is continued in the white matter.

Axons of secondary order neurons from laminae I and II target different specific areas of the brain, providing a mechanism by which information relating to nociception can be integrated with information from the autonomic nervous system and the hypothalamic–pituitary-adrenal axis (HPA axis). This integration allows the activation of other physiological systems that can be linked to pain such as changes in heart rate, respiratory rate, and blood pressure.

The Cerebral Cortex

Pain is recognized to be a complex multidimensional phenomenon and the cerebral cortex is considered to be the seat of pain perception in mammals. Electrophysiological and functional imaging (such as functional magnetic resonance imaging) studies inform us that no one single structure is responsible for the processing of pain, instead the experience of pain is thought to arise from co-activation of a number of different structures within the cerebral cortex.

Two functionally distinct parallel systems are recognized to contribute to pain processing: (1) the medial pain system that results in the affective motivational aspects of pain, causing aversion, fear, and anxiety; (2) the lateral pain system that leads to the sensory-discriminative aspects of pain, providing information about stimulus location and intensity.

Different brain structures are involved in these two systems although functional interconnectivity between them

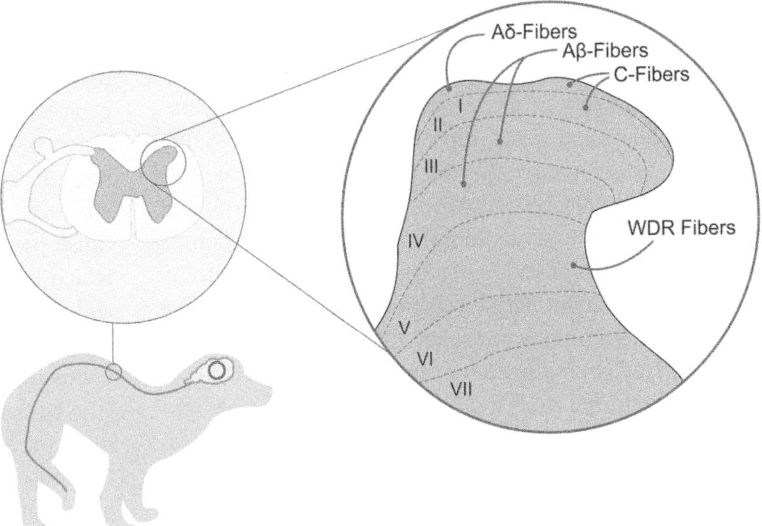

Figure 3.2 Laminae of the dorsal horn of the spinal cord, showing key locations of nerve fiber synapses. Aδ and C fibers are the most important nociceptors, terminating predominantly in laminae I and II. WDR, wide dynamic range neurons.

ensures that the two systems do not function independently of each other. For example, information about the intensity of pain is likely to determine, in part, how aversive the experience is likely to be. The anterior cingulate cortex (ACC) and insular cortex are recognized to be key structures in the medial pathway, receiving significant input from medial thalamic nuclei and also contributing to the descending control of pain. In contrast, the primary and secondary somatosensory cortices are important structures in the lateral pain pathway, receiving input from the lateral thalamic nuclei.

Pain and the Autonomic Nervous System

Pain also induces specific changes in the autonomic nervous system. These changes are critical to adaptation and survival and ensure that pain results in appropriate modulation of the cardiovascular and respiratory systems to facilitate a change in behavioral state.

The central autonomic nervous system network is widely distributed throughout the brain, including the ACC and insular cortices, central nucleus of the amygdala, hypothalamus, periaqueductal gray (PAG), parabrachial nucleus (PBN) of the pons, and nucleus tractus solitarius (NTS). These brain regions are also intimately involved in the processing of nociceptive stimuli and the perception of pain such that pain generates stimulus-specific patterns of autonomic nervous system activation. Sympathoexcitation, characterized by hypertension and tachycardia, is commonly associated with noxious stimulation in unconscious (e.g., anesthetized) animals and pain in conscious individuals, but bradycardia and hypotension can also occur.

The PAG is particularly important for integration of the nociceptive and autonomic nervous systems. Somatic nociceptive stimuli cause activation of the lateral PAG that initiates flight-or-fight responses by sympathoexcitation, causing tachycardia, hypertension, and redistribution of blood to muscles, representing an active coping response to escapable stimuli. The ventral lateral PAG predominantly receives input from muscle, visceral, and poorly localized somatic stimuli and initiates responses such as bradycardia and hypotension, and hyporeactivity to the environment. These reflect adoption of a passive coping strategy in the presence of inescapable stimuli characterized by quiescence and decreased vigilance where the animal does not try to elicit a flight-or-fight response. Outputs from the lateral and ventral lateral PAG project to different regions of the medulla to allow the appropriate modulation of cardiovascular responses according to stimulus type.

Visceral Pain

Visceral pain is common and difficult to manage pharmacologically. The sensation of visceral pain differs markedly from somatic pain, reflecting differences in the processing of visceral and somatic stimuli. Generally, sufferers of visceral pain attribute a greater negative emotional component to it than somatic pain and this is also associated with exaggerated autonomic nervous system responses. Cardinal features of visceral pain are: (1) its poorly localized and diffuse nature; (2) it may not be evoked from all internal organs as not all viscera are innervated by sensory afferent fibers; (3) it is not always linked to tissue injury, and functional disturbances of the viscera may also result in pain; and (4) it is referred to the "body wall."

The sensations that can arise from visceral organs are very different than those arising from somatic stimuli. Visceral pain results from direct inflammation of a visceral organ, occlusion of bile or urine flow, or functional visceral disorders. It is associated with sensations such as distention, bloating, nausea or dyspnea, a marked contrast to the sensations of heat, touch, pinch, and crush that are elicited by somatic stimuli.

Central and Peripheral Sensitization

A unique feature of the pain pathways is that they are not hard-wired. Instead, they show marked plasticity; the sensitivity and responsiveness of pain pathways is modulated by the peripheral noxious sensory input into the system. This plasticity is responsible for the changes in pain sensation that occur following nerve damage and inflammation. Clinically it is apparent that following tissue injury pain sensitivity is increased, which can make provision of effective analgesia more challenging. Increased sensitivity is thought to serve a protective function, with enhanced pain resulting in greater protection of the damaged tissue. However, it can also lead to persistent pain that is maladaptive. The changes in pain sensation that accompany tissue injury are typically hyperalgesia, allodynia, and spontaneous pain. Hyperalgesia is enhanced pain sensation from stimuli that would normally cause pain and can be divided into primary hyperalgesia, which is enhanced sensitivity in the area of tissue damage, and secondary hyperalgesia, which is present in the area of surrounding uninjured tissue. Primary hyperalgesia results in increased sensitivity to both thermal and mechanical stimuli whereas secondary hyperalgesia is generally considered to be mechanical stimuli only. It is important to detect secondary hyperalgesia during pain assessment (e.g., by looking for an exaggerated response to firm pressure in the area of uninjured tissue surrounding a wound or surgical site) because this may be a cardinal indicator that central sensitization is present. Allodynia is pain due to a stimulus that does not normally cause pain such as touch. Pain does not normally arise spontaneously without stimulation of the tissue; therefore spontaneous pain is also an aberrant sensation that accompanies central and peripheral sensitization. Sensitization is a feature of both somatic and visceral pathways, but the mechanisms of central and peripheral sensitization will be discussed with reference to the somatic pathway only.

Peripheral Sensitization

Peripheral sensitization, triggered by inflammation, results in primary hyperalgesia, allodynia, and spontaneous pain. When tissue damage occurs it stimulates the release of inflammatory mediators from damaged cells, the endothelial cells of local blood vessels and white blood cells that migrate into the area. Inflammatory mediators include prostaglandin E_2, leukotrienes, cytokines, bradykinin, platelet activating factor, glutamate, nerve growth factor, endothelin, and Substance P. Collectively, these mediators enhance sensory neuron background activity and lower thermal and mechanical thresholds (allodynia) and increase responses to suprathreshold stimuli (hyperalgesia), all features of peripheral sensitization.

Peripheral sensitization, as well as mediating primary hyperalgesia, also contributes to the development and maintenance of central sensitization by increasing C fiber afferent activity into the dorsal horn of the spinal cord.

Central Sensitization

Central sensitization, a phenomenon that occurs in the spinal cord but also in higher brain centers, is critical to the development of enhanced pain sensitivity after injury and the development of secondary hyperalgesia and chronic maladaptive pain. Understanding key mechanisms that underpin central sensitization is essential for knowledge of pain pathophysiology and analgesic drug action. These mechanisms are extremely complex and only key points are given here (see Further Reading).

Central sensitization is a manifestation of the functional and morphological plasticity in the central nervous system (CNS). It comprises both acute and long-term changes in nociceptive processing. As a result of central sensitization, there is an increase in synaptic strength, and change in the receptive field properties of dorsal horn neurons and reduced inhibition of nociceptive processing in the spinal cord, collectively enhancing nociceptive transmission from the peripheral sensory system to the brain and manifesting clinically as increased pain sensitivity.

Under basal conditions, glutamate is the most common excitatory neurotransmitter in the dorsal horn of the spinal cord. It is released from the presynaptic membrane of primary afferent sensory fibers (first-order neurons) and primarily binds to α-amino-3-hydroxy-5-methyl-4-isoxazelpropionic acid (AMPA), kainate, and G-protein-coupled metabotropic receptors on the post-synaptic membrane of dorsal horn cells. The N-methyl D-aspartate (NMDA) receptor, also present on the post-synaptic membrane, does not participate in nociceptive transmission under normal conditions due to blockade of the glutamate binding site by magnesium ions (Mg^{2+}) found in nervous tissue. Although glutamate is the most prevalent excitatory neurotransmitter, other neurotransmitters also play a role, including Substance P and calcitonin-gene-related peptide (CGRP). Substance P is released by petidergic C fibers and binds to the NK-1 (neurokinin) receptor, and CGRP, synthesized by small diameter sensory neurons, binds to the CGRP receptor, both found on the post-synaptic membrane of dorsal horn cells. Central sensitization is only induced by sustained and intense noxious stimuli that are sufficient to increase C fiber activity and thereby cause prolonged depolarization of the post-synaptic membrane of dorsal horn cells. Membrane depolarization removes the Mg^{2+} block of the NMDA receptor allowing activation by glutamate and influx of calcium into the dorsal horn cell. This initiates a cascade of events resulting in heightened activity of dorsal horn neurons. Many of these events involve receptor phosphorylation, mediated by protein kinases. Substance P and CGRP also potentiate central sensitization by causing long-lasting depolarization of the dorsal horn post-synaptic membrane and temporal summation.

Normally, only a small percentage of synaptic inputs to dorsal horn neurons contribute to generation of an action potential in the dorsal horn cell. However, nociceptive-specific neurons in the dorsal horn laminae I and II receive many synaptic inputs from low threshold sensory afferents as well as inputs from nociceptors that lie outside the receptive field of the cell and do not contribute to the output of the cell under normal resting conditions. Following central sensitization, the receptive field of dorsal horn neurons increases so that these subthreshold inputs contribute to cell output and nociceptive-specific neurons start to adopt the electrophysiological properties of wide dynamic range neurons. These modifications contribute to allodynia because Aβ activity (resulting from stimulation of low threshold receptors) becomes interpreted as pain.

This is a brief overview of some of the mechanisms that produce central sensitization. Mechanisms are multiple, but all result in increased membrane excitability of dorsal horn neurons, increased synaptic efficacy in the nociceptive pathway, and reduced inhibition. Consequently, nociceptive processing in the spinal cord is facilitated, increasing the barrage of noxious information that is relayed to the brain where it is interpreted as pain.

Descending Control of Nociception

The understanding of descending control pathways and their role in nociceptive processing has significantly increased recently, and the concept that it functions only as an inhibitory system has been disproven. Modulation of these pathways offers a potential target in the therapeutic management of chronic pain.

Descending control of nociception is the modulation of nociceptive processing by supraspinal (brain) centers and it is an important survival mechanism, allowing implementation of appropriate behavioral responses to life-threatening stimuli by decreasing afferent nociceptive input to higher brain centers. However, it can also be maladaptive, contributing to the development of chronic pain states. Therefore, although descending control was previously considered to be inhibitory only, the importance of facilitation of nociceptive processing by supraspinal centers is now accepted. The balance between inhibition and facilitation is dynamic and a switch between a predominance of inhibition to facilitation is likely to underlie chronic inflammatory or neuropathic pain states leading to the development of maladaptive pain.

The superficial dorsal horn is the primary target for descending pathways. Pathways emerge from different areas of the brain, one of the most important being the periaqueductal gray–rostral ventromedial medulla (PAG–RVM) system (Figure 3.3). This system is recognized to be pivotal to descending control. In turn, the PAG receives multiple inputs from other brain structures, including the hypothalamus and limbic system, acting as a center for integration of nociceptive, autonomic nervous system and cognitive, emotional, and behavioral responses.

The descending control of dorsal horn neurons is selective for noxious stimuli, and activation of dorsal horn cells by non-noxious stimuli undergo limited modulation by descending pathways. Evidence is also emerging that descending control differentiates between C and A fiber nociceptive input in the deep dorsal horn such that C fiber input is inhibited to a much greater extent than A fiber input. The evolutionary advantage of this phenomenon is that A fiber input predominantly provides information on the sensory-discriminative aspects of pain, such as intensity and location. Preservation of this information is important for survival, whereas C fiber input is aversive and distracting, suppression allows a more effective behavioral and cognitive response to the threat, increasing chances of survival.

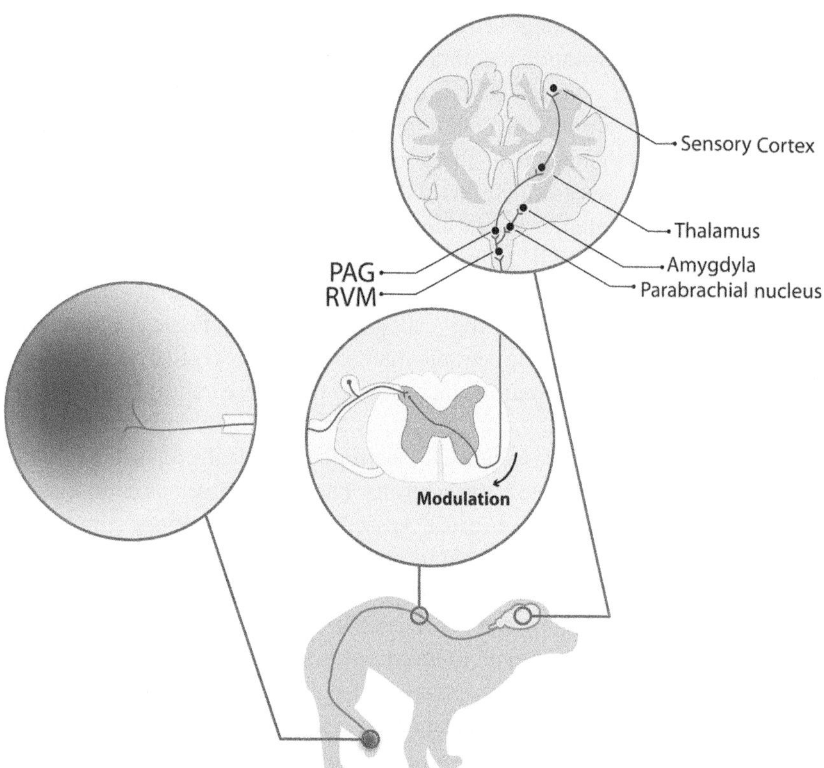

Figure 3.3 Modulation of nociception by descending control from the brain. PAG, periaqueductal gray; RVM, rostral ventromedial medulla. The PAG–RVM system plays a central role in descending control, receiving input from other brain centers.

The Development of Maladaptive Pain

Until recently, the terms "acute pain" and "chronic pain" were broadly used to define different pain states, with *chronic pain* usually defined as pain that lasts more than three months, although this definition is taken from the human field and may not be appropriate for animals that have shorter life spans than humans. However, more recently, the terms "adaptive" and "maladaptive" pain have been used to differentiate between different pain states. Adaptive pain refers to nociceptive or inflammatory pain that has a protective purpose because it stops the animal from using the injured body part and allows healing. However, it is important to note that nociceptive pain and inflammatory pain are different from each other, with inflammatory pain associated with central and peripheral sensitization. Nociceptive pain should also not be confused with nociception, where nociception is the neural process of encoding of noxious stimuli and nociceptive pain is the conscious perception of a tissue-damaging stimulus. Both nociceptive and inflammatory pain are reversible, although it is important to note that despite having a protective function it is still important to treat these pain states with analgesia.

Maladaptive pain is not protective, serves no benefit to the animal, and is primarily due to plastic changes in the pain processing system (central and peripheral sensitization and a switch from descending inhibition of pain to descending pathway facilitation). It can be divided into neuropathic pain, where there is damage to the nervous tissue itself, and functional pain, where there is no evidence of pathology in the nervous system or inflammation, but pain persists due to dysfunction of the nociceptive system. Neuropathic pain states are likely numerous in animals and include spinal cord injury, osteoarthritis (which also has an inflammatory component), and many cancers. Functional pain states in animals are less clearly defined but may include feline hyperesthesia syndrome as an example. In humans there is good evidence that poorly managed acute pain, for example pain after surgery, can lead to the development of maladaptive pain and this is another reason to treat acute adaptive pain promptly and aggressively with analgesia.

Pain Assessment and Scoring Systems

Importance of Pain Assessment in the Management of Pain

Recognizing and quantifying pain is critical to the adequate management of pain in all species. Unless pain is recognized and quantified, it is impossible to balance the provision of analgesia to give adequate pain relief against the risks of over-analgesia and the potential for analgesic-drug-related adverse effects. Tools to quantify pain are available for different species and can be helpful in recognizing and quantifying both acute and chronic pain. It is important to choose a tool that has been validated for the target species and the type of pain (e.g., acute or chronic) that the animal is likely to be experiencing in order to reduce the likelihood of error in the scoring system. It is also important to apply the tool in a sensible manner. For example, acute pain scoring tools do not take into account sedation, i.e., sedated animals may score highly on pain scoring tools because immobility or dullness/depression due to pain can be confused with immobility or dullness/depression due to sedation. Therefore, the acute pain scoring tools for all species should be applied once the animal is fully recovered from anesthesia and conscious. Stress can also confound acute pain scoring tools, with animals that are very stressed potentially scoring highly on the tool due to stress rather than pain-related behaviors. Therefore, animals should be assessed for pain in a quiet environment away from potential stressors.

Validating Pain Assessment Tools

Validity provides evidence that an instrument is measuring what it is designed to measure – for example, that a pain assessment tool is actually measuring pain, and it is a fundamental property of a tool that needs to be ensured before a tool is put forward for use in clinical practice.

Validity can be divided into a number of different elements as follows:

Criterion Validity

This is the agreement of a new instrument with an existing gold standard instrument designed to measure the same thing; however, this can be problematic for pain assessment tools because currently no "gold standard" tool is recognized. For example, in the adult human field, the gold standard for pain may be taken as a person's self-report of pain, but this is obviously not possible in animals.

Content Validity

This relates to the appropriateness of the items comprising the instrument with a judgment being made about whether the items comprising the instrument comprehensively sample the items being measured. Content validity is usually measured using subjective expert judgment to rate the contents of the instrument and their relevance.

Construct Validity

This describes whether changes in assessed scores fit with a hypothetical construct. For example, for a pain assessment tool, whether the scores increase after surgery and decrease with the administration of analgesia.

Reliability of an Instrument

Reliability can be divided into intra-rater reliability and inter-rater reliability. Intra-rater reliability is when the same person produces the same score with the instrument when the assessment is made at two time points (for example two weeks apart) in an unchanging subject (e.g., when the pain level is stable). Inter-rater reliability is when two (or more) assessors score the individual at the same time point and come up with similar scores. Obviously, both forms of reliability are important for a pain assessment tool, but inter-rater reliability is particularly important when the tool is used in a multi-user setting.

Responsiveness of an Instrument

This is an important property of a pain assessment tool and relates to the ability of an instrument to measure clinically relevant differences in pain state (e.g., to be able to differentiate between mild, moderate, and severe pain).

Clinical Utility

Clinical utility refers to how "user-friendly" an instrument is, and good clinical utility is fundamental to a pain scoring tool being adopted in clinical practice. For example, the tool needs to be easy to understand and quick to apply in order to make it feasible for use to pain score a large number of animals.

Acute Pain

How to Apply Tools in Practice

Most validated pain scoring tools are termed "composite tools." This is important because it implies that they try to measure both the sensory and emotional components of pain. Choose a tool that has been validated in the target species that works for your practice. Ideally, choose a tool that can be completed within about five minutes to increase the likelihood that the tool will be used frequently to score as many animals as possible during the day; tools that are lengthy to complete are unlikely to be widely adopted by the practice team. It does not matter who carries out the pain assessments in your practice as long as the people carrying out the pain assessments have been adequately trained to use the pain assessment tool. The authors believe that veterinary nurses or technicians are ideally positioned to carry out pain scoring in practice as these individuals spend more time with the animals than veterinarians during the day. As noted in the preceding text, it is important that pain assessment is carried out in a quiet environment when the animal is fully conscious and as relaxed as possible. If possible, it is helpful to carry out a baseline pain assessment before surgery or painful intervention so that animals that score highly (e.g., due to stress and anxiety, in the absence of a preexisting painful condition) before intervention can be detected. In this circumstance, it is helpful to deduct the baseline pain score from the post-intervention score to obtain a better idea about the animal's true pain state.

Validated Scoring Tools for Acute Pain in Dogs

Although a number of tools to assess pain have been developed for dogs, very few of these have undergone rigorous validation. The only validated scales to measure acute pain in dogs are the Composite Measure Pain Scale developed by researchers at the University of Glasgow (Morton et al. 2005) and its Short Form (Reid et al. 2007). The Short Form of the Glasgow Composite Measure Pain Scale – Canine – is probably the most widely used pain scoring tool in English-speaking countries. It is quick to complete (less than five minutes) and has a defined validated intervention score to guide administration of analgesia which is very helpful for the clinical management of painful dogs. The main limitation of this tool is that it is confounded by sedation; therefore it is important to score dogs when they are fully conscious.

Validated Scoring Tools for Acute Pain in Cats

There are currently three tools that have been validated to score acute pain in cats. The first to be validated was the UNESP-Botucatu Multidimensional Pain Scale (Brondani et al. 2011). This tool was only validated for cats undergoing ovariohysterectomy so it may not be that applicable to cats undergoing different painful procedures. It is also fairly time-consuming to complete. However, there is a validated intervention score for administration of rescue analgesia which is helpful for the management of painful cats. A short version of this scale (UNESP-SF) has since been validated using a range of orthopedic and soft tissue surgeries and found to be comparable to the full version of the scale and the Glasgow Composite Pain Scale - Feline (Belli et al. 2021). The next tool to be validated was the Glasgow Composite Pain Scale – Feline (Calvo et al. 2014). This tool has a very similar "look and feel" to it as the Short Form of the Glasgow Composite Pain Scale – Canine. It is quick to complete and has a validated intervention score for rescue analgesia. Finally, more recently, a grimace scale has been validated for cats (Evangelista et al. 2019). This scale also has a validated intervention score for administration of rescue analgesia.

Table 3.1 Tools developed to assess acute pain in horses.

Name of scale	Authors	Type of pain	Validated?	Time to complete the scale
Composite pain scale	Bussières et al. (2008) and van Loon et al. (2014)	Acute orthopedic pain; post-operative pain after emergency gastrointestinal surgery	Yes	Relatively quick to complete although includes measurement of some physiological variables
Equine acute abdominal pain scale-1	Sutton et al. (2013)	Acute colic pain	Yes	Quick, completion time around two minutes
EQUUS-COMPASS	van Loon and van Dierendonck (2015) and van Dierendonck and van Loon (2016)	Acute colic pain	Yes	Quick, completion time around five minutes
UNESP-Botucatu	Taffarel et al. (2015)	Post-castration pain	Yes	Quick, completion time around five minutes
Horse Grimace Scale	Dalla Costa et al. (2014) and Dalla Costa et al. (2016)	Post-castration pain; pain associated with laminitis	Yes – but only from photographs of horses rather than direct observation or from video footage	Quick to complete
EQUUS-FAP	van Loon and Dierendonck (2015) and van Loon and van Dierendonck (2017)	Acute colic pain and acute post-operative head-related pain	Yes	Quick, completion time around two minutes

Validated Scoring Tools for Acute Pain in Horses

There are a number of different tools to score acute pain that have been developed for horses. These tools are presented in Table 3.1.

Validated Scoring Tools for Acute Pain in Other Species

Cattle (de Oliveira et al. 2014), sheep (Silva et al. 2020), and pigs (Luna et al. 2020) also have validated pain scoring tools for acute pain. The UNESP group in Brazil has been pivotal in validating scales in these species, developing scales mainly based on behavioral changes. Grimace scales have been validated for numerous species, including rats (Sotocinal et al. 2011), mice (Langford et al. 2010), and rabbits (Keating et al. 2012), which are particularly helpful to improve the management of pain in experimental animals (see Mogil et al. (2020) for a review of grimace scales).

Tools to Assess Chronic Pain

The majority of tools that have been developed to assess chronic pain in companion animals are clinical metrology instruments (CMIs) that are completed by the owner. This is based on recognition that owners spend more time with their pets than veterinarians and are therefore perhaps better placed to detect subtle changes in behavior associated with chronic pain states. Similarly to tools to measure acute pain, it is important that the CMI is validated for the species and type of pain that it is measuring (e.g., pain caused by osteoarthritis). Generally, to avoid bias, it is recommended that CMIs are completed by only one owner (rather than by consensus) and that when sequential questionnaires are completed over time (e.g., before and after starting analgesic treatment), the more recent questionnaire is filled in without looking back at older questionnaires (termed "independent interviewing"). A concept called "Client-Specific Outcome Measures" (CSOMs), developed by Lascelles and colleagues (Lascelles et al. 2007), has also been widely used to measure chronic pain in dogs and cats. With this strategy, the owner and veterinarian together identify behaviors that are important to the dog or cat that are impaired by pain and monitor a change in the frequency with which these behaviors are performed with analgesic medication.

The importance of measuring Health-Related Quality of Life (HRQL) is also being increasingly recognized in dogs and cats, particularly in animals with chronic pain conditions. This is a difficult concept to measure with continuing discussion around what Quality of Life actually means in companion animals. In humans, HRQL is defined as the effect of the condition (e.g., osteoarthritis or cancer) on body function and well-being. This definition can also be applied to animals by considering the effect of pain on the global well-being of the animal; for example, in a cat with pelvic limb osteoarthritis it might take into account the effect of pain on the animal as well as the impact of not being able to use the litter tray to toilet.

Clinical Metrology Instruments for Dogs

Many of the CMIs to measure chronic pain in dogs have been validated to measure pain caused by osteoarthritis. Examples include the Liverpool Osteoarthritis in Dogs (LOAD) (Walton et al. 2013) and Helsinki Chronic Pain Index (Hielm-Bjorkman et al. 2009). The Canine Brief Pain Inventory (CBPI) has been validated for both osteoarthritis and bone cancer pain (Brown et al. 2008). This makes it a useful instrument to measure pain associated with more generalized and less specific pain conditions, although it has not been validated for other pain states such as neuropathic pain. The CBPI has notably been used in analgesic drug regulatory studies for the Food and Drug Administration (FDA) to prove analgesic drug efficacy for the management of chronic orthopedic pain. The Canine Osteoarthritis Staging Tool (COAST; Cachon et al. 2018) has been validated to stage osteoarthritis in dogs and therefore help with decision-making about analgesic drug management and includes application of a clinical metrology instrument as part of the grading process.

Clinical Metrology Instruments for Cats

The Feline Musculoskeletal Pain Index (Benito et al. 2013) is a questionnaire that has been developed and validated to measure pain in cats with degenerative joint disease. It asks the owner to rate what their cat can do in terms of activity and mobility compared to a normal cat and also includes a question about Quality of Life. It is quite quick to complete and therefore a practical tool to use in the clinical environment. Although the scale is less widely accessible than the Feline Musculoskeletal Pain Index, another group have developed a separate tool for owners and veterinarians to assess pain in cats with osteoarthritis (MI-CAT (C) and MI-CAT (V)) (Klinck et al. 2015, 2018). The veterinarian tool contains 25 items involving body posture, gait, willingness and ease of horizontal movements, jumping, and a general lameness score. A commercial company has also initially validated a tool to measure HRQL in cats (Noble et al. 2019) although this tool requires payment of a fee to use it which may limit widespread uptake of the scoring system.

There are no CMIs that have been developed for horses or other species to measure chronic pain.

Unidimensional Pain Scoring Tools

Unidimensional pain scoring tools focus on the measurement of the sensory-discriminative aspect of pain and do not take into account the emotional component of pain and have largely been replaced with composite pain scoring tools in veterinary practice. The types of unidimensional pain scoring tools that have been developed for the measurement of pain are detailed in Table 3.2.

Principles of Treating Pain

Concept of Pre-emptive and Preventive Analgesia Strategies

Pre-emptive analgesia is the principle of giving analgesics early, before the onset of pain, with the aim of preventing development of peripheral and central sensitization and thereby facilitating pain control in the post-operative period. There are very few clinical studies on the effectiveness of pre-emptive analgesia strategies in dogs and cats. Lascelles and colleagues investigated the pre-emptive analgesic effects of pethidine (meperidine) in dogs undergoing ovariohysterectomy and hypothesized that pre-operative pethidine blocked central sensitization to a greater extent than post-operative pethidine administered after surgery (Lascelles et al. 1997). Importantly, although pre-emptive analgesia has not turned out to be the "holy grail" in the prevention of post-operative pain, it has been shown to have a few disadvantages and may improve post-operative pain management; therefore, pre-emptive strategies are to be encouraged. Currently, the concept of preventive analgesia has superseded pre-emptive analgesia (Katz et al. 2011). Preventive analgesia acknowledges that in order to prevent central and peripheral sensitization nociceptive signals must be blocked from the start of skin incision, intra-operatively and post-operatively until tissue healing is complete. A *preventive analgesic effect* is defined as when "post-operative pain and/or analgesic consumption is reduced relative to another treatment, a placebo treatment, or no treatment as long as the effect is observed at a point in time that exceeds the expected duration of action of the intervention. The intervention may or may not be initiated before surgery" (Katz et al. 2011). Therefore, the major difference with pre-emptive analgesia is that instead of only considering the pre-operative phase it considers that all peri-operative phases (pre-operative, intra-operative, and post-operative) can contribute to the development of central sensitization. The requirement that the reduced pain and/or analgesic consumption be observed after the duration of action of the target drug ensures that the preventive effect is not simply an analgesic effect. Thus, preventive analgesia relies on both early and sustained analgesic administration until tissue healing is complete. Therefore, even though data are lacking to support duration of analgesic administration in cats and dogs and other species after surgery, preventive analgesia strategies are encouraged to improve pain management in the post-operative period.

Table 3.2 Unidimensional pain assessment tools.

Name of the scoring tool	Brief description of the tool	Advantages	Disadvantages
Simple Descriptive Scale (SDS)	There is a brief description of the pain state accompanied by a score (e.g., 1–3) or classification of the pain state as mild, moderate, or severe	Simple to use and quick to complete	Insensitive to different severities of pain No defined intervention level for requirement for additional analgesia Not validated
Numerical Rating Scale (NRS)	The pain is rated typically at a level between 0 and 10 with 0 being no pain and 10 being worst possible pain	Simple to use and quick to complete	No defined intervention level for requirement for additional analgesia Not validated
Visual Analog Scale (VAS)	There is a line that is typically 100 mm long with two anchors: 0 at one end indicating no pain and 100 mm at the other end indicating worst possible pain for that procedure. The assessor makes a mark on the line that corresponds to their assessment of pain in the individual animal	Simple to use and quick to complete Very sensitive to different severities of pain Intervention levels for requirement for additional analgesia have been suggested (but not validated)	Large inter-rater variability therefore not useful in a multi-user setting Not validated
Dynamic Interactive Visual Analog Scale (DIVAS)	Similar to a VAS but the score is awarded after interaction with the animal	See above for VAS	See above for VAS

Multimodal Analgesia

The pain pathway is complex with multiple different neurotransmitters and receptors involved in nociception and the perception of pain. Multimodal analgesia is the principle of administering different classes of analgesic drug, which attack the pain pathway at different sites, in combination, with the aim of producing better analgesia than could be achieved by using uni-modal (single drug) analgesia therapy. There is good evidence to support the use of multimodal analgesia strategies in dogs and cats. Many of these studies have compared a combination of an opioid and a nonsteroidal anti-inflammatory drug (NSAID) compared to either drug alone and found the combination therapy to be superior. Therefore, when designing analgesic regimens for animals, it is important to aim for a multimodal approach in order to maximize analgesic benefit.

Concept of Adjunctive Therapeutic Approaches

Although opioids, NSAIDs and local anesthetic techniques usually form the backbone of analgesic therapy in animals; in some circumstances, additional analgesics in the form of adjunctive drugs are required in order to provide adequate pain relief. Adjunctive drugs such as ketamine, lidocaine, and (dex)medetomidine usually have less evidence to support their use as an analgesic in different companion animal species. Nonetheless, there is evidence from laboratory animal studies that these drugs are analgesic and there is a growing body of literature to support their use in companion animal and food-producing species. Combining adjunctive drugs with more traditional analgesics also plays to the principle of multimodal analgesia. Pain scoring the individual animal is fundamental to identifying those animals that would benefit from adjunctive analgesic therapy. It is also important to distinguish the strategic use of adjunctive drugs from polypharmacy. Ideally, introduce adjunctive drugs one at a time so that their effectiveness can be evaluated in the individual animal (using validated pain scoring tools) and refer to the literature for optimal dose rates and dose intervals. Although analgesic mixtures such as morphine/fentanyl, lidocaine, and ketamine combined in a single fluid infusion bag have become popular, the stability of these drugs combined together in solution has not been tested and giving them via one infusion line means that the dose rates of individual drugs cannot be adjusted, and all drugs must be started and stopped at the same time.

Opioids

"Opioid" is the term used to broadly describe all compounds that work at the opioid receptors whereas opiates are naturally occurring alkaloids such as morphine or codeine (Chapter 7). In many parts of the world, opioids are central to the management of acute peri-operative pain in companion animals. However, it is important to be aware that opioid availability differs in different parts of the world, predominantly due to restrictions in prescription due to opioid misuse in man. Opioids are subject to controlled drug legislation in all parts of the world, meaning that their use in animals must be recorded in a log book and that opioids must be kept in a locked cabinet. It is important to be aware of the legislation surrounding opioid use in the country where you are working.

Principally, three different opioid receptors have been identified: *mu* (μ), *delta* (δ), and *kappa* (κ), although subtypes of these receptors also exist (e.g., *mu 1* and *mu 2* receptors). There are naturally occurring endogenous peptides in the body that bind to these receptors (e.g., enkephalins, beta-endorphins, and dynorphin A). *Mu* opioid receptors are found at widespread sites within the CNS and in the periphery (following the onset of inflammation). In the CNS, they are found at pre- and post-synaptic sites in the dorsal horn of the spinal cord particularly, where the primary afferent fiber (primary order neuron) synapses with the dorsal horn neuron, and in the brainstem, thalamus, and cerebral cortex. *Mu* opioid receptors are also found in brain areas that comprise the descending inhibitory system (midbrain peri-aqueductal gray, the nucleus raphe magnus, and the rostral ventral medulla), which modulate spinal cord pain transmission. *Kappa* opioid receptors are found in the limbic system, brain stem, and spinal cord while Delta receptors are located largely in the brain and their effects are not well studied. Mechanistically, at a cellular level, opioids have a number of different actions.

Traditionally, opioids have been classified as agonists, partial agonists, agonists–antagonists, and antagonists. Agonists, such as morphine, methadone, and fentanyl, create their effect by stimulating opioid receptors. Partial agonists have high affinity but low efficacy at the *mu* receptor creating a "ceiling effect" so that higher doses do not provide greater analgesia but may increase adverse effects. Buprenorphine has long been considered at partial agonist but this has more recently been called into question, with some evidence suggesting that buprenorphine may act as a full-*mu* receptor agonist for analgesia. Nalbuphine and butorphanol may be considered partial agonists, but, because they have poor efficacy at the *mu* receptor, they can act as *mu* receptor antagonists. For example, butorphanol is sometimes used to partially antagonize the effects of a full-*mu* agonist (such as hydromorphone). Nalbuphine and butorphanol also provide some analgesia through *kappa* receptor agonist activity. *Mu* receptor agonists provide the most efficacious analgesia, followed by partial agonists and then agonists–antagonists. The opioid receptor antagonists such as naloxone are competitive antagonists with a high affinity for *mu*, *kappa*, and *delta* receptors but no receptor efficacy.

Opioids are predominantly metabolized in the liver through oxidation (by a CYP enzyme expressed from the cytochrome P450 gene, phase I of biotransformation) and conjugation (usually by gluconidation, phase II of biotransformation), see Chapter 6 for further details, with the kidney an important route of excretion.

The major reason for the administration of opioids is for the provision of analgesia, although in some species (e.g., dogs) the concurrent sedation provided by some opioids makes them a useful adjunct for premedication and sedation regimens. Opioids have a number of adverse effects, although these rarely limit use. Behavioral side effects such as sedation or dysphoria can be problematic. They also have a tendency to reduce heart rate although this is via stimulation of the vagal nerve (parasympathetic branch of the autonomic nervous system) and can be managed by the administration of anticholinergics. Nausea and vomiting may occur although this is species and opioid dependent. Suggested opioid doses are presented in Table 3.3.

Opioid-free Analgesia

Opioids are becoming more and more restricted in some countries and difficult to obtain for use in animals due to an "opioid epidemic" or "crisis" reflecting increasing numbers of hospitalizations and deaths of humans due to prescription or illicit opioid drugs. This has led to the development of "opioid-free" analgesia or anesthesia techniques. These techniques generally heavily rely on the use of local anesthetic techniques, ketamine and NSAIDs to provide analgesia. They may also allow opioid-related adverse effects such as nausea and regurgitation to be avoided in patients at a high risk of side effects from these adverse events such as dogs undergoing laryngeal tie-back surgery for laryngeal paralysis, where regurgitation or vomiting is associated with a high risk of aspiration. However, it has also been shown that adequate pain management cannot be achieved in cats undergoing ovariohysterectomy without the concurrent use of opioids in the peri-operative analgesia protocol (Diep et al. 2020); therefore, opioid-free techniques should be used with caution in the presence of adequate pain assessment.

Nonsteroidal Anti-inflammatory Drugs

Traditional NSAIDs are cyclo-oxygenase (COX) enzyme inhibitors, thereby reducing the production of prostaglandins that are major mediators of pain, inflammation, and pyrexia. In the first step of the prostaglandin cascade,

Table 3.3 Examples of primary drugs and their dose ranges (mg/kg unless otherwise stated) administered intravenously (IV), intramuscularly, subcutaneously (SC), or oral, as per drug package insert, used to treat pain in animals.

Drug name	Dogs	Cats	Horse	Cattle	Sheep and goats	Pigs
Opioid class of drugs						
Morphine	0.1–0.5	0.1–0.5	0.1–0.2	0.05–0.1	0.1–0.2	0.1–0.2
Methadone	0.1–0.5	0.1–0.5	0.22		0.2	–
Pethidine (meperidine)	2–5	2–5	4.4	3.3–4.4	–	–
Hydromorphone	0.025–0.2	0.025–0.2		–	–	–
Oxymorphone	0.025–0.2	0.025–0.2	0.033	–	–	–
Fentanyl	2–5 mcg/kg bolus, 1–10 mcg/kg/h CRI	2–5 mcg /kg bolus, 1–7 mcg/kg/h CRI	1–4 mcg /kg/h	–	–	50 mcg/kg 30–100 mcg/kg/h CRI
Alfentanil	20–50 mcg/kg bolus, 10–60 mcg/kg/h CRI	20–50 mcg/kg bolus, 10–60 mcg/kg/h CRI	–	–	–	–
Sufentanil	0.2–0.5 mcg/kg bolus, 0.1–0.6 mcg/kg/h CRI	0.2–0.5 μg/kg bolus, 0.1–0.6 mcg/kg/h CRI	–	–	–	–
Remifentanil	4–12 mcg/kg/h CRI	4–12 mcg/kg/h CRI	–	–	–	–
Buprenorphine	10–20 mcg/kg	10–20 mcg/kg	10 mcg/kg	5–10 mcg/kg	20 mcg/kg	–
Butorphanol	0.2–0.4	0.2–0.4	0.01–0.1	0.02–0.04	–	–
Nalbuphine	0.2–0.5	0.2–0.5	0.3	–	–	–
Pentazocine	1–2	1–2	–	–	–	–
Naloxone (IV)	0.04	0.04	–	–	–	0.5 mg/kg
Local anesthetics						
Lidocaine (infiltration)	6–10	3–5	2	10	4	8
Bupivacaine (infiltration)	2	1–1.5	2	3	1	2
Ropivacaine (infiltration)	3	1.5	2	–	1	–
Mepivacaine (infiltration)	5–6	2–3	5–6	–	–	–
NSAIDs						
Carprofen	4 once daily (or 2 twice daily)	Not recommended for use in cats	Not licensed in horses in USA but 0.7 mg/kg once daily in EU	1.4 once daily	Not licensed in sheep or goats	Not licensed in pigs
Cimicoxib	2 once daily	Not licensed in cats	Not licensed in horses	Not licensed in cattle	Not licensed in sheep or goats	Not licensed in pigs
Firocoxib	5 once daily	Not licensed in cats	57 mg tablet per 450–600 kg horse	Not licensed in cattle	Not licensed in sheep or goats	Not licensed in pigs
Flunixin	Not licensed in dogs	Not licensed in cats	1 once daily	2 once daily	Not licensed in sheep or goats	2 mg/kg once daily

(*Continued*)

Table 3.3 (Continued)

Drug name	Dogs	Cats	Horse	Cattle	Sheep and goats	Pigs
Meloxicam	0.2 loading dose followed 24 h later by 0.1 once daily	For acute post-operative pain a single dose of 0.3 SC maybe given. For acute musculoskeletal disorders the loading dose is 0.2 followed 24 h later by 0.05 once daily. For chronic musculoskeletal disorders the loading dose is 0.1 followed by 0.05 once daily.	0.6 once daily	0.5 once daily	Not licensed in sheep or goats	0.4 daily
Robenacoxib	2 once daily	2 once daily	Not licensed in horses	Not licensed in cattle	Not licensed in sheep and goats	Not licensed in pigs

CRI: constant rate infusion; –: no recommendations found.

membrane phospholipids are broken down by phospholipase A_2 in response to cellular damage to arachidonic acid. Arachidonic acid is converted via COX and lipoxygenase (LOX) enzymes to lipid mediators known as "eicosanoids." The initial COX reaction converts arachidonic acid to prostaglandin G_2. This is subsequently converted to prostaglandin H_2, which in turn is converted to five biologically active prostaglandins (including PGE_2 and PGI_2) by cell-specific isomerases and synthases. Prostaglandins are important drivers of peripheral sensitization, sensitizing peripheral nociceptors to inflammatory mediators and lowering thresholds for activation.

There are two isoforms of cyclo-oxygenase enzyme (COX-1 and COX-2). COX-1 is constitutively expressed in most tissue types and activity results in the production of so-called "housekeeping prostaglandins" that are important for normal cellular function. COX-2 enzyme, although constitutively expressed in some tissues such as the brain and kidney, is also rapidly induced by tissue damage and results in the production of inflammatory prostaglandins that drive peripheral sensitization. The beneficial antipyretic, anti-inflammatory, and analgesic effects of NSAIDs come through a reduction in the production of PGE_2 and PGI_2 in the periphery and in the CNS. NSAID-related adverse effects result from a reduction in the production of housekeeping prostaglandins that are essential for normal organ function. However, it is important to realize that the COX-1/COX-2 story is often oversimplified and, for example, some prostaglandins produced by COX-2 are also important for essential functions, such as the healing of gastrointestinal ulcers.

Grapiprant is a nontraditional piprant class of NSAID that acts differently to the traditional NSAIDs. It is an EP4 receptor antagonist, one of the receptors that is bound by PGE_2 to mediate pain and inflammation associated with osteoarthritis (Kirkby Shaw et al. 2015). Therefore, grapiprant decreases peripheral sensitization by blocking the action of PGE_2 on one of the receptors important in the pain pathway. The potential advantage of grapiprant over traditional NSAIDs is that by acting as a receptor antagonist the production of housekeeping prostaglandins is unaffected and this may lead to a reduction in NSAID-related adverse effects.

Local Anesthetic Drugs

Local anesthetic drugs, such as lidocaine and bupivacaine, block action potential propagation in nerve fibers by inhibiting the influx of sodium ions through voltage-gated channels or ionophores within the neural membrane. There is a hierarchy in nerve fiber sensitivity to local anesthetics with small rapidly firing autonomic neurons being the most sensitive (a smaller volume of local anesthetic is sufficient to block the number of sodium channels to prevent impulse transmission), followed by sensory fibers and then by somatic motor fibers.

By blocking action potential propagation in peripheral sensory nerves, local anesthetic drugs reduce noxious input to the spinal cord and higher brain centers thereby reducing central sensitization and upregulation of the pain pathways, as well as providing analgesia. During anesthesia, the reduction in sensory input to higher brain centers through application of local anesthetic techniques, can have a significant positive benefit to stabilize anesthetic depth, prevent or limit autonomic responses to tissue damage, and reduce the concentration of inhalational anesthetic required to maintain anesthesia ("MAC-sparing").

Different types of neuronal blockade can be achieved using the application of local anesthetic drugs. Starting most simply, topical or surface application can be used to apply local anesthetics to mucous membranes or to surgically exposed nerves. An example is topical desensitization of the larynx in cats before endotracheal intubation. Surface application of local anesthetics to the skin is not normally successful because local anesthetic solutions are not readily absorbed across the skin unless special topical formulations are used (e.g., EMLA cream). Infiltration anesthesia involves infiltration of local anesthetics into surgical sites, for example along wound edges after closure. Regional anesthesia is the injection of local anesthetic solution in the vicinity of a peripheral nerve to temporarily block sensory and or motor nerves to provide peri-operative pain control. An example of regional anesthesia is a brachial plexus nerve block or a femoral/sciatic nerve block. Neuraxial anesthesia is application of local anesthetics either into the epidural space (epidural/extradural anesthesia) or into the subarachanoid space (spinal or intrathecal anesthesia). Intravenous regional anesthesia (IVRA) involves administering local anesthetic (almost exclusively lidocaine [lignocaine]) into a peripheral vein in a distal limb after application of a tourniquet to the proximal limb. This prevents rapid systemic absorption of the local anesthetic and systemic toxicity.

Adjunctive Drugs

Ketamine

Ketamine, at sub-anesthetic doses, is becoming increasingly popular as an adjunctive analgesic agent. Its analgesic effects are mainly attributed to its noncompetitive and nonspecific antagonism of NMDA receptors. These receptors are usually activated by the excitatory neurotransmitters glycine and glutamate. NMDA receptor activation is pivotal to the development of central sensitization in the dorsal horn of the spinal cord. The NMDA receptor does not contribute to nociceptive transmission in individuals without central sensitization because the NMDA receptor ion channel is normally blocked by an Mg^{2+}. Therefore, ketamine may not be effective as an analgesic unless there is central sensitization and presence of maladaptive pain. Ketamine is also considered to act at *mu* opioid receptors that may contribute to its analgesic effects (Zanos et al. 2018).

In human medicine, ketamine (administered by continuous rate infusion) is most commonly used as an adjunct to opioid-mediated analgesia in patients with moderate-to-severe pain as part of a multimodal analgesia technique. Evidence for ketamine analgesia in dogs and cats is limited but extrapolation of data from humans suggests that it is also best used as part of a multimodal analgesia regimen in patients with moderate-to-severe pain. It is usually used as a continuous rate infusion (preceded by a loading dose) because intermittent bolus doses are thought to be minimally effective as ketamine is rapidly excreted from the body.

Alpha-2 Adrenergic Receptor Agonists

Alpha-2 adrenergic receptor agonists (α_2 agonists) are a class of drug that are widely used for premedication and sedation of many different species of animals. In addition to their profound sedative properties, α_2 agonists are also potent analgesic drugs. Specific α_2 receptor subtypes mediate the different pharmacodynamic effects of α_2 agonists with α_{2A} and α_{2B} receptors implicated in mechanisms of analgesia. The analgesic sites of action of α_2 agonists are complex and both supraspinal and spinal mechanisms are considered to contribute to analgesia. Alpha-2 agonists depress C-fiber-mediated input to the spinal dorsal horn suggesting that selective inhibition of nociceptive input to the primary afferent terminal occurs pre-synaptically. In addition, α_2 receptor activation decreases spontaneous activity in nociceptive dorsal horn neurons suggesting a post-synaptic inhibitory contribution. A site of analgesic action in the brain (locus coeruleus) has also been proposed. Antinociceptive synergism between α_2 agonists and opioids is also recognized which may be particularly important in mechanisms of analgesia involving descending modulatory systems from the brainstem. There are a number of studies that have investigated the analgesic and antinociceptive effects of α_2 agonists in a variety of species although in these studies it can be difficult to separate analgesia from sedation. Analgesia from a single dose of an α_2 agonist is considered to be relatively short-lived, necessitating administration by continuous rate infusion for sustained effects. Importantly, the duration of analgesia from a single dose of an α_2 agonist such as dexmedetomidine 10 mcg/kg intramuscularly is significantly shorter (approximately 1 h) than the duration of sedation (approximately 3–4 h).

Lidocaine

Lidocaine is a local anesthetic drug that can be given systemically (intravenously) by continuous rate infusion to provide analgesia. Other local anesthetics, such as bupivacaine, must not be given systemically because of the risk of cardiotoxicity. The mechanisms by which systemic lidocaine provide analgesia are complex, with effects mediated through different ion channels and receptors. The evidence for an analgesia effect of systemic lidocaine in cats, dogs, and horses is relatively weak although there is stronger evidence for an effect, particularly in the management of neuropathic pain, in man. For the most part, studies in humans involve use of lidocaine as part of a multimodal analgesia technique highlighting the importance of using systemic lidocaine as an analgesia adjunct rather than as a stand-alone therapy. However, it is important to note that lidocaine and its metabolites can accumulate in the course of multiple IV infusions given for many hours, resulting in sedation.

Paracetamol (Dogs, Horses, and Ruminants)

Paracetamol (acetaminophen) is widely used for the long-term management of pain in dogs with osteoarthritis. There are, however, no studies investigating the safety or efficacy of this preparation for management of osteoarthritis pain. It cannot be administered to cats because of toxicity. Paracetamol is also being increasingly used to manage acute pain and human-injectable preparations are used in the peri-operative period. There appears to be the general perception that paracetamol is better tolerated by dogs than NSAIDs, but there are no data to support this contention. Furthermore, in humans, the use of paracetamol for five days or longer can cause a type B hyperlactatemia (plasma lactate >3 mmol/L; Gillespie et al. 2017) and, through clinical observation, has been identified in dogs with long-term (>10 days) use. The clinical relevance of this has not been investigated or reported on but could result in paracetamol poisoning and liver injury as reported in experimental animal research models (Shah et al. 2011). Due to the lack of information, monitoring liver enzyme and plasma lactate (at least every three months) in dogs given prolonged courses of paracetamol appears prudent.

Tramadol

Tramadol is a centrally acting synthetic analog of codeine that has two different analgesic modes of action. Tramadol principally exerts an agonist effect to inhibit norepinephrine and serotonin reuptake in the CNS, thereby modulating descending analgesia pathways. In addition, the first metabolite (M1) of tramadol (the O-desmethyl metabolite) acts at opioid receptors to provide analgesia, although this metabolite is made in very low concentrations in dogs. There is an increasing body of evidence showing that tramadol provides negligible analgesia in the majority of dogs. Therefore, if used in this species, pain assessment must be performed. Cats make higher concentrations of the M1 metabolite and therefore tramadol may provide greater analgesia in cats than dogs, although tramadol administration to cats may be more associated with opioid-mediated adverse effects such as sedation and dysphoria because of the higher concentrations of M1. Furthermore, cats find the taste of tramadol very aversive so it can be extremely difficult to dose cats effectively in the long term with this drug orally. There has been a huge increase in the popularity of tramadol as a longer-term analgesic for dogs and cats with acute and chronic pain, probably because it is perceived to be safe and devoid of NSAID-related adverse effects. However, due to the lack of efficacy data, particularly for oral tramadol, it is not advised to use tramadol in preference to NSAID therapy in dogs and cats, unless NSAIDs are contraindicated or poorly tolerated by an individual patient.

Oral Opioids

The oral administration of opioids to cats and dogs for the management of acute or chronic pain is generally not recommended because of poor oral bioavailability in these species. This is due to a large first pass metabolism effect in the liver. The bioavailability of oral methadone is increased in dogs when given in combination with a cytochrome p450 inhibitor (which decreases the expression of oxidizing enzymes of phase I of liver biotransformation of drugs; see Chapter 6) such as fluconazole (KuKanich et al. 2019), but there are no clinical pharmacodynamic studies investigating this combination in dogs. Codeine is available as an oral preparation for administration to humans and is available in some countries as a product combined with oral paracetamol. It has poor oral bioavailability in dogs although codeine-6-glucuronide was formed in high concentrations after oral administration of codeine to dogs, which may provide some analgesia. Data are lacking in cats and other species although it is likely that the analgesic effect of oral codeine is low in all species compared to parenteral opioids. The oral administration of other opioids to species such as horses, cattle, and pigs has not been widely investigated.

Amantadine

Amantadine is an oral NMDA receptor antagonist that may therefore be effective in limiting or reversing central sensitization that occurs as a result of osteoarthritis. Lascelles et al. (2008) investigated the analgesic efficacy of amantadine combined with an NSAID (meloxicam) in dogs with spontaneous osteoarthritis and pain that was refractory to NSAID therapy alone and found that pain scores were decreased compared to dogs that continued on meloxicam therapy only. No behavioral, biochemical, or hematological abnormalities were noted after 42 days of treatment, although amantadine is excreted by the kidneys and caution is advised when using amantadine in human patients with kidney disease. These limited data suggest that amantadine may be a useful adjunct to NSAID therapy in dogs with pain caused by osteoarthritis. There are no studies investigating the efficacy of amantadine in cats with osteoarthritis, but a similar dosing schema is used in cats as for dogs. The drug is relatively expensive which can limit use in some patients.

Gabapentin

Gabapentin is a structural analog of gamma-aminobutyric acid (GABA), but its analgesic action is attributed to binding to the alpha-2/delta subunit of the voltage-gated calcium channel, thereby decreasing the release of excitatory neurotransmitters in the dorsal horn of the spinal cord. It is licensed in humans for the treatment of some neuropathic pain conditions and may therefore have a role in the treatment of neuropathic pain in animals. However, despite being widely used for the management of many chronic pain conditions, including osteoarthritis, there are limited data describing efficacy of gabapentin for these conditions. Adverse effects of gabapentin include sedation and drowsiness that may limit use in some animals. It is also not recommended to stop the drug abruptly after chronic administration due to the risk of seizures, with the recommendation to reduce the dose of the drug over a period of approximately one week.

Pregabalin

Similarly to gabapentin, pregabalin binds to the alpha-2/delta subunit of the voltage-gated calcium channel decreasing the release of several neurotransmitters including glutamate and Substance P. In contrast to gabapentin, which has a short terminal half-life in dogs and cats, in dogs, the terminal half-life is longer (approximately 7 h) making it amenable to twice daily dosing which may be better for owner compliance compared to gabapentin. It is also well absorbed orally compared to gabapentin that may make it a preferred drug over gabapentin. A recent study showed that pregabalin 5 mg/kg twice daily improved signs of neuropathic pain in dogs with syringomyelia (Sanchis-Mora et al. 2019). Similarly to gabapentin, adverse effects such as sedation and drowsiness may preclude use in some animals. Clinically, pregabalin may be easier to use in animals under 10 kg because of the available tablet strengths in some countries compared to gabapentin.

Cannabinoids

Although worldwide there are no cannabinoids that are licensed for administration to animals, cannabinoids are being increasingly widely used for the treatment of pain in cats and dogs. This is being largely driven by pet owners who are probably following the trend for increased publicity and awareness of the use of cannabinoids in humans. Cannabinoid receptors (CB1 and CB2) are found in plasma membranes and are activated by endogenous ligands called "endocannabinoids," and both CB1 and CB2 receptors are involved in the pain pathway. Cannabinoid products marketed as supplements are unregulated and are not standardized, so there is a wide and unpredictable variation in the concentration of active ingredients between different products. It is also important to be aware that the law with respect to cannabis use varies from country to country. A few small studies have been conducted investigating the use of cannabidiol in the management of pain caused by osteoarthritis in dogs. Generally, these studies show an improvement in owner assessed pain (using CMIs) although there is no consistency between studies in the dose/formulation of cannabidiol administered or route of administration. Further robust, well-controlled studies are needed to fully evaluate the role of cannabidiol in pain management in animals.

Nonpharmacological Methods to Treat Pain

A variety of nonpharmacological methods to treat pain such as ice, heat, massage, acupuncture, laser therapy, transcutaneous electrical nerve stimulation (TENS), and physiotherapy are increasingly used as sole or adjunctive (with pharmacotherapy) methods to treat both acute and chronic pain. Generally, the evidence base to support these methods is poor, with few randomized, blinded, appropriately controlled studies evaluating their efficacy. However, proponents of these techniques often report good outcomes, particularly when used in combination with pharmacotherapy where they may allow the required dose of drugs to be reduced. The use of cold therapy in dogs and cats was recently reviewed (Wright et al. 2020). Cold therapy decreases activation of tissue nociceptors and slows conduction along peripheral neurons as well as having an effect to decrease edema formation, all mechanisms that can contribute to analgesia. There is increasing recognition of the importance of physiotherapy and hydrotherapy as part of rehabilitation protocols after surgery, particularly orthopedic surgery, and there is an increasing evidence base of its value in this context. Other modalities such as acupuncture are less well studied, but many owners and practitioners are convinced of the benefits of acupuncture, particularly as a part of a multimodal approach to the management of osteoarthritis-related pain.

Questions and Answers

There are more practice questions and answers available for this chapter on the website. Please visit http://www.wiley.com/go/VeterinaryAnesthesiaZeiler.

Questions

1) What type of surgery is most likely to give rise to neuropathic pain in a cat?
   a) Ovariohysterectomy
   b) Diaphragmatic rupture repair
   c) Amputation of the hind limb
   d) Castration

2) Define pre-emptive analgesia
   a) Any analgesic treatment initiated before the onset of nociceptive stimulation
   b) Any analgesic treatment initiated during the peri-operative period
   c) Any analgesic treatment initiated in the post-operative period
   d) An opioid analgesic treatment initiated before the onset of nociceptive stimulation
3) Why is it helpful to use a formal tool to assess pain in companion animals?
   a) It promotes more frequent assessment of pain
   b) It increases variability in pain assessment between different observers
   c) It is a legal requirement to use a formal assessment tool
   d) It allows an intervention criterion to be set for administration of rescue analgesia

Answers

1) c
2) a
3) d

Further Reading

Belli, M., de Oliveira, A.R., de Lima, M.T. et al. Clinical validation of the short and long UNESP-Botucatu scales for feline pain assessment. *PeerJ* 9: e1125.

Benito, J., Hansen, B., Depuy, V. et al. (2013). Feline musculoskeletal pain index: responsiveness and testing of criterion validity. *J Vet Intern Med* 27: 474–482.

Brondani, J.T., Luna, S.P.L., Beier, S.L. et al. (2009). Analgesic efficacy of perioperative use of vedaprofen, tramadol or their combination in cats undergoing ovariohysterectomy. *J Feline Med Surg* 11: 420–429.

Brondani, J.T., Luna, S.P., and Padovani, C.R. (2011). Refinement and initial validation of a multidimensional composite scale for use in assessing acute pain in cats. *Am J Vet Res* 72: 174–183.

Brown, D.C., Boston, R.C., Coyne, J.C., and Farrar, J.T. (2008). Ability of the Canine Brief Pain Inventory to detect response to treatment in dogs with osteoarthritis. *J Am Vet Med Assoc* 233: 1278–1283.

Bussières, G., Jacques, C., Lainay, O. et al. (2008). Development of a composite orthopaedic pain scale in horses. *Res Vet Sci* 85: 294–306.

Cachon, T., Frykman, O., Innes, J.F. et al. (2018). Face validity of a proposed tool for staging canine osteoarthritis: Canine Osteoarthritis Staging Tool (COAST). *Vet J* 235: 108.

Calvo, G., Holden, E., Reid, J. et al. (2014). Development of a behaviour-based measurement tool with defined intervention level for assessing acute pain in cats. *J Small Anim Pract* 55: 622–629.

Dahl, J.B. and Moiniche, S. (2004). Pre-emptive analgesia. *Br Med Bull* 71: 13–27.

Dalla Costa, E., MInero, M., Lebelt, D. et al. (2014). Development of the horse grimace scale (HGS) as a pain assessment tool in horses undergoing routine castration. *PLoS One* 9: e92281.

Dalla Costa, E., Stucke, D., Dai, F. et al. (2016). Using the horse grimace scale (HGS) to assess pain associated with acute laminitis in horses (*Equus caballus*). *Animals (Basel)* 6: 47.

de Oliveira, F.A., Luna, S.P., Barras do Amaral, J. et al. (2014). Validation of the UNESP-botucatu unidimensional composite pain scale for assessing post-operative pain in cattle. *BMC Vet Res* 10: 200.

Diep, T.N., Monteiro, B.P., Evangelista, M.C. et al. (2020). Anesthetic and analgesic effects of an opioid free, injectable protocol in cats undergoing ovariohysterectomy: a prospective, blinded, randomized clinical trial. *Can Vet J* 61: 621–628.

Evangelista, M.C., Watanabe, R., Leung, V.S.Y. et al. (2019). Facial expressions of pain in cats: the development and validation of a feline grimace scale. *Sci Rep* 13: 19128.

Gillespie, I., Rosenstein, P.G., and Hughes, D. (2017). Update: clinical use of plasma lactate. *Vet Clin N Am: Sm Anim Prac* 47: 325–342.

Hielm-Bjorkman, A.K., Rita, H., and Tulamo, R.M. (2009). Psychometric testing of the Helsinki chronic pain index by completion of a questionnaire in Finnish by owners of dogs with chronic signs of pain caused by osteoarthritis. *Am J Vet Res* 70: 727–734.

Katz, J., Clarke, H., and Seltzer, Z. (2011). Preventive analgesia: quo vadimus? *Anesth Analg* 113: 5.

Katz, J. and McCartney, C.J.L. (2002). Current status of pre-emptive analgesia. *Curr Opin Anesthesiol* 15: 435–441.

Keating, S.C.J., Thomas, A.A., Flecknell, P.A., and Leach, M.C. (2012). Evaluation of EMLA cream for preventing pain during tattooing of rabbits: changes in physiological, behavioural and facial expression responses. *PLoS One* 7: e44437.

Kirkby Shaw, K., Rausch-Derra, L.C., and Rhodes, L. (2015). Grapriprant: an EP4 prostaglandin receptor antagonist and novel therapy for pain and inflammation. *Vet Med Sci* 2: 3–9.

Klinck, M.P., Railland, P., Guillot, M. et al. (2015). Preliminary validation and reliability testing of the

Montreal instrument for cat arthritis testing, for use by veterinarians, in a colony of laboratory cats. *Animals (Basel)* 5: 1252–1267.

Klinck, M.P., Gruen, M.E., Del Castillo, J.R.E. et al. (2018). Development and preliminary validity and reliability of the Montreal instrument for cat arthritis testing, for use by caretaker/owner, MI-CAT (C), via a randomized clinical trial. *Appl Anim Behav Sci* 200: 95–105.

KuKanich, B., KuKanich, K., Rankin, D., and Locuson, C.W. (2019). The effect of fluconazole on oral methadone in dogs. *Vet Anaesth Analg* 46: 501–509.

Langford, D.J., Bailey, A.L., Chanda, M.L. et al. (2010). Coding of facial expressions of pain in the laboratory mouse. *Nat Methods* 7: 447–449.

Lascelles, B.D.X., Cripps, J.P., Jones, A., and Waterman, A.E. (1997). Post-operative central hypersensivity and pain: the pre-emptive value of pethidine for ovariohysterectomy. *Pain* 73: 461–471.

Lascelles, B.D.X., Gaynor, J.S., Smith, S.C. et al. (2008). Amantadine in a multimodal analgesic regimen for alleviation of refractory osteoarthritis pain in dogs. *J Vet Intern Med* 22: 53–59.

Lascelles, B.D., Hansen, B.D., Roe, S. et al. (2007). Evaluation of Client-Specific Outcome Measures and activity monitoring to measure pain relief in cats with osteoarthritis. *Vet Intern Med* 21 (3): 410–416.

Luna, S.P.L., de Araujo, A.L., da Nobrego Neto, P.I. et al. (2020). Validation of the UNESP-botucatu pig composite acute pain scale (UPAPS). *PLoS One* 15: e0233552.

Mogil, J.S., Pang, D.S.J., Silva Dutra, G.G., and Chambers, C.T. (2020). The development and use of facial grimace scales for pain measurement in animals. *Neurosci Biobehav Rev* 116: 480–493.

Moiniche, S., Kehlet, H., and Dahl, J.B. (2002). A qualitative and quantitative systematic review of preemptive analgesia for postoperative pain relief – the role of timing of analgesia. *Anaesthes* 96: 725–741.

Morton, C.M., Reid, J., Scott, E.M. et al. (2005). Application of a scaling model to establish and validate an interval level pain scale for assessment of acute pain in dogs. *Am J Vet Res* 66: 2154–2166.

Muller, C., Gaines, B., Gruen, M. et al. (2016). Evaluation of clinical metrology instrument in dogs with osteoarthritis. *J Vet Intern Med* 30: 836–846.

Noble, C.E., Wiseman-Orr, L.M., Scott, M.E. et al. (2019). Development, initial validation and reliability testing of a web-based, generic feline health-related quality-of-life instrument. *J Feline Med Surg* 21: 84–94.

Ossipov, M., Harris, S., Lloyd, P. et al. (1990). Antinociceptive interaction between opioids and medetomidine: systemic additivity and spinal synergy. *Anaesthes* 73: 1227–1235.

Reid, J., Nolan, A.M., Hughes, J.M.L. et al. (2007). Development of the short-form Glasgow Composite Pain Scale (CMPS-SF) and derivation of an analgesic intervention score. *Anim Welf* 16: 97–104.

Sanchis-Mora, S., Chang, Y.M., Abeyesinghe, S.M. et al. (2019). Pregabalin for the treatment of syringomyelia-associated neuropathic pain in dogs: A randomized, placebo-controlled, double-masked clinical trial. *Vet J* 250: 55–62.

Shah, A.D., Wood, D.M., and Dargan, P.I. (2011). Understanding lactic acidosis in paracetamol (acetaminophen) poisoning. *Br J Clin Pharmacol* 71: 20–28.

Silva, N., Trindade, P.H., Oliveira, A.R. et al. (2020). Validation of the UNESP-botucatu composite scale to assess acute postoperative abdominal pain in sheep (USAPS). *PLoS One* 15: e0239622.

Sotocinal, S.G., Sorge, R.E., Zaloum, A. et al. (2011). The rat grimace scale: a partially automated method for quantifying pain in the laboratory rat via facial expressions. *Mol Pain* 7: 55.

Staffieri, F., Centonze, P., Gigante, G. et al. (2013). Comparison of the analgesic effects of robenacoxib, buprenorphine and their combination in cats after ovariohysterectomy. *Vet J* 197: 363–367.

Sutton, G.A., Dahan, R., Turner, R., and Paltiel, O. (2013). A behaviour-based pain scale for horses with acute colic: scale construction. *Vet J* 196: 394–401.

Taffarel, M.O., Luna, S.P.L., de Oliveira, F.A. et al. (2015). Refinement and partial validation of the UNESP-Botucatu multidimensional composite pain scale for assessing postoperative pain in horses. *BMC Vet Res* 11: 1–12.

van Dierendonck, M.C. and van Loon, J.P. (2016). Monitoring acute equine visceral pain with the Equine Utrecht University Scale for Composite Pain Assessment (EQUUS-COMPASS) and Equine Utrecht University Scale for Facial Assessment of Pain (EQUUS-FAP): a validation study. *Vet J* 216: 175–177.

van Loon, J.P., Jonckheer-Sheehy, V.S., Back, W. et al. (2014). Monitoring equine visceral pain with a composite pain scale score and correlation with survival after emergency gastrointestinal surgery. *Vet J* 200: 109–115.

van Loon, J.P.A.M. and van Dierendonck, M.C. (2015). Monitoring acute equine visceral pain with the Equine Utrecht University Scale for Composite Pain Assessment (EQUUS-COMPASS) and the Equine Utrecht University Scale for Facial Assessment of Pain (EQUUS-FAP): a scale-construction study. *Veterinary* 206: 356–364.

van Loon, J.P.A.M. and van Dierendonck, M.C. (2017). Monitoring equine head-related pain with the Equine Utrecht University Scale for facial assessment of pain (EQUUS-FAP). *Vet J* 220: 88–90.

Walton, M.B., Cowderoy, E., Lascelles, D., and Innes, J.F. (2013). Evaluation of construct and criterion validity for the "Liverpool Osteoarthritis in Dogs" (LOAD) clinical metrology instrument and comparison to two other instruments. *PLoS One* 8: e58125.

Wright, B., Kronen, P.W., Lascelles, D. et al. (2020). Ice therapy: cool, current and complicated. *J Small Anim Pract* 61 (5): 267–271.

Zanos, P., Moaddel, R., Morris, P.J. et al. (2018). Ketamine and ketamine metabolite pharmacology: insights into therapeutic mechanisms. *Pharmacol Rev* 70: 621–660.

4

Principles of Anesthetic Monitoring and Monitoring Equipment

H. Nicole Trenholme and Daniel Pang

Overview of Patient Monitoring and Standard of Practice

The ability to have veterinary patients monitored continuously is vitally important, not only under general anesthesia but also in the peri-anesthetic period. This allows for early detection of physiologic derangements that have the potential to cause morbidity and mortality. Through early detection, the anesthetist is able to take corrective steps to alleviate negative sequelae. A variety of resources can be used, from hands-on physical assessment of the patient to physiologic monitoring equipment. Many individual monitors have been combined into a multiparameter monitor, some of which are made specifically for veterinary patients and others that are intended for human use have been adapted to various degrees for veterinary species. This chapter covers options for monitoring veterinary patients, the appropriate use of monitoring, and key principles of function.

At minimum, monitoring of sedation and general anesthesia should include signs that are imperative for the life and vitality of the patient. In sedated patients, this should include heart rate and rhythm, respiratory rate, oxygenation, and temperature. Multiparameter monitors that offer electrocardiography, pulse oximetry, and a temperature probe are available. Alternatively, these modalities are offered as separate units. Additionally, ventilation parameters should ideally be assessed, which may include subjective parameters, such as appropriate chest excursion and ventilatory effort. However, there are also methods of monitoring capnography, even without intubation, when attached to a wye-piece (y-piece) and oxygen is administered with a tight-fitting facemask. There are also some nasal oxygen cannulas that also allow for ventilation monitoring in nonintubated patients via capnography. In some instances, more specialized monitoring may be required, such as monitoring blood glucose in neonatal, juvenile, or septic patients, or evaluating electrolyte balance in cats with urethral obstruction or uroabdomen in foals. Good clinical judgment is required when considering what monitoring is appropriate for each patient to minimize the risk of adverse events and reduce peri-anesthetic morbidity and mortality.

Principles and Techniques of Hands-on Monitoring

Monitoring the Central and Peripheral Nervous System

One of the key elements of anesthesia is ensuring that the patient is unconscious and at an appropriate "depth" (plane) of anesthesia for diagnostic and therapeutic interventions. It is a welfare imperative to prevent nociception/pain that might result from these procedures. Although some patient monitoring devices, such as bispectral index (BIS) and patient state index systems, have theoretical benefits in patient monitoring, they do not yield consistent results with regard to monitoring patient anesthetic depth and risk of arousal. Therefore, it continues to be necessary to use physical examination to determine if a patient is at an adequate anesthetic depth and provide timely intervention if they require further analgesia or anesthesia. Clinical signs that indicate the need for intervention are determined mainly by drug choice. Inhalant anesthetic protocols have different criteria for determining depth of anesthesia compared to total injectable anesthesia protocols.

Regardless of anesthetic protocol used, markers of inadequate analgesia and/or light anesthetic plane may include development of tachycardia, hypertension, tachypnea, and purposeful movements. By contrast,

Fundamental Principles of Veterinary Anesthesia, First Edition. Edited by Gareth E. Zeiler and Daniel S. J. Pang.

Companion Website: www.wiley.com/go/VeterinaryAnesthesiaZeiler

Table 4.1 Evaluation of anesthetic depth with volatile anesthetics and total intravenous anesthesia (TIVA) based on physical monitoring parameters.

Depth	Anesthesia	Jaw tone	Eye position	Palpebral reflex	Corneal reflex	Heart rate and blood pressure	Respiratory rate
Light	Inhalant	Very tight[1]	Central	Present	Present	High	Rapid
	TIVA	Very tight	Central	Present	Present	High	Rapid
Medium light	Inhalant	Moderate	Ventromedial	Slow	Present	Moderate	Even
	TIVA	Tight	Central	Present	Present	Moderate	Even
Medium	Inhalant	Moderate	Ventromedial	Slow	Present	Moderate	Even
	TIVA	Moderate	Central	Present	Present	Moderate	Even
Medium deep	Inhalant	Mild	Ventromedial	Absent	Present	Slightly low	Slow to absent
	TIVA	Mild to moderate	Central	Slow	Present	Slightly low	Slow to irregular
Deep	Inhalant	Absent	Fixed[2], central	Absent	Absent	Low	Absent
	TIVA	Absent	Fixed, central	Absent	Absent	Low	Absent

1) tight; increased muscle tone increasing resistance to opening the mouth.

2) Eyes often have a glassy appearance as tear production is reduced.

normal or unchanging vital parameters indicate an adequate anesthetic depth. Patients that are too deeply anesthetized are often bradycardic and hypotensive, and exhibit bradypnea or apnea. However, similar complications can also occur in patients who are at an adequate anesthetic depth as a result of adverse effects of the anesthetic drugs being used, sequelae of the procedure being performed, or due to underlying pathology. Therefore, it is important to also consider the physical examination findings of the patient alongside other monitoring devices.

Where inhalational anesthetics are the primary source of anesthesia, an adequate anesthetic depth in most species is characterized by minimal or no palpebral reflexes, ventromedial rotation of the eye, minimal or no jaw tone, and relaxed skeletal musculature. When patients become too deep, the eye is central, there is no palpebral reflex, no corneal reflex (rarely tested due to risk of damaging cornea), and no jaw tone. Notably, a patient at a light anesthetic plane can also have a central eye position, but combined with an obvious, possibly brisk palpebral reflex (may also blink spontaneously), and have significant jaw tone. When using injectable anesthetic agents for maintenance of anesthesia (i.e., total intravenous anesthesia, TIVA), there are slightly different physical signs. Patients often maintain palpebral reflexes and spontaneous blinking may occur until they are too deeply anesthetized. Eye position varies depending on the protocol in use. As an example, a ketamine-based protocol is likely to maintain a central eye position whereas a propofol-based TIVA is more likely to be associated with ventromedially rotated eyes. Additionally, the assessment of muscle tone can be very useful for patients being maintained with TIVA. Further details are provided in Table 4.1.

There are some species variations that may also alter physical signs observed during general anesthesia. Equidae tend to have increased lacrimation when they are at a light anesthetic plane. Camelids often maintain palpebral reflexes even with deep anesthetic planes. Similarly, the assessment of jaw tone is impractical and not useful in Equidae and Bovidae. In these species, individual eyes can exhibit different signs (see Chapter 2; Figure 4.1). Whenever possible, both eyes should be examined to avoid missing

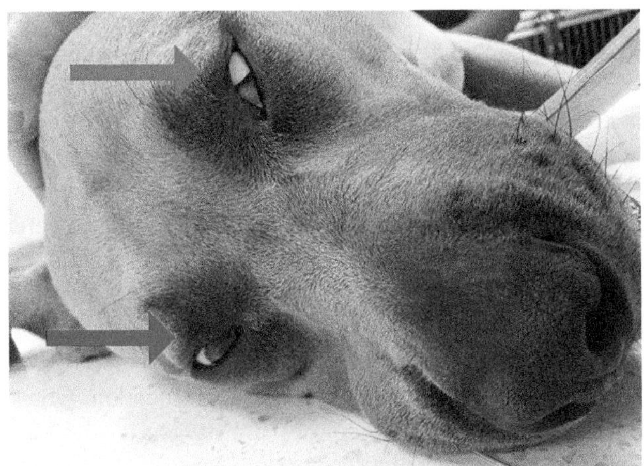

Figure 4.1 Eye rotation in dogs, cats, and ruminants can help assess depth of anesthesia. Occasionally, each eye will show a different position. As shown in the figure, one eye is rotated ventromedially (ventrorostrally; blue arrow) and the other eye is central (red arrow). This could indicate a light plane of anesthesia. Sometimes, a recent change in recumbency (e.g., from dorsal to lateral) can transiently (for a few minutes) alter eye rotation.

signs consistent with inadequate depth of anesthesia. If one eye indicates a light plane of anesthesia, it is recommended to assume this reflects overall anesthetic depth (Figure 4.1).

While the preceding description provides general guidance, individual variation in physical signs occurs, especially in Equidae, so serial evaluations at regular intervals are important to ensure an adequate and appropriate depth of anesthesia and analgesia is maintained. Depth of anesthesia can be altered by the procedure performed and should be adjusted accordingly. For example, the degree of stimulation during an imaging study performed is far less than during surgical manipulation, so it is recommended to always reassess a patient when noxious stimulation or patient manipulation is changing (e.g., moving onto another table, placement of towel clamps, initial incision, etc.).

Monitoring of the Cardiovascular System and Perfusion

Although we heavily rely on monitoring equipment to aid evaluating cardiovascular status and perfusion, physical examination can also provide key information. Mucus membrane color and capillary refill time should be monitored serially during anesthesia to ensure adequate perfusion, which can be inferred through the presence of pink mucus membranes and a normal capillary refill time (Figure 4.2). With reduced cardiac output, pallor may be observed, and there may be a delay in capillary refill time. Oxygenation may also be inferred based on mucus membrane color, with cyanosis (blue discoloration) of the mucus membranes associated with hypoxemia. Patients that are profoundly anemic will have pale mucous membranes and may not appear cyanotic despite being hypoxemic. This is because 5 g/dL of hemoglobin have to be desaturated before overt cyanosis occurs. Therefore, if a patient has a hematocrit of 21% (estimate 7 g/dL hemoglobin), then >70% of its hemoglobin would have to not be carrying oxygen for cyanosis to occur. Though a useful sign to include in monitoring, mucous membrane color is relatively insensitive as evaluation is subjective. Therefore, it should not be relied upon in place of pulse oximetry and PCV measurement. Notably, a very recently dead animal will maintain capillary refill for a short time, highlighting the insensitivity of this monitoring method.

Thoracic auscultation identifies new or progressive cardiac murmurs and alteration in pulmonary sounds (e.g., development of crackles in a volume-overloaded patient). Physical examination can be used to help identify poor perfusion, based on distal extremity temperature. Patients with adequate cardiac output should have warm extremities. However, patients with diminished cardiac output may begin to centralize their circulation via arteriolar vasoconstriction, leading to cold extremities.

Palpation of peripheral pulses, such as the dorsal pedal artery or the femoral artery in small animals, or the facial artery or metatarsal artery in large animals, is useful for evaluating heart rate. In small animal patients, palpation of the femoral artery, compared with other peripheral pulses, has been shown to yield the most accurate heart rate. Pulse palpation may also aid in identifying poor cardiac output. However, this is neither a sensitive nor a specific measure of arterial blood pressure (ABP) or perfusion. Remember that when a peripheral pulse is palpated, it is the difference between systolic and diastolic pressures (pulse pressure) that is palpated. So, the pulse pressure of a normotensive patient (e.g., systolic blood pressure 120 mmHg and diastolic blood pressure 80 mmHg) and a profoundly hypotensive patient (e.g., systolic blood pressure 60 mmHg and diastolic blood pressure 20 mmHg) could be the same. This is because they both have a pulse pressure of 40 mmHg. This highlights the risk of drawing conclusions regarding ABP, cardiac output, and perfusion based on peripheral pulse palpation alone.

Monitoring of the Respiratory System

A physical examination can be key in assessing the respiratory system in the peri-anesthetic period. Evaluation of respiratory patterns, even when intubated and anesthetized, can give insight into pulmonary function and anesthetic depth. If there is a sudden change in respiratory rate or pattern of breathing, it can indicate an alteration in anesthetic depth, acute drop in oxygenation, or inadequate analgesia. Although it must be combined with other findings on examination and on monitoring equipment, the evaluation of the ventilatory pattern can be very revealing. Additionally, if there is concern for volume overload, auscultation of the thoracic field for crackles may help guide next steps with diagnostics and treatments. In patients who may have pneumonia and other lung pathology, auscultation may allow for an observant anesthetist to identify lung fields that are affected, which may aid in decision-making for patient positioning. As with auscultation for cardiac murmurs, there is a steep learning curve, and the new clinician is encouraged to listen serially to patients to identify subtle changes.

Assisted positive pressure ventilation by closing the adjustable pressure limiting (APL) valve and squeezing the reservoir bag gives the anesthetist subjective information about *pulmonary compliance*, which is defined as the change in volume divided by the change in pressure within the lungs. A patient that has developed "stiffer" lungs characterized by reaching a higher pressure with a lower tidal volume could have pulmonary infiltrates (worsening edema and progressive pneumonia), fibrosis, worsening pleural space disease (e.g., pneumothorax and pyothorax), or accidental one lung intubation. Evaluating compliance

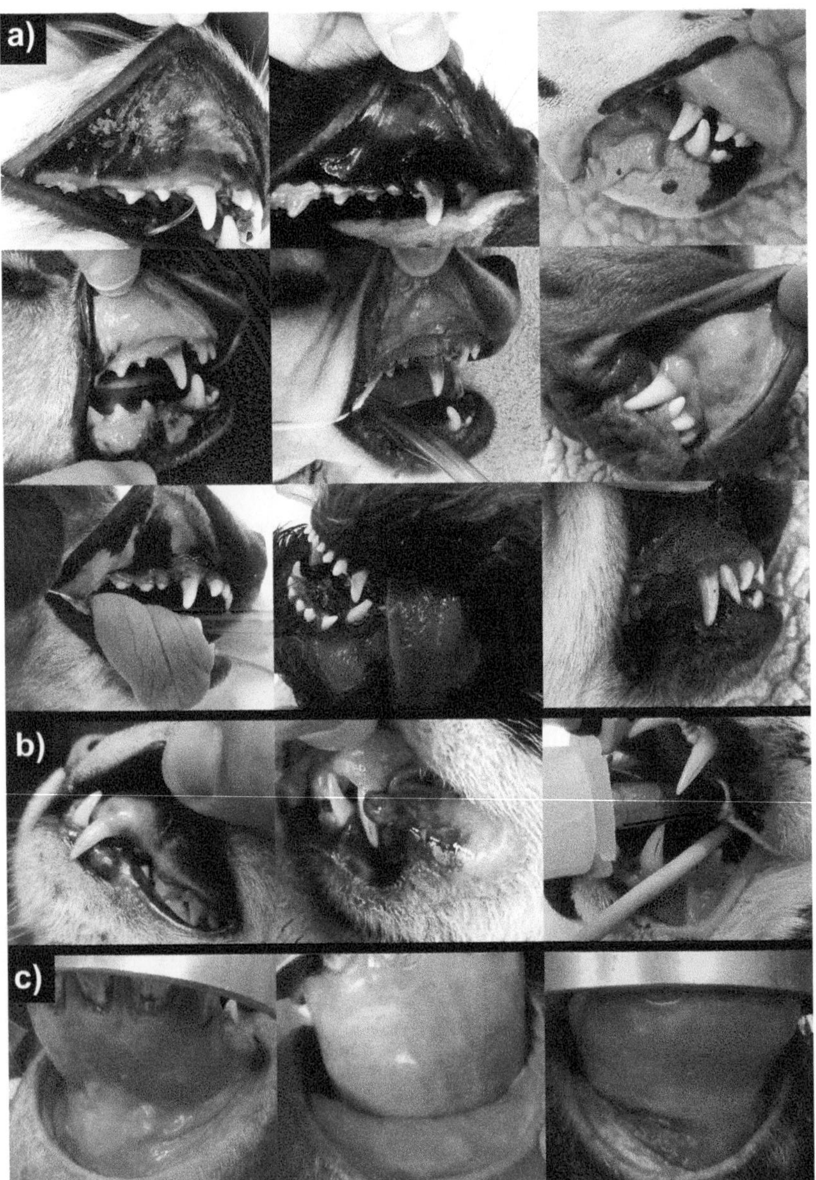

Figure 4.2 Different mucous membrane colors in dogs (a), cats (b), and horses (c). In dogs, from top left to right, top row: normal pink, normal pigmented color (some breeds, like the Chow Chow have pigmented mucous membranes), and pallor (pale pink); second row: severe pallor (very pale pink to white), mild icterus (notice yellow tinge), and obvious icterus; third row: cyanosis (blue hue), congested (brick red), and congested (brick red, "injected") with periodontal disease. In cats: Normal pink, cyanotic or blue (methemoglobinemia), and obvious icterus. In horses: Normal pink, pallor (pale pink), hyperemic and verging on congested (bright red).

should also be combined with visualizing the rise and fall of the thoracic cavity in combination with tidal volume and the peak inspiratory pressure being delivered to the patient. If there is inadequate thoracic wall movement with ventilation, steps should be taken to correct the underlying cause to ensure adequate ventilation and oxygenation. For example, in cases of suspected one lung intubation, the anesthetist may only hear lung sounds on one side of the thorax with assisted ventilation. If the endotracheal tube (ET tube) is retracted so that the distal tip lies in the trachea, then lung sounds should be audible bilaterally.

If breathing system pressure cannot be maintained during the inspiratory phase of ventilation, there may be a leak. By listening to the patient while delivering a breath, with a peak inspiratory pressure of up to 20 cmH_2O, the anesthetist can listen for a hissing sound indicative of a leak around the ET tube cuff. Inflating the cuff with air will establish an airway seal, protecting the airway from aspiration risk and reducing personnel exposure to inhalants. Observing the reservoir bag allows basic monitoring of spontaneous ventilation. A definitive determination of ventilatory status cannot be determined simply by looking at the reservoir bag, as doing so does not provide quantitative information on tidal volume (both rate and volume are necessary to evaluate ventilation). As volume measurement requires spirometry, it is more common to assess ventilation with capnography (see section on Capnography).

Types of Patient Monitors

Monitoring equipment should not take the place of patient observation and physical evaluations (as described in the preceding text). However, they do aid in improving the quality of care. There are numerous types of monitoring equipment available, some of which are marketed for veterinary medicine, while others have been adapted from the human medical field. Veterinary monitors often have pre-set alarm limits that may pertain to specific species. Although these typically have a lower price point, there is often less rigorous testing and greater potential for electrical interference with some models. Those monitors that are made in accordance to human standards are frequently available with more advanced features, such as inhalant anesthetic concentration monitoring, but are more expensive. Some monitoring equipment is available as stand-alone unit (e.g., Doppler, pulse oximeter, capnography, and electrocardiography), while others have multiple modalities combined into a multiparameter monitor. The goals of using monitoring equipment are to facilitate continuous assessment of vital parameters, to provide more information than can be obtained by observation and physical examination alone, and to improve safety of the anesthetic event (when applied and interpreted correctly).

Principles and Techniques for Monitoring Equipment

Cardiovascular System

Monitoring the cardiovascular system requires evaluating multiple variables. These include heart rate and rhythm, which may give insights into levels of consciousness, pain control, arrhythmogenic potential, electrolyte imbalances, and shock states. Additionally, ABP monitoring is important as a means of indirectly evaluating tissue perfusion. A more direct method of assessing tissue perfusion and oxygen delivery is with cardiac output monitoring, but this is not commonly performed in clinical practice.

Heart Rate and Rhythm

Management of hypotension is important in the peri-anesthetic period, and a main component of that is evaluation of heart rate and rhythm as both contribute to cardiac output (see Chapter 16). Tachycardia and bradycardia can both have negative consequences. Patients that are tachycardic may have inadequate filling of the heart ventricles (secondary to reduced time in diastole as heart rate increases), thereby reducing stroke volume. Patients who are profoundly bradycardic may have reduced cardiac output simply due to the low number of heart beats per minute. Patients with arrhythmias may also have reduced stroke volume, dependent upon the type of arrhythmia present (see Chapter 17).

Electrocardiograph (ECG)

When evaluating heart rate and rhythm in the peri-anesthetic period, using an ECG allows for continuous evaluation of cardiac electrical activity. When performing a three-lead ECG, which is typical for peri-anesthetic monitoring, electrodes are placed in accordance with Einthoven's triangle (Figure 4.3). Leads can be attached to the patient with metal "alligator" clips with ECG gel or alcohol applied to improve conductance of the electrical signal. Alternatively, commercially available adhesive ECG pads that snap onto ECG leads can be purchased. In accordance to the American Heart Association (AHA), the white lead is placed on the right thoracic limb, the black lead is placed on the left thoracic limb, and the red lead is placed on the left pelvic limb, to act as a ground. However, in other countries that follow the International Electrotechnical Commission guidelines, the red lead is placed on the right thoracic limb, the yellow lead is placed on the left thoracic limb, and the green lead is placed on the left pelvic limb. It is widespread practice to display and read an ECG in the lead II configuration. This reflects the signal obtained between the right thoracic limb (negative electrode) and left pelvic limb (positive electrode). Lead II usually provides the most robust complexes, and this is the view commonly used to identify arrhythmias. This gives the classic appearance of a depolarizing P wave followed by a QRS complex and then a T wave repolarization.

In horses and other large animal species, a different electrode configuration is usually applied: a base–apex configuration. In this arrangement with the AHA color scheme, the red ground electrode is placed on the neck (or on the shoulder) alongside the white electrode (within the right jugular groove; base lead), while the black electrode is

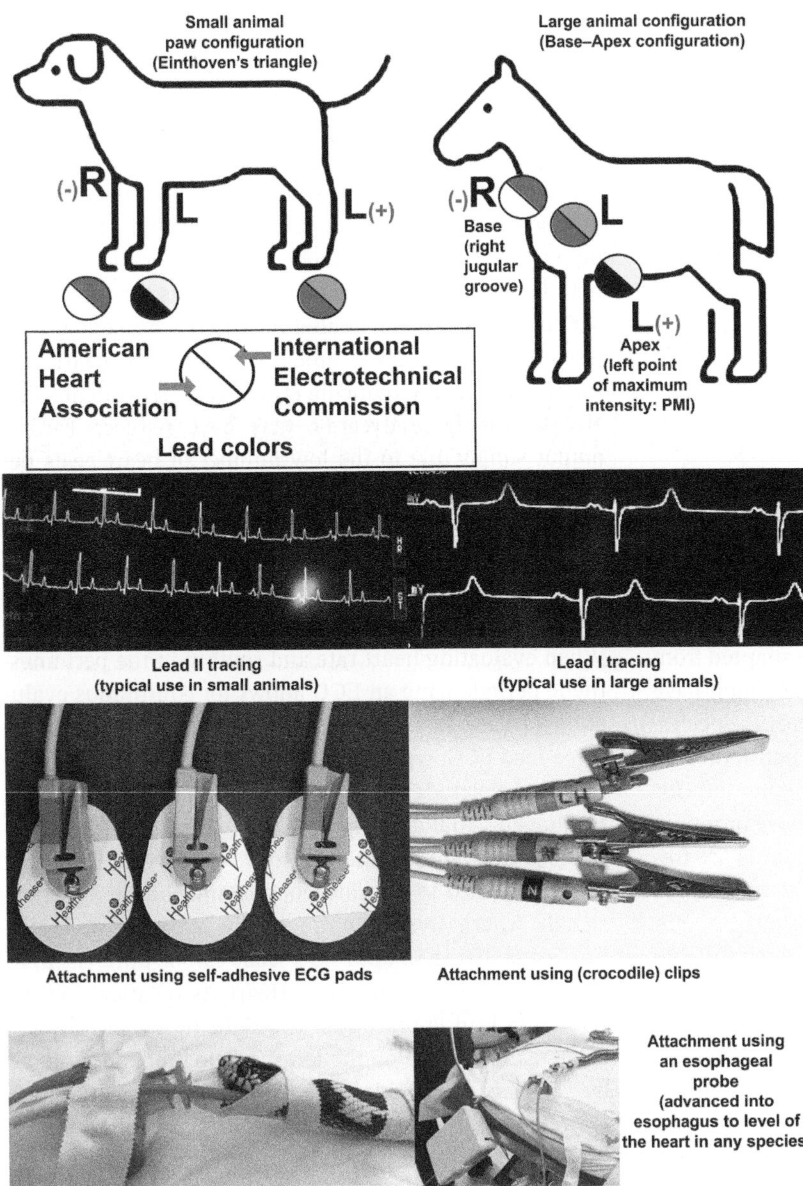

Figure 4.3 Placement of electrocardiogram (ECG) leads in small and large animals during anesthesia (top row), typical tracings of a lead II and lead I configuration seen on physiologic monitors (second row), and different methods of attaching leads to animals (third row). The esophageal ECG probe has the electrode encased within a tube that is advanced into the esophagus. An esophageal ECG can be used in most species; however, it is particularly useful in exotic animals, such as snakes (bottom row).

placed caudal to the elbow (on the thorax at the level of the point of maximum intensity of the heartbeat; apex lead). In this arrangement, lead I is used to evaluate the tracing and the QRS complex begins with the first negative deflection after the P wave and is noted by a prominent negative S wave.

With some species, such as birds or reptiles, it may be difficult to obtain good electrode contact due to their presence of feathers or scales, respectively. For avian species, using ECG pads trimmed down to a smaller surface area reduces the number of feathers that need to be removed to ensure good skin contact. Similar adaptations can be made to affix ECG pads on the paws of other exotic companion animals. Alternative options, such as esophageal ECG probes, allow monitoring of cardiac electrical activity in these species. These devices have a probe that is inserted into the esophagus with the distal end positioned at the level of the heart. The proximal end of the probe (outside the patient) is then connected to ECG electrodes. A recently available device incorporates ECG monitoring (along with respiratory rate and temperature) into a wearable harness that transmits a wireless signal to a monitor for display.

It is important to note that the ECG only gives information about the electrical activity of the heart. It does not give insight into ABP or tissue perfusion. Therefore, an ECG should be considered a good adjunctive monitor, for use with other monitoring equipment to gather information on perfusion and cardiovascular stability. Most ECGs used in veterinary anesthesia practice are not stand-alone units, but are combined in multiparameter monitors that include capnography, oscillometric blood pressure, pulse oximetry, and temperature monitoring. Users can often select some of the monitoring modalities included in a monitor at the time of purchase.

Esophageal Stethoscope

Another means of assessing heart rate is with an esophageal stethoscope, which is a probe that is placed into the esophagus and advanced to the level of the heart. This connects to an adapted stethoscope, with which the anesthetist can hear the heartbeat. Breath sounds are also audible. Although an esophageal stethoscope does not give information about ABP or perfusion, it can provide continuous information that a heartbeat is present, from which a heart rate can be calculated. It is minimally invasive, cheap, and can be useful in noisy working environments.

Doppler Ultrasound Probe Device

Using a Doppler ultrasound device is a low-cost and efficient means to continuously hear the pulse wave generated by the heartbeat (Figure 4.4). As opposed to the ECG, this method of assessment confirms that the heart is contracting sufficiently to generate a pulse. As pulsatile blood flow moves past the Doppler ultrasound probe, the shift in frequency (Doppler effect) of reflected sound waves is converted into an audible signal. Most commonly, the probe is taped in place over a peripheral artery to provide hands-free monitoring. In small animal patients, the probe is typically placed over the metatarsal, metacarpal, dorsal pedal, or coccygeal arteries. In exotic companion animals, such as small rodents and fish, the probe may be placed directly over the heart and taped into place. In avian species, the probe may be placed on the roof of the mouth or over the brachial artery of the wing, with two tongue depressors fashioned to keep the probe in place. Snakes can have the probe taped over their heart (cranial 1/3 of body). Different probe shapes are available for reptiles that can be placed under the carapace and directed toward the heart. In larger species, such as pigs, large ruminants, and horses, the coccygeal artery is often a convenient and easily accessible location for Doppler probe application.

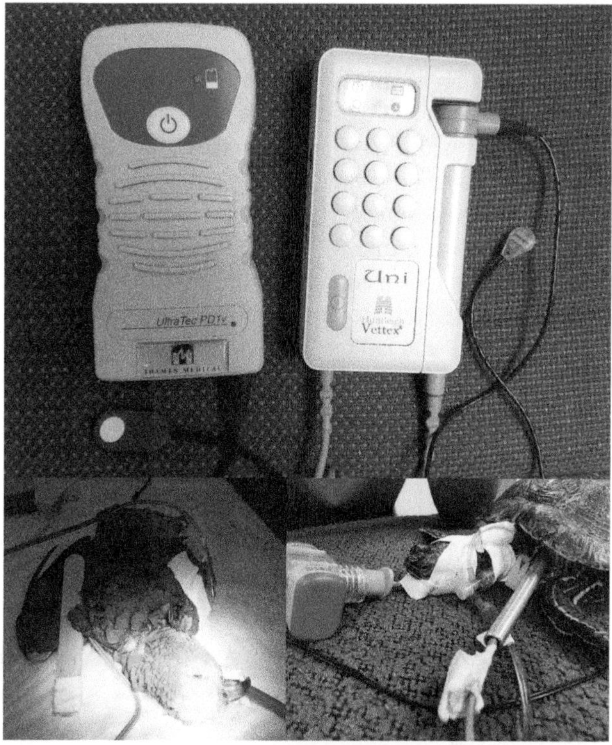

Figure 4.4 Doppler probe attached to a device with a speaker so that blood flow can be heard (top). It is commonly used in exotic species to hear a pulse wave or the heartbeat. Bottom left: The pulse wave is monitored in a bird with the Doppler placed over brachial artery (held in place with tongue depressors). Bottom right: Pencil style Doppler probe in a Chelonian, with probe directed toward the heart.

Arterial Blood Pressure

Although heart rate and rhythm are important determinants of cardiac output, monitoring ABP is necessary to infer the quality of tissue perfusion. In order to perfuse organs, it is necessary to have adequate blood pressure (see Chapter 16 for more details). Although our targets for blood pressure may vary according to species and age group, the same basic principles apply to all species.

Doppler Ultrasound Probe, Pressure Cuff, and Sphygmomanometer

When using a Doppler device (as described in the preceding text), it is commonly combined with a pressure cuff and sphygmomanometer to allow for measurement of ABP. This requires a circumferential inflatable pressure cuff to be placed proximal to the Doppler probe, which may be impractical in some species, depending on Doppler probe location. For example, it is not feasible to obstruct arterial flow proximal to the probe when it is placed directly over the heart, on the hard palate, or on a wing. However, in many species (including small and large companion animals), where the Doppler probe can be placed on an extremity, it is possible to obtain an ABP reading. Cuff size is selected for the extremity being used, aiming for a cuff width that is approximately 40% of the circumference of the placement site (Figure 4.5). When using the tail in horses, a cuff width of approximately 60% of the tail circumference is recommended. If the cuff is too small, the true value of ABP will be overestimated. Conversely, if it is too large, the measured ABP will underestimate the true ABP value. If an ideal cuff size is unavailable, it is considered better to select a larger cuff, reducing the risk of overestimating ABP and failing to recognize hypotension.

When using a Doppler and sphygmomanometer for blood pressure evaluation, the limb should be in a relaxed position (i.e., no occlusion to arterial blood flow). The Doppler crystal will require a contact medium (alcohol or ultrasound gel). Ensure that there is an audible signal before inflating the cuff. Once this is heard, inflate the cuff with a sphygmomanometer until the audible signal disappears. When this occurs, cuff pressure exceeds systolic ABP. In healthy animals, this is usually >120 mmHg. However, a higher level may be necessary in hypertensive patients. Once the audible signal disappears, stop inflation of the cuff and slowly release pressure (approximately 5–10 mmHg per second) and listen for return of the audible signal. Note the pressure on the sphygmomanometer at which the sound returns. This is an approximation of ABP. In healthy dogs, this has been shown to most closely approximate systolic ABP. However, in cats, this approximates the mean ABP. Further research is still needed to assess ABP approximation in other species and for different sizes of patients.

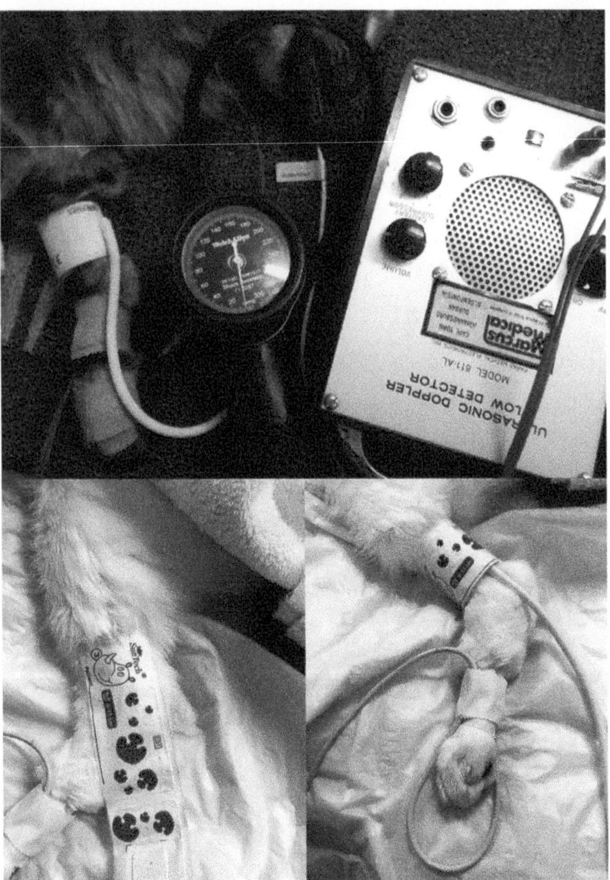

Figure 4.5 A Doppler probe can be used, in combination with a sphygmomanometer (hand held manometer) and cuff, to measure blood pressure (top). The width of the blood pressure cuff must be 40–50% of the limb circumference (bottom left). Appropriate Doppler probe placement on the metatarsal artery of a cat, with the probe positioned distal to the blood pressure cuff (bottom right).

Doppler blood pressure measurement allows for continuous measurement of heart rate and intermittent assessment of blood pressure. Although it is not an automated process, it does allow for repeated measurement in a short period of time. The device does require charging between use and pressure cuffs will need to be replaced as they wear with use (cuff material eventually tears), but it is a cost-effective means to monitor heart rate and ABP in a variety of species.

Oscillometric Devices

The oscillometric ABP monitor can be set to automatically measure ABP at predetermined intervals. This is the most commonly employed method of ABP measurement in small animal veterinary practice. In general, these monitors are sold with various size cuffs to accommodate a variety of patient sizes. The blood pressure cuff is selected to fit to the limb/appendage to which it will be attached (as described in the preceding text). Each manufacturer uses a proprietary algorithm to identify or calculate the systolic, diastolic, and mean ABP. In contrast to the Doppler method, where cuff inflation is performed manually by the user (using a sphygmomanometer, as described in the preceding text), oscillometric devices use a pump to inflate the cuff (Figure 4.6). Additionally, oscillometric devices provide three values of ABP (systolic, diastolic, and mean) in contrast to the single value obtained with the Doppler technique. In general, the most accurate value is the mean ABP.

Unfortunately, many oscillometric devices do not meet the reliability and accuracy standards established by the American College of Veterinary Internal Medicine Consensus Statement on validation of blood pressure measurement devices. Based on clinical experience, oscillometric devices work well in the normotensive patient; however, the greater the deviation in ABP from normal, the less accurate the values provided. At extremes of body size and in patients with oddly shaped appendages (e.g., conical limbs of pigs and chondrodystrophic limbs), there is some concern about accuracy of generated ABP values.

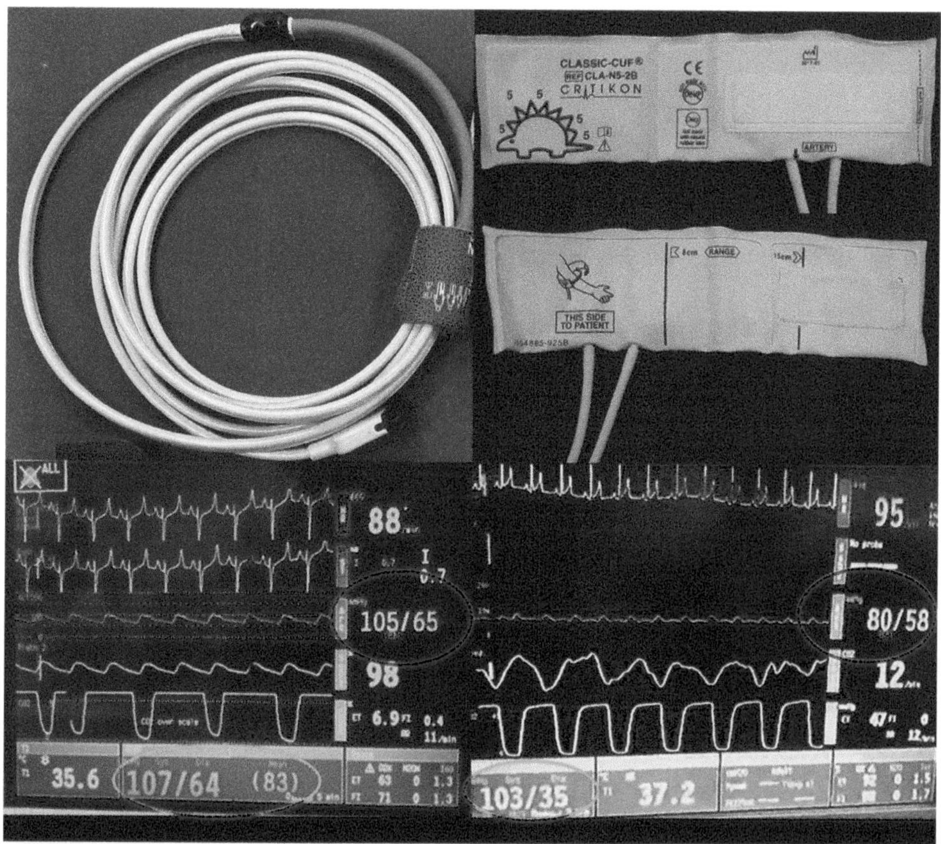

Figure 4.6 Oscillometric method of noninvasive blood pressure monitoring uses a blood pressure cuff attached to a monitor via a proprietary tube (top left). The cuffs (mostly for human use) have many indicator markings, the most important being the artery indicator (top right). The artery indicator should be position over the artery of the limb where the cuff will be placed. The width of the cuff should be between 40 and 50% of the circumference of the limb attachment site. Note: Oscillometric devices are not continuous monitors of blood pressure. Values from invasive blood pressure monitoring is visible within the blue circles (second row) and the oscillometric readings (obtained every five minutes) are within the green circles. These readings are similar in the bottom left figure, but blood pressure can change rapidly during anesthesia and surgery as highlighted by the different blood pressure values in the bottom right figure.

Additionally, there can be aberrant readings in the face of some brady- and tachyarrhythmias. Despite these concerns, this method of assessment of ABP remains widely used in the peri-anesthetic period. There are a large number of devices on the market; some are stand-alone units, while others are incorporated into multiparameter monitors.

Invasive Blood Pressure Monitoring

Although this is the most accurate method of obtaining continuous monitoring of blood pressure during anesthesia, it is invasive, requires expensive, specialized equipment, is technically more challenging, and therefore impractical for routine use in small companion animals. A catheter is placed aseptically within a peripheral artery (e.g., dorsal pedal, coccygeal, or femoral arteries in small animals, and facial or metatarsal arteries in horses) and connected to a pressure transducer. The transducer is placed at the level of the heart and zeroed to the atmosphere. Once this calibration has been performed, the transducer can be connected to the arterial catheter and allows for continuous beat-to-beat monitoring of blood pressure and pulse rate. To minimize the risk of clot formation within the arterial catheter, heparinized saline is used as a flush. Invasive ABP monitoring is the preferred method for monitoring blood pressure in Equidae and other large animal patients (Figure 4.7). No medications should ever be injected through the arterial catheter. There are certain risks associated with intra-arterial catheters, including risk of hemorrhage, thrombosis and reduced perfusion of tissue distal to the catheter, infection, and pain with insertion. Invasive ABP monitoring requires additional equipment, not usually included with standard veterinary multiparametric monitors, and additional technical skills. Therefore, noninvasive ABP monitoring methods as discussed in the preceding text are more commonly used.

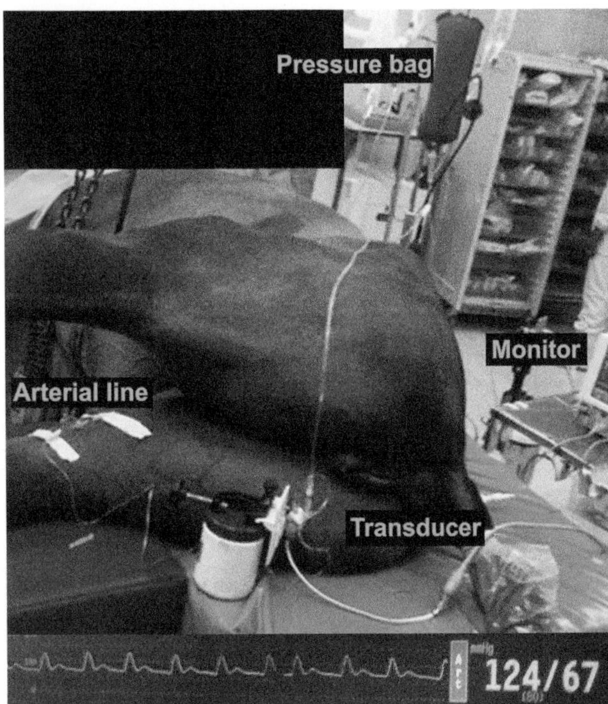

Figure 4.7 Invasive blood pressure monitoring is used in horses, especially if the surgery is longer than 45 minutes. In this example, an artery on the medial aspect of pelvic limb (branch of the medial saphenous artery) is cannulated. A noncompliant fluid filled (isotonic crystalloid) tube that is held under constant pressure (300 mmHg; set by the pressure bag) is connected to the arterial cannular and the electronic transducer. The transducer is connected to a physiologic monitor and an arterial wave form is displayed (bottom figure).

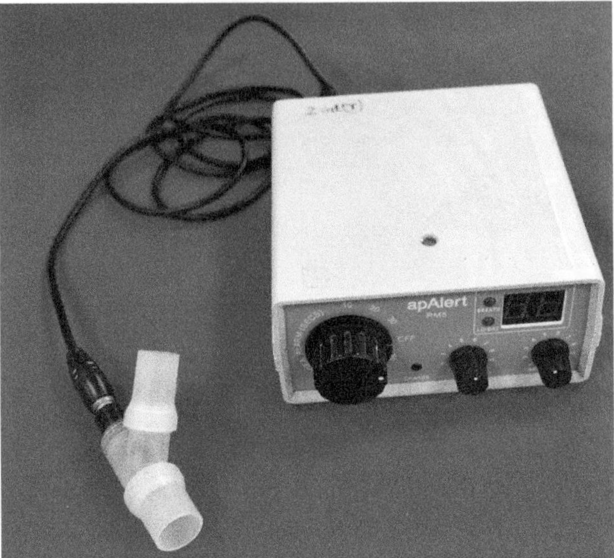

Figure 4.8 An affordable stand-alone device can be used to detect apnea in animals. With this device, an alarm can be set to 10, 20, or 30 s of apnea before an audible beeping is heard. Device sensitivity can also be set and this should be adjusted according to the patient size, where patients >20 kg should have a low sensitivity and those <3 kg have a high sensitivity, with sensitivity for intermediate weights set in between. If sensitivity is not set correctly, then false positive or false negative alarms will occur.

Monitoring of the Respiratory System, Airway Gases, and Oxygenation

While monitoring heart rate, rhythm, and blood pressure are important to use as surrogate markers of oxygen delivery and tissue perfusion, the respiratory system is primarily monitored through ventilation and oxygenation, and anesthetic gas concentrations may also be monitored.

Respiratory System

Apnea Alarm

Maintenance of ventilation during anesthesia is vitally important to ensure adequate oxygenation, avoid hypercapnia, and deliver inhalant anesthetics. Steps should be taken immediately to investigate and manage unintended apnea.

Many machines that include capnography (see later) will also have an apnea alarm that will inform the anesthetist when the patient is apneic. This is often an audible alarm combined with a visual alert on the monitoring screen. Stand-alone monitors that detect apnea are available. These rely on hot-wire aerometry (Figure 4.8). The wire is heated to a fixed temperature and when the animal exhales it cools the wire, which is detected as a breath. The monitor emits an audible alert (usually a "beep") to accompany each breath. When no breath is detected for a pre-set time interval (usually 30 s), then the monitor will sound an alarm. A common user error with this device is to use the monitor with a very sensitive setting so that a "breath" is detected with very gentle manipulation of the thorax or abdomen. Operators should resist the temptation of using a very sensitive setting to reduce the risk of false positives (i.e., indication of a breath when one has not occurred).

Respiratory Gases

Capnography

Carbon dioxide is continuously produced as a byproduct of metabolism, and the primary means of removal from the body is by ventilation; therefore, the ability to noninvasively measure expired carbon dioxide reflects the balance between production and removal. As production of carbon dioxide is relatively constant during general anesthesia, measuring this gas in the airway serves as a monitor of ventilation (capnography).

The capnograph sampling chamber is placed between the patient end of the anesthetic breathing system and the ET tube. Infrared light is passed through the gas to measure the concentration of carbon dioxide present in inhaled and exhaled gas. Normally, patients should have an end-tidal carbon dioxide tension ($PETCO_2$) between 35 and 45 mmHg and an inhaled carbon dioxide tension ($PiCO_2$) of 0 mmHg. Capnography has many uses, including the ability to monitor ventilation (i.e., $PETCO_2$) and respiratory rate and identify various respiratory system pathologies and some anesthetic machine problems. A normal capnograph trace will always return to a baseline close to 0 mmHg and have an identifiable plateau (Figure 4.9). During exhalation, the waveform rises from baseline to generate a plateau, which reflects alveolar emptying. At the end of exhalation, as

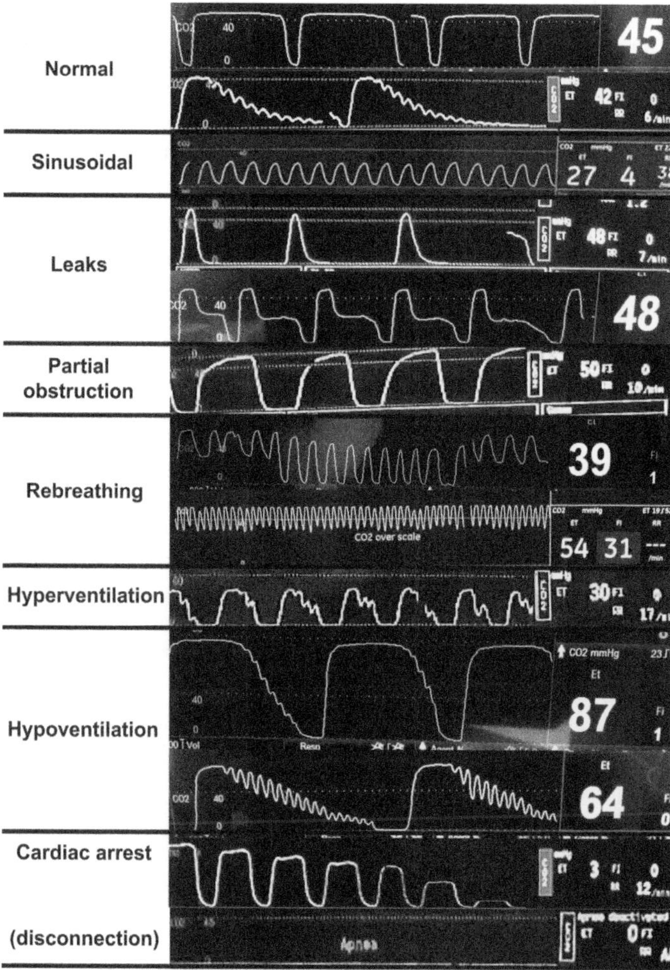

Figure 4.9 Capnograph waveforms and their interpretations. Normal: Top trace is typical for mechanically ventilated animals; the one immediately beneath is common in spontaneously breathing patients with a low respiratory rate. The oscillations visible in the downstroke are called "cardiac" (cardiogenic) oscillations and are normal. The *sinusoidal* graph is often a normal appearance and is common when high fresh gas flow rates are used in nonrebreathing circuits. Leaks: Top trace is typical for leaks at the ET tube; trace beneath is common in cats with uncuffed ET tubes, where exhaled gases pass around the ET tube instead of through it during peak exhalation. Partial obstruction: Identified by the "shark fin" appearance, which can indicate a partially bent or occluded ET tube or bronchoconstriction. Rebreathing: Top traces from left to right; fresh gas flow was not started when the patient was initially connected to the breathing circuit, then it was started (trace reaches baseline), before being stopped again (to demonstrate the elevated baseline). An elevated baseline is diagnostic for rebreathing when the inspired carbon dioxide increases >3–5 mmHg. The bottom trace is from an animal connected to a nonrebreathing circuit that was panting. Note the marked rebreathing (fraction of inspired carbon dioxide [Fi] is 31 mmHg). Hyperventilation: When the end-tidal carbon dioxide is <35 mmHg, it can be due to minute ventilation being higher than normal. Hypoventilation: When the end-tidal carbon dioxide is >45 mmHg; however, this is common under anesthesia and is often tolerated if there is no specific contraindication (e.g., raised intracranial pressure), up to a level of approximately 50–55 mmHg (called "permissive hypercapnia"). If >60 mmHg, hypoventilation is usually addressed, such as by starting mechanical ventilation, reducing the plane of anesthesia, etc. Top trace indicates severe hypoventilation and the bottom trace moderate hypoventilation (notice the cardiac oscillations). Cardiac arrest: Top trace is from a mechanically ventilated patient who was euthanized while under general anesthesia. Note the precipitous drop in end-tidal carbon dioxide with each mechanically delivered breath. Bottom trace is of apnea. One of the many reasons for apnea is cardiac arrest and this should be rapidly investigated. Other reasons (nonexhaustive list) for apnea include a deep plane of anesthesia, decrease in blood pressure, administering drugs that can depress ventilation during anesthesia (e.g., opioids and ketamine), or a disconnection of the capnograph or breathing circuit.

inhalation begins, the waveform trace returns to baseline. This depicts a respiratory cycle, from which respiratory rate can be calculated (by the anesthetist or the monitor). If the capnograph waveform does not return to zero, this indicates the presence of carbon dioxide in inhaled gas (i.e., rebreathing is occurring). This results from failure to completely remove exhaled carbon dioxide. This should be addressed as it can lead to hypercapnia and respiratory acidosis. When using a circle breathing system, rebreathing can be caused by exhausted carbon dioxide absorbent or a unidirectional valve stuck in the open position within the circle breathing system. Rebreathing can also occur in patients connected to a nonrebreathing system (e.g., Bain system) when fresh gas flow is inadequate or during hyperventilation: in either of these cases, the fresh gas flow is insufficient to remove carbon dioxide. Additionally, a patient with increased dead space ventilation (e.g., very long ET tube) may exhibit rebreathing. Some respiratory pathologies can also be appreciated using capnography. With bronchospasm, the capnograph trace will appear as a shark fin shape, resulting from delayed emptying of lower airways during exhalation. The loss of a well-defined steep inspiratory slope can be associated with a leak in the system, most commonly around the ET tube cuff. Acute loss of the capnograph waveform is indicative of apnea. A sudden decrease in $PETCO_2$ (especially when seen on a normal square waveform tracing) can indicate a fall in cardiac output. As cardiac output decreases, less blood (carrying carbon dioxide) is delivered to the lungs, resulting in less carbon dioxide available for exhalation (measured by the capnograph). This clinical picture suggests an impending cardiac arrest. This also explains why $PETCO_2$ is low during cardiopulmonary resuscitation (CPR) as cardiac output remains below normal levels with CPR efforts. Capnography can be used as a tool for the assessment of return of spontaneous circulation in dogs ($PETCO_2 > 15$ mmHg) and cats ($PETCO_2 > 18$ mmHg) during CPR: the increase in $PETCO_2$ values reflects an increase in cardiac output.

The two types of capnograph used in veterinary medicine are mainstream and sidestream (Figure 4.10). With

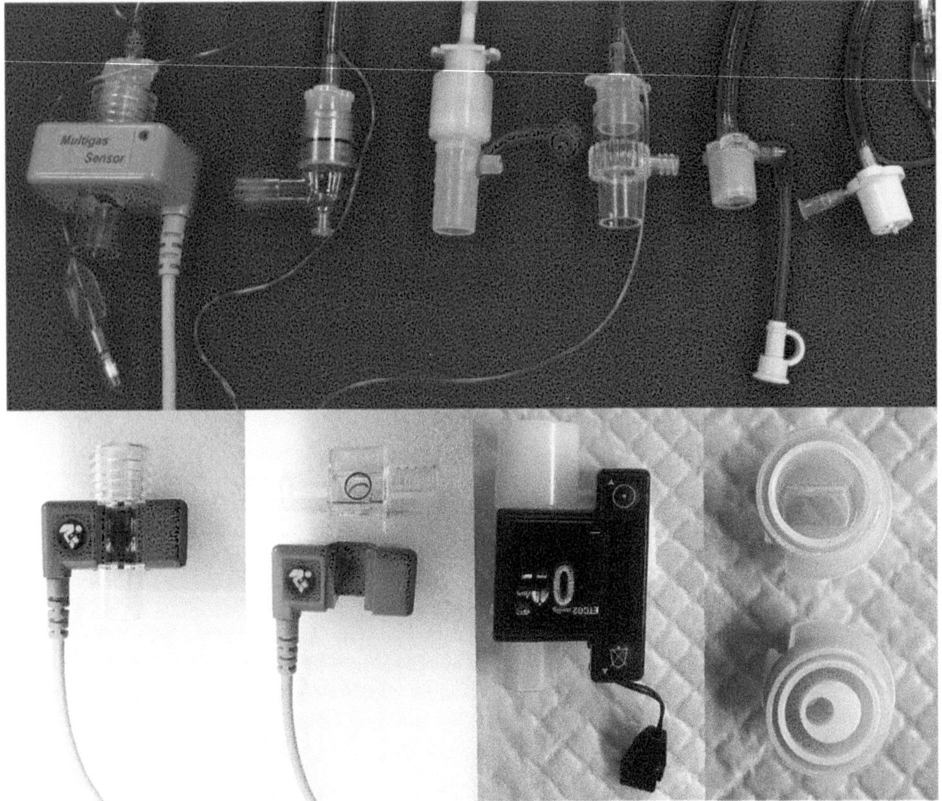

Figure 4.10 Examples of capnograph sampling chambers. Top: Left is an example of a mainstream sampling chamber, the five to the right are examples of sampling chambers for a sidestream capnograph. With sidestream capnography, a thin sampling tube links the sampling chamber to the physiologic monitor. Note: The two examples furthest to the right have a very low dead space volume because they are incorporated into the ET tube breathing circuit connector. Second row: Left two figures show a mainstream capnograph with the sampling chamber in position and removed (done for cleaning or to swap between adult and pediatric chambers). Two right figures are of a battery-operated mainstream capnograph, showing adult and pediatric chambers alongside one another.

both devices, a sampling chamber is connected between the patient end of the breathing system and the ET tube. The devices differ in site of carbon dioxide measurement. The mainstream capnograph is connected around the sampling chamber and measures carbon dioxide tension here. Because measurement takes place locally, mainstream capnographs provide near-instantaneous carbon dioxide readings as there is no delay for sampled gas to be delivered to a distant location for measurement. However, the connection of a mainstream capnograph to the breathing system adds bulk and weight to the end of the ET tube. This can pose an inadvertent ET tube extubation risk in smaller patients and may result in twisting of the ET tube if the patient's head and capnograph are not supported. If these devices are battery powered, then frequent battery changes may be necessary. The airway adaptor (sampling chamber) incorporated in mainstream capnographs is usually interchangeable. This allows for changing adaptors if it becomes contaminated with condensation of expired gases, fluid, or secretions. Different adaptor sizes may be available. Pediatric adaptors will provide a more accurate $PETCO_2$ and waveform in smaller patients, but care should be taken that the adaptor inner diameter is not smaller than the ET tube diameter or it will increase resistance to airway gas flow and work of breathing. There are mainstream capnographs that do not require frequent battery changes and use a main electrical supply instead.

The sidestream capnograph operates by drawing airway gases from the sampling chamber (via a sample line) and delivering them to the infrared analyzer for carbon dioxide measurement. Gas sampling rates range from 75 to 400 mL/min. Due to this transit, there is a delay from the time of sampling to the reading displayed on the monitor. However, this delay is typically only a few seconds. This method of capnography is less prone to damage and breaking, though the sampling line can be accidentally occluded by kinking or with respiratory secretions, so they may occasionally need to be replaced. Regardless of capnograph type, their use increases dead space (mechanical dead space) ventilation, which may pose a problem in very small patients, especially when a pediatric adaptor is not available.

Readers should be aware of differences in capnograph waveforms caused by use of nonrebreathing systems. With these systems, the relatively high fresh gas flow causes gas mixing within the capnograph sampling chamber. This results in sample dilution, causing a further underestimation of arterial partial pressure of carbon dioxide (P_aCO_2) by $PETCO_2$ and transforms the waveform to a more rounded "hill top" shape, in contrast to the ideal square waveform tracing seen with circle breathing systems. As described in the preceding text, the use of a pediatric sampling chamber, when appropriate, will improve $PETCO_2$ accuracy and the waveform appearance by reducing the dilution effect. There are numerous types of adapters in both pediatric and adult sizes.

Alveolar Dead Space

In a healthy patient, there is a fixed amount of dead space present within the trachea and bronchi, called "anatomical dead space" (see Chapter 18). This is because the trachea takes gases in but does not have a capillary bed to engage in gas exchange. Alveolar dead space occurs when gas flows in/out of alveoli that are not perfused. Any reduction/obstruction to alveolar blood flow contributes to alveolar dead space, including pulmonary thromboembolism and poor cardiac output.

When alveolar dead space is present there is a lack of gas exchange. Gas exiting the alveoli contains a low concentration of carbon dioxide. This gas has a dilutional effect on gas exhaled from alveoli where ventilation and perfusion are better matched. The net effect of this is to produce a $PETCO_2$ value that underestimates the patient's true arterial partial pressure of carbon dioxide (P_aCO_2). This discrepancy can be confirmed with arterial blood gas (ABG) analysis (see later), if available. Quantifying the percentage of total dead space ventilation can be performed by calculating the dead space to tidal volume ratio (V_d:V_t) via the Engoff method, where the inspired carbon dioxide (P_iCO_2) should be equal to zero in an appropriately functioning anesthetic circuit, and P_eCO_2 is the mixed expired carbon dioxide.

$$V_d : V_t = (P_aCO_2 - P_eCO_2) \div (P_aCO_2 - P_iCO_2) \qquad (1)$$

In this equation, in most of our small animal patients, normal values are 20–35% under general anesthesia. However, some horses can have a normal V_d: V_t of 50%.

Inhalational Anesthetic Gas Monitoring

Many multiparameter monitors now also include the ability to monitor the concentration of inhalational anesthetic in the breathing system. As with capnography, both inhaled and exhaled anesthetic concentrations are displayed, confirming agent delivery and reflection of alveolar concentration, respectively (Figure 4.11). Although anesthetic depth must

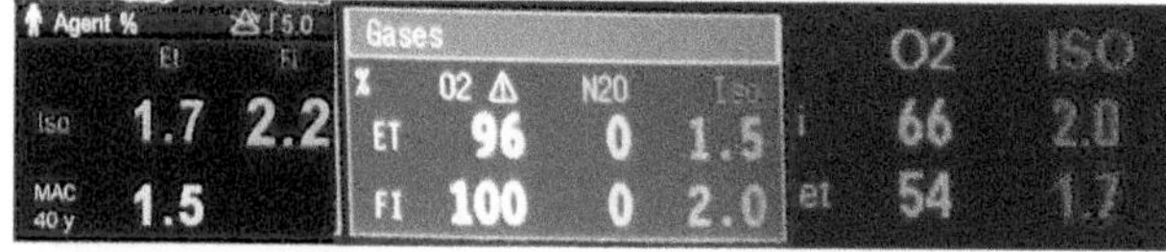

Figure 4.11 Some physiologic monitors will have anesthetic agent analyzer or ability to monitor other gases than CO_2. In these examples, the inspired (Fi, FI, and i) and expired (Et, ET, and et) concentrations of isoflurane are shown. Clinically, the most important value is the expired value because it reflects the concertation within the patient.

still be assessed, as previously described, inhalational anesthetic gas monitoring is a useful additional tool for patient care. Using the minimum alveolar concentration (MAC) value as a guideline (Chapter 8), this can be a starting target for end-tidal anesthetic concentrations. Nevertheless, inhalant anesthetic administration should be titrated to the patient's response and assessment of anesthetic depth.

Oxygenation

Pulse Oximetry

During sedation and anesthesia, it is also important to closely monitor oxygenation as the majority of our anesthetic drugs alter the body's natural response to increase ventilation in the presence of hypoxemia. The least invasive method of monitoring hypoxemia is with a pulse oximeter. Pulse oximeters are placed on peripheral tissue (i.e., tongue, digit, skin flap, vulva, etc.). They transmit a combination of infrared and red light through tissue. The fraction of light absorbed by hemoglobin in the arterial blood is used to calculate the percentage (%) saturation of hemoglobin carrying oxygen. Patients under general anesthesia should have a pulse oximeter reading (SpO_2) close to 100% (usually 97–100%). When the fraction of inspired oxygen (FiO_2) is 100%, as is the case for most anesthetized patients, the PaO_2 should be approximately 500 mmHg (PaO_2 can be estimated by multiplying FiO_2 by 5).

However, due to the shape of the oxygen–hemoglobin dissociation curve (see Chapter 18), an SpO_2 reading of 100% indicates a PaO_2 value anywhere between 100 and 500 mmHg. *Hypoxemia* is defined as PaO_2 <60 mmHg, which equates to an SpO_2 value <90%. Once the PaO_2 falls to 60 mmHg, there is a precipitous drop in oxygen–hemoglobin saturation (Table 4.2). Although there are some species variations resulting from differences in hemoglobin structure and affinity for oxygen, this general guideline applies across species. Care should be taken to not confuse SpO_2 and PaO_2 values.

There are numerous versions of pulse oximeters available with different probes (Figure 4.12). The most common form of pulse oximeter probe is the transmission probe, which consists of a clamp (clip) system. Light emitters on one side of the clamp are positioned opposite detectors on the other side. The clamp is attached to a patient so that light passes through tissue sitting between the light emitters and detectors. An alternative arrangement is the reflectance probe (similar in arrangement to a transflectance probe). This houses both the light emitters and detectors in the same plane and requires a flat surface to reflect emitted light back to the receiver. Reflectance probes are usually placed rectally, on the ventral surface of the tail or on the gingiva. Paddle-shaped, transflectance probes are usually placed over a superficial artery, enabling

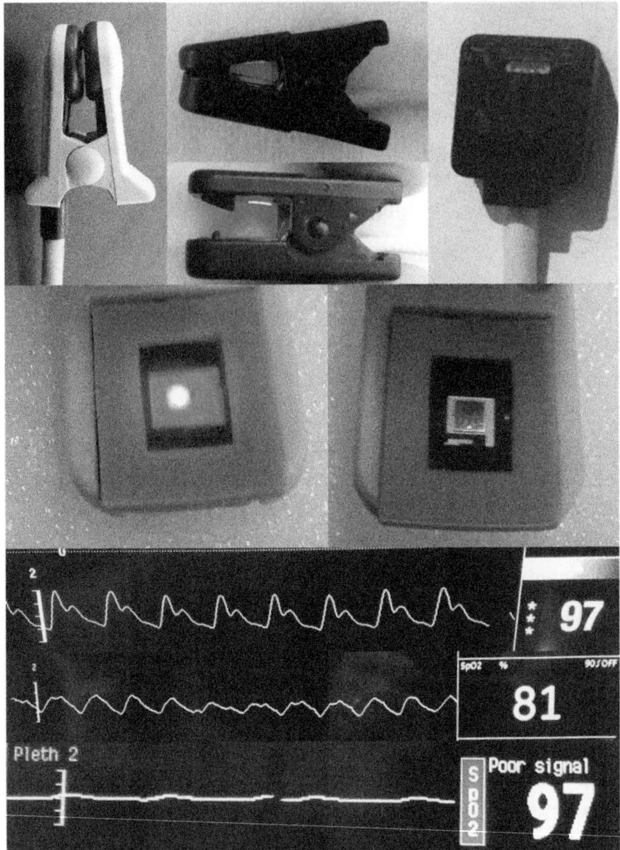

Figure 4.12 Peripheral oxygen–hemoglobin saturation (SpO_2) monitors are available with different probes. These include transmission probes (top left and middle) and reflectance probes (top right). For transmission probes (most common type in small animal practice), the light emitting diodes emit light (red and infrared light) that is transmitted through tissue and detected by photodetectors located on the opposite probe (top middle and second row). Reflectance probes rely on the emitted light reflecting from the mucosa, with emitted light returning to the photodetector, which is located alongside the light emitters. With all types, a plethysmograph, based on pulsatile light absorption, is calculated and displayed (bottom three traces). The top trace the patient is not hypoxemic (97% saturation), the middle trace is of a hypoxemic animal (81% saturation), and the bottom graph indicates adequate saturation (97%) but the pulse wave is poorly detected.

Table 4.2 Pulse oximetry (SpO_2) readings and corresponding estimated partial pressure of arterial oxygen (PaO_2).

SpO_2 (%)	PaO_2 (mmHg)
100	100–500
95	80
90	60
70	40
60	30

continuous pulse oximeter readings even with subtle movements. Different probe types operate using the same basic principles, with variation in the method by which light is transmitted and detected. Paddle-shaped probes can be extremely useful in patients where there is concern that they may become hypoxemic on extubation, as the anesthetist can affix it over a superficial artery with vet wrap or tape, which is easier than trying to maintain a transmission probe on the tongue.

Hypoxemia is a life-threatening complication and requires urgent investigation and treatment. The intervention will depend on the cause. Examples of causes of hypoxemia and potential interventions are listed (Table 4.3).

Shunt

There are naturally occurring shunts in the body, such as the Thebesian veins and bronchial circulation, through which blood bypasses the pulmonary circulation and does not participate in gas exchange but is returned to the left side of the heart as poorly oxygenated blood. An intrapulmonary shunt is an area where blood flows into the alveolar capillary beds but there is no ventilation to allow gas exchange. When this happens inappropriately under anesthesia, such as with one lung ventilation (because the ET tube is passed into a mainstem bronchus), compression atelectasis, or a mucus plug in an alveolus, air is not able to enter an alveolus despite blood flowing to that capillary bed (see Chapter 18). If the shunt is >20% it can lead to hypoxemia. If the shunt is >30%, then the response to supplemental 100% oxygen therapy to treat the hypoxemia starts to diminish. The amount of shunting in a patient can be calculated with an arterial and mixed venous blood gas; however, this technique is beyond the scope of this chapter. If hypoxemia is present, then the possibility of intrapulmonary shunting as a cause should be considered, and steps taken to address this. Such steps may include repositioning the ET tube so that it is not advanced into a mainstem bronchus, performing an alveolar recruitment maneuver to expand collapsed alveoli and to apply positive end expiratory pressure (PEEP) to reduce the likelihood of repeated alveolar collapse. Some ventilators have some inherent PEEP, while others allow the user to set the desired level of PEEP.

Anesthetic Machine and Safety Equipment

ET Tube Cuff Inflation Devices

When placing an ET tube in most animals, it is important to create a seal within the trachea by inflating the ET tube cuff with air. The most common method to do this is by auscultation, where air is injected into the cuff of the ET tube with a syringe while simultaneously giving the patient a positive pressure breath up to a peak inspiratory pressure of 15–20 cmH_2O. Listening at the patient's mouth identifies any leak around the cuff as a hissing sound. It is important to use the least amount of air needed to achieve a seal because high pressures within the cuff increase the risk of tracheal mucosal damage and pressure necrosis. An adequate airway seal reduces the risk of aspirating liquid present in the caudal oropharynx (e.g., from regurgitation) and prevents workplace pollution with anesthetic gases.

Table 4.3 Examples of etiologies of hypoxemia and potential corrective interventions during anesthesia.

Cause	Example	Potential intervention
Diffusion impairment	Congestive heart failure	Treatment with furosemide
	Volume overload	Discontinuation of intravenous fluids
Decreased inspired oxygen	Oxygen cylinder not opened/empty	Replace oxygen cylinder
	Medical air flow with no oxygen flow into a breathing circuit of an anesthetic machine	Connect to pipeline oxygen
Right-to-left shunt	Compression atelectasis	Mechanical ventilation and PEEP
	Reversed blood flow/end-stage PDA	Phenylephrine for reversed PDA[1]
Hypoventilation	Cervical disc causing spinal cord compression at C2–3	Mechanical ventilation
	Neuromuscular blocking agent use	
***V/Q* mismatch**	Hypoperfusion/diminished cardiac output	Improve cardiac output (reduce delivered inhalant anesthetic, fluids, and vasopressors as appropriate)

1) Phenylephrine is a vasoconstrictor and increases systemic blood pressure. If the systemic blood pressure is greater than the pulmonary blood pressure, then the shunt will be in a left-to-right direction which decreases the development of hypoxemia (see Chapters 17 and 18). *V/Q*: ventilation to perfusion ratio; PDA: patent ductus arteriosus; PEEP: positive end expiratory pressure; MAC: minimum alveolar concentration.

For low-pressure, high-volume cuffed ET tubes, there are also devices that allow for the anesthetist to determine the appropriate pressure to place within the cuff to create a seal (Figure 4.13). Other handheld devices take the place of a traditional cuff syringe and give a target range for appropriate pressure (20–30 cmH_2O).

Anesthetists should be aware that a leak can develop around the ET tube cuff despite an initial seal being created if the ET tube is moved (e.g., during patient repositioning) or as the patient's anesthetic depth becomes deeper.

Breathing System and Anesthetic Machine

The APL valve is designed to allow excess breathing system pressure to be relieved. Some anesthetic machines can be fitted with a high breathing system pressure alarm that emits an audible alarm when a predetermined pressure is exceeded. These devices are usually battery operated, commonly fitted between the common gas outlet and breathing system (other sites may be used depending on machine design), and the trigger pressure can be adjusted by the user (commonly set between 20 and 30 cmH_2O). Anesthetic machines and breathing systems are discussed in more detail elsewhere (Chapter 5).

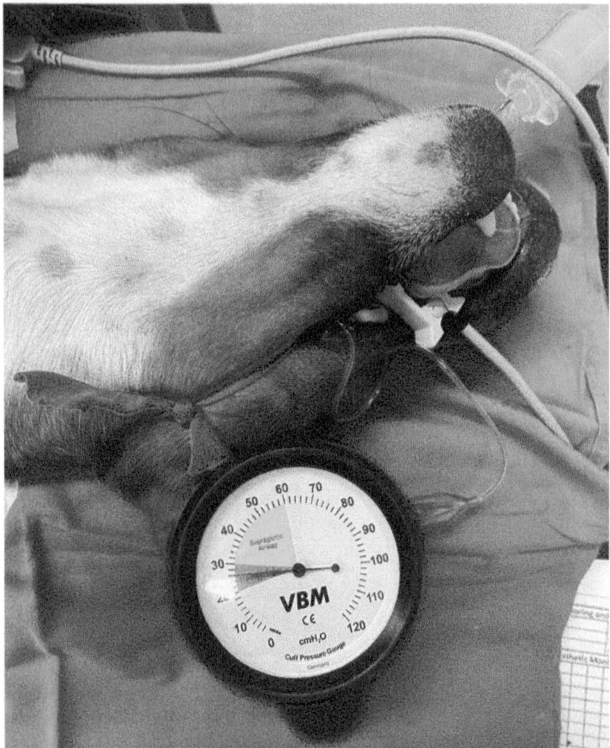

Figure 4.13 A dog under general anesthesia with an ET tube in place. The cuff of the ET tube is filled with room air using a cuff inflating device.

Laboratory Analyses

Traditional Blood Gas Analysis

The most accurate method to determine ventilation and oxygenation is by analysis of an arterial blood sample for blood gases, known as an "arterial blood gas analysis." While traditionally limited to referral clinics and university hospitals, this diagnostic modality has become relatively affordable and portable blood gas analyzers are increasingly available. Additionally, with both arterial and venous blood samples, acid–base status can be evaluated.

Assessing oxygenation and ventilation is based on the PaO_2 and $PaCO_2$, respectively. With most veterinary patients receiving an FIO_2 of 100%, the expected PaO_2 should be close to 500 mmHg (as described in the preceding text). While *hypoxemia* is defined as PaO_2 <60 mmHg, values lower than expected for the FiO_2 delivered, or downward trends in PaO_2, should be investigated. A PaO_2:FiO_2 (P:F) ratio can also be evaluated by dividing the PaO_2 by FiO_2:

$$P:F\ ratio = PaO_2 \div FiO_2 \tag{2}$$

This method was originally developed for the evaluation of human patients with acute respiratory distress syndrome to determine severity of disease. However, it can be applied to estimate oxygen dependence. A P:F ratio >300 is interpreted as minimum risk of hypoxemia without oxygen supplementation, while <200 indicates moderate, and <100 indicates severe dependence on oxygen supplementation.

To evaluate the acid–base status of the patient, an arterial or jugular venous blood sample can be used. The minimum necessary components for assessment are pH, partial pressure of carbon dioxide (PCO_2), and concentration of bicarbonate (HCO_3^-).

A useful mnemonic for approaching acid–base evaluation is the "rule of fours." Normal physiologic pH is 7.4, normal $PaCO_2$ is 40 mmHg, and normal bicarbonate is 24 mmol/L. Although there is variation between species, this is a good approximation for starting to analyze blood gases. pH is tightly regulated and managed in the short term by the respiratory system (i.e., ventilation) and more chronically with the buffering capacity of the kidneys (i.e., conservation of bicarbonate).

A useful tip to remember is that physiologic systems will never overcompensate; therefore, a compensatory change will never make the pH return to normal. If HCO_3^- and PCO_2 change in opposite directions, then a mixed acid–base disturbance is present.

The first step for the evaluation of the acid–base status of a patient based on a blood gas is to determine if the pH is high, low, or normal. If pH is decreased from normal, then it is consistent with an *acidemia* (and likely acidosis at tissue level). This can be caused by an excess of acid (e.g., elevated carbon dioxide) or a lack of base (e.g., decreased bicarbonate). If pH is increased from normal, then it is consistent with an *alkalemia* (and likely alkalosis at tissue level). This can be caused by a decrease of acid (e.g., reduced carbon dioxide) or an elevation of base (e.g., increased bicarbonate). If the pH is normal, this indicates one of two things – either there is no acid–base abnormality or there is a mixed acid–base status.

Following evaluation of pH, the respiratory and metabolic components must then be evaluated to determine which of these is the primary disturbance. In other words, does the alteration in analyte (HCO_3^- and PCO_2) move in the same direction as the pH? Remember that carbon dioxide is an acid, and it is regulated at the level of the lungs. Bicarbonate is a base and is regulated by the kidneys. There can also be compensatory/adaptive changes or multiple acid–base disturbances occurring simultaneously, so the evaluation of both HCO_3^- and PCO_2 is necessary.

For example, an elevated carbon dioxide (e.g., 60 mmHg) represents an increase in acid content within the blood. If the pH is 7.15 (acidemia), then the pH change is readily explained by the increase in PCO_2. Therefore, it is likely to be the primary disturbance. However, as mixed acid–base disturbances can occur, one should always evaluate bicarbonate. If bicarbonate is elevated (e.g., 28 mmol/L), this indicates an excess of base. This does not explain the pH change, so it is likely a compensatory change. It is possible to estimate the expected compensatory change that is expected given the change in the primary abnormality (Table 4.4).

Blood Analytes

Evaluation of electrolytes during the peri-anesthetic period can be an important aspect of patient management, especially with acute changes, such as hyperkalemia. This may be most pertinent in cats with feline idiopathic cystitis, horses with hyperkalemia periodic paralysis, and goats with urethral obstruction requiring anesthesia. In these cases, it can be useful to obtain a baseline potassium concentration before anesthesia and serially monitor the potassium concentration throughout the anesthetic episode. However, if there is an abrupt change in ECG rhythm (such as the appearance of tall, tented T waves; Figure 4.14) or slowing of the heart rate that is unexplained by other interventions, then checking the potassium level is recommend. There are numerous portable analyzers available with the ability to evaluate electrolyte concentrations in bodily fluids as well as blood gas measurement capabilities. Alternatively, benchtop analyzers can be used. Regardless of analyzer type, the ability to generate results rapidly is important to ensure that timely intervention is possible.

There may be instances that it is recommended to also monitor serial blood glucose in patients prone to abnormalities. Blood glucose should ideally be maintained between 80 and 180 mg/dL (4.4–10 mmol/L). Hypoglycemia (<80 mg/dL; <4.4 mmol/L) can be associated with neurological impairment, hypotension, seizures, and arrest. Some healthy patients, such as neonates and fasted

Table 4.4 Methods of estimation of acid–base compensation in response to primary metabolic disturbances.

		Primary change	Compensatory change
Metabolic acidosis		Each 1 mEq/L *decrease* in HCO_3^-	pCO_2 *decreases* by 0.7 ± 0.3 mmHg
Metabolic alkalosis		Each 1 mEq/L *increase* in HCO_3^-	pCO_2 *increases* by 0.7 ± 0.2 mmHg
Respiratory acidosis	*Acute*	Each 1 mmHg *increase* in pCO_2	HCO_3^- *increases* by 0.15 ± 2 mEq/L
	Chronic	Each 1 mmHg *increase* in pCO_2	HCO_3^- *increases* by 0.35 ± 2 mEq/L
Respiratory alkalosis	*Acute*	Each 1 mmHg *decrease* in pCO_2	HCO_3^- *decreases* by 0.25 ± 2 mEq/L
	Chronic	Each 1 mmHg *decrease* in pCO_2	HCO_3^- *decreases* by 0.55 ± 2 mEq/L

HCO_3^-: bicarbonate ion; pCO_2: partial pressure of carbon dioxide.

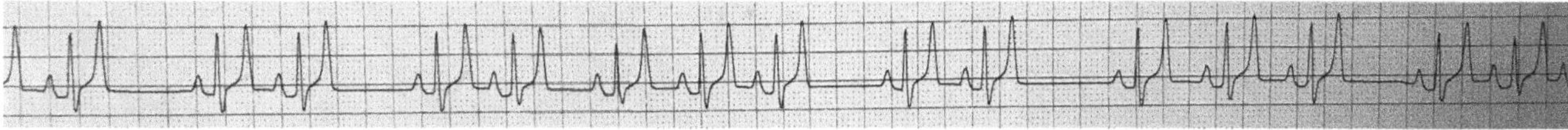

Figure 4.14 A nine-year-old, male, castrated Greyhound was anesthetized and developed hyperkalemia (K^+ = 7.98 mmol/L) during the anesthesia. The first indication of an abnormality was noted on the ECG, where T waves became tall and tented. The heart rate also began to slow.

juveniles, may need dextrose supplementation in their fluids if they become hypoglycemic. Patients with comorbid conditions, such as liver failure or insulinoma, may also become hypoglycemic and require immediate intervention. By contrast, hyperglycemia can induce diuresis and promote dehydration, as well as lead to a negative energy state (e.g., ketosis in diabetics). Depending on the level of hyperglycemia, these patients may need peri-operative management of blood glucose to maintain it close to that patient's normal range for the species. Remember that some drugs that we administer, such as alpha-2 adrenergic receptor agonists and catecholamines (e.g., norepinephrine), can induce a mild hyperglycemia. This should be considered when interpreting blood glucose concentrations in patients receiving these drugs.

Lactate is another analyte that can be measured by some blood gas analyzers or separately, with a lactate meter. Elevations of blood lactate may indicate hypoperfusion and subsequent anerobic metabolism. Hyperlactatemia is often associated with acidosis. Serial evaluations following fluid administration in hypovolemic patients can help track if tissue perfusion has improved. This is discussed in more detail elsewhere (Chapter 16).

Miscellaneous Monitoring

Body Temperature

There are numerous sites used for monitoring body temperature. Traditionally, a rectal temperature is obtained before premedication. This can be continued in most patients, unless contraindicated by the procedure. Approximate core body temperature can also be monitored during anesthesia by placing a temperature probe into the esophagus in small animals, small ruminants, pigs, and camelids. Often, a temperature probe will be placed into the nasal cavity of horses and large ruminants under anesthesia. For avian species, a cloacal probe can be placed. The goal is usually to maintain normothermia. Hypothermia is a commonly observed anesthetic complication, occurring in over 85% of dogs and cats. Adverse effects depend on the severity of hypothermia, ranging from slowed anesthetic recovery to altered enzymatic processes and protein function. Bradyarrhythmias and risk of cardiac arrest will occur with severe hypothermia (<89.6 °F; <32 °C). Shivering also increases oxygen consumption by 2–4 ×, which may necessitate oxygen supplementation in these patients. Other adverse effects, associated with hypothermia in humans, but not yet shown in animal species, include increased rates of surgical site infections, increased post-operative analgesic requirements, increased coagulopathies, and longer hospital stays.

Hyperthermia is generally less common than hypothermia during the intra- and post-anesthetic periods. However, care should be taken to not overheat patients when active warming is used during long procedures (e.g., in dentistry, when it is possible to cover a large area of the body surface with a warming device). Though rare, a sudden increase in temperature, accompanied with increased carbon dioxide production and tachycardia, may indicate malignant hyperthermia, an often fatal condition triggered by exposure to inhalational anesthetics.

There are various types of thermometers and temperature probes available, including resistance thermometers, thermistors, thermocouple devices, and infrared devices. There are numerous products of each type on the market. Other methods of obtaining body temperature have been evaluated, such as axillary or aural temperatures. However, agreement between these and rectal/esophageal temperature can be poor and exhibit user variability. Therefore, they are not recommended when accuracy is important but may be used for serial monitoring for evaluation of changes in temperature with trends over time.

Fluid Administration

It is important to closely monitor fluid administration throughout anesthesia. Fluids should be considered a medication and can have adverse effects if administered too rapidly, or if too much or too little is given. Continuous monitoring of not only both the fluid volume administered (as displayed on an electronic pump, if available) but also the volume of fluid left in the fluid bag is important (what has actually gone into the patient), as pumps can malfunction. All fluids, including analgesic and vasopressor constant rate infusions, should be included when calculating the total volume of fluids administered to minimize the risk of volume overload.

Tips on Purchasing Patient Monitoring Devices

Unfortunately, the ideal veterinary anesthetic monitoring device does not exist. Even monitors that are designed specifically for the veterinary field are often adapted from human technology. We have the unique challenge of having a less uniform patient population compared with the humans so we often have to use multiple monitoring devices in order to provide appropriate care for our patients. Decisions on purchasing monitoring equipment will depend on the patient population being treated, anticipated frequency of anesthesia/sedation, diagnostic modalities being used, and the available budget.

Determining the most easily accessible method of monitoring appropriate parameters for the relevant patient population is crucial. For example, the practitioner who predominantly anesthetizes in small exotic species will likely benefit from a combination of a mainstream capnograph, pulse oximeter, and a Doppler unit with various probes. Whereas a clinic that anesthetizes predominantly dogs and cats may benefit from a single multiparameter monitor, as it would serve the majority of their patients. An equine practitioner who practices anesthesia primarily for field castrations will be well served by physical monitoring techniques, along with a stethoscope and pulse oximeter. These simple examples underline the importance of considering the likely patient population and planned procedures in guiding the choice of anesthetic monitoring equipment to use in practice.

To conclude, peri-anesthetic monitoring is vitally important to the successful management of both sedated and anesthetized patients. There are many tools available to improve the quality of care that can be given to veterinary patients, and their use varies by type of patient and style of practice. Although monitoring equipment is very helpful, it is important to remember that physical monitoring of a patient is a core skill to ensure safety of both the patient and caregivers.

Questions and Answers

There are more practice questions and answers available for this chapter on the website. Please visit http://www.wiley.com/go/VeterinaryAnesthesiaZeiler.

Questions

1) When using a mechanical ventilator on veterinary patients, what is the most important variable to monitor serially throughout anesthesia to limit the risk of iatrogenic barotrauma to the lungs?
   a) Oxygen flowmeter
   b) Tidal volume administered
   c) Cufflator manometer
   d) Pressure manometer
2) The Doppler blood pressure is being used on a dog under general anesthesia, and the most recent value was 190 mmHg. When the anesthetic depth is checked, the eyes are ventromedial, mandibular tone is loose, and there is no change heart or respiratory rates. The blood pressure cuff is evaluated, it is proximal to the probe and the width measures approximately 20% of the limb circumference. What should be the next step to appropriately measure the blood pressure on this patient?
   a) Obtain a larger blood pressure cuff
   b) Obtain a smaller blood pressure cuff
   c) Move the cuff lower on the limb
   d) Place the cuff distal to the probe
3) You are anesthetizing a two-year-old quarter horse stallion for castration in the field. Following induction of anesthesia, you note that he has moderate cervical muscle tone, is tachypneic, and has moderate lacrimation of his eye. He shows a pulse oximeter reading of 98% with the probe on his tongue. Is he at an adequate anesthetic plan to safely begin surgery? Why or why not?
4) What configuration would the electrodes of an electrocardiograph be placed onto a small animal patient? What about an equine patient?

Answers

1) d – Iatrogenic barotrauma can occur when the peak inspiratory pressure (PIP) becomes elevated, which is measured on the pressure manometer on the anesthetic machine. Ensuring that the PIP is appropriate for the size and age of the patient being anesthetized aids in reducing complications from delivery of too much pressure into the lungs.
2) a – The blood pressure cuff is too small, giving an erroneously elevated blood pressure (overestimation of true blood pressure). Choosing a cuff whose width is 40–50% the circumference of the limb is recommended for a more accurate blood pressure reading.
3) No – The patient is exhibiting signs of being at a light anesthetic plane, with having increased muscle tone, rapid breathing, and increased ocular tearing. Especially since the surgical site is between the two pelvic limbs, administration of additional injectable anesthetics is recommended to allow for safe surgical manipulation.
4) By convention, small animal patients have electrodes placed according to Einthoven's triangle, which stipulates that the white lead is placed on the right thoracic limb, black lead on the left thoracic limb and red ground lead on the left pelvic limb. In contrast, equine electrodes are placed in a base–apex arrangement, with the red ground lead placed in the cervical region, the white lead alongside or more cranial on the neck, and the black lead on the thorax, caudal to the olecranon.

Further Reading

Balakrishnan, A. and Tong, C.W. (2020). Clinical application of pulmonary function testing in small animals. *Vet Clin North Am Small Anim Pract* 50: 273–294.

Cichocki, B., Dugat, D., and Payton, M. (2017). Agreement of axillary and auricular temperature with rectal temperature in systemically healthy dogs undergoing surgery. *J Am Anim Hosp Assoc* 53: 291–296.

Dagnall, C., Wilson, H., and Khenissi, L. (2022). An investigation into the detection of the pulse in conscious and anaesthetized dogs. *Vet Anaesth Analg* 49: 589–596.

Skelding, A. and Valverde, A. (2020a). Non-invasive blood pressure measurement in animals: part 1 – techniques for measurement and validation of non-invasive devices. *Can Vet J* 61: 368–374.

Skelding, A. and Valverde, A. (2020b). Review of non-invasive blood pressure measurement in animals: part 2 – evaluation of the performance of non-invasive devices. *Can Vet J* 61: 481–498.

5

Inhalation Anesthetic Delivery Apparatus

Eugene P. Steffey and Gareth E. Zeiler

An advantage of inhalation anesthesia is the ability to deliver known concentrations of inhalation anesthetics, oxygen (O_2), and perhaps other gases such as medical air, nitrogen (N_2), and carbon dioxide (CO_2) to patients and the ability to rapidly, precisely, and variably regulate that delivery. The *Inhalation Anesthetic Delivery Apparatus* (IADA) (Figure 5.1a, b) is used to improve safety and efficiency of anesthetic delivery and support optimal anesthetic care. Advantages and disadvantages of an IADA are provided in Table 5.1. We intend the term "IADA" to include only the basic pneumatic devices historically defined as the *anesthetic machine* and the patient breathing circuit, i.e., the anesthetic machine reliably delivers medical gases and inhaled anesthetics to the patient via a breathing circuit. The term "IADA" is in contrast to "Anesthesia Workstation," which is more commonly used in contemporary human health-care-focused textbooks to describe a substantially more costly and complex, multicomponent (including, e.g., a ventilator, monitors of multiple respiratory and anesthetic gases, and fail-safe devices), computer-controlled unit used in modern human operating rooms (Figure 5.1c). Anesthesia Workstations are not commonly used in veterinary clinics but may be found in some large multi-specialty private- or university-based veterinary hospitals. Standards have been established at both national and international levels and they are periodically upgraded to provide guidelines to manufacturers regarding minimum performance expectations, design characteristics, and safety requirements for equipment designed for inhaled anesthetic delivery. This information is of specific importance and guidance to manufacturers of machinery for anesthetic management of human patients. Manufacturing requirements for machinery directed specifically to animal patient use may or may not closely follow standards for human patient use.

The IADA is available in a variety of forms and from numerous manufacturers. Importantly, they all must have the same fundamental elements (Table 5.2) and these are shown in a schematic format in Figure 5.2. Knowledge of the fundamental elements that comprise an IADA is essential to understanding how they function for safe anesthetic management. Beyond the basic elements, optional equipment is added at the needs and discretion of the anesthetist, i.e., moving toward the concept of an Anesthetic Workstation.

Fresh Gas Sources

The gases used in anesthetic practice are commercially supplied in containers in liquified (e.g., O_2 and N_2O) or compressed gas form (e.g., O_2 and medical air). More recently, O_2 may also be obtained by on-site generation via commercially available O_2 concentrating (from ambient air) devices.

Compressed Gases in Cylinders

Compressed gases are stored in cylinders of various sizes. Typical medical grade gas cylinders are identified as B, D, E, M, G, and H (smallest to largest in size and gas volume). The E and H size cylinders are the two most common sizes used in current veterinary practice and are further characterized in Table 5.3. The E-cylinders are usually attached directly to the IADA and serve as the primary gas source in many veterinary applications. Regardless of the primary gas source, in the case of O_2, an E-cylinder should also be available for emergency backup gas supply.

Evaluating Cylinder Gas Volume

Gases that are stored in cylinders (e.g., O_2 and medical air) as a compressed gas have an important pressure to volume relationship (Figure 5.3a). As these gases escape from the cylinder, the pressure within the cylinder decreases in a

Fundamental Principles of Veterinary Anesthesia, First Edition. Edited by Gareth E. Zeiler and Daniel S. J. Pang.

Companion Website: www.wiley.com/go/VeterinaryAnesthesiaZeiler

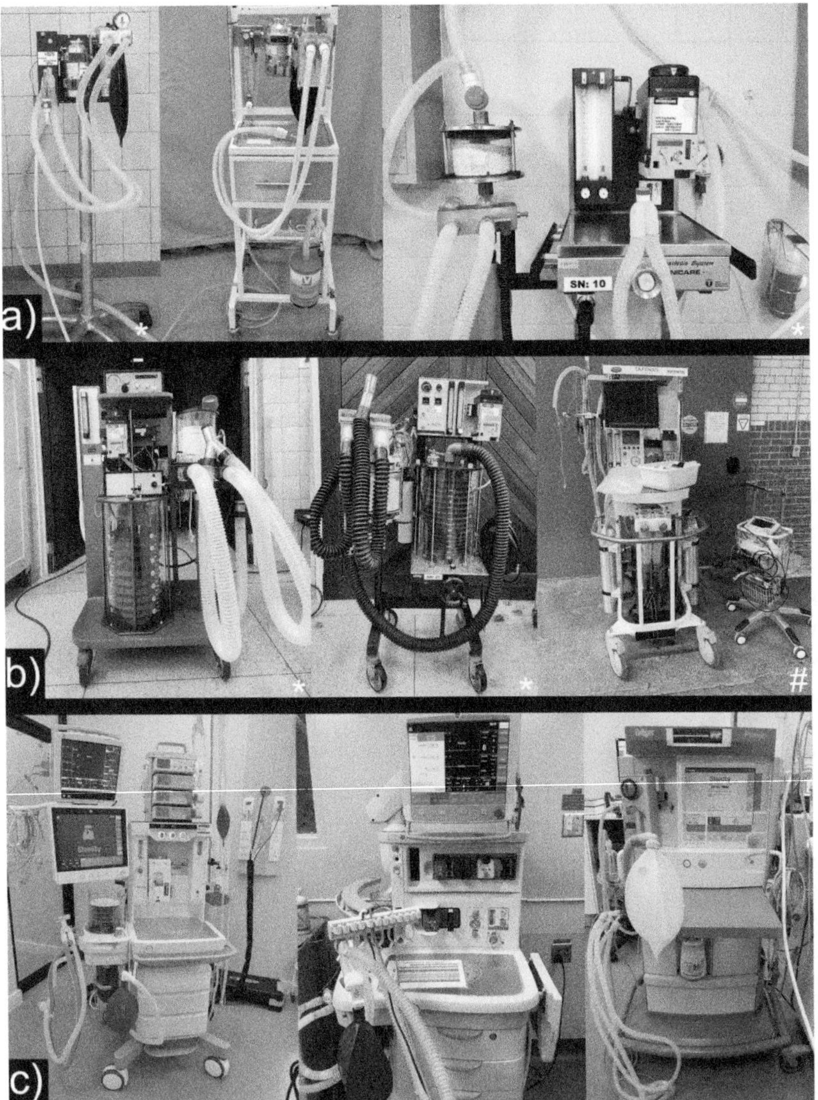

Figure 5.1 Examples of Inhalational Anesthetic Delivery Apparatuses (IADAs): all assembled with a circle circuit breathing circuit that is used in small animal (row (a)) and large animal (row (b)) anesthesia. Examples of contemporary Anesthesia Workstations are presented in row (c). (*Source:* Courtesy of *Dr Abdur Kadwa and #Dr Roxanne Buck.)

Table 5.1 Advantages and disadvantages of an Inhalation Anesthetic Delivery Device (IADA).

Advantages

- Delivers a gas mixture that may be of variable composition; the components are known and precisely regulated
- Permits easy regulation of patient inspired oxygen tension
- Facilitates the monitoring and control of patient ventilation
- Eliminates expired carbon dioxide

Disadvantages

- System complexity
- Cost

Table 5.2 The fundamental components of an Inhalational Anesthetic Delivery Apparatus (IADA).

Essential basic components

- Fresh gas source(s)
- Gas-regulating device(s)
- Breathing circuit (system)
- Vaporizer(s)
- Waste gas scavenge device
- Delivery device(s) (e.g., facemask, endotracheal tube, and/or induction chamber)

Optional components

- Ventilator
- Vigilance aids, e.g., O_2, CO_2, and/or anesthetic analyzers; pulse oximeter, respirometer, etc.

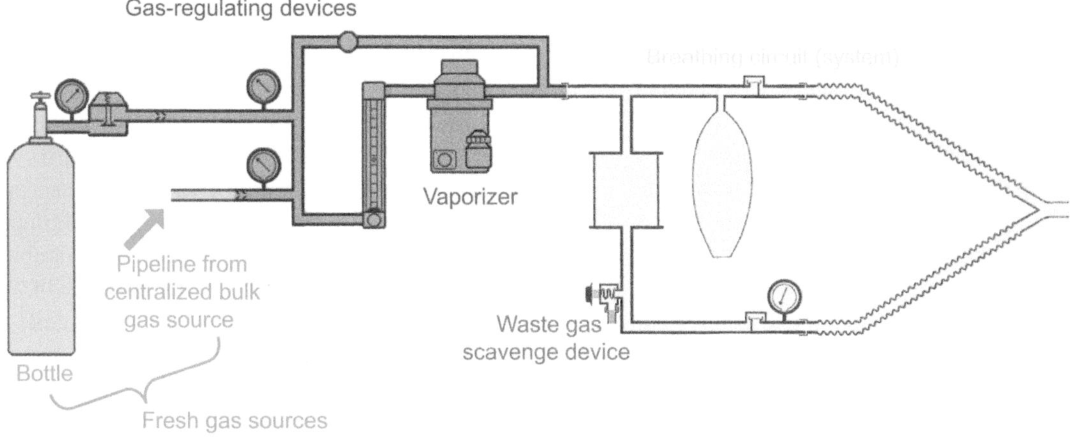

Figure 5.2 Schematic of the fundamental components of an Inhalational Anesthetic Delivery Apparatus (IADA).

Table 5.3 Characteristics of the cylinders containing compressed medical gas commonly used in veterinary anesthesia.

Cylinder size	Empty cylinder weight	Capacities and pressures (at 21 °C/70 °F)	Oxygen	Air
E	6.4 kg	Liters	400	625
	(14 lb)	kPa	13 100	13 100
		psi	1900	1900
H	54 kg	Liters	6900	6550
	(119 lb)	kPa	15 168	15 168
		psi	2200	2200

kPa: kilopascal; psi: pounds per square inch.

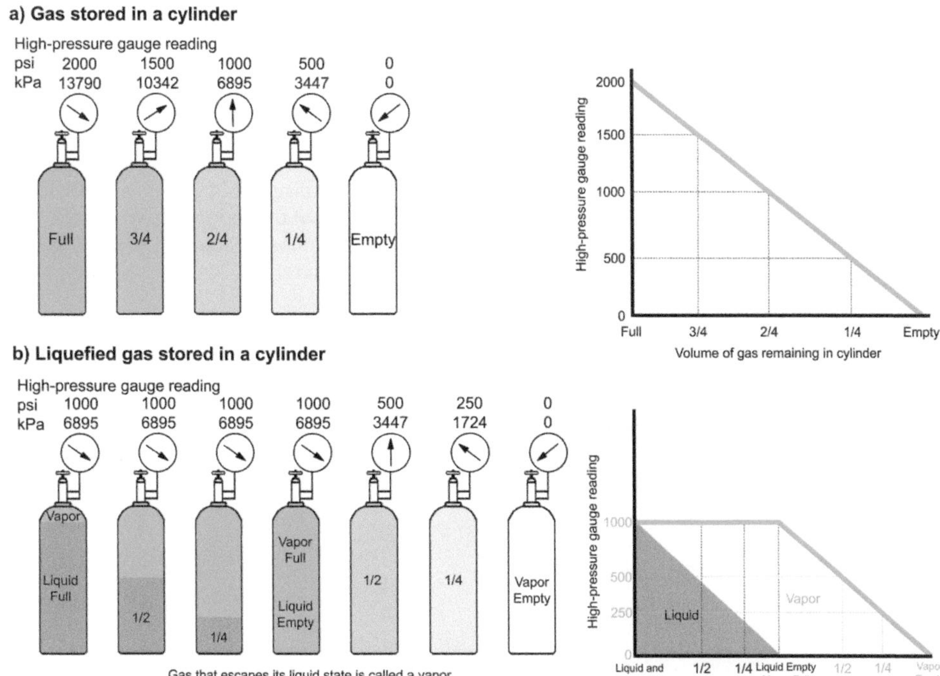

Figure 5.3 The relationship between the high-pressure gauge reading and the remaining volume of gas within a cylinder when stored as (a) a compressed gas or as (b) a liquified gas.

linear fashion (i.e., the graphical plot of the remaining gas volume versus pressure is a straight line) and thus remaining cylinder gas volume is judged by measured pressure. This relationship differs from liquefied gases, such as liquid O_2 or N_2O, that are stored in cylinders (Figure 5.3b). Nitrous oxide is used much less frequently than in the past and liquid oxygen tanks are primarily used by larger clinics and hospitals. A simplified explanation of a liquified gas (i.e., a vapor) released from the cylinder is that the gas pressure will remain relatively constant until all the liquid is vaporized. Up to this point, estimating remaining agent volume or use time is, at best, difficult and more precision would entail either weighing the cylinder and its contents or keeping an accurate record of each cylinder's time of use. Once there is no liquid remaining in the cylinder, the gas pressure within the cylinder will drop in proportion to the volume of gas escaping from the cylinder and some sense of remaining time of use is possible. This simplified explanation for liquified gases is reasonablein clinical settings under typical conditions (i.e., room temperature of about 20 °C) and anesthetic management of small companion animals. However, extreme conditions of veterinary practice, such as environmental temperatures (high and low) or high-flow-rate use of liquified gases, especially N_2O (e.g., large animal use), compromise this explanation, and readers are referred elsewhere for further information and accuracy (see Further Reading).

Physical characteristics of pressure, volume, and flow are commonly used in discussions of gas use. Within the North American medical community gas pressure is commonly discussed using units of *pounds per square inch* (psi), and elsewhere in the world *kilopascals* (kPa) or *millimeters mercury* (mmHg) are used. For safety considerations, it is important to recall the following pressure relationships to ambient or sea level pressure, i.e., 1 atmosphere at sea level = 14.7 psi = 760 mmHg = 29.92 inches Hg = 101 kPa = 1034 cmH_2O.

Centralized Bulk Gas Source

In addition to gas cylinders attached directly to the IADA, gas (especially O_2) may be supplied from large reservoirs (e.g., a collection of manifold-connected individual H-cylinders or a single very large tank type container containing liquid O_2) usually positioned remotely and some distance from patient use. The use of liquid O_2 is the common source for most human hospitals but can also be found in some larger veterinary hospitals (Figure 5.4). The gases from the centralized bulk gas source are carried within the hospital via a pipeline to standardized color-coded wall outlets (Table 5.4), and these outlets are then connected to the IADA via flexible pressure tubing with special gas-specific fittings (the Diameter Index Safety System [DISS]) that attach the wall source to the IADA. The DISS connection format is designed to prevent misconnection of pipeline gases and resultant delivery of

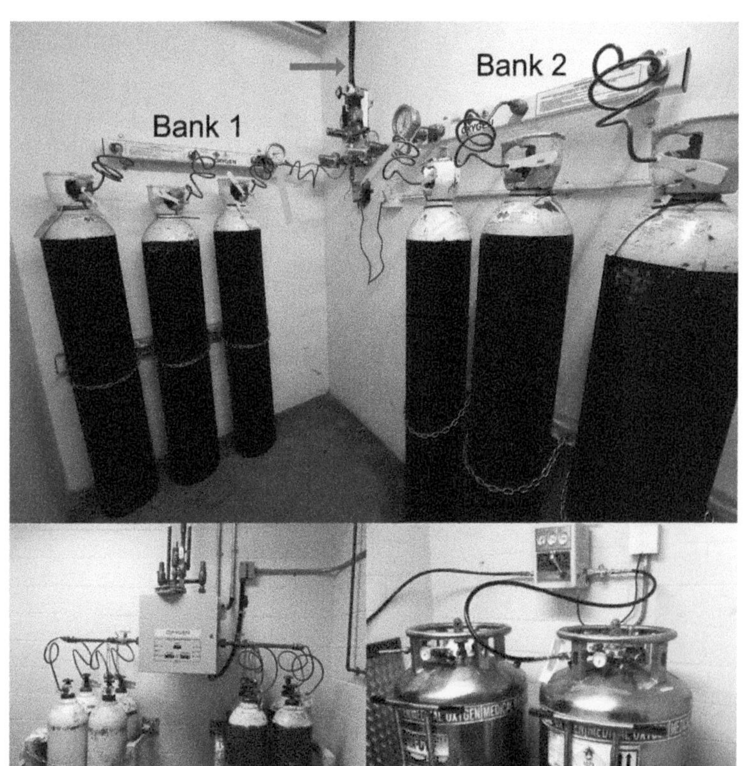

Figure 5.4 Centralized bulk gas source made up of oxygen stored in cylinders (color varies by country) as a compressed gas (top and bottom left) or liquified gas (bottom right). There are two banks with an electronic automated switch that changes the supply from an empty bank to a full bank. Each bank has their own high-pressure gauge (green arrows). The gas is distributed via a hospital-wide pipeline (blue arrow) that originates within the store room and terminates at a wall socket (not depicted in this figure).

Table 5.4 Color conventions of flexible utility hoses (gases and vacuum lines) and safety features (DISS and plugs and sockets) to ensure safe use.

Component	ISO color scheme	USA color scheme
Oxygen		
Cylinder	White	Green
Flexible hose	White	Green
Medical air		
Cylinder	Black and white	Yellow
Flexible hose	Black and white	Yellow
Vacuum		
Flexible hose	Yellow	White

Connects the IADA (via the DISS connector) to the central gas pipeline (via a plug that fit into a corresponding socket or directly to a gas cylinder)

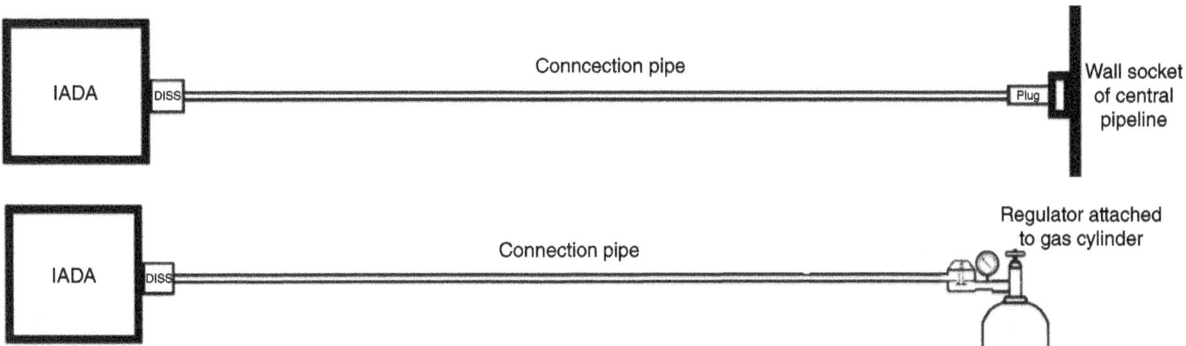

Photographs of DISS connectors on the oxygen pipe (white) and medical air pipe (black). A vernier caliper was used to measure the diameters of the connectors.

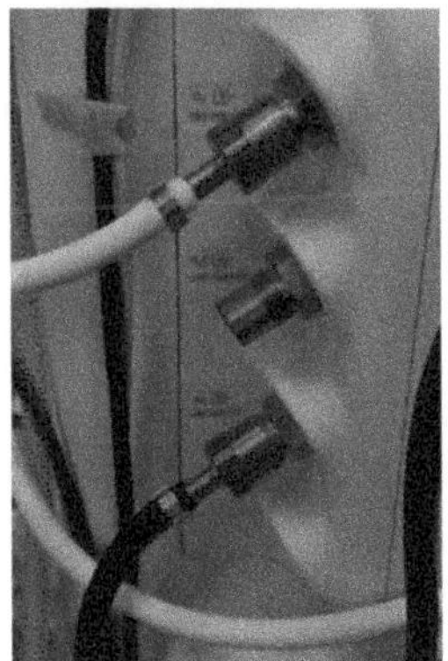 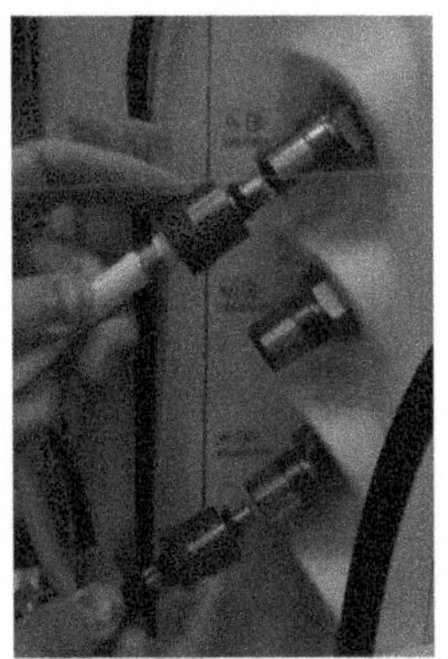 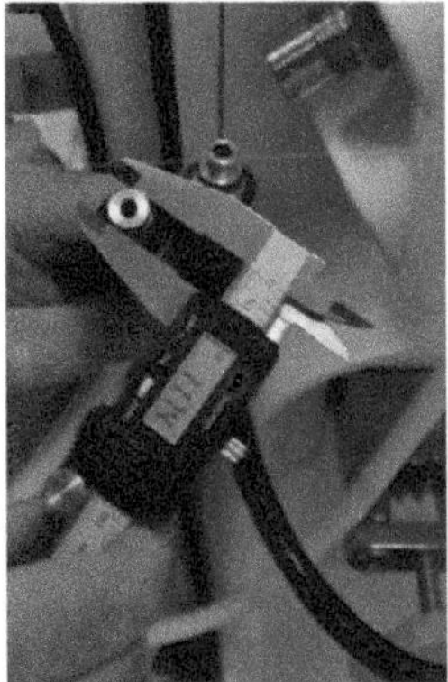 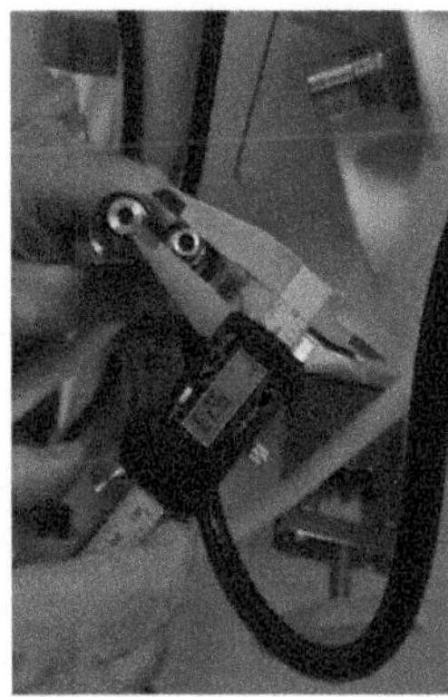

hypoxic gas mixtures to patients. The gas from the central supply is delivered to the IADA at about 50 psi (345 kPa) pressure for proper flowmeter function.

Oxygen Concentrator Source

An O_2 concentrator is a device that removes nitrogen from entrained air. The result is a gas that is 90–96% oxygen. Large-scale O_2 concentrators can be found in human hospitals; however, in veterinary hospitals, smaller portable O_2 concentrators are often used. As with a liquid O_2 source, the large-scale O_2 concentrator is usually positioned some distance from the IADA, and patient use and delivery is usually via a hospital gas pipeline system. By contrast, portable O_2 concentrators are directly connected to an IADA as the gas source (Figure 5.5). The advantage of using a portable O_2 concentrator is that the production of O_2 is continuous and limitless for its life expectancy compared to stored gas sources that need regular replacement. However, there are disadvantages that require careful consideration within context of its intended application. For example, the portable O_2 concentrator can typically only deliver a maximum gas flow of around 5 L/min at low

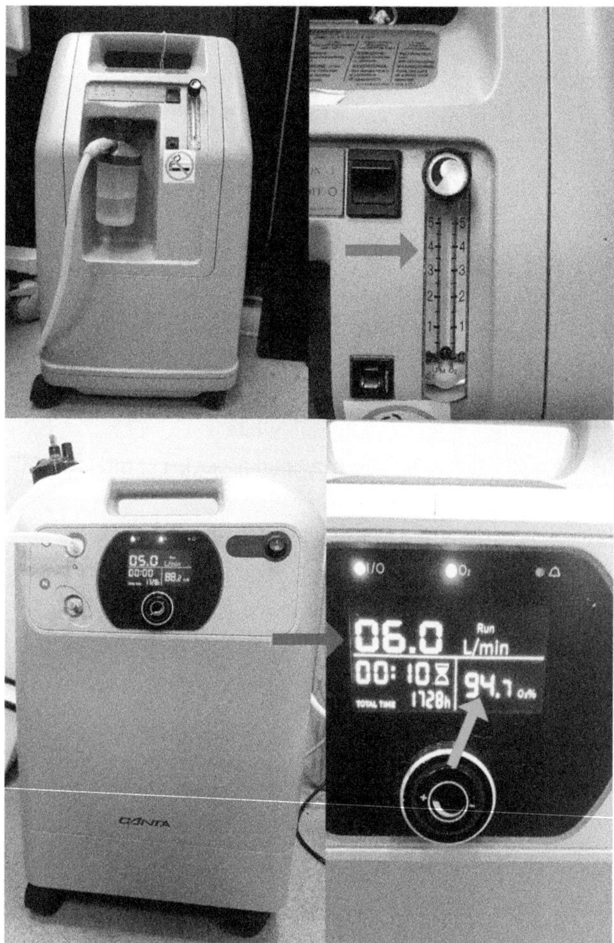

Figure 5.5 Examples of portable oxygen concentrators that are used as a gas source for an IADA. The top example uses a rotameter-type flowmeter (blue arrow; maximum flow rate is 5 L/min) to set the flow rate and the bottom example uses an electronic flowmeter (red arrow; maximum flow rate is 6 L/min). The advantage of some electronic systems is the inclusion of an oxygen sensor to detect the output percentage of oxygen (green arrow).

driving pressure (see the section on pressure reduction valve in the following text). Therefore, if large demands for O_2 are required such as activation of the O_2 flush control, then O_2 delivery performance will be poor since demand exceeds the concentrator output. In addition, because O_2 concentrators draw in air to function, it is important that they are located in areas in which air supply to the concentrator is not contaminated by atmospheric pollutants, including infectious agents.

With O_2 concentrator use, routine monitoring of O_2 concentration to, or within, the breathing circuit is recommended and there needs to be an O_2 reservoir supply available should there be a mechanical or electrical malfunction of the concentrator. Finally, regular servicing of the concentrator, by a certified technician, supports safe anesthetic practice.

Gas Delivery and Regulation Devices

The gas circuitry of the IADA is discussed based on the gas pressure as gas progresses downstream from its source (specifically O_2 stored as a compressed gas) to the patient breathing circuit; the parts considered are the high-, intermediate-, and low-pressure components (Figure 5.6).

The High-pressure System

The high-pressure system is that part of the IADA that is exposed to gas at pressures greater than 50 psi (345 kPa). The pressure within the gas cylinders is, of course, the location of the highest pressure associated with the IADA and depends upon the gas and its volume contained within the cylinder. While contemporary small animal practice increasingly relies on O_2 delivered from a centralized bulk gas source through pipelines, the IADA is usually equipped with gas cylinder attachments. Directly attached cylinders provide flexibility for location of IADA use, and in the case of O_2 provide patient safety should delivery from a central source fail for any reason.

Yoke and Other Bottle Attachments

Gas cylinders (e.g., E-cylinders) are safely attached to the IADA with yokes, each equipped with a *pin indexing system* (Figure 5.7a). The yoke provides a tight seal and includes a check valve to ensure unidirectional downstream flow of gas into the components of the IADA. Check valves also prevent reverse flow from the IADA as might occur during replacement of a cylinder during anesthetic management. Check valves are also integral to hose attachments when gases are supplied from a centralized bulk gas source, as discussed in the preceding text.

The pin indexing system is characterized by two pins that are positioned within the gas-specific yoke that is arranged so that they project into the valve assembly of a gas cylinder. Each gas has a specific arrangement of pins on the yoke and pin holes on the valve assembly of the cylinder (Figure 5.7b). The pin indexing system is designed to prevent a gas cylinder different from that intended being attached to the yoke (e.g., placement of an N_2O cylinder on a yoke intended for O_2). Each yoke or group of interconnected yokes supplying a specific gas must be provided with a high-pressure gauge.

In some countries, a single large (i.e., H-cylinders) oxygen cylinder is attached to an IADA via an oxygen-gas-specific regulator (see the following text). These regulators are attached by a bullnose or a pin index system connector. These regulators are fitted with a reduction valve and high-pressure gauge (Figure 5.7c).

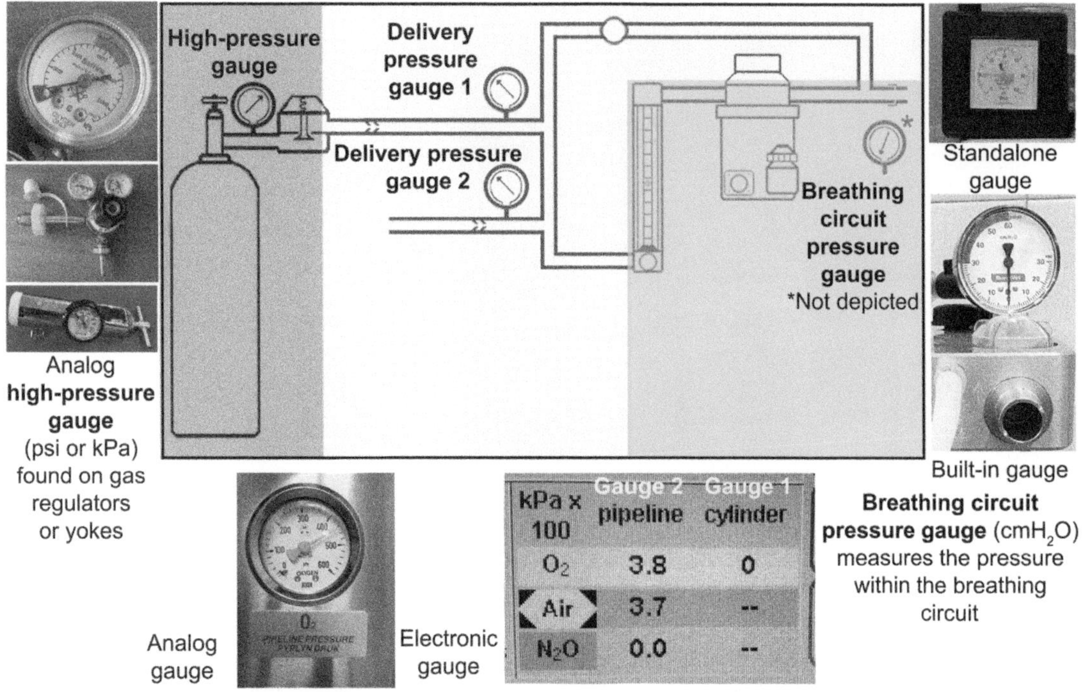

The **delivery pressure gauges** (psi or kPa) are usually built into an IADA and its purpose is to measure the pressure that gas is supplied to the machine. This allows the anesthetist to ensure the supplied pressure is within a safe "working pressure." This is the intermediate pressure system of the IADA

Figure 5.6 The gas circuitry of an IADA can be separated into high-pressure (red), intermediate-pressure (yellow), and low-pressure (green) regions. Appreciating the different pressure regions ensures safe use.

High-pressure Gauge

There must be a gauge for each different gas type that is attached to the IADA. Accordingly, there will always be one for O_2, but many repurposed human patient IADAs found in veterinary practice often come with gauges for N_2O and medical air on their independent yokes. The purpose of the high-pressure gauge is to indicate cylinder gas volume, as previously noted.

Pressure-reducing Valve

The pressure-reducing valve or gas regulator is the terminal portion of the high-pressure system of the IADA. The pressure-reducing valve serves two functions: (1) it decreases the gas pressure from the cylinder pressure to a lower intermediate pressure and (2) it converts the upstream cylinder pressure (drive pressure) from a variable pressure to a downstream pressure that remains constant at the intermediate pressure. This intermediate pressure is the standard "working" pressure for medical gas apparatus and is about three times atmospheric pressure at sea level. For example, the pressure-reducing valve decreases O_2 pressure of a full E-cylinder from approximately 2000 psi (13 790 kPa or 137 times ambient sea level pressure) to a constant working pressure of about 50 psi (345 kPa). This action facilitates a constant downstream gas flow despite a time-variable upstream gas pressure at its source. One regulator is required for each gas source available to the IADA.

The Intermediate-Pressure System

The components of the IADA that receive gases at the intermediate pressure are the oxygen flush control and the gas flowmeters.

Oxygen Flush Control

The O_2 flush control (or O_2 bypass) is usually a button that, when pressed, causes O_2 to flow from the O_2 source (e.g., downstream from the cylinder regulator) bypassing the flowmeter assembly and any "out-of-circuit" (explained in the following text) vaporizers. The O_2 then enters the common gas outlet, at high, unmetered flow rates (35–75 L/min), for direct delivery to the patient breathing circuit.

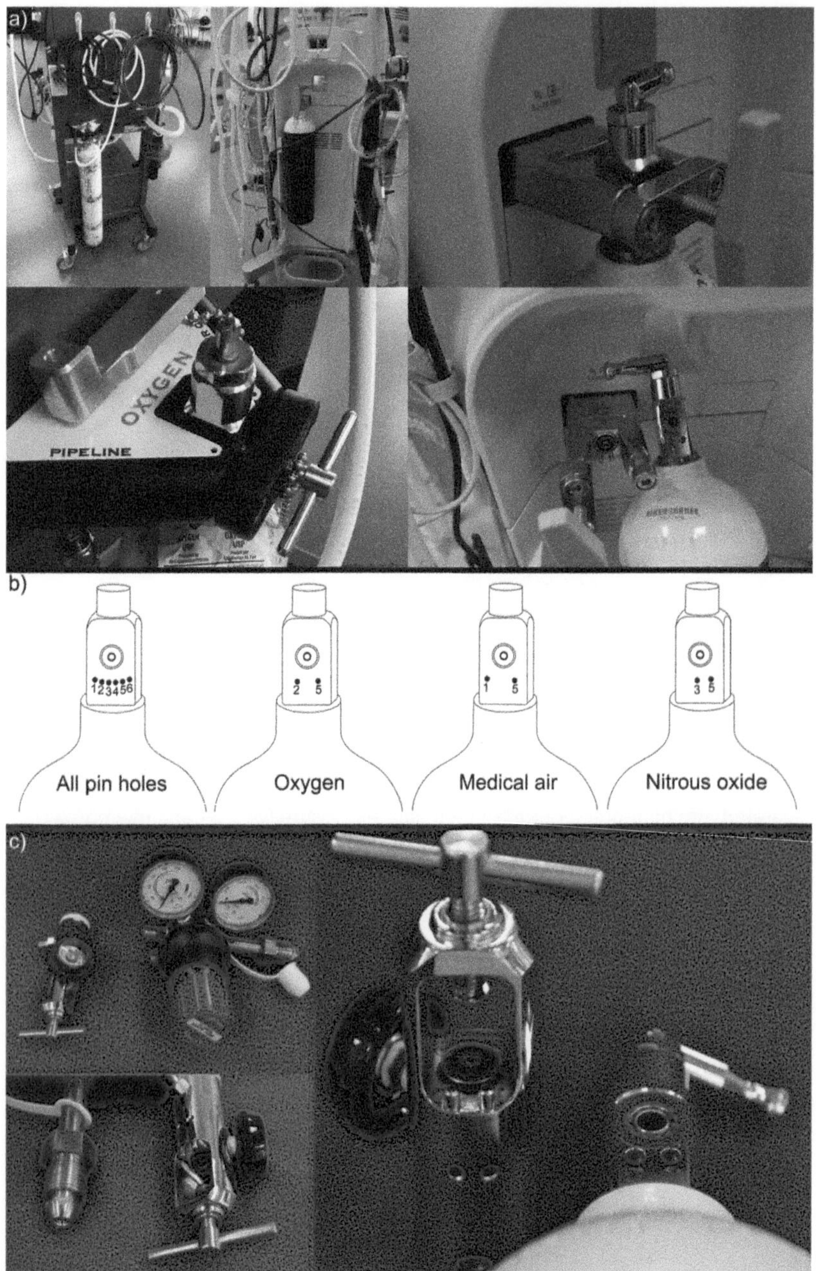

Figure 5.7 An oxygen bottle attached to an IADA by a yoke attachment (a) with close-ups of an attached and then unattached oxygen bottle to demonstrate the pin index system. The pin index system uses two pins on a yoke or gas regulator that fits into corresponding holes on the bottle attachment and (b) is a schematic representation of the holes and their position for the gases described in the text. Bottles storing compressed gas can be attached to the IADA by gas-specific regulators with either a bullnose (screw-like attachment) or a pin index system (c).

Care should be taken if using the oxygen flush while a patient is connected to the breathing circuit, with the following considerations:

- High rate of oxygen flow can result in pressure increase in the breathing circuit particularly in circuits with low volumes such as those used in smaller patients. As pressure builds in the circuit it will eventually also increase in the patient's lungs, with a risk of trauma to the airway and lungs.
- The oxygen flush bypasses the vaporizer so that any inhalational anesthetic will be diluted. This can be problematic or beneficial depending on the intent of using the oxygen flush.

The Low-pressure System

For simplicity, the low-pressure system is that portion of the IADA downstream of the flowmeter which includes the patient breathing circuit. Recognize that the flowmeter assembly accounts for most of the substantial drop in gas pressure after the pressure-reducing valve and that the gas pressure downstream of the flowmeters is closer to, but still slightly above, ambient pressure.

Flowmeter

Flowmeters (Figure 5.8) precisely measure and maintain the constant pre-set flow of gas passing through them and onto downstream IADA components. Flowmeters are calibrated for a specific gas under usual ambient conditions, generally considered 20 °C (68 °F; a common operating room temperature), at sea level pressure, and with an upstream gas driving pressure of about 50 psi

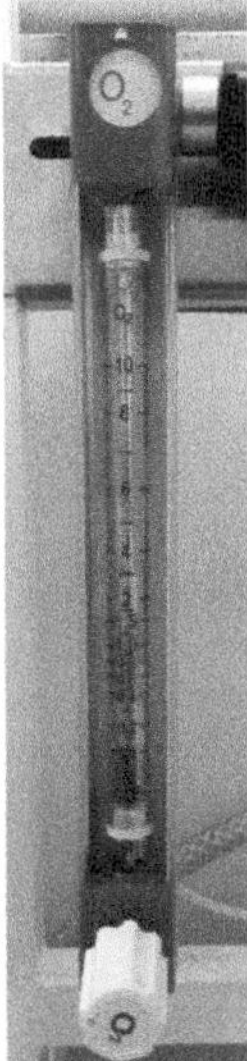

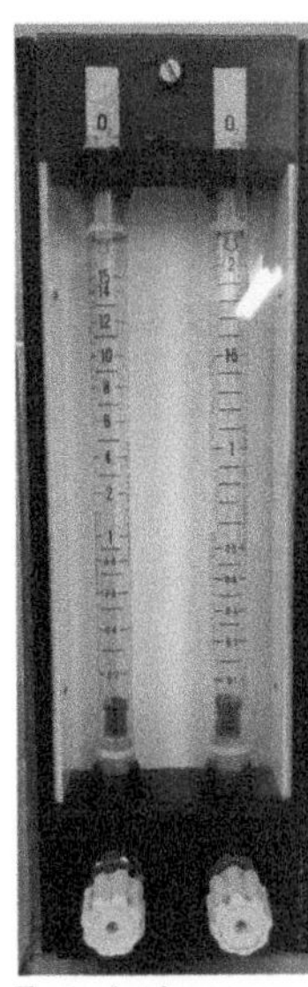

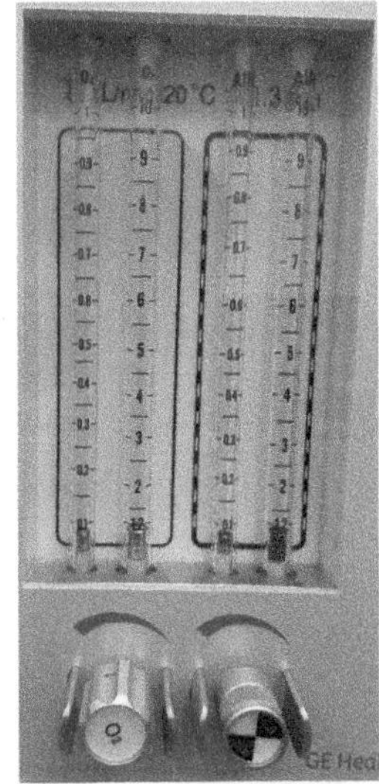

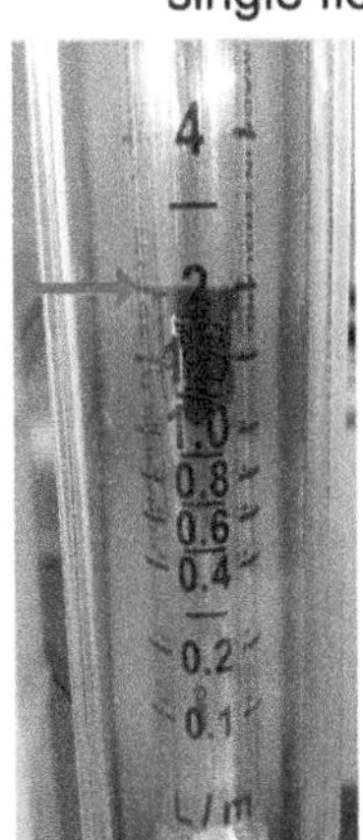

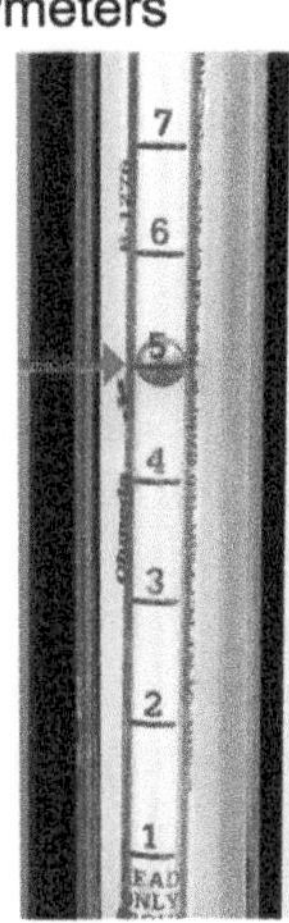

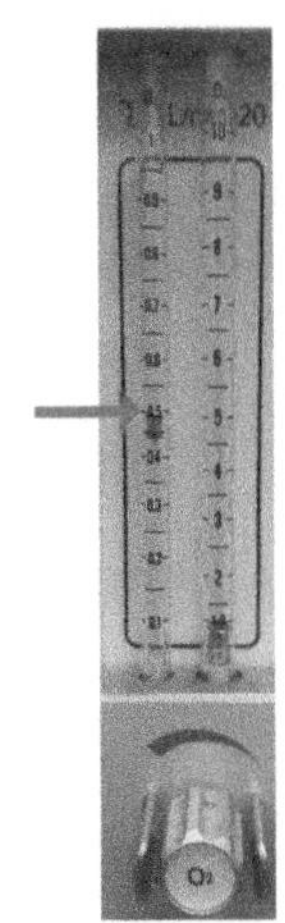

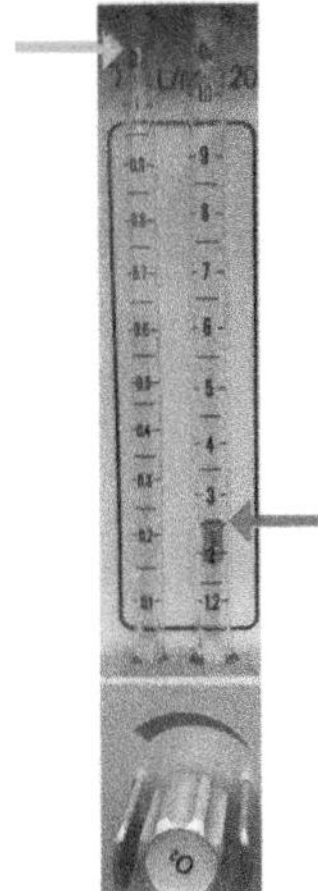

Figure 5.8 Various types of flowmeter assemblies (a) and how to read the rotameter (bobbin or ball) flow rate (b). The blue arrows indicate where to read the flow rate and the green arrow indicates the highest position of the rotameter in the first tube of a cascade assembly.

(345 kPa). Large changes in temperature and pressure from usual operating room conditions will affect both gas density and viscosity and thereby influence the accuracy of the measured gas flow rate. While small changes in these conditions may vary with little clinical consequence, the extremes of veterinary practice settings (e.g., altitude and climatic conditions) may require additional consideration for safe clinical practice, especially in circumstances where two or more gases are used simultaneously and/or at low gas flow rates.

Flowmeters are individually calibrated to read in mL/min or L/min, or both. Safety standards dictate that the scale should be marked on the tube or alongside the tube. Clinical practice dictates which style is appropriate. For example, to use a style calibrated in only L/min for a "low flow rate" in a patient <5 kg or a style calibrated only in mL/min for the "high flow rate" required for a larger animal, such as a horse, is not desirable and most importantly may not be safe clinical practice.

There are different styles or types of flow indicators, e.g., bobbin and ball float. Gas flow rate readings are usually taken from the upper rim (edge) of the bobbin style and from the midpoint of the sphere with the ball style. Flowmeters for different gases are usually grouped together, side by side on a common manifold assembly. Sometimes there are two flowmeters for the same gas. One example of this is when one of the flowmeters is calibrated in mL/min and the other is calibrated in L/min. Another example is the addition of a second flowmeter calibrated for O_2 delivery to a special type of anesthetic vaporizer (e.g., a measured-flow or copper kettle style; neither of these is in common use).

Common Gas Outlet

The common gas outlet (sometimes identified as the fresh gas outlet) receives the gas mixture (O_2 and all other gases, such as medical air and anesthetic vapor from the vaporizer) and delivers them to the patient breathing circuit.

Accessory, Safety, and Other Optional Components

Accessory, safety, or other optional components (before the patient breathing circuit) may also be included. Examples of such are highlighted in the following text.

Pipeline Supply and Machine Gas Inlet

In hospital settings with a central gas storage/supply facility, this is the primary gas source for O_2 and perhaps medical air. The gas from the pipeline supply source arrives at the IADA gas inlet at a pressure of about 50 psi (345 kPa). The pipeline supply pressure is reduced (to the intermediate pressure) upstream at its source (as liquid O_2 or from a bank of H-cylinders) to a pressure that accounts for plumbing and distance from the central gas source to the IADA intake (see Figure 5.6). Accordingly, this O_2 source enters the IADA separate from O_2 delivered from a cylinder attached directly to the IADA.

O_2 Supply Pressure Failure Alerting Devices

These are devices intended to minimize the possibility of delivering hypoxic gas mixtures to the patient. They include pneumatic and electronic alarms and "fail-safe" systems. Pneumatic and electronic alarms activate at an O_2 supply pressure less than about 30 psi (206 kPa). Fail-safe systems are usually associated with all of the gases of an IADA *except* O_2. This type of system is activated to shut off or proportionally decrease the supply of gases other than O_2 (e.g., N_2O) when the O_2 pressure is decreased.

Ventilator Power Outlet

This is a connection on the IADA to supply O_2 to power a ventilator, thus only one O_2 source pressure reduction assembly is necessary.

Breathing Circuits (Systems)

The breathing circuit is a gas pathway that interfaces between the source of the inspired gas and the patient. In most cases, the circuit receives anesthetic, O_2, and, when desired, other gases from the common gas outlet of the IADA (see the preceding text) and delivers a tidal flow of gas of appropriately managed composition, volume and pressure to a mask or endotracheal tube fitted to the patient.

Breathing Circuit Function

The functions of the patient breathing circuit are to (1) deliver a controlled composition of O_2 and anesthetic to the patient, (2) eliminate patient expired CO_2, and (3) provide a means to monitor and assist (or control, as necessary) the patient's ventilation. The circuit should not add to the patient's breathing effort or in other ways jeopardize the health or welfare of the patient.

A suitably functioning patient breathing circuit has the several following favorable characteristics.

Minimal Rebreathing

Rebreathing means to inhale some amount of alveolar gas that had previously been expired. The metabolically produced CO_2 contained in just expired (alveolar) gas may or may not have been removed. In the context of respiratory physiology and anesthesiology discussions, *rebreathing* *usually implies an accumulation of CO_2* with a resultant increase in the arterial partial pressure of carbon dioxide (P_aCO_2), i.e., inspired gas contains previously expired alveolar gas high in CO_2 and lower in O_2 than fresh gas, with resultant increase in P_aCO_2 and potential for hypoxemia. However, with properly selected and applied anesthetic equipment, it is possible to have partial or total rebreathing without CO_2 buildup in arterial blood (e.g., a circle breathing circuit [see the following text]). The amount of rebreathing depends on the design of the breathing circuit and the amount of fresh gas inflowing (i.e., fresh gas flow rate) into the circuit from the common gas delivery outlet.

Designs of breathing circuits include those intended to permit rebreathing of expired gas and those in which rebreathing of expired gas should not normally occur. Further characterization of these two basic types of circuits appears later in this chapter. Designs influence the amount of added *mechanical dead space*. Recall from knowledge of respiratory physiology that respiratory dead space is space within the respiratory system (physiologic dead space made up of anatomic and alveolar dead space; see Chapter 18) that is occupied by gas that is rebreathed, without undergoing alveolar gas exchange and thus there is no change in composition. In this case, once again the implication is an associated increase in P_aCO_2. Mechanical dead space potentially contributes to existing patient physiologic dead space, complicating anesthetic care.

The amount of fresh gas flowing into the circuit is an important modifier of mechanical dead space. In general, the higher the fresh gas inflow to the circuit, the effect of the mechanical dead space volume is reduced (the lower limit being zero additional dead space).

Minimal Equipment or Mechanical Resistance to Breathing

The authors consider a simple review of the physics of resistance helpful at this point. Recall that resistance (R) is equal to a change in pressure relative to a change in flow. Pressure difference ($\Delta P = P1 - P2$) is usually expressed in cmH_2O or mmHg and, in this case, respiratory gas flow (abbreviated as $\dot{V}$) is expressed as units of volume (mL or L) per unit of time (s or min). Rearranging the equation gives $\dot{V} = \Delta P/R$. According to Poiseuille's equation for resistance to laminar flow in straight tubes: $R = 8\eta l/\pi r^4$, where η is the gas viscosity, l is the tube length, and r is the tube radius. Consequently, other things considered equal, an excessively long tube, e.g., an inappropriately long endotracheal tube, increases resistance to gas flow, and a small breathing tube (i.e., small radius of opening relative to tracheal diameter) markedly increases resistance to breathing (by a factor of the fourth power). Therefore, added resistance to breathing by equipment decreases gas flow (inspired, expired, or both). A decrease in gas flow results in a decrease in tidal breath volume or an increase in the duration of a breath or both. Consequently, the healthy, spontaneously breathing patient usually attempts to compensate for this condition by increasing its work of breathing to establish a greater pressure difference to maintain adequate alveolar ventilation, arterial partial pressure of oxygen (P_aO_2), and P_aCO_2. Increased resistance to breathing is usually not desired. However, in some patients with respiratory system disease, added respiratory resistance is carefully used as a component of therapy.

Minimal Respiratory System Loss of Patient Heat and Water

This third desired characteristic of a breathing circuit is especially important in smaller animals (<5 kg).

Breathing Circuit Classification

Anesthesia breathing circuits have been historically classified in numerous ways with no single classification having universal agreement. The classification in the following text is used with the intent of trying to simplify, as much as possible, the description and categories of anesthetic equipment used in veterinary medicine. For a detailed review, see Further Reading. Two major classifications are emphasized here: *nonrebreathing* and *rebreathing* circuits. The intention when using a nonrebreathing circuit is that there is no rebreathing of exhaled gas. By contrast, with a rebreathing circuit there is partial or total rebreathing of exhaled gas.

Nonrebreathing Circuits

Nonrebreathing circuits may be further classified into open and semi-open styles. Their general characteristics include simple construction, inexpensive to purchase, provide for no chemical absorption of CO_2, but instead rely on a high fresh gas inflow to the circuit for CO_2 removal, and contribute no or minimal added resistance and mechanical dead space to the patient's breathing.

Open Style

With the open style of circuit, anesthetic gases and O_2 are directly supplied to the patient's nose or deeper airways and are mixed to varying degrees with atmospheric air. Exhaled gases flow into the surrounding atmosphere. This style is the simplest of all methods of inhalation anesthetic and O_2 delivery. There is no airway isolation (e.g., endotracheal tube), equipment valves, or gas reservoirs. There is also no direct ability to assist or control the patient's ventilation. Examples are the open drop or "ether mask," "insufflation," and an induction box. With open drop, in its simplest form a porous mask is applied over the mouth and/or nose. The patient breathes air through the mask and volatile anesthetic is "dripped" onto the mask; the anesthetic vapors then join the air on inspiration (i.e., anesthetic is brought to the lungs and diluted only with atmospheric air). With insufflation, anesthetic gases and O_2 are directly delivered to the patient's airway via, for example, a hose connection to the common gas delivery outlet of the IADA. Examples of this form of delivery are "nasal pongs" or "facemask" (see Chapter 14) or a hose delivering O_2 to the horse's endotracheal tube during recovery from anesthesia. The more common example of the open style is the "induction box." In this case, the animal is placed within box with ambient air and a cotton ball or piece of absorbent cloth moistened with volatile anesthetic liquid. Anesthesia is induced as the animal breathes the anesthetic infused air. Alternatively, anesthetic gases and O_2 are delivered with greater control and precision directly to the box from the IADA's common gas delivery hose.

Semi-open Style

With this style of nonrebreathing circuit, the inspired gas comes from a circuit that includes tubes and connecting parts. The circuit may also include a reservoir bag and unidirectional valve(s). Exhaled gases flow into the atmosphere and into the inspiratory limb of the apparatus. There is no chemical removal of exhaled CO_2. The amount of rebreathing of exhaled gas is directly dependent upon the fresh gas inflow rate to the circuit. Equipment components of this style include breathing tubes, a reservoir bag, and associated connectors.

The purpose of the breathing tubes is to conduct gases to and from the patient and connect circuit components. They also serve as a gas reservoir, either completely, when a reservoir bag is absent, or in part when a reservoir bag is present. The tubes need to be of large bore, i.e., at least as large in diameter as the patient's trachea and nonrigid. They are usually made of corrugated rubber or plastic. The corrugation adds flexibility without adding to collapsibility and gas flow obstruction.

Connectors are usually made of metal or rigid plastic. They serve to extend and/or connect components. If not carefully considered, connectors may add to undesirable equipment-added breathing resistance (lumen diameter too small) or mechanical dead space (volume of lumen too large).

The reservoir bag is also known as the "breathing bag" or simply as "the bag." It serves as a reservoir of gas for inspiration and provides a means to assist or control the patient's ventilation. Tactile or visual observation also provides a subjective measure of breath (tidal) volume and breathing rate. Finally, it also serves to buffer breathing circuit pressure fluctuations. The size of the bag depends on the patient's tidal volume and personal preference, although it ordinarily should be at least 1.5 times the patient's usual awake tidal breath volume. A useful rule of thumb in smaller patients (dogs and cats) is a bag size of 1 L per 10 kg of body mass (e.g., 27 kg dog = 3 L bag). Excessive bag volume serves to confound the rate of change of delivered anesthetic concentration. The pressure–volume characteristics of the bag are important in that adding volume to the bag should cause virtually no increase in gas pressure until the limits of the bag's volume are reached. At this point, gas pressure within the bag increases steeply (Figure 5.9). This is important because it represents the pressure developed within the entire breathing circuit and is potentially transmissible to the patient's airway and lungs.

Many types of semi-open circuits have been historically available. They are classified according to a system described by Mapleson (see Further Reading and Figure 5.10). There were five basic types originally described, Types A through E. A sixth type (F) was added later. Each type has its advantages and disadvantages. The Mapleson Type A circuit is often referred to as the "Magill circuit." The Bain circuit (described in detail in the following text) is a more recent addition. As shown in Figure 5.10, the Mapleson classification arranges breathing circuits according to their differing configurations. These differences influence performance and use. Some, but not all, of these circuits include one-way valves to facilitate reduced fresh gas inflow rates and economy of use. For purposes of this introductory text, the focus of this chapter is on two of the Mapleson types, and both of these circuits are without valves. These are the most commonly, if not exclusively, used styles in veterinary medicine in most parts of the world. They are (1) the *Mapleson Type F*, commonly referred to as the "Jackson-Rees Modification of the Ayre's T-piece" (simplified to "Modified T-piece") and (2) the *Mapleson Type D*, its coaxial version is known as the "Bain circuit." Both circuits are most often used with small animals up to about 5–10 kg in size. Their advantages include minimal contributions to mechanical dead space and breathing resistance, and they are relatively inexpensive to purchase. Disadvantages include a requirement for high fresh gas flows that are wasteful of inhalational anesthetic and O_2, and contribute to environmental pollution. In addition, if the gas escape vent is obstructed, the high gas flow rapidly increases airway pressure with potential for respiratory system trauma. These circuits also lack humidification of inspired air and contribute to reduction in the animal's core body temperature since warm expired gas is not rebreathed.

The *Modified T-piece* circuit is composed of fresh gas in-port and endotracheal tube connection, corrugated tubing, and a breathing bag with a mechanism for venting excess gases

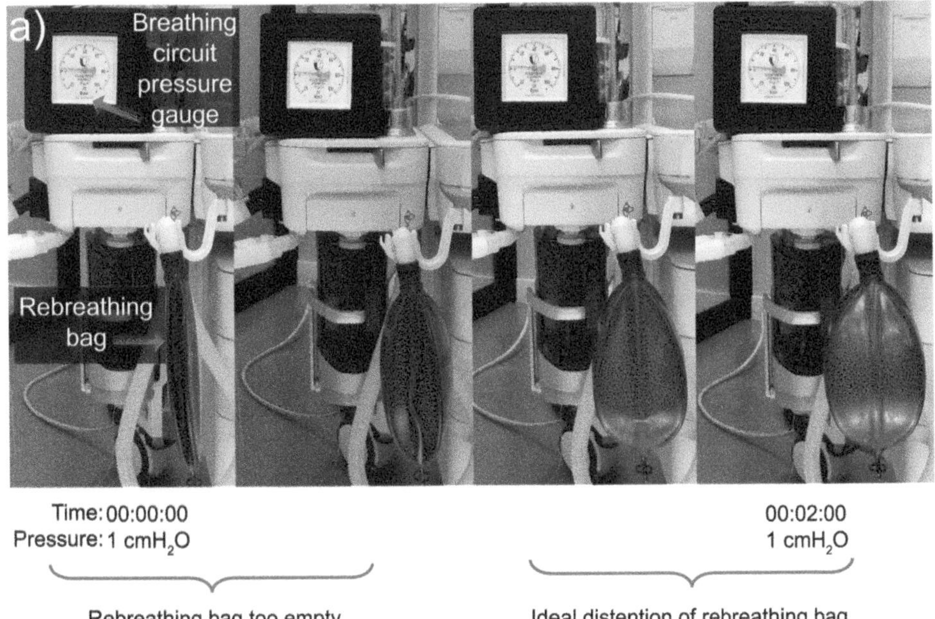

b)

00:02:05
3 cmH$_2$O

00:02:30
76 cmH$_2$O

Limit of the bag's volume is reached and gas pressure within the bag (and entire breathing circuit) increases rapidly. Causes, such as a closed pop-off valve, require immediately investigated to prevent injury to the respiratory system.

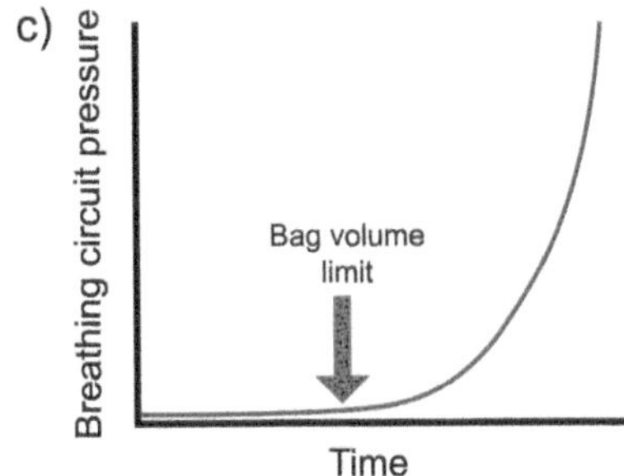

Figure 5.9 Serial photographs demonstrating the rebreathing (or reservoir) bag pressure–volume relationship. The principles apply to all types of breathing circuits. In this example, the bag is part of a circle circuit and the pop-off valve has been screwed closed to demonstrate how quickly pressure can develop within the bag. The fresh gas flow rate is set to 2 L/min and the bag volume is 2 L. The bag is increasing in volume (a), but there is no increase in breathing circuit pressure until the volume limit has been reached (b). Once the volume limit is reached and gases cannot be vented via the pop-off valve, for example, the pressure within the breathing circuit rises rapidly (c).

(Figure 5.11). Excess gas venting is commonly accomplished by a hole on the side of the rebreathing bag or at the end of the bag's tail. A waste gas scavenging device should be fitted to the hole. Mechanical ventilation may be used with the bag in position, or the bag removed, and the T-piece connected to a ventilator. This breathing circuit is commonly used in exotic companion mammals and birds, see Chapter 14.

Before summarizing the functioning of this circuit recall there are usually three phases of gas flow during a normal spontaneous breathing cycle. These are inspiration, expiration, and the expiratory pause (with no bulk gas flow in the respiratory tree before the next inspiration). During exhalation, gas exhaled from the patient moves into the breathing circuit (along with fresh gas from the IADA common delivery hose) toward and into the rebreathing bag. Overflow gas exits the bag via the bag hole. During the expiratory pause, fresh gas flow continues (remember a constant gas flow rate has been set via the flowmeter assembly). This fresh gas displaces the exhaled gas down the tubing. During the next inspiration, inspired gas comes from gas contained in the corrugated tubing plus that coming from the common fresh gas delivery (i.e., continuous inflow of fresh gas). Rebreathing of exhaled gas (with, of course, CO_2) can occur if the fresh gas inflow rate is too low to sufficiently "wash out" the previous breath from the corrugated tubing. Therefore, the amount of CO_2 rebreathed is related to the fresh gas inflow rate. Our usual guideline for fresh gas inflow to prevent rebreathing is 200 mL/kg/min. This guideline is based on a requirement of 2–3 times minute ventilation to prevent rebreathing under normal circumstances (normal tidal volume and respiratory rate). Because the high fresh gas flow required is wasteful, the usefulness of these circuits is limited as patient body size increases.

The Mapleson Type D is very similar in construction to the Modified T-piece, with the exception of having a complete reservoir bag and a unidirectional expiratory valve that vents excess gases into the waste gas management (scavenging) system. Our usual guideline for fresh gas inflow to prevent rebreathing is 150–200 mL/kg/min. The *Bain circuit* is a coaxial modification of the Mapleson Type D circuit (Figure 5.12). The modification is that the fresh gas supply tube runs inside the corrugated tubing in a coaxial fashion, hence an alternative name of this circuit is "Bain Coaxial Circuit." If lower fresh gas inflow rates are used, the inspired concentration of CO_2 needs to be monitored to verify that no rebreathing is occurring. This circuit

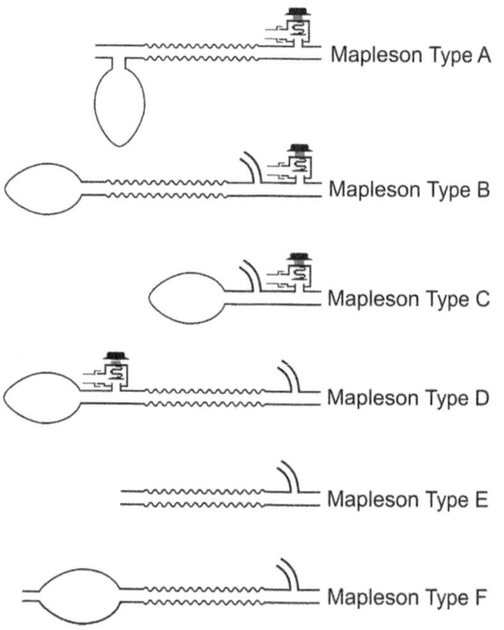

Figure 5.10 Schematic drawings of the Mapleson classification of nonrebreathing circuits. (*Source:* Redrawn from Mapleson (1954)).

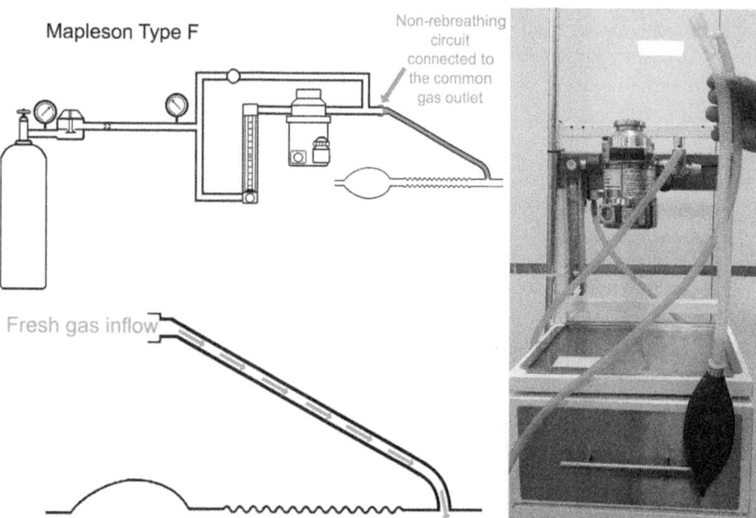

Figure 5.11 Mapleson Type F nonrebreathing circuit. All breathing circuits connect to the common gas outlet of the IADA, as indicated in the schematic drawings (blue arrow). This nonrebreathing circuit relies on a continuous delivery of fresh gas inflow (green arrows) to vent the exhaled carbon dioxide; please consult the text for a description of gas flow within this nonrebreathing circuit.

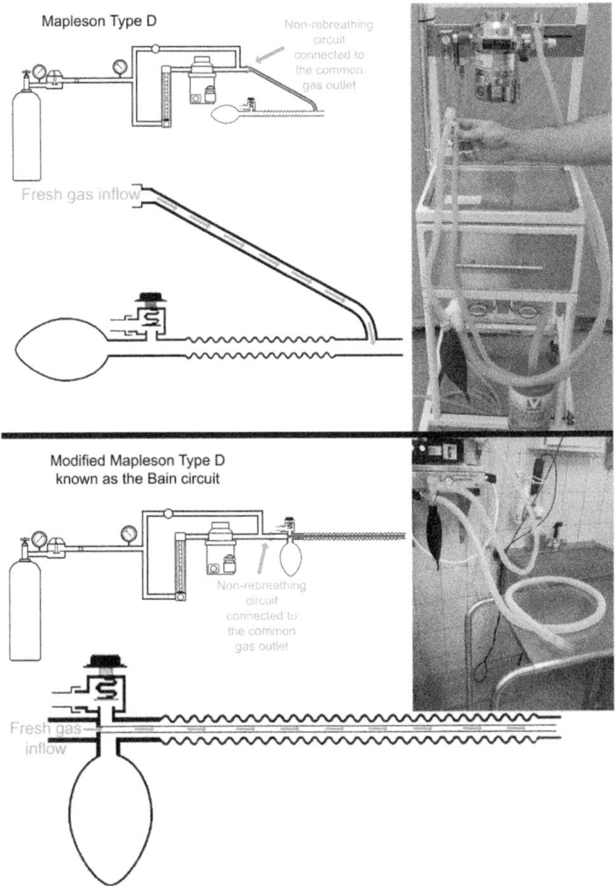

Figure 5.12 The Mapleson Type D (top) and the modified coaxial version (bottom). All breathing circuits connect to the common gas outlet (blue arrows) of the IADA, as indicated in the schematic drawings. These nonrebreathing circuits rely on a continuous delivery of fresh gas inflow (green arrows) to vent the exhaled carbon dioxide; please consult the text for a description of gas flow within these nonrebreathing circuits.

is also recommended for small animals under 5–10 kg. The Bain circuit has some advantages over the Modified T-piece. With the Bain circuit, unlike the Modified T-piece, the inspired limb (and thus the delivered gas) is warmed somewhat by the exhaled gas in the coaxial expiratory circuit. In addition, the circuit is lightweight, not bulky and unlikely to cause excessive drag on the tracheal tube and thereby contribute to tracheal tube disconnection or tracheal extubation. Finally, because of the coaxial tube arrangement it is less likely that the fresh gas delivery hose will become kinked and result in reduced fresh gas delivery.

Rebreathing Circuits

Rebreathing circuits are composed of many parts (Figure 5.13) and are therefore more expensive to purchase than nonrebreathing circuits, more complex to set up and operate, and more difficult to clean following use. Improper assembly can cause malfunction, which may be life-threatening. In these circuits, carbon dioxide is chemically removed from exhaled gases that are then rebreathed. Removal is accomplished by directing exhaled gases through a canister that contains CO_2 absorbent granules. Carbon dioxide removal is based on the chemical principle of a base neutralizing an acid. The acid is carbonic acid formed by CO_2 reacting with water, and the neutralizing process end products are water, heat, and carbonate salts (which vary depending on the absorbent composition). Indicators are added to the absorbent granules to indicate capacity of absorption capability. The original color of the absorbent and the change in color when the CO_2 absorption capability is exhausted vary with commercial preparations. Accordingly, the anesthetist must be aware of the associated colors of the product in use. "Regeneration" of a fresh color from an exhausted color may occur with some formulations. For example, soda lime partially reactivates with a period of disuse. Therefore, soda lime previously used to the point of color change may not initially show an exhausted color change following a period of disuse. Then, when used again, the exhausted soda lime shows reappearance of the exhaustion color after only a brief exposure to CO_2.

There are numerous CO_2 absorbents available today and there is some variability internationally. Soda lime is a traditional absorbent but contains large amounts of potassium and/or sodium hydroxide (amounts vary with commercial formulations). If these formulations become desiccated, they react with volatile anesthetics (most notably, desflurane) to form carbon monoxide. In addition, sevoflurane can react with soda lime to form Compound A (a vinyl ether), which is potentially nephrotoxic. As a result, a variety of new CO_2 absorbents are commercially available that do not have this disadvantageous property, replacing soda lime in many parts of the world. Further review of absorbents is available elsewhere (see Further Reading).

The CO_2 absorbent is a consumable item of rebreathing circuits and the authors suggest it should be changed when (1) two-thirds to three-quarters of the absorbent has changed color in systems that are used daily, or (2) when the fraction of *inspired* CO_2 measured using a capnograph increases to greater than 3 mmHg (and is not secondary to another cause; see Chapter 4), or (3) if the breathing circuit is not regularly used and has been opened to room air for protracted periods of time (risk of desiccation and potential for consequent inhalation anesthetic agent reaction), then it should be changed at a monthly interval (Figure 5.14).

Relatively low fresh gas flows are possible with rebreathing circuits because of the presence of one-way valves directing gas flow within the circuit and because of chemical removal of exhaled CO_2 by absorbents. Use of

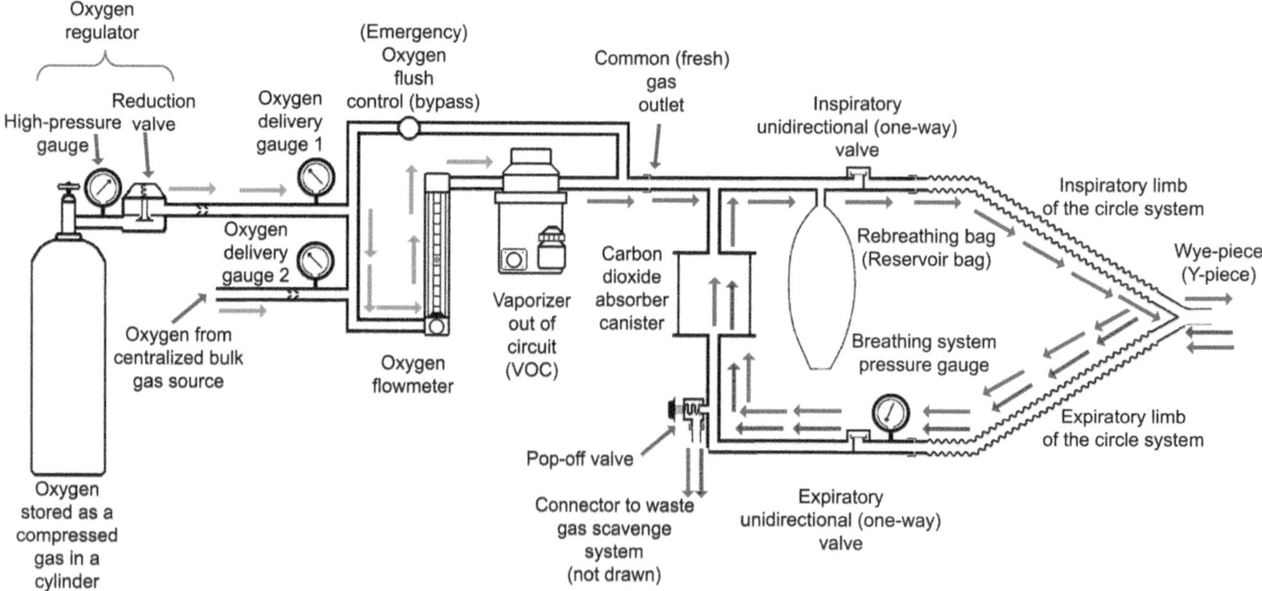

Figure 5.13 The rebreathing circuits are made up of many components as demonstrated in the labeled IADA where a circle circuit is attached to the common gas outlet. The oxygen flow (green arrows) is set by the flowmeter and as it passes the vaporizer it forms a gas mixture with an inhalational anesthetic which is the fresh gas mixture (blue arrows) that continuously enters the circle circuit via the common gas outlet. The animal will exhale gases that include carbon dioxide (red arrows), which is absorbed by special absorbents placed in a canister. Circuit gas flow is managed by unidirectional valves. Excess gas within the rebreathing circuit is vented via the pop-off valve. Oxygen is the most common carrier gas and can be delivered to the IADA via an oxygen cylinder or a centralized bulk source or preferably both. Delivery pressure gauges (insert) measure the pressure of the intermediate pressure system.

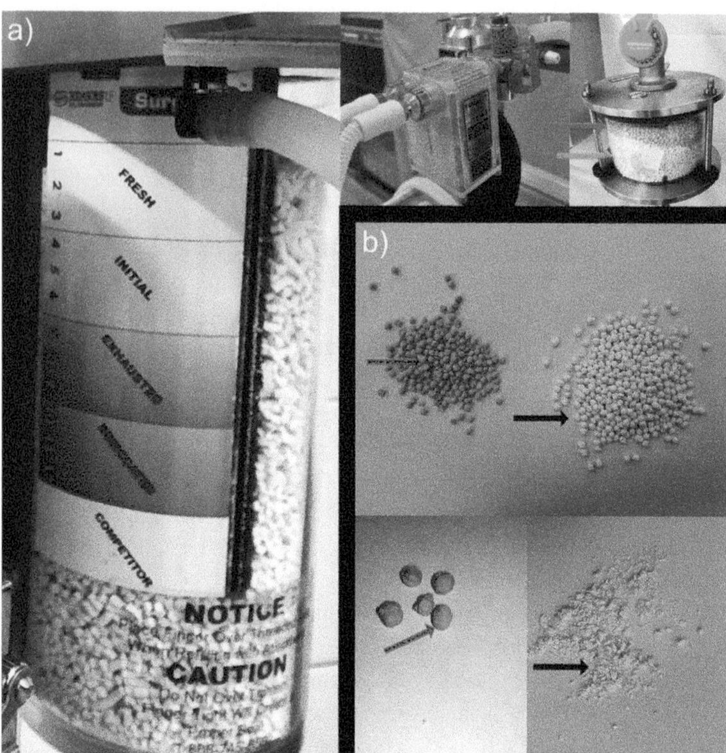

Figure 5.14 Examples of carbon dioxide absorbent canisters (a); note that the example on the left has a color chart insert to indicate the various color changes that the recommended absorbent undergoes. The exhausted absorbent is purple in color (blue arrow) and the fresh is a cream to white color (green arrow). If the indicator dye is not working (desiccated, open to room air for prolonged period of time not in use), then using a gloved hand to feel the granules is helpful (b). Exhausted granules (red arrows) turn to stone (calcium carbonate) and do not easily crush into powder as fresh granules do (black arrows). This is generally true for exhausted "contemporary" or "commercially available" absorbent regardless of a color change.

lower flows results in less waste of anesthetic gases and O_2, reducing the cost of anesthetic management. There is also pollution of the atmosphere with anesthetic gases. Furthermore, as a result of rebreathing of exhaled gases, there is some conservation of airway moisture and body heat. By contrast to nonrebreathing circuits, use of lower gas flows means that patient and circuit denitrogenation (i.e., rise of the inspired O_2 concentration) occurs more slowly, changes in anesthetic depth are delayed compared to nonrebreathing circuits, and the concentration of any potentially toxic by-products of inhaled anesthetics (e.g., Compound A) may be increased.

Rebreathing circuits can be used two ways: semi-closed and closed modes. The main difference between these is the fresh gas inflow rate required and, as a result, the amount of rebreathing of exhaled gas.

Semi-closed Mode

The most commonly used mode of rebreathing circuit for delivery of anesthetic gases and O_2 in clinical veterinary practice is a partial rebreathing or semi-closed mode. Fresh gas is supplied to the breathing circuit in excess of the patient's metabolic and anesthetic needs (ranges from 10 to 100 mL/kg/min, i.e., less than the patient's minute ventilation; see Chapter 8). Excess gas is eliminated from the circuit via an overflow or "pop-off" valve. That is, exhaled gas passes either into the atmosphere or returns to the rebreathing bag with the incoming fresh gas and is rebreathed. Rebreathing is acceptable because CO_2 is chemically removed from the circuit.

Closed Mode

The closed mode of rebreathing circuit use is a complete rebreathing mode. In this case, fresh gas is supplied to a level that matches the patient's metabolic O_2 and anesthetic needs (ranges from 3 to 10 mL/kg/min). The closed mode is more often used with large domestic (e.g., horses) or nondomestic (e.g., captive zoological) species to reduce cost, but the principle can be applied to smaller species. Regardless of these factors, a prominent disadvantage of this mode is the delay in developing a desired inspired O_2 and anesthetic concentration, and longer time to change the circuit anesthetic concentration.

As O_2 delivery is matched to patient metabolic requirement and CO_2 is removed, there is no excess gas to vent from the circuit. Consequently, the overflow (pop-off) valve can be "closed" with a result of no net change in circuit characteristics (i.e., no net change in breathing bag volume). In contrast, if the pop-off valve is closed with the semi-closed mode and associated higher gas inflows, the volume of gas contained within the breathing circuit (as manifested by bag volume) will increase with time (the rate of change dependent on fresh gas inflow; see Figure 5.9). If the pop-off valve closure remains uncorrected, this situation results in a rapidly developing, potentially life-threatening elevated airway pressure, lung expansion, and associated intrathoracic pressure with reduced venous blood return to the heart. In an extreme situation, airway and/or lung barotrauma, hemodynamic collapse or pressure-induced rupture of some portion of the anesthetic circuit, or some combination of these conditions are a likely, undesirable outcome.

On the one hand, closed mode anesthesia delivery is more economical (i.e., makes use of some inhaled anesthetics more affordable), but on the other hand this delivery mode is technically more demanding to ensure safety to the patient. For example, in the absence of gas monitoring devices, amounts of required O_2 are unpredictable and concentrations of potent inhaled anesthetics are unknown. There is also greater possibility of accumulation of undesirable and potentially toxic gases in the breathing circuit (e.g., methane and reaction products of some inhaled anesthetics with CO_2 absorbents; see the preceding text) especially during prolonged anesthesia.

Types of Rebreathing Circuits

Two types of rebreathing circuits are available, and both may be used in either the semi-closed or closed mode. The *to-and-fro circuit* (Figure 5.15), while of historical importance, is seldom used in clinical practice and will not be discussed further. The *circle circuit* is the most popular breathing circuit in most veterinary facilities, especially for animals greater than 5–10 kg in size. It is so named because gas flow follows a circular pathway through separate inspiratory and expiratory limbs. Essential components of a generic circle circuit are shown in Figure 5.13.

Important components of breathing circuits, not previously discussed, are the unidirectional valves, pressure relief valve, the circuit pressure gauge, and the Y-piece (wye-piece; circle). Two unidirectional valves (also referred to as "flutter" or "one-way" valves) provide for unidirectional gas flow within the circuit. One ensures fresh gas flows toward the patient, and the other that exhaled gas flows away from the patient. These valves can be displaced and/or stick, contributing to excessive increase in breathing resistance (if stuck in the closed position) or added mechanical dead space (if stuck in the open position). The pressure relief valve, also known as the "pop-off valve" or "adjustable pressure limiting" (APL) valve, is a variable vent for circuit gases. Its purpose is to release excess gas from the circuit to prevent airway gas pressure gas buildup. It is designed to allow a one-way nonreturnable gas flow out of the circuit, i.e., allow gas to escape from the circuit to the atmosphere (or waste gas scavenge device) and not allow ambient gas to enter the circuit and dilute resident gases. If fresh gas inflow exceeds patient uptake and gas

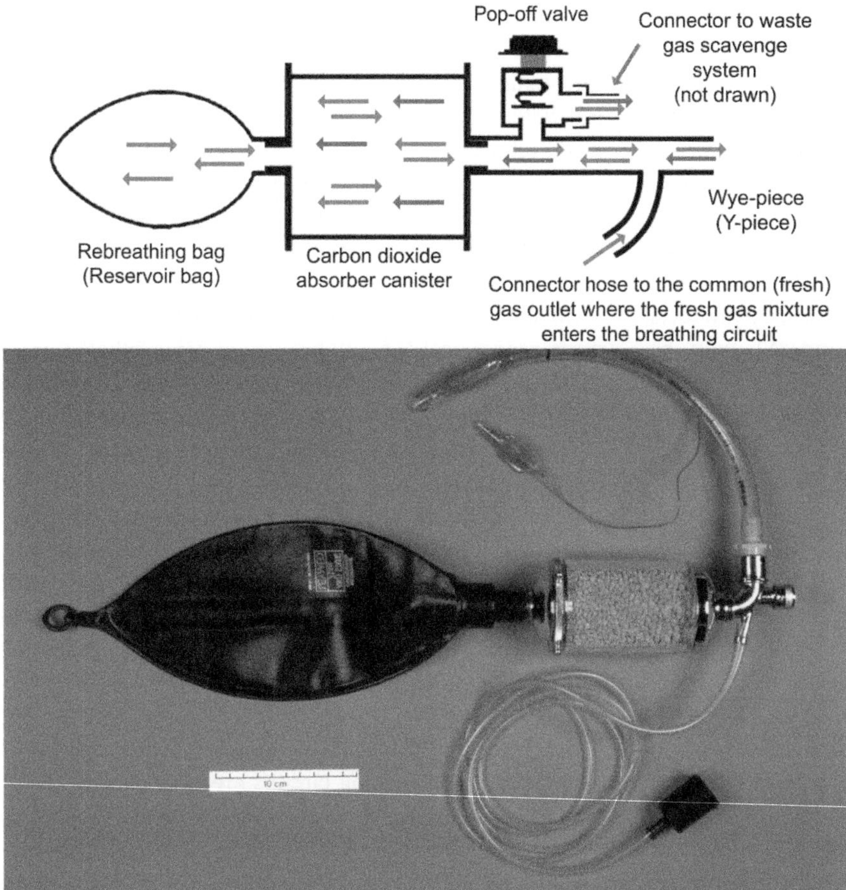

Figure 5.15 A schematic of a to-and-fro rebreathing circuit that is also known as a "Waters' canister." Fresh gas enters the breathing circuit via the common gas outlet (blue arrows). Exhaled carbon dioxide (red arrows) is removed by the carbon dioxide absorber within a canister. The patient rebreathes exhaled gases from the rebreathing bag and excess gases within the breathing circuit are vented via the pop-off valve.

outflow from this valve, the rebreathing bag size, and eventually circuit and airway pressures, increases. The pop-off valve may be closed when the circuit is used in a complete rebreathing (i.e., closed) mode and partially or fully open in a partial rebreathing (i.e., semi-closed) mode. The latter is more common. Note that at least partial closure is required for intermittent positive pressure ventilation (IPPV). As an aside, and of practical value here, is that a distended bag does not always imply an undesirable elevated airway pressure. Check the pressure gauge (or squeeze the bag to see how easy it is to empty) and the magnitude of opening of the pressure relief valve (e.g., pop-off valve) to determine whether this situation is of immediate clinical importance. Bags that are hard to empty with the gentle squeeze could indicate that the pressure relief valve is "sticky" or partially or completely closed and needs to be opened more to allow venting of breathing circuit gases. The circuit pressure gauge provides a means of determining gas pressure within the circuit. This pressure gauge is different to that used in the high-pressure portion of the IADA (described earlier). Calibration of the gauge is usually in cmH_2O but occasionally in mmHg (1 mmHg = 1.3 cmH_2O). This gauge is used to detect the magnitude of airway pressure above ambient pressure during spontaneous breathing or to aid control of ventilation during various mechanical maneuvers. Examples of use include ventilating the patient to a specific peak inspiratory pressure (for additional information, refer to Chapter 18), to detect an unwanted positive end expiratory pressure (commonly referred to by its acronym "PEEP"), or to monitor a therapeutic amount of PEEP. Finally, the wye-piece (Y-piece) is a metal or plastic three-way tubular connector that connects the two breathing hoses to the endotracheal tube or patient facemask.

Optional components that may be attached or placed within the circle circuit include filters, respirometers, humidifiers, and switches. A filter is sometimes added to protect the patient from pathogens and airborne particulate matter. A respirometer can be used to measure and monitor the patient's tidal breath and minute ventilation volumes. A humidifier will add moisture to the inspired breath. Some circuits include a ventilator-rebreathing bag selector switch that permits rapid switching between the rebreathing bag and mechanical ventilator. If the IADA is not equipped with a ventilator, then a stand-alone anesthesia ventilator can be attached, usually at the site of rebreathing bag attachment. Placement of components of the circle circuit influence function and many different designs are possible and available, each with their advantages and disadvantages. Historically, circle circuits for inhalation anesthetic management have been commercially available for small and large animals. Circuits for small animals are copies of circuits for human patients and, in general, are considered for use in animals up to about 150 kg in body mass. Large animal circuits are designed with similar principles but of course with a larger internal diameter of the circuit tubing (and larger rebreathing bag and CO_2 absorbent canister) to satisfy gas volume and flows associated with the larger species such as adult horses. Recently, it has been suggested that an intermediate size circuit would be helpful to improve management of animals between about 100 and 350 kg (see Further Reading).

Vaporizers

Most of the inhalation anesthetics in use today are liquids at room temperature and sea level pressure and must be converted to their vapor state before they are administered. In addition, the saturated vapor concentration of most volatile anesthetics at usual vaporizing temperatures is far greater than needed to provide a safe range for clinical delivery (Table 5.5). A working knowledge of the physical principles of gas vaporization and vaporizer function is important to safe anesthetic practice given the breadth of application in veterinary medical practice, which often includes extremes of ambient temperature and pressure.

A vaporizer is a device that permits the conversion of a liquid into its vapor state and permits the delivery of a controlled amount to the breathing circuit. The vaporizer provides a means of diluting the saturated vapor concentration

Table 5.5 The relationship of vapor pressure and saturated vapor concentration for inhalational anesthetics (according to 1 atmosphere pressure [101 kPa, 760 mmHg] at sea level).

Inhalational anesthetic	Vapor pressure (mmHg at 20 °C)	Saturated vapor pressure (%)	Common maximal vaporizer dial settings (%)
Halothane	244	32	5
Isoflurane	240	32	5
Sevoflurane	160	21	7
Desflurane	664	87	18

with, for example, O_2 so that the concentration of anesthetic emerging from the vaporizer is within a known range. The ideal vaporizer should ensure a constant, known anesthetic output concentration for a prolonged period and under varying conditions of carrier gas flow, compressed gas pipeline pressure fluctuations, and ambient temperature. The precision of controllability of the delivered anesthetic concentration depends on the degree of sophistication of vaporizer design.

The first volatile anesthetics that were developed for clinical use (e.g., diethyl ether and chloroform) were inhaled from open drop masks (e.g., "ether mask" and the Cox and Hobday masks for horses) or from containers. Air was drawn over the surface of the liquid agent and the gas mixture inhaled. This simple method is still used in certain circumstances in veterinary (and human) medicine, e.g., "an induction box" for small animals. However, a major disadvantage of this method is that vapor concentrations of the agent are erratic and sometimes unpredictable. High concentrations can lead to overdose and low concentrations to insufficient anesthesia.

Some physical characteristics of volatile anesthetics fundamental to vaporizer design and performance will be briefly reviewed. More in-depth reviews are available elsewhere (Chapter 8).

Vapor pressure (VP) is a characteristic of volatile anesthetics and, under usual circumstances, primarily varies according to temperature. The VP describes the maximum partial pressure of a volatile liquid that can be attained in the vapor phase at a given temperature. Consequently, it is meaningless to consider specific concepts of VP without specifying the environmental temperature. The VP at a given environmental temperature relative to the associated atmospheric pressure (VP/P_{bar}), multiplied by 100, equals the *saturated vapor concentration* at that temperature. The boiling point of a liquid is the temperature at which VP equals P_{bar}. Therefore, the lower the P_{bar}, the lower the boiling point. Within the wide range of environmental pressures typical of clinical circumstances in veterinary practice, VP does not meaningfully vary with P_{bar} and therefore is not further considered in this discussion. In summary, as temperature decreases for a given volatile anesthetic, VP for that agent decreases. This results in a predictable decrease in vapor concentration. The reverse occurs with a temperature increase.

Energy in the form of heat is necessary for molecules in the liquid phase to break their mutual attraction (intermolecular forces) and for them to enter the gaseous phase. *Heat of vaporization* is defined as the number of calories necessary to convert 1 g or 1 mL of liquid into vapor. Heat for vaporization is derived from the liquid, with the result that liquid temperature decreases as vaporization takes place. With an unopposed decrease in liquid temperature, VP and, in turn, vapor concentration decrease. A temperature gradient is established between the liquid and that of the surroundings until a new equilibrium is established. Therefore, thermal conductivity and thermal stabilization of the material used for vaporizer construction is an important consideration. Examples of poor conductors of heat are glass and air while examples of relatively good conductors are copper and aluminum.

When the vaporizer is in use, carrier gas flow (set by the flowmeter(s)) to the vaporizer is split. Part of this flow is directed to the vaporizing chamber and the remaining flow bypasses the vaporizing chamber (the diluent flow; see later). The two gas paths meet once again just before leaving the vaporizer. A flow of gas (agent carrier gas) through the vaporizing chamber is necessary to collect anesthetic vapor for patient delivery and to continue the vaporizing process, i.e., as gas-carrying anesthetic molecules exits the vaporizing chamber, the vaporization equilibrium shifts in favor of more anesthetic molecules moving from liquid to the vapor phase. Therefore, carrier gas-anesthetic liquid surface contact is very important. Contact time is limited due to the continuous flow of carrier gas through the vaporizing chamber; therefore, a large gas–liquid surface interface is important to promote efficiency of the vaporization process. Recall that, presuming appropriate working conditions, the concentration of anesthetic in the vaporizing chamber depends upon the saturated vapor pressure (SVP) and therefore substantially above clinical use. Accordingly, the vaporizer bypass flow serves to dilute the gas emerging from the vaporizing chamber before delivery downstream.

The vaporizer is commonly positioned at one of two locations with respect to the patient breathing circuit: either within the circuit (vaporizer-in-circuit or VIC) or outside of the circuit (vaporizer-out of-circuit or VOC) (Figure 5.16). Since vaporizer positioning relative to the breathing circuit influences the inspired anesthetic concentration in addition to the selected dial setting of the vaporizer, knowledge of this bears on clinical decision-making.

The breathing circuit used with a VIC positioning is the circle circuit. In this case, the animal's respiratory tidal volume in whole or part (depending on the fresh flow rate) is used to collect anesthetic from the vaporizing chamber. Because of the reliance on the anesthetized animal's respiratory efforts to add anesthetic to inspired gas only low resistance vaporizers (see the following text) are used with this circuit-related positioning. While VIC was popular decades ago in small animals, its safe clinical use, especially in inexperienced hands, heavily relied on use in healthy animals, and with volatile anesthetics of moderate to high blood solubility (such as diethyl ether and methoxyflurane). Most current use of the VIC style is

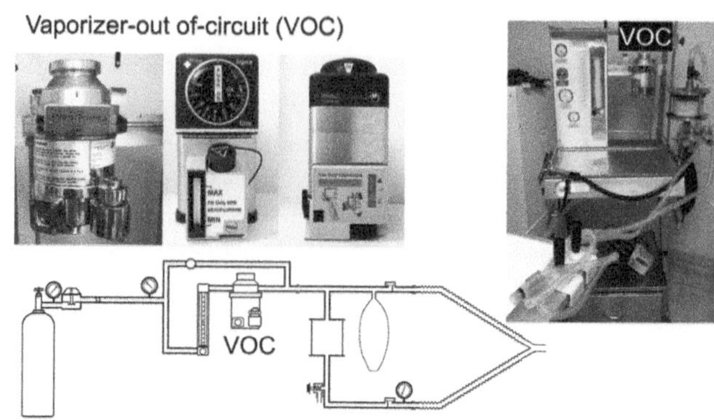

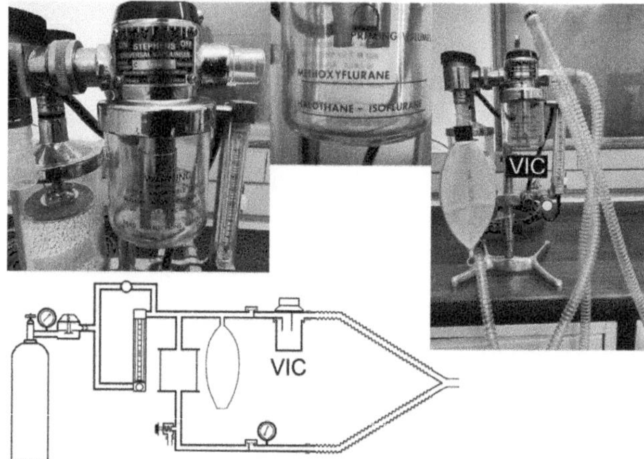

Figure 5.16 Examples of vaporizers classified by position within an IADA. The vaporizer-out-of-circuit (VOC) are precision vaporizers that are inhalational anesthetic specific and color coded. The VOC has a dial that is used to deliver an accurate percentage of inhalational anesthetic vapor to the fresh gas mixture. The vaporizer-in-circuit (VIC) are nonprecision (i.e., does not have a percent calibrated dial) and a version still used in some countries is the Stephens machine that can accept different inhalational anesthetics.

geographically limited (e.g., Australia and South Africa; see Further Reading).

Anesthetic vaporizers in contemporary use are most commonly positioned VOC. Unlike VIC positioning, only fresh gas (carrier gas) from the gas source(s) is directed to and through the vaporizer and there are no restrictions on the type of breathing circuit used with this arrangement. The VOC positioning is a safer and more versatile arrangement compared to VIC because it permits finer control of delivered anesthetic concentration and a change in ventilation has no effect on vaporizer output. Consequently, assisted and controlled ventilation can be used with greater safety with the VOC versus the VIC arrangement.

Vaporizer Classification and Design

Anesthetic vaporizers can be classified into nonprecision and precision designs.

Nonprecision Design

This category of vaporizer includes several design styles. Anesthetic concentrations with this delivery style are erratic and skill is necessary to avoid overdose, especially with anesthetic agents in current use, which have vapor pressures greatly exceeding minimal effective anesthetic doses.

The *glass jar* (Figure 5.17a), historically, was introduced because there was a need for greater safety in the delivery of inhaled anesthetics, compared to an open system. As understanding of the physics of anesthetic delivery improved, early anesthetists devised means of delivering more predictable and uniform anesthetic concentrations. Volatile anesthetics were placed in glass containers, and O_2 or O_2-enriched air (carrier gas) was introduced into the container. As a result, controllable mixtures of carrier gas and anesthetic vapor were possible. There are three different styles of glass jar. With the carrier gas flow-, or draw-over type, the carrier gas flows over the surface of the liquid anesthetic picking up anesthetic molecules as they vaporize (Figure 5.17a). The wick style incorporates a cotton wick that is inserted part way into the liquid anesthetic allowing anesthetic to migrate up the wick by capillary action. Carrier gas is directed through the wick, resulting in greater exposure of anesthetic to carrier gas (Figure 5.17b). Finally, with the bubble through style, the carrier gas is directed through a fenestrated disc that is positioned some distance below the liquid surface and in turn bubbled through the liquid anesthetic (Figure 5.17c). This technique increases the surface area between carrier gas and liquid anesthetic, thereby improving efficiency and controllability of vaporization.

The final nonprecision style to mention is the dropper or injection style in which liquid anesthetic is dripped or injected directly into the breathing circuit of the IADA.

The advantages of nonprecision vaporizers are their very simple nature. They are relatively inexpensive to add to the IADA and they can be used with a variety of volatile anesthetics. However, there are several important considerations impacting safe use. The actual delivered concentration is usually unknown and widely varies depending on ambient conditions (e.g., ambient temperature and pressure). In addition, the controllability of delivered concentration for a given vaporizer dial setting widely varies with duration of use. An exception to this is the injection technique that can be quite precise with care and understanding of the principles of use. Finally, there is a greater potential for error, e.g., inadvertent mixing of two or more volatile anesthetics within a jar or delivery of the incorrect agent.

Precision Style

Precision style vaporizers are characterized by their ability to control delivered inhaled anesthetic concentration.

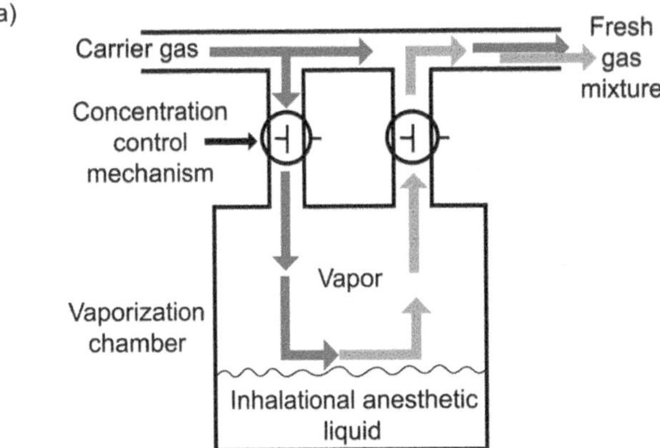

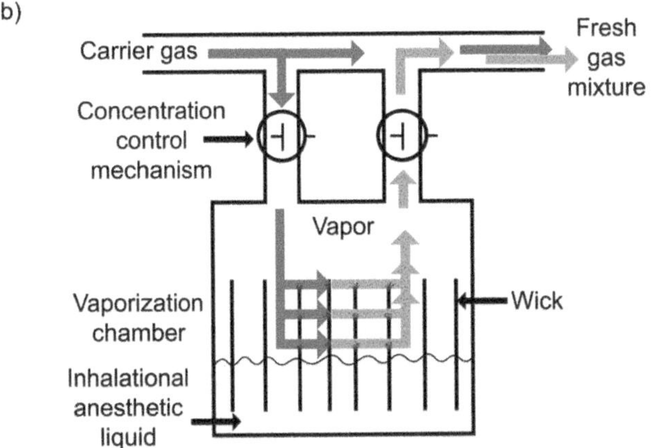

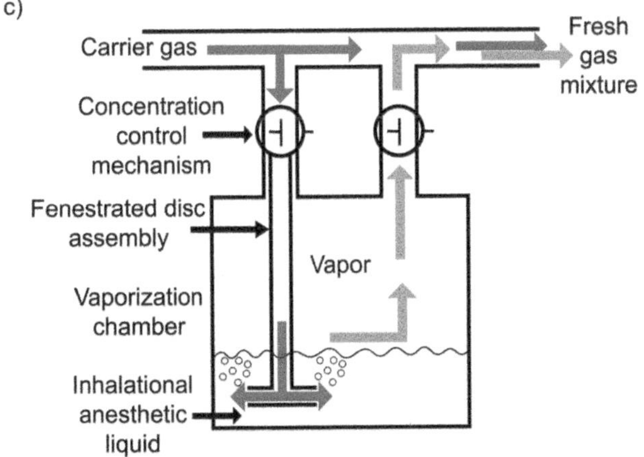

Figure 5.17 Three different configurations of a nonprecision glass jar vaporizer, an earlier form of vaporizer technology where all modern forms originate. The different configurations are (a) draw-over (e.g., "present-day" Stephens universal vaporizer), (b) addition of wicks to increase contact surface area of the liquid anesthetic, and (c) the bubble through configuration. The carrier gas is split into two channels (blue arrows): the bypass gas that does not enter the vaporizer and the vaporizer gas that enters the vaporization chamber to "collect" anesthetic vapor (green arrows). The vaporizer gas rejoins the bypass gas that is called the "fresh gas mixture" (carrier gas + inhalational anesthetic vapor).

Most of them can be further classified according to a variety of characteristics (Table 5.6) but are most commonly described as agent-specific, variable-bypass, flow-over, temperature-compensated vaporizers. The one exception to this description is the desflurane vaporizer, which is engineered so that both temperature and pressure of the vaporizing chamber are *actively* controlled to create an environment for predictable volatility. A precision vaporizer is always positioned in the VOC arrangement.

A precision vaporizer is usually calibrated at sea level atmospheric pressure. If its use is substantially above sea level (e.g., Denver, Mexico City, and Johannesburg; >5000 feet [1524 m] above sea level), the influence of altitude should be considered. A decrease in ambient pressure from sea level conditions does not significantly alter the anesthetic *partial pressure* (i.e., agent vapor-pressure–temperature relationship) emerging from a calibrated vaporizer. However, a decrease in ambient pressure from sea level conditions results in an increase in vapor *concentration* (vol%). The anesthetic concentration emerging from a vaporizer at an ambient pressure change, compared to the marked dial setting, can be calculated from $C' = C(P/P')$, where C' is the new anesthetic concentration, C is the marked concentration on the dial of the vaporizer, P is the ambient pressure for which the vaporizer is calibrated (usually at sea level or 760 mmHg), and P' is the new pressure (in mmHg), for which C' is being calculated. For example, for a vaporizer in use at the top of Mount Kinabalu (Malaysia, 13 435 feet [4095 m] above sea level, P_{bar} around 465 mmHg), with the dial set to 2%, the effect of altitude would result in an output of 3.3%.

A contemporary IADA may include one or multiple agent-specific vaporizers depending on its considered use. If two or more precision vaporizers are present, a commercial safety interlock mechanism is recommended in place so that only one vaporizer may be used at a time. In addition, an anesthetic-specific filling device should be used to transfer an agent from its container to the agent-specific vaporizer (Figure 5.18). Such a device prevents

Table 5.6 Classification of precision vaporizers.

Method	Classification
Method of regulating vaporizer output concentration	a. Concentrated calibrated b. Measured flow
Method of vaporization	a. Flow-over (with or without wick) b. Bubble through c. Injection
Temperature compensated	a. Thermocompensated b. Supplied heat
Specificity	a. Agent specific b. Multiple agent
Resistance	a. High (Plenum) b. Low

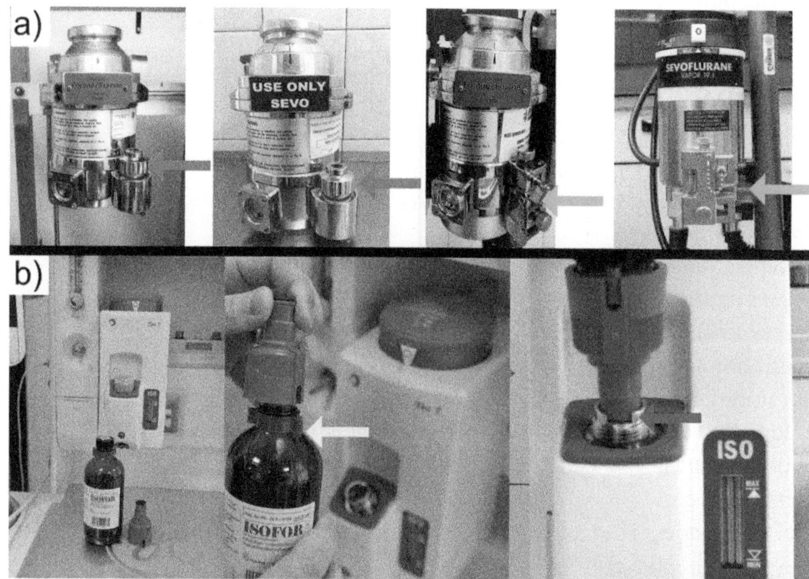

Figure 5.18 Examples of vaporizers (a) that do not (blue arrows) require an anesthetic-specific filling device to fill an agent-specific vaporizer. These vaporizers are unsafe in that they could accidentally be filled with the incorrect anesthetic agent for which the vaporizer is specifically calibrated. To increase operational safety, older vaporizers can be fitted with aftermarket anesthetic-specific filling ports that require these filling devices (green arrows). The filling of an agent-specific vaporizer (b) involves attaching the anesthetic-specific filling device to the bottle containing the anesthetic agent by lining up the keys (yellow arrow) and then attaching this assembly to the keyed filling port on the vaporizer (red arrows).

mistakenly filling a vaporizer with an anesthetic that differs from that for which the vaporizer was calibrated. For additional safety reasons, it is recommended that individual vaporizers are commercially serviced, including anesthetic vapor output calibration confirmation or re-calibration, on a regular schedule appropriate to conditions of use. At minimum, annual servicing should be performed.

Precision vaporizers can be sub-classified into numerous ways; however, in-depth discussion of this matter is beyond the scope of this chapter, and readers are referred elsewhere for further information (see Further Reading). The *variable-bypass vaporizer* (Figure 5.19) is the most widely used vaporizer in veterinary medicine and therefore briefly discussed in the following text. Other types include *dual circuit*, *cassette*, and *injection* vaporizers. The relatively inexpensive, multiple-agent, *measured-flow* (e.g., copper kettle) style vaporizer is considered by physician and veterinary anesthesiologists of only historical clinical interest but is useful in teaching how the carrier gas it split through the vaporizer and as bypass gas because two independent flowmeters needed to be set.

Variable-bypass vaporizers are calibrated for a specific volatile anesthetic (i.e., characterized as an agent-specific vaporizer) and include several proprietary styles with the most common being the *Tec*, *Vapor*, and *Penlon* (Figure 5.20). The Tec and Vapor style vaporizers were introduced in the late 1950s to deliver halothane (e.g., Fluotec Mark 2 and Halothane Vapor) and updated over time to incorporate engineering and safety improvements, and the introduction of new volatile agents. For example, a recent Tec model, the Tec-6, is designed for use only with desflurane. Tec-7 vaporizers are available for halothane, enflurane,

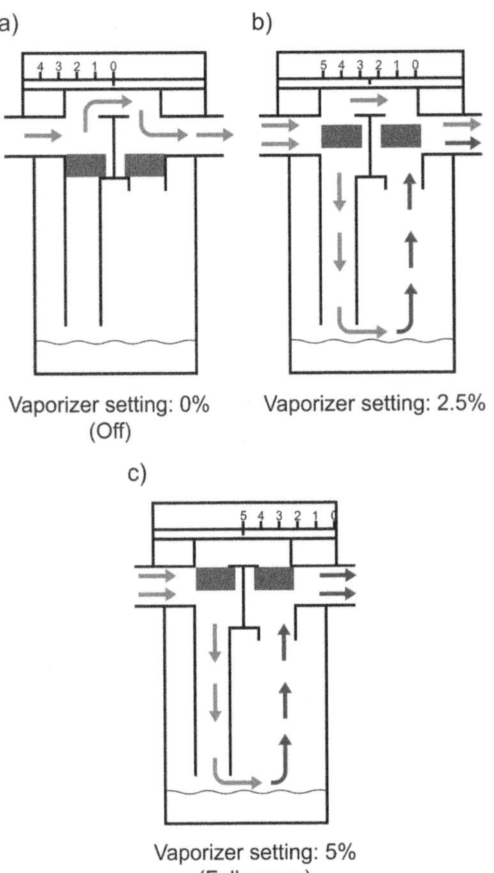

Figure 5.19 A schematic representation of the workings of a variable-bypass vaporizer (i.e., a procession vaporizer-out-of-circuit) where its concentration dial is set to 0% (a), 2.5% (b), and the maximum setting of 5% (c). The carrier gas (blue arrows) is either channeled through the bypass channel, as in (a), or it is split to go through the bypass channel and enter the vaporizing chamber where inhalational anesthetic gas is mixed (purple arrows) to an accurate concertation set by the dial as in (b), or the dial is set to maximum whereby none of the carrier gas enters the bypass channel and all moves through he vaporizing chamber.

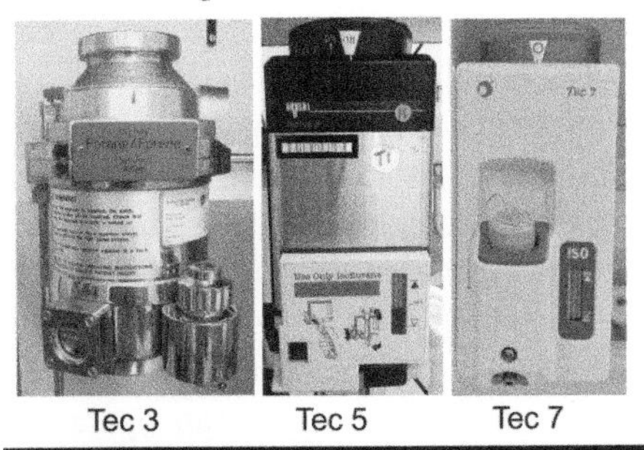

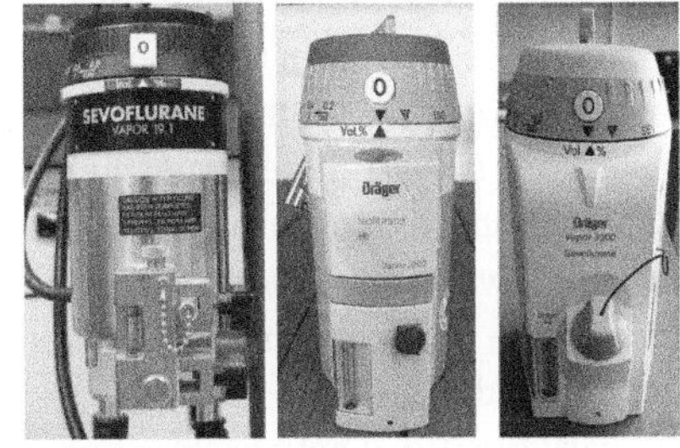

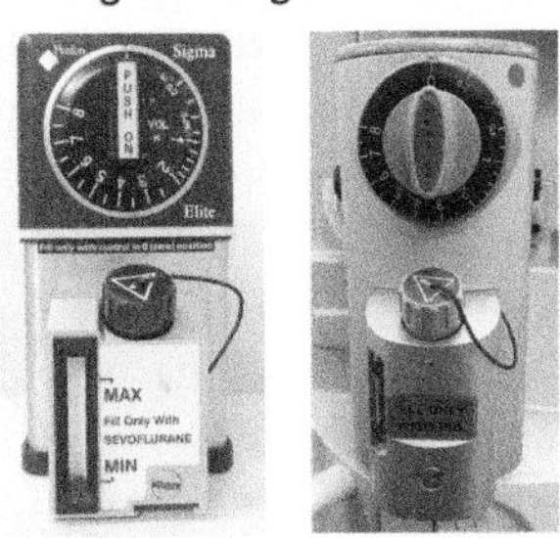

Figure 5.20 Photographs of precision vaporizers commonly used in clinical veterinary practice.

isoflurane, and sevoflurane. Vapor style vaporizers have different compensatory technology to the Tec style but are designed for similar use and the more recent available versions are the Vapor 19.1, the Vapor 19.2, and the Vapor 2000; the Drager D-Vapor is only used for desflurane delivery. Because of their durability and economic considerations, many of the early types of both Tec (e.g., Fluotec Mark 3) and Vapor (Halothane Vapor) styles remain in veterinary use. Specific performance characteristics such as the measured output of the anesthetic for a given dial setting of the agent-specific vaporizers are available from the manufacturers and specialized texts (see Further Reading).

Scavenging Waste Anesthetic Gases

Chronic exposure to low or trace concentrations of inhalation anesthetics may pose a human health hazard. With the possible exception of reproductive problems in women, evidence of health hazards is suggestive rather than conclusive. Collection and removal (i.e., scavenging) of waste inhalation anesthetic agents is prudent and mandatory in many jursidictions. In the United States of America, the Occupational Safety and Health Administration (OSHA) presently has no required exposure limits for inhalation anesthetics; however, their long-standing published recommendations for handling waste inhalation anesthetic gases in human operating room and dental suites remain in use. These guidelines should be followed in veterinary practice, i.e., waste anesthetic gases should be scavenged from the anesthetic machine and the immediate working environment of an operating room. In addition, since inhaled anesthetics are potent greenhouse gases, additional simple strategies (e.g., control of fresh gas flow, with appropriate monitoring) can reduce the volume of these emissions to the environment (see Further Reading).

Scavenging systems vary greatly. Their basic components include a means for collecting excess gas venting from the patient breathing circuit, connecting tubing and some means for final disposal. Most commonly in veterinary medicine, scavenged gases from the breathing circuit are vented to the external atmosphere. Volatile anesthetics can be chemically adsorbed, though this practice is less popular because the cannisters are not reusable, do not remove N_2O, and add to the cost of anesthetic management. Scavenging systems may be active (i.e., use of a surgical vacuum source) or passive (Figure 5.21).

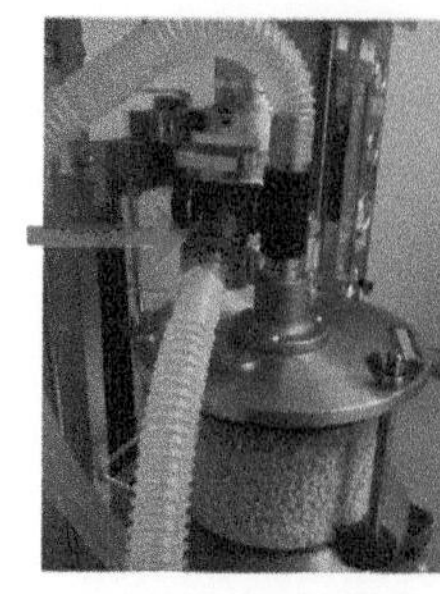

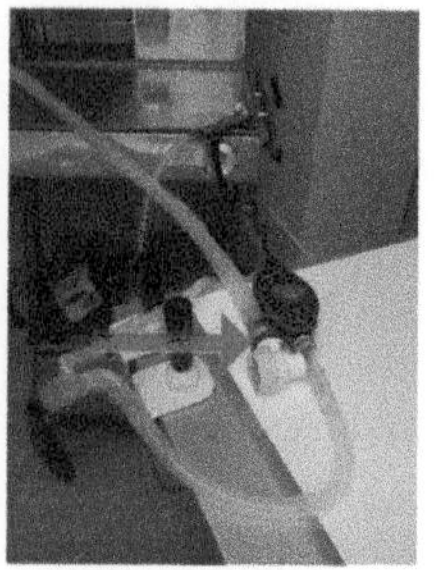
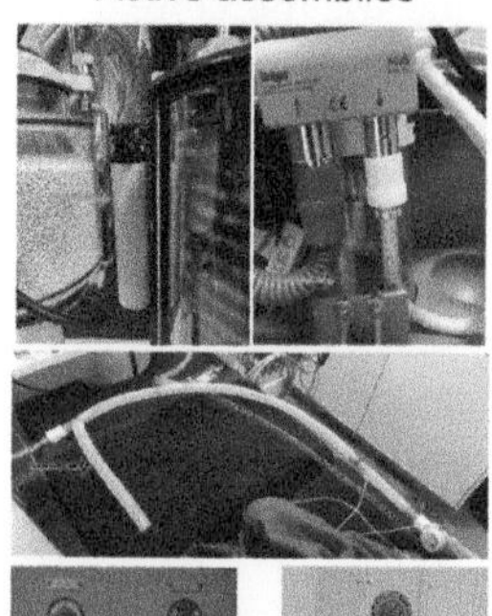

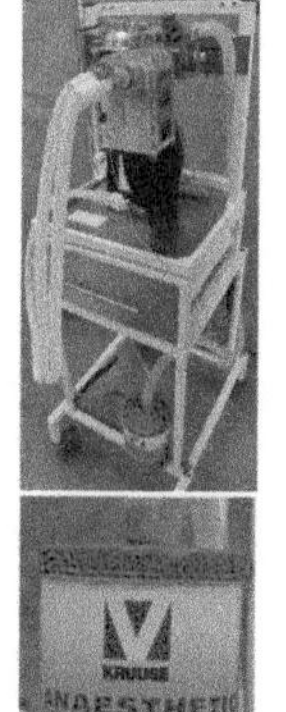

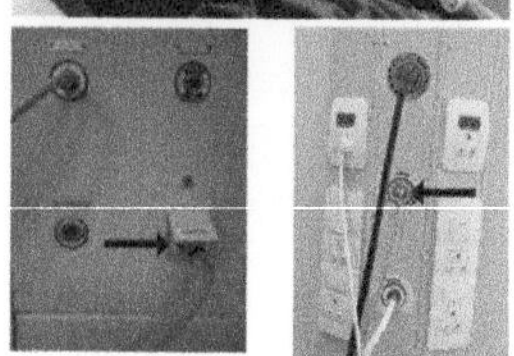

Figure 5.21 All waste gas management (scavenging) systems are attached via a connector (blue arrows) to the pop-off valve (a). There are active and passive assemblies of these systems (b). For active assemblies, there are either proprietary collection devices (green arrows) that allow the free flow of room air into the collection unit where active suction is applied by the hospital-wide vacuum line (black arrows). If the IADA does not have a specialized collection unit, one can be built using 22 mm hosing and a T-piece connector attached to a hose that will continuously allow room air into the system (orange arrow below in (b), "Active assemblies"). If room air is not allowed to enter the active assembly, then a negative pressure will be created, and this will interfere with the proper functioning of the pop-off valve. Passive assemblies are made up of a scavenger hose that is placed in an area away from the working area (maximum 5 m in length; not depicted); if this is not possible, then an activated charcoal collection canister may be used, as depicted.

Pre-use Function Check of the IADA

A checkout of the IADA must be conducted before administering each anesthetic. The checkout process is much like that performed by an airplane pilot prior to takeoff. A guideline for anesthetists to use before anesthesia induction ("takeoff") is provided as example in Table 5.7. The guideline should be modified to suit individual clinical practice.

Table 5.7 Checkout procedures for the Inhalation Anesthetic Delivery Apparatus (IADA).

Inspect the anesthetic machine for general presence of:
Gas source (compressed gas tanks attached to the machine)
Gas delivery hoses(s)
Vaporizer(s)
Patient breathing circuit
Turn on any electrical equipment that may be associated with anesthetic management
Check
For the presence of cylinder wrench
Flow controls are in OFF position
Vaporizers are off
For presence of waste gas scavenging system
Inspect and verify operational
Gas source(s) (oxygen, medical air, etc.)
Open O_2 cylinder, check pressure, close cylinder, and observe high-pressure gauge for a high-pressure leak
Use O_2 flush valve to bleed line
Repeat check of all compressed gas cylinders
Replace any cylinders with low pressure (e.g., less than 200–600 psi, circumstances dependent)
Open less full cylinder(s)
Piped gas line(s) attached and pressurized (source volume/pressure adequate)
Test flowmeters
Rotameter bobbins at zero flow
Gas flow through correct flowmeter
Flowmeter operational through its full flow range
Rotameter bobbin rotation with gas flow; no sticking
No apparent gas leaks
Vaporizers
Vaporizers for desired agents securely and properly positioned on machine; no gas leaks
Vaporizers are filled and filling caps sealed tightly
Controls freely movable
Controls in OFF position
Breathing circuit
Assemble functional circuit
Nonrebreathing circuit
Presence of necessary components and their competence
Bain circuit; patency of inner gas delivery tube
Rebreathing circuit
Proper filling of carbon dioxide absorbent in canister
Carbon dioxide absorbent at a suitable state for anticipated time of use
Valves present and competent, i.e., one-way gas flow
Presence of clean and patent breathing hoses should not be cracked or badly worn
Presence of breathing hose to endotracheal tube connecter (Y-piece) and endotracheal tube to Y-piece connector
Presence of appropriate size breathing bag
Pressure relief (pop-off) valve checked and competent

(Continued)

Table 5.7 (Continued)

Inspect the anesthetic machine for general presence of:
Check breathing circuit for leaks. To do this, screw the pop-off valve closed and occlude the Y-piece with hand/thumb, close the pop-off valve and turn the fresh gas flow to 2 L/min until the breathing circuit pressure gauge has reached 30 cmH2O pressure. Then turn off the fresh gas flow and watch the gauge to confirm the pressure holds steady. If the pressure drops, increase the fresh gas flow to a maximum of 250 mL/min and watch the gauge to confirm the pressure holds. If the pressure does not hold then there is a relevant circuit leak that requires investigation (leaks < 250 mL/min are generally considered acceptable). Once the positive pressure check is finished, the pop-off valve is opened while the Y-piece remains occluded to release the gas within the circuit. As the gas escapes, the needle of the pressure gauge should fall to 0 cmH2O. This confirms the pop-off valve is functional.
Inspect components of waste gas scavenging system
Verify presence of functional adsorber, if use intended
Attach vacuum/passive flow line
Verify operation of any associated valves
Additional tests
Test ventilator, if applicable
Check availability and readiness of other equipment, e.g., laryngoscope, endotracheal tubes, syringes, needles, adequate supply of appropriate drugs, monitoring devices, etc.
Check final position of all controls
Set up anesthetic plan and record

Questions and Answers

There are more practice questions and answers available for this chapter on the website. Please visit http://www.wiley.com/go/VeterinaryAnesthesiaZeiler.

Questions

1) To which component do you connect the breathing circuit to when assembling an IADA?
   a) Back bar
   b) Common gas outlet
   c) Vaporizer
   d) Oxygen flowmeter
2) The one-way valves found on IADA are located before the common gas outlet.
   a) True
   b) False
3) Which component of the IADA is essential and used to reduce the cylinder pressure to a normal working pressure (intermediate pressure)?
   a) Regulator
   b) Oxygen flowmeter
   c) Vaporizer
   d) Back bar
4) List 2 components that are found in a rebreathing system that is not found in a nonrebreathing system

Answers

1) b
2) False
3) a
4) Carbon dioxide absorbent canister and unidirectional (one-way) valves

Further Reading

Axelrod, D., Bell, C., Feldman, J. et al. (2017). Greening the operating room and perioperative arena: environmental sustainability for anesthesia practice. Schaumberg, IL: American Society of Anesthesiologists. https://www.asahq.org/about-asa/governance-and-committees/asa-committees/environmental-sustainability/greening-the-operating-room.

Dorsch, J.A. and Dorsch, S.E. (1975). *Understanding Anesthetic Equipment: Construction, Care & Complications*. Philadelphia: The Williams & Wilkins Co.

Fowler, M.E., Parker, E.E., McLaughlin, R.F. Jr., and Tyler, W.S. (1963). An inhalation anesthetic apparatus for large animals. *J Am Vet Med Assoc* 143: 272–276.

Hall, L.W. (1971). Equine anesthesia. In: *Textbook of Veterinary Anesthesia*, 1e (ed. L.R. Soma), 318–343. Baltimore: Williams & Wilkins Co.

Heath, R.B. (2019). Veterinary anesthesia intermediate rebreathing circuits. *Vet Anaesth Analg* 46: 407–408.

Manley, S.V. and McDonell, W.N. (1979a). A new circuit for small animal anesthesia: the Bain coaxial circuit. *J Am Anim Hosp Assoc* 15: 61–66.

Manley, S.V. and McDonell, W.N. (1979b). Clinical evaluation of the Bain breathing circuit in small animal anesthesia. *J Am Anim Hosp Assoc* 15: 67–72.

Mapleson, W.W. (1954). The elimination of rebreathing in various semi-closed anaesthetic systems. *Brit J Anaesth* 26: 323–332.

Mosley, C.A. (2015). Anesthetic equipment. In: *Veterinary Anesthesia and Analgesia*, 5e (ed. K.A. Grimm, L.A. Lamont, W.J. Tranquilli et al.), 23–85. Iowa: Wiley-Blackwell.

Roth P (2011). Anesthetic delivery systems. In: Basics of Anesthesia, 6e (ed. R.D. Miller and M.C. Pardo, Jr.), 198–218. Philadelphia: Saunders.

Soma, L.R. (1971). Systems and techniques for inhalation anesthesia. In: *Textbook of Veterinary Anesthesia*, 1e (ed. L.R. Soma), 201–228. Baltimore: Williams & Wilkins Co.

Steffey, E.P., Hodgson, O.S., and Kupershoek, C. (1984). Monitoring oxygen concentrating devices. *J Am Vet Med Assoc* 184: 626–638.

Steffey, E.P. and Howland, D., Jr. (1977). Rate of change of halothane concentration in a large animal circle anesthetic system. *Am J Vet Res* 38: 1993–1996.

Steffey, E.P., Mama, K.R., and Brosnan, R.J. (2015). Inhalation anesthetics. In: *Veterinary Anesthesia and Analgesia*, 5e (ed. K.A. Grimm, L.A. Lamont, W.J. Tranquilli et al.), 297–331. Iowa: Wiley-Blackwell.

Venticinque, S.G. and Andrews, J.J. (2015). Inhaled anesthetics: delivery systems. In: *Miller's Anesthesia*, 8e (ed. R.D. Miller), 752–820. Philadelphia: Saunders.

6

Introduction to Pharmacology and Pharmacotherapy

Gareth Zeiler and Daniel Pang

This chapter provides an overview of pharmacology, including terminology and aspects of pharmacotherapy that are important to understanding the fundamental principles of anesthesia and analgesia.

Terminology and Drug Classification Conundrum

The classification of drugs according to their clinical effect (e.g., sedatives, hypnotics, and dissociative anesthetics) is largely extrapolated from human pharmacology. The clinical effects of drugs can vary among species. This means that applying human-based classifications to animal species may not be appropriate and can cause confusion. For example, diazepam, a benzodiazepine, is classified as a hypnotic-sedative in human anesthesia, which means the more drug you administer the sleepier the human patient becomes. By contrast, when diazepam is given to healthy dogs, cats, and horses they do not become reliably sedated and there is the potential for an increase in arousal, and even excitement. Conversely, when diazepam is administered to ruminants and pigs, it causes sedation. Therefore, in this text, certain terms are defined in the context of veterinary use and not based on human medicine definitions. Many of the key terms defined in the following text are also listed in the glossary.

Anxiolysis: This is the reduction of anxiety. There are many drugs used in anesthesia that have anxiolytic effects. Anxiety is a normal physiological and emotional response to stressors. When a patient is admitted to hospital, there can be numerous stressors present: new surroundings, other animals, being caged, handling by unfamiliar people, etc. This situation creates stress and is often termed "anxiety." When anxiety is treated pharmacologically with an anxiolytic, the physiological responses of increased heart rate, arterial blood pressure, and arousal (manifested as behaviors associated with fear, nervousness, or aggression) tend to decrease, and the patient becomes calmer. This change in behavior from an anxious state to a calm and relaxed (less anxious) state is frequently confused with sedation. Anxiolysis can be applied over both the short and long terms (e.g., using behavior modification drugs) depending on the situation and goals. Tranquilization is the same as anxiolysis but with the aim of providing short-term anxiolysis for a specific situation (arrival at a veterinary facility, transportation, etc.).

Sedation: Sedation describes a decreased level of consciousness, from an awake state to a sleepy, but rousable, state. All sedative drugs also have anxiolytic properties. The key difference between sedation and anxiolysis is that sedation reflects a decrease in level of consciousness. Sedatives have been classified into two subgroups. (1) The hypnotic-sedatives cause a dose-related decrease in the level of consciousness so that, if given at high enough doses, they result in loss of consciousness (general anesthesia). (2) The tranquilizer-sedatives cause limited dose-dependent sedation so that loss of consciousness is not usually achievable.

Key Points on Pharmacology for Anesthetists

Drug formulation and how it relates to pharmacokinetic (what the body does to the drug) and pharmacodynamic (what the drug does to the body) effects are important concepts.

Fundamental Principles of Veterinary Anesthesia, First Edition. Edited by Gareth E. Zeiler and Daniel S. J. Pang.

Companion Website: www.wiley.com/go/VeterinaryAnesthesiaZeiler

Drug Formulation

There are many pharmaceutical companies that make licensed drugs. In some countries, there are also compounding pharmacies that will formulate (compound) a drug, often to a requested specification (e.g., addition of flavors to improve palatability and more concentrated solution for injection). Drugs used in the peri-anesthetic period are usually formulated for oral administration (capsules, tablets, pills, and syrups) or for injection (already constituted or requires reconstitution). Importantly, the same active ingredient (active pharmaceutical ingredient [API]) may be formulated in different concentrations. For example, in some countries, morphine is available in concentrations of 1, 5, 10, and 15 mg/mL. In addition to the active ingredient, drugs are formulated with other ingredients, called "excipients." These may include stabilizers (lactose, mannitol, and glycerol), preservatives (benzyl alcohol and phenol), chelators (ethylenediaminetetraacetic acid [EDTA], calcium, and zinc), and buffers (acetate, citrate). Therefore, despite purchasing the same active ingredient, there can be differences in the final drug product, underscoring the importance of reading the label. For example, propofol, a drug commonly used to induce general anesthesia, is available with or without a preservative. Some of the preservatives used in propofol, such as benzyl alcohol, if given at a high enough dose, can cause delayed recovery or ataxia in some species, such as cats. While it is common in some situations to combine drugs in the same syringe for injection, not all drugs are miscible and reference texts should be consulted before mixing an unfamiliar combination. With regard to oral drug formulations, they contain active ingredient(s) with fillers added to provide bulk. This means that splitting tablets not intended to be split can result in under/overdosing as it is unknown if the active ingredient is uniformly distributed throughout the tablet. Also, because pH can dramatically affect the uptake of the drug, some oral drugs are coated to prevent early breakdown in the stomach. If these drugs are crushed for administration (e.g., via a nasogastric tube or to add to a liquid), it can alter the pharmacokinetics of the drug.

Pharmacokinetics

This can be thought of as "what the body does to the drug." Drug formulation needs to be linked to this concept because drugs can be administered via several routes and absorption may be affected. The fundamental processes of pharmacokinetics are described by the acronym "ADME": Absorption (applies to drugs that are not given intravenously [IV]), Distribution, Metabolism, and Excretion. An important concept is that these processes occur simultaneously, beginning once a drug is administered, rather than one after another.

Absorption

Absorption is the process of a drug being taken up into the blood stream from the site of administration. No absorption takes place when the drug is administered intravenously because it is administered directly into the blood stream. Bioavailability of a drug is calculated by comparing a fixed dose of the drug given by the route of interest (e.g., intramuscular injection) and comparing this to intravenous administration. Plasma concentration of the drug is determined at intervals and plotted on a concentration–time graph. Bioavailability is calculated by comparing the area under the curve (AUC) for each route of administration studied against that of intravenous administration (Figure 6.1). While it may be common practice to mix drugs within a single syringe, users should be aware that not all combinations are miscible and mixing can also lead to changes in pH, with consequences for absorption.

Distribution

Distribution of a drug within the body occurs when it exits the central compartment (circulation and highly perfused organs: central nervous system [brain and spinal cord], heart, lungs, liver, and kidneys) to enter peripheral compartments. There are generally two peripheral compartments described: the muscle tissue compartment and the fat tissue compartment. A drug, when in the central compartment, will be either free or bound to plasma proteins. It is only the free fraction of drug that can move from one compartment to the other. Drug size and ionization (dependent on plasma pH) will determine how easily it moves into other compartments. Generally, drug in the free, ionized, form is highly water soluble and tends to remain within the plasma. Whereas drug in the free,

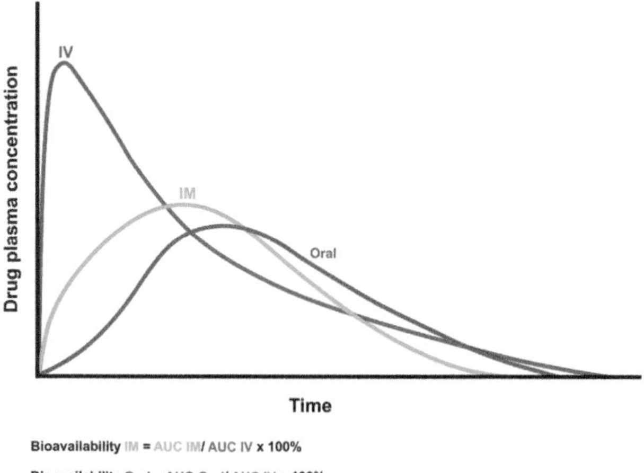

Figure 6.1 A concentration–time graph for a drug administered intravenously (IV), intramuscularly (IM), and orally (oral). The area under the curve (AUC) for each route of administration is used to calculate the bioavailability (%).

unionized, form is highly lipid soluble and can easily cross cell membranes. Furthermore, free drug is available to interact with its effect site (usually a receptor) to elicit its clinical effect. Drugs should be administered at the recommended dose to achieve a desired effect, reflected by the plasma concentration within the therapeutic window (Figure 6.2). This process of drug distribution from the plasma takes time, especially with anesthetic drugs, which must cross the blood–brain barrier before being able to interact with the target site of action (central nervous system). The time from when a drug is administered to the onset of clinical signs is called the "time to onset of action." In anesthesia, we often administer multiple drugs within a short period of time. These drugs can potentially influence drug distribution and alter the onset time of other drugs being administered. For example, alpha-2 adrenergic receptor agonists (e.g., medetomidine) decrease cardiac output, leading to a slowing in the onset of action of intravenous induction drugs (e.g., propofol) compared to when an induction drug is administered alone. Understanding the concept of time to onset of action helps in avoiding accidental drug overdoses. This explains why sufficient time should be given for a drug to take effect before deciding to administer further doses.

Metabolism

Metabolism of most drugs used during the peri-anesthetic period involves two phases of biotransformation. The liver is the major organ of biotransformation; however, biotransformation can also occur in other organs, such as the kidneys and lungs. Phase 1 (oxygenases) of liver biotransformation is the active drug undergoing oxidation to become an ionized molecule. Ionized molecules are water soluble, which allows excretion by the kidneys. Oxidation is mostly driven by specific oxygenase enzymes (CYP enzymes) manufactured by the cytochrome P450 system. These cause oxidation of carbon or oxygen within the drug molecule or dealkylation. Some breeds of animals are deficient in cytochrome P450 genes and thus cannot produce the correct enzymes required for this phase of drug metabolism. In these animals, lower doses of drugs are often required to achieve the desired clinical effect, or drugs that can be metabolized by other organs should be used. Other oxygenases also play a role in drug metabolism but often to a lesser degree than CYP enzymes. These include flavin-containing monooxygenases (oxidation of nitrogen, sulfur, or phosphorus atoms within the drug molecule) and epoxide hydrolases (hydrolysis of epoxides). Phase II (transferases) of liver biotransformation is when the ionized drug undergoes conjugation via various transferase pathways to create an unionized form of the drug. The most common pathway of conjugation is glucuronidation (UDP-glucuronosyltransferases), but other pathways, such as sulfation (sulfotransferases), acetylation (N-acetyltransferases), and glutathione (glutathione-S-transferases) conjugation, also occur. Importantly, in cats, glucuronidation is exhausted rapidly and has been suggested as the mechanism for delayed metabolism of some drugs in this species. The conjugated drug is unionized and is readily excreted with bile via the gastrointestinal tract. Drugs can be metabolized into active metabolites or inactive metabolites. Some anesthetic drugs, such as ketamine and diazepam, are metabolized into active metabolites (see Chapter 7). This needs to be considered in situations when drug excretion may be compromised or limited (e.g., renal failure).

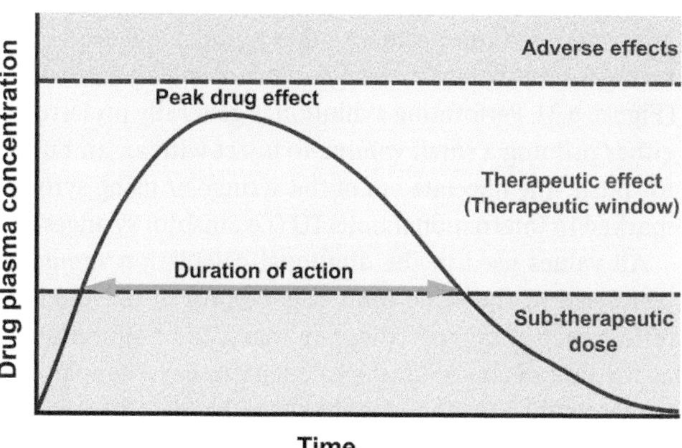

Figure 6.2 A concentration–time graph of a drug. In this example, the drug plasma concentration is enough to achieve the desired effect because it peaks within the zone of therapeutic effect without entering the adverse effect zone of the graph. When the plasma concentration enters the therapeutic effect zone, this can be considered as the onset time of effect for the drug.

Excretion

Excretion is defined as removal of drug compound from the body (including active metabolites), either via the kidneys (urine) or the liver (bile). Excretion of drug from the central compartment decreases its concentration over time as it is removed from the body. This needs to be differentiated from distribution, where the concentration of drug in the central compartment decreases but drug is not yet permanently removed from the body. As plasma concentration of the drug decreases to concentrations lower than the therapeutic window, drug effects will be reduced. "Elimination," a term sometimes incorrectly used interchangeably with "excretion," relates to how long the plasma concentration of the drug remains within the therapeutic window, able to exert the desired clinical effect. This is the "duration of action" of a drug.

Pharmacodynamics

This can be considered as "what the drug does to the body." Drugs are selected based on the ability of the active ingredient to cause a desired effect in a target organ system, such as using propofol to induce general anesthesia by interacting with gamma-aminobutyric acid A ($GABA_A$) receptors in the central nervous system. Most drugs used in veterinary anesthesia interact with more than one organ system. This manifests as both desirable and undesirable (adverse) clinical effects. For example, when propofol is administered at a recommended dose to induce general anesthesia (desired response), it also causes vasodilation (undesirable cardiovascular effect) and hypoventilation (undesirable respiratory effect). One aspect of safer provision of anesthesia is understanding both desirable and undesirable effects. Applying clinical judgment, which generally improves with practice and experience, allows users to refine drug and dose selection for different patients and contexts. The drugs that are commonly used in veterinary anesthesia, their site of action and their desirable and undesirable effects are presented in Chapters 7–10.

Important Aspects of Pharmacotherapy Related to Anesthesia

Veterinarians play a key role in the pharmaceutical value chain because they are responsible for stocking, prescribing, dispensing, and administering many drugs (see Further Reading). Briefly, the pharmaceutical value chain includes all activities that occur between the point when a medicine is manufactured and shipped from a production or import facility until it is used to treat a patient. Pharmacotherapy requires an understanding of drugs and how they meet the desired goals of the anesthetic event, combined with an understanding of the patient and its response to the drugs. Additionally, veterinarians should understand the effects of drug mixing. Other aspects of pharmacotherapy, such as pharmacogenomics and pharmacovigilance, should also be considered.

Alterations to Drugs

Three common alterations to drugs are diluting, altering dose form (reformulating), and dividing. These are frequently performed to facilitate accurate administration because animals range in size from a few grams to hundreds of kilograms. Veterinarians must observe local laws and regulations in the region of practice because altering a commercial (or compounded) drug may be illegal under certain circumstances. Drug alteration is an act of compounding (tailoring a drug to patient needs), and the responsibility (and risks associated with adverse reactions) rests with the prescribing veterinarian. Therefore, fundamental principles of compounding should be followed to minimize the occurrence of adverse effects or decreased efficacy.

Dilution of a Drug

Dilution of injectable drugs is a common practice when treating smaller patients. Examples of different techniques of dilution will be presented. Understanding the orders of magnitude and percentage concentration facilitates swift and accurate calculations. It is assumed readers are familiar with the following:

- 1000 mcg in 1 mg
- 1000 mg in 1 g
- 1000 mL in 1 L
- a 1% solution of drug is equivalent to 10 mg/mL

Note that to covert a % solution (i.e., "how many parts per 100") to mg/mL simply multiply the % value by 10.

Before diluting a drug, every effort should be made to ensure that an existing formulation of the desired concentration is not already available (from a pharmaceutical company or compounding pharmacy) or that an acceptable alternative drug is unavailable. As a general guideline, dilution of a drug should only be performed if the injection volume of the undiluted drug is less than 0.1 mL. If dilution is required, then consider using appropriately graduated (ideally in 0.01 mL increments) syringes with concentric plungers (or other types of low dead space syringes) or tuberculin syringes, with a small gauge needle (Figure 6.3). Performing a dilution is generally preferred to either priming a small volume to inject with an air bubble to "push" the injectate out of the syringe or using syringes marked in international units IU (i.e., insulin syringes).

All values used in the dilutional calculation should be converted to the same unit. It is helpful to use the dose (either mcg or mg) per kilogram that is to be administered as the unit of choice for the calculation. For example, dexmedetomidine is often dosed in mcg/kg (e.g., 10 mcg/kg), but the injectable drug is presented in mg/mL. Therefore, before calculating the volume to inject, one of the two units must be converted. As per the recommendation in the preceding text, if the dose per kg is used as the unit of choice, then the drug concentration must be converted from mg/mL to mcg/mL (i.e., multiply mg/mL by 1000 to get mcg/mL). If a dilution of an injectable drug is performed, then a 10× dilution is a useful technique to facilitate calculations.

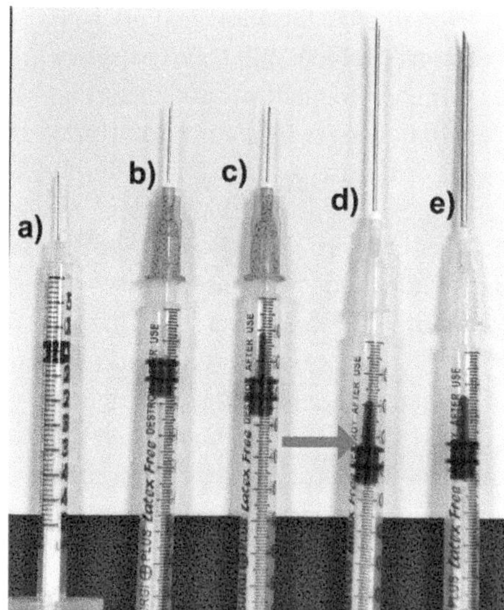

Figure 6.3 Different 1 mL syringes that can be used for diluting injectable drugs: (a) a tuberculin syringe with a 26 G (gauge) needle already affixed, (b) a 1 mL syringe with no concentric plunger and a 25 G needle attached, (c) a 1 mL syringe with a concentric plunger and a 25 G needle attached, (d) a 1 mL syringe with a concentric plunger (blue arrow) and a 21 G needle attached, and (e) a 1 mL syringe with concentric plunger with an 18 G needle attached. The correct selection for mixing small volumes of drugs and to perform a 10× dilution would be either syringe (b) or (c). The needle from syringe (a) cannot be removed, preventing the dilution procedure described in the text. Syringes (d) and (e) are the correct volume syringes, but the needles are inappropriate for puncturing multidose vials (breakdown of the rubber stopper) and injecting small patients. (*Source:* Photos prepared by Pebble Rock Media.)

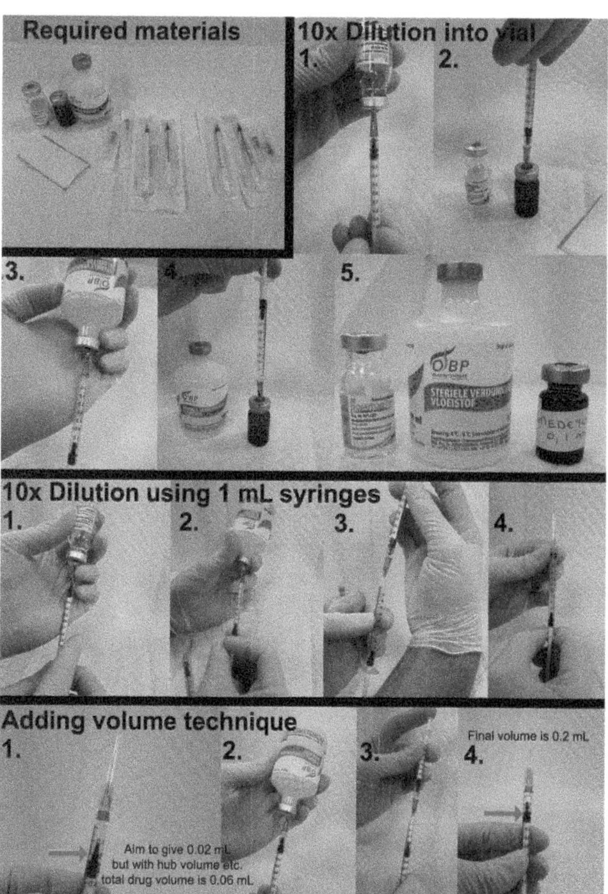

Figure 6.4 A stepwise photo guide to diluting an injectable drug using the "10× dilution" technique or the "adding volume" technique. See text for description.

Worked Example of Injectable Drug Dilution

Case: A healthy, six-month-old, Yorkshire terrier of 2 kg body mass presents for ovariohysterectomy. A combination of methadone (dose of 0.2 mg/kg, intramuscularly [IM]) and medetomidine (dose of 10 mcg/kg, IM) is prescribed for pre-anesthetic sedation. Figure 6.4 demonstrates the dilution techniques discussed in this worked example.

Step 1: Calculate the volumes to be injected using the following drug information: methadone, 10 mg/mL; medetomidine, 1 mg/mL.

Methadone dose: 0.2 mg/kg × 2 kg = 0.4 mg

Methadone volume to inject: 0.4 mg/10 mg/mL = 0.04 mL

Medetomidine dose: 10 mcg/kg × 2 kg = 20 mcg

Convert drug concentration to dose unit: 1 mg/mL × 1000 mcg/mg = 1000 mcg/mL

Medetomidine volume to inject: 20 mcg/1000 mcg/mL = 0.02 mL

Step 2: Decide if dilution is required.
Both drug volumes are under the recommended 0.1 mL injection volume. As discussed later, these drugs are mixed into a single syringe for IM injection. Thus, the methadone volume of 0.04 mL could be considered high enough that once the diluted medetomidine is added to the methadone syringe the total injectate volume would be above 0.1 mL. Therefore, in this example, only medetomidine requires dilution.

Step 3: Performing the dilution.
There are two commonly used techniques: a "10× dilution" or "adding volume." The preferred technique is a simple 10× dilution. The diluent that is used can be sterile water for injection or normal saline (i.e., 0.9% NaCl). Other isotonic crystalloids used for intravenous injection (e.g., lactated Ringer's solution) are generally not recommended for drug dilution because they can contain ions (e.g., ionized calcium or magnesium) that can react with the drug (see Further Reading). Good practice standards should be followed by using aseptic technique when performing the dilution.

Procedure for performing a "10× dilution" using a rubber top sterile vial (or any suitable container, such as a 1 mL syringe):

1) Withdraw 0.1 mL of medetomidine (1 mg/mL) using a 1 mL syringe and small gauge needle (24–26 G) and inject into vial.

2) Withdraw 0.9 mL of diluent (preferably sterile water for injection) using a separate 1 mL syringe and small gauge needle (24–26 G) and inject into vial.
3) With both, the injectate should not be "forced" or "blown" out of the syringe because additional volume (up to 0.1 mL) could inadvertently be added to the mixture.
4) Gently swirl or roll the vial on a flat surface to mix well.
5) Mark the date of when the dilution is prepared, the drug name, and new concentration (0.1 mg/mL or 100 mcg/mL).

A further method, described here for completeness, but not recommended, is the practice of "adding volume" to create a dilution. In this technique, the calculated drug volume is drawn into a 1 mL syringe (e.g., 0.02 mL of medetomidine in the preceding example). A second syringe is used to withdraw a small volume of diluent (e.g., 0.1 mL). Then, the plunger of the syringe containing medetomidine is pulled back to about the 0.4 mL mark and the needle is removed. The diluent is then slowly injected into the medetomidine syringe. Finally, the syringe is held vertically (plunger at the bottom) and air bubbles expelled. This technique is not recommended because (1) 1 mL syringes are not accurate enough when withdrawing volumes of less than 0.1 mL, (2) a large amount of dead space in the hub of the needle and lure of the syringe (can amount to 0.1 mL) can make the dilution inaccurate, and (3) while moving the plunger of the drug syringe the small volume of drug can be accidently lost.

Step 4: Calculating the new volume of injection based on the diluted drug.

Medetomidine dose: 10 mcg/kg × 2 kg = 20 mcg

Drug dilution concentration: 0.1 mg/mL

Convert drug to dose unit: 0.1 mg/mL × 1000 mcg/mg = 100 mcg/mL

Medetomidine volume to inject: 20 mcg/100 mcg/mL = 0.2 mL

The new total injection volume is 0.24 mL (0.2 mL medetomidine + 0.04 mL methadone), which is below the maximum recommended 0.25 mL/kg volume for IM injection in dogs. A good tip is to calculate the maximum recommended volume for injection (see later) and then to ensure that the 10× dilution does not exceed this recommendation. If the new volume of injection exceeds this recommendation, then a 5× dilution could be used instead (i.e., 0.1 mL drug and 0.4 mL of diluent is added). Doing this with the worked example: a 5× dilution would give a concentration of 0.2 mg/mL and an injectate volume of 0.1 mL.

Altering Dose Form (Reformulation)

Drugs for oral administration are mainly presented as tablets, pills, capsules, pastes, or syrups. Pastes and syrups are generally in a low enough concentration that altering the dose form is unnecessary. Tablets, pills, and capsules are often presented as a higher concentration per unit and if used in animals less than 5 kg may require some form of alteration. These oral drugs are usually altered to liquid, syrup, or paste form using a diluent. This can be sterile water for injection, edible oils (sunflower oil), syrups (cherry or raspberry flavored), or pastes (liver pâté). Another reason for altering the dose form is not to create a manageable dose but to change the presentation to allow administration through a feeding tube (nasogastric, esophagostomy, gastric, etc.). Sometimes, crushing a tablet and mixing it into a syrup is a method used to try to increase patient compliance in accepting an oral medicine. Before attempting reformulation, a pharmacist (or a pharmaceutical textbook on compounding) should be consulted to select an appropriate diluent. Any change in the presented drug form is essentially creating a new drug. A change may alter palatability (animals will foam from the mouth or hypersalivate after administration, especially cats) or pharmacokinetics (especially the absorption characteristic, which can render the drug ineffective). Any oral drug that is specifically designed to be slow (or sustained or steady) release should not be altered because under- or overdosing can occur. Generally, water-soluble drugs can be diluted in water-based diluents (water for injection or syrups that have a high water content), and lipid-soluble drugs can be diluted in edible oils.

When performing reformulation, aseptic technique should be followed, and accurate equipment should be used to measure diluent (i.e., use a syringe for liquids and a scale for syrups and pastes). Before dilution is performed, the final administration volume must be considered to ensure it is appropriate for the patient (see later). An excessive volume will be difficult to administer, especially if the palatability of the medication is altered. Therefore, calculating the total volume should be determined when planning reformulation. When crushing tablets, pills, or opening capsules, the entire amount should be included in the reformulation or dilution. Once the reformulation is complete, the bottle should be labeled with key information: patient details, date of reformulation, expiry date, contents, concentration per mL, and any information required in the region of practice. Compounding an oral drug must be done for an individual patient. It is illegal to mass compound drugs for multiple patients in most countries.

Division of a Drug

This applies to oral drugs that are presented in a solid form such as tablets (pills) and capsules (see Further

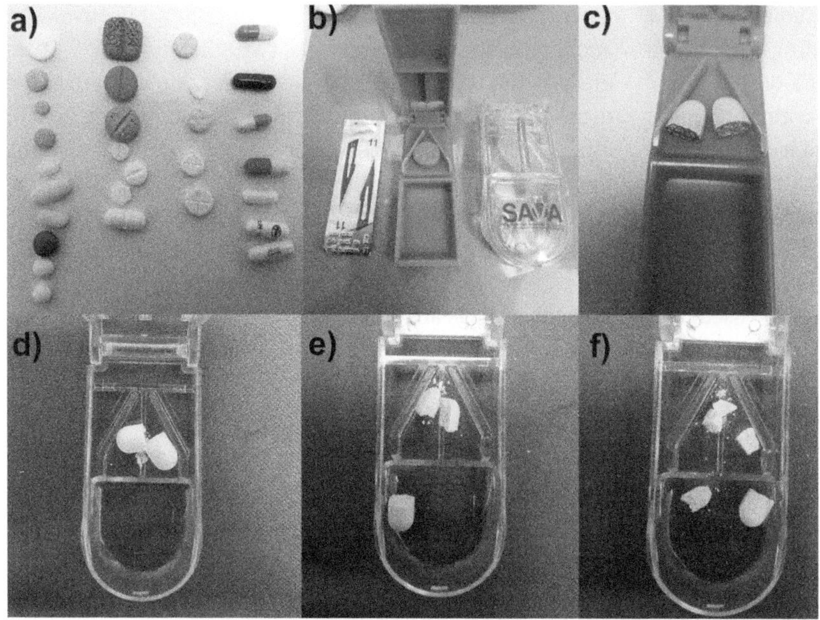

Figure 6.5 A collection of different pills, tablets, and capsules that can be used for oral administration of drugs (a). From the left-hand column are examples of unscored pills and tables, the second column are tablets and pills with one score line, the third column are tablets with two score lines, and the fourth column are examples of capsules. (b) Different tools to divide a pill or tablet. Left is a scalpel blade, and middle and right are examples of pill cutters. (c) An unscored pill being divided using a pill cutter; note that this is a coated tablet and that the content is brown. This is one of the reasons to not divide a tablet or pill that is not scored because the loss of coating can alter pharmacokinetic properties (especially absorption) that can result in altered pharmacodynamic response. (d) A pill is cut along its score line. (e) Half the pill is cut but not along a score line. (f) The quarter pill is cut. Note how it is starting to crush and become powder; therefore, pills and tablets should not be cut more times than there are score lines. (*Source:* Courtesy of Valley Farm Animal Hospital).

Reading). Tablets may be scored to facilitate splitting (Figure 6.5). Using a divider (blade encased in a hardened shell) is the preferred method of dividing a tablet or pill. Other methods include using a scalpel blade or knife. The aim is to minimally handle the drug while performing division. If there is no score line marked, this could indicate that the drug is sugar-coated or enterically coated and should not be divided. Doing so might alter the palatability or absorption kinetics, or both. Scoring can indicate the smallest division that ensures predictable drug distribution within each defined section (i.e., splitting into smaller segments may not result in even drug distribution). Pills and tablets that require further division than the indicated scoring should perhaps be reformulated (see the preceding text).

Division of capsules is more complex because the active ingredient is mixed with a filler and they are often in powder form of the same color, so it is impossible to differentiate drug from filler (Figure 6.6). Therefore, in these cases, referral to a pharmacy for capsule division is recommended. However, as a last resort, performing a reformulation (see the preceding text) may be a better approach than trying to divide capsule contents.

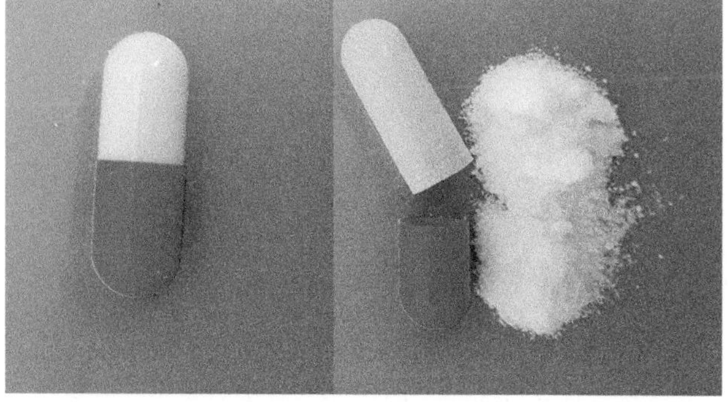

Figure 6.6 A capsule before opening (left-hand figure) and after opening to reveal its content (right-hand figure). Note that the powder is white. This is made up of active drug, excipients, and fillers to provide bulk. Capsules cannot be reliably divided into smaller doses because the active drug cannot be differentiated from excipients and fillers. (*Source:* Courtesy of Valley Farm Animal Hospital.)

Drug Mixing

The mixing of two or more drugs into a single syringe (or vial or infusion) is an act of compounding. An important consideration with this practice is the relative lack of pharmacokinetic and pharmacodynamic studies of drug mixtures. For practical reasons, mixing of drugs will continue to be practiced in veterinary medicine despite this limitation. In anesthesia, for example, it is a common practice to mix drugs used during the pre-anesthetic period into a single syringe for IM injection; or a combination of drugs may be infused IV during anesthesia maintenance and recovery; or drugs may be infused (or injected as boluses) IV together with an isotonic crystalloid fluid. There are common drug combinations that have been used in veterinary anesthesia that are (seemingly) effective. The stability of these drug mixtures (whether combined drugs are miscible, if combining drugs causes one or more of the drugs to come out of solution) has not been investigated for almost all combinations and it is unknown for how long they can be stored. Similarly, little is known about solution stability of drugs presented in a vial for reconstitution. In some cases, instead of using the diluent recommended on the package insert (often sterile water for injection), other injectable drugs are used (Table 6.1).

Table 6.1 Examples of injectable drug combinations used during the peri-anesthetic period.

Peri-anesthetic period	Drug combination	Notes
Drug mixtures in common use		
Premedication	Opioid + acepromazine	Mixed in a syringe before injection
	Opioid + alpha-2 adrenergic receptor agonist	Mixed in a syringe before injection
	Opioid + benzodiazepine	Mixed in a syringe before injection
Induction (IM)	Ketamine + alpha-2 adrenergic receptor agonist (+opioid)	Common drug combinations for intramuscular injection to chemically immobilize or anesthetize a companion animal
	Tiletamine–zolazepam + alpha-2 adrenergic receptor agonist (+opioid)	
	Alfaxalone + alpha-2 adrenergic receptor agonist (+opioid)	
Induction (IV)	Ketamine + diazepam	Mixed in a syringe before injection
	Propofol or alfaxalone + lidocaine	Lidocaine (2 mg/kg) is usually given first, at least a minute before injecting the induction drug. Flushing the IV port using 0.9% saline is used. Avoid this combination in dogs that are bradycardic.
	Propofol or alfaxalone + benzodiazepine	The benzodiazepines (diazepam or midazolam; 0.2–0.4 mg/kg) can cause increased arousal in dogs, cats, and horses. Many users will give a small dose of induction agent (one-quarter of calculated dose), followed by full calculated dose of benzodiazepine, to minimize risk of excitement, then induction drug to effect. Flushing the IV port with 0.9% saline between different drug administration is recommended
	Propofol or alfaxalone + fentanyl or hydromorphone	Fentanyl (5–10 mcg/kg) or hydromorphone (0.1–0.2 mg/kg) are administered 2–5 min before the induction drug. Flushing the IV port with 0.9% saline between different drug administration is recommended
Maintenance	Propofol + fentanyl (+midazolam)	Total or partial intravenous combinations mixed in syringes for infusion or in intravenous fluid solution like 0.9% saline
	Alfaxalone + fentanyl (+midazolam)	
	Ketamine + fentanyl (+midazolam)	
Recovery	Morphine + lidocaine + ketamine	MLK and FLK can also be used during maintenance as part of balanced anesthesia
	Fentanyl + lidocaine + ketamine	
Drug mixtures reported for inducing general anesthesia		
Induction	Propofol + ketamine	Mixed into a single syringe and injected to effect
	Propofol + thiopental	
Powdered drugs for reconstitution		
Induction	Ketamine, or tiletamine–zolazepam powder for reconstitution, is mixed with medetomidine (+midazolam), (+butorphanol), and (+other opioid)	Many mixtures have been proposed, especially for mass sterilization campaigns in dogs and cats. The advantage is simple dosing of a fixed volume/kg. The disadvantage is that the combination does not allow alterations in drug dosing and stability of the mixture is unknown

Fundamental Principles of Drug Mixing

- Drug mixing should not be considered a routine practice but used when necessary, and the benefit to the animal outweighs the risk of an adverse effect or lack of efficacy (e.g., a single IM injection of a drug combination is better than repeated injections; if the drugs are administered IV, then, instead of mixing, they can be injected separately, flushing the IV injection port between injections).
- Most drugs are not readily miscible.
- Only mix drugs with a similar pH. Mixing an acidic drug with an alkaline drug will cause the mixture to precipitate (e.g., atropine and thiopentone, and furosemide and midazolam). Lack of macroscopic evidence of a precipitate forming (such as a cloudy appearance) does not guarantee that no microscopic crystallization has occurred.
- If drugs are mixed into a single syringe for premedication by IM injection (for example), then each individual drug should be drawn into their own syringe before mixing into the final syringe for injection. This is performed to prevent contamination of vials whereby drugs drawn one after the other can be accidently injected into the subsequent vials. Furthermore, dosing errors are more common, especially if three (or more) drugs are drawn into a single syringe one after the other.
- Only reconstitute powered drugs to concentrations known to be stable (e.g., ketamine is stable up to 150 mg/mL at room temperature).
- If powered drugs are reconstituted with a diluent other than that indicated, then the solution contents should be listed on the labeling with the date of formulation.
- Only mix drugs that are at room temperature and, before administration, examine the mixture for precipitate formation.
- Once drugs are mixed, they should be administered within 15 minutes. Evidence that some mixtures remain stable when kept refrigerated is largely anecdotal.
- While it is common for drugs to be added to isotonic crystalloid solutions being delivered IV, this is best avoided with polyionic solutions, especially those containing calcium (a common cause of precipitation). In many instances, 0.9% sodium chloride (NaCl) solution is the only acceptable crystalloid fluid for this purpose. In general, it is preferable to either deliver a drug infusion IV in the appropriate diluent (e.g., sterile water) or, if 0.9% NaCl is to be used as the diluent, to prepare a small volume (e.g., 100 mL bag) to minimize the risk of creating hyperchloremic acidosis (associated with large volumes of 0.9% NaCl).
- To reliably deliver a small-volume IV drug infusion, it is simplest to use an electronic infusion pump or syringe driver.

Principles of Drug Administration During the Peri-anesthetic Period

During the peri-anesthetic period, animals are given a number of drugs in a short period of time. Before selecting which drugs to use, some principles need to be considered. (1) The animal may have already been given other drugs (not necessarily related to anesthesia, e.g., antimicrobial, behavior modifiers) that could cause a drug–drug interaction (DDI). (2) Consider the most appropriate route of drug administration, taking into account the time of onset of effect, desired outcome, and animal temperament. (3) The total volume of drug administered should be considered, especially if drugs are prepared for very small animals (as discussed in the preceding text).

Drug Interactions

Drug interactions that are important in veterinary anesthesia encompass drug–drug interactions, and this should not be confused with drug mixing as discussed in the preceding text. DDIs are when two or more drugs are given and there is some form of interaction. There are four types of DDI that can occur: (1) alteration in physicochemical properties, (2) alteration in pharmacokinetics (mainly absorption, distribution, and metabolism), (3) alteration in pharmacodynamics (mainly antagonism, synergism, and additive effects), and (4) creation of toxicity. In anesthesia, intentional DDIs are mostly pharmacodynamic interactions. These include an intent to decrease the amount of drug used to induce and maintain anesthesia (synergistic and additive effects), and antagonizing (reversal) the effects of drugs with an antagonist. DDIs may occur from other substances administered around the time of anesthesia. In some instances, these may not be considered drugs (e.g., herbal treatments, nutraceuticals, and unusual diet items, such as grapefruit), emphasizing the importance of a full history. Common examples of DDIs relevant to the peri-anesthetic period are summarized in Table 6.2.

Drug Administration Volumes

Drugs that are administered orally, subcutaneously, intramuscularly, intraperitoneally, and intravenously need to be given at volumes that are safe and effective for the species. If the volume is too small it may be lost during administration (accidently pushing a syringe plunger and discharging the drug before the needle has been positioned

Table 6.2 Examples of drug–drug interactions that can occur during the peri-anesthetic period.

Drug A	Drug B	Comment
Alterations in physicochemical properties		
Thiopentone	Atropine	Cannot mix because of an acid–base pH reaction causing macroscopic precipitation of crystals. Adequate flushing of IV injection port is required between drug administration
Pentobarbital	Penicillin (most formulations)	Cause precipitate to form, and do not mix or use same IV injection port
Calcium gluconate	Many	Can clause microthrombus formation if injected with citrated blood products. Causes chelation and possible crystallization (fluroquinolone antimicrobials, dobutamine, metoclopramide, methylprednisolone, etc.)
Lactated Ringer's solution	Ciprofloxacin, cyclosporine, diazepam, ketamine, lorazepam, nitroglycerin, phenytoin, propofol, and citrated blood products	Cause precipitate or microthrombus formation with citrated blood products
Oral antacids or chelating agents	Many oral drugs	Cause chelation and decreased absorption or altered absorption if gastric pH is different that intended for the drug
Heparin	Aminoglycoside or beta-lactam antimicrobials, benzodiazepines, and morphine	Cause precipitate formation. Do not use "heparin saline flushes" if administering these drugs intravenously
Altered pharmacokinetics		
Alpha-2 adrenergic receptor agonist	Any other drug given IV during the peri-anesthetic period	Decreased cardiac output and blood flow through organs responsible for drug distribution and metabolism. Must account for this to avoid risk of overdose
Cimetidine	Theophylline	Cimetidine causes inhibition of P450 system activity, specifically CYP 2EI and 2C9, which slow substrate phase I biotransformation. A potential concern in patients treated for respiratory illness being given theophylline
Chloramphenicol	Phenobarbital or propofol	Chloramphenicol causes inhibition of P450 system activity, specifically CYP 3A4 inhibition, which can prolong the elimination half-life of both these drugs
Fluroquinolone antimicrobials	Theophylline	Fluroquinolone antimicrobials cause inhibition of P450 system activity, specifically CYP 1A2 inhibition, which slows substrate phase I biotransformation. A potential concern in patients treated for respiratory illness with theophylline
Ketoconazole	Midazolam	Ketoconazole causes inhibition of P450 system activity, specifically CYP 3A12, which can prolong the half-life of midazolam (and possibly other benzodiazepines)
Phenobarbital	Many drugs	Phenobarbital causes induction of P450 system, which can accelerate metabolism of many drugs
Altered pharmacodynamics		
Examples presented here are to highlight unintended/undesirable combinations. This contrasts with desired synergistic, additive, and antagonist effects (see text and Chapter 7).		
Alpha-2 adrenergic receptor agonist	Anticholinergic drug	Anticholinergic administration causes further hypertension and increased myocardial work, with the risk of cardiac arrhythmias
Angiotensin-converting enzyme inhibits	Acepromazine, propofol, and inhalational anesthetics	Can cause profound vasodilation that results in hypotension that can be difficult to manage
Butorphanol	*Mu* opioid receptor agonists (e.g., morphine, methadone, and fentanyl)	If butorphanol is administered first, then the effect of a subsequent dose of a *mu* opioid receptor agonist is diminished. Either a higher dose of the *mu* opioid receptor agonists needs to be administered or a dose given 60–90 min after butorphanol administration
Creation of toxicity		
NSAID	Corticosteroid	Can result in gastrointestinal ulcerations and perforation, especially in dogs

NSAID: nonsteroidal anti-inflammatory drug.

Table 6.3 Acceptable and maximum (in parentheses) volumes (mL/kg) for drug administration.

Species	Oral	Subcutaneous	Intraperitoneal	Intramuscular	Intravenously
Companion animals					
Dog[a]	5 (15)	1 (2)	1 (20)	0.25 (0.5)	2.5 (5)
Cat[b]	10 (15)	2 (5)	5 (20)	0.25 (0.5)	5 (10)
Horse	–	<15 (20)[c]	–	<10 (20)[c]	<10 (20)[c]
Production animals					
Cattle	–	–	–	<10 (20)[c]	<10 (20)[c]
Small ruminants	–	–	–	<10 (20)[c]	<10 (20)[c]
Pig	–	–	–	<10 (20)[c]	<10 (20)[c]
Exotic or small laboratory mammals					
Rat[a]	10 (40)	5 (10)	10 (20)	0.1 (0.2)	5 (20)
Mouse[a]	10 (50)	10 (40)	20 (80)	0.05 (0.1)	2 (25)
Rabbit[a]	10 (15)	1 (2)	5 (20)	0.25 (0.5)	2 (10)

[a] Petrie and Wallace (2015).
[b] Recommended dose volumes for common laboratory animals; IQ 3Rs Leadership Group–Contract Research Organization Working Group (https://iqconsortium.org/initiatives/leadership-groups/3rs-translational-and-predictive-sciences).
[c] Total milliliters per injection site.

for injection), and if the volume is too large it could inadvertently cause physiological changes (e.g., hemodilution) or cause harm (e.g., muscle damage if a large volume is injected at a single IM site). Acceptable and maximum daily cumulative volumes are reported in Table 6.3.

Principles of Induction of General Anesthesia Using an Intravenous Drug

Traditionally, a single intravenous induction drug is administered to achieve an unconscious state (anesthesia) and allow tracheal intubation. Another induction technique is to use two (or more) drugs in combination, known as a "co-induction technique" (described later). Following induction, anesthesia is most commonly maintained with an inhalational anesthetic. Achieving a smooth transition from intravenous induction of anesthesia to maintenance with an inhalational anesthetic requires a sufficient concentration of inhalational drug in the brain to maintain anesthesia before the anesthetic effects of injectable drugs dissipate. Chapters 8 and 5 cover inhalational anesthetics and their delivery methods, respectively.

The IV induction drug must cross the blood–brain barrier to reach the target receptors within the brain to induce anesthesia; therefore, these drugs are highly lipid soluble. Drugs that move across this barrier and interact with their target receptor more quickly, such as thiopental, require one or two blood volume circulations to reach their peak effect. In a resting patient with normal cardiac output, the entire circulating blood volume will travel throughout the body 2–4 times per minute which is every 15–30 s. This means, for these drugs, after a single bolus, 15–30 s should be allowed to pass before deciding on administering additional boluses. Drugs that have a slower interaction at their target receptor, such as propofol or alfaxalone, require more time to take effect, up to 40–60 s for an induction bolus to take effect. Changes in cardiac output will alter the onset of action of the IV drugs: a low cardiac output results in a slowed circulation so that more time is required for drug to reach the brain (and vice versa for a high cardiac output state). Alpha-2 adrenergic receptor agonists, which are commonly used for premedication, profoundly decrease cardiac output, meaning that the time to desired effect of the IV induction drug bolus will be significantly delayed (approximately two times longer). Speed of induction is an important aspect to consider. Animals that are at a high risk of regurgitation and aspirating, or when rapid control of the airway is desired, require a faster induction, with the aim of securing the airway quicker.

The time to allow tracheal intubation when using common induction drugs are:
Thiopentone ≪ propofol, etomidate, and alfaxalone ≪ ketamine

In a co-induction technique, two or more drugs are given within a short space of time (usually less than 1–2 min) or, less preferred, mixed together for administration. A primary induction drug (e.g., propofol, alfaxalone, and ketamine) is administered and followed by a second drug. The additional drug(s) is selected because it (1) has muscle relaxation properties, (2) lowers the overall dose of the primary drug, or (3) minimizes the response to tracheal intubation (e.g., cough, increased intracranial pressure, increased intraocular pressure, and increased arterial blood pressure).

In some cases, two primary induction drugs are mixed into a single syringe (thiopentone + propofol, colloquially known as "thiofol"; ketamine + propofol, colloquially known as "ketofol"). This practice is not advocated until good-quality evidence of mixture stability is available. A further concern with mixing two induction drugs together is the lack of evidence for how much of each drug is added to the mixture.

Principles of Using Injectable Drugs During Maintenance of Anesthesia

When the goal is to prolong the anesthetic period beyond that of the effect of the induction drug, additional drug(s) is given to maintain anesthesia. Maintenance of anesthesia begins once drug(s) used for induction of anesthesia has decreased in plasma concentration to a level below the therapeutic window. The simplest approach is a single drug to be administered. This can be an inhalational drug (see Chapter 8) or an injectable drug (see Chapter 7). Additionally, the concepts of "balanced anesthesia" and "multimodal analgesia" are important to understand when planning a general anesthetic. These concepts are discussed again in species-specific chapters and the chapter on pain (see Chapter 3). Understanding these concepts facilitates rational drug selection.

Balanced Anesthesia

Balanced anesthesia is the concept of using more than one drug, each at a lower dosage than required if used alone, to achieve one or more of the goals of general anesthesia. The intent is to reduce adverse effects and the potential accumulation or toxicity produced by large doses of a single anesthetic drug, while still providing all the desirable effects of general anesthesia. Drugs administered during the premedication period can have an effect during the anesthetic maintenance period, thus contributing to balanced anesthesia. For example, premedicating with dexmedetomidine and methadone will decrease the requirement of both the injectable induction agent (e.g., propofol) and the inhalational anesthetic for maintaining anesthesia (e.g., isoflurane), by providing CNS depression and analgesia.

Multimodal Analgesia

Multimodal analgesia is the concept of using two or more drugs that act through different mechanisms to produce analgesia (see Chapter 3). For example, a dog undergoing ovariohysterectomy could be given a nonsteroidal anti-inflammatory drug to decrease the inflammatory response at the incision site and an opioid, which modulates the pain signal as it enters the spinal cord and alters the perception of pain in the brain. Multimodal analgesia also has the benefit of decreasing anesthetic drug requirement though its use is not restricted to during anesthesia.

Concept of Minimum Alveolar Concentration and Minimum Infusion Rate

Minimum alveolar concentration (MAC) is defined as the expired alveolar concentration of an inhalational anesthetic drug, when administered alone, that produces immobility in 50% of patients undergoing a standard supramaximal nociceptive stimulus at a pressure of 1 atmosphere (see Chapter 8). Similar in concept to MAC, *minimum infusion rate* (MIR) is defined as the minimum infusion rate (the dose of drug administered over a time period, usually in mg/kg/min or mg/kg/h) of an injectable anesthetic drug, when administered alone, that produces immobility in 50% of patients undergoing a standard supramaximal nociceptive stimulus.

Techniques of Administering Drugs to Maintain Anesthesia

There are three different techniques that can be used to maintain anesthesia: (1) inhalational, (2) partial intravenous anesthesia (PIVA), and (3) total intravenous anesthesia (TIVA) techniques.

The inhalational technique is where an inhalational drug is administered alone to maintain anesthesia. To achieve balanced anesthesia, the animal is given drugs during the premedication period to decrease the MAC and provide analgesia (not a property of inhalational drugs in current use).

The PIVA technique was originally described with anesthesia maintained using a combination of an inhalational anesthetic and an injectable anesthetic (i.e., propofol, alfaxalone, ketamine, etc.) infused intravenously to reduce the required concentration of the inhalational drug (MAC reduction). Reducing inhalational drug concentration has the benefit of reducing its adverse effects. PIVA has also come to include the IV infusion of analgesic drugs throughout the anesthetic maintenance period in order to achieve MAC reduction (see Further Reading). In most species, opioids, alpha-2 adrenergic receptor agonists, benzodiazepines, and lidocaine are used alone, or in various combinations, as an infusion. If an infusion is not possible, then boluses of these drugs can be given. This latter method is less preferred because of the pharmacodynamic response during fluctuations in plasma concentration. For example, a bolus of ketamine can result in a transient period of apnea; a bolus of medetomidine can cause a baroreceptor-mediated bradycardia secondary to decreased cardiac output; and a bolus of an opioid can cause a vagally mediated bradycardia and apnea.

The TIVA technique is, in its simplest form, delivery of an injectable anesthetic drug (e.g., propofol, alfaxalone, or ketamine) to maintain general anesthesia. There are three methods of delivering TIVA: (1) a bolus technique (with intermittent injections), (2) an IV infusion (continuous infusion of the primary anesthetic, or drug combination, with the infusion rate adjusted according to depth of anesthesia), and (3) a target-controlled infusion (TCI) (continuous infusion of primary anesthetic drug according to targeted plasma or effect site concentration). As with the inhalational technique, a combination of drugs is commonly used to decrease the MIR of the primary anesthetic drug and provide analgesia.

Intermittent Hand Bolus Technique

Intermittent hand boluses to "top-up" the primary anesthetic drug are administered when the plane of general anesthesia is deemed too light (see Chapter 2) or at set time intervals. Generally, one-quarter to one-third of the initial induction dose is used as a "top-up" dose. The advantage of this technique is that it is simple and does not require an infusion pump. The disadvantage of this technique is that the desired and adverse effects of the drug wax and wane according to fluctuations in plasma concentration. Generally, this technique is acceptable for short-term anesthesia that is not expected to last longer than 30 min. Endotracheal intubation is recommended in most cases for the many advantages associated with a secure airway.

Intravenous Infusion Technique

An IV infusion is when a drug is administered continuously, initially at a predetermined infusion rate. The initial rate is adjusted according to the response of the animal in achieving the desired anesthetic depth. Ideally, the primary anesthetic drug should be infused alone, via a dedicated IV catheter, to allow for titration to clinical response. Drugs that are added to provide analgesia and decrease the MIR can be infused either alone (preferably) or as a mixture (practical, but limits individual drug titration), preferably via a second intravenous catheter (often the one through which peri-anesthetic fluids are administered). Ideally, electronic infusion devices or electronic syringe drivers should be used to ensure an accurate continuous infusion of drugs. However, gravity fluid administration sets can be used when necessary. See Concept Box 5.1 for an example of how to calculate and plan for a propofol–fentanyl TIVA in a dog.

Concept Box 5.1

Worked example of a total intravenous anesthesia (TIVA) drug protocol administered by infusion in a dog.

The first consideration is drug selection. A primary drug that can induce and maintain anesthesia is required. Then, additional drugs can be infused to decrease the infusion rate of the primary drug. In dogs, propofol is a common primary anesthetic drug that is administered by infusion to maintain anesthesia. The infusion dose range of propofol is 0.1–0.6 mg/kg/min (6–36 mg/kg/h). Fentanyl is an example of an additional drug that could be infused to decrease the propofol requirement. In this example, a propofol–fentanyl combination will be used for infusion.

Step 1: Decide if the drugs can be mixed together or in a solution for administration.

The advantage of mixing drugs in a single syringe or infusion bag is that less equipment is required. However, the major disadvantages are that the drugs are administered at a fixed dose ratio and cannot be individually titrated to effect, and the stability of drug mixtures is not known. These disadvantages often outweigh the advantages. Another important consideration is whether a drug will be used in other periods of the peri-anesthetic event. In this case, providing continued analgesia in the recovery period can be desirable; therefore fentanyl should be administered separately. In this example, fentanyl will be infused using an electronic syringe driver and propofol will be mixed into an isotonic crystalloid fluid for infusion to demonstrate the mathematics of both types of commonly used infusion techniques.

Step 2: Calculating infusion rates and volumes to be drawn up for administration.

The patient's body weight is 15 kg. There are 3 equations that are required to calculate drug volume:

$$\text{Volume to be infused per hour} = \text{Body weight} \times \text{dose rate per hour/drug concentration} \quad (1)$$

$$\text{Volume of drug that should be drawn up} = \text{Volume to be infused per hour} \times \text{hours of constant rate infusion} \quad (2)$$

It is common to prepare additional drug anticipating that the procedure may take longer than expected e.g., 30–50% additional.

Equation (3) can be used to calculate the additional drug volume.

$$\text{Volume of drug that should be drawn up} = \text{Volumeto be infused per hour} \times \text{hours of variable rate infusion} + 30\%\ (\text{x}1.3) \text{ to } 50\%\ (\times 1.5) \quad (3)$$

(Continued)

Box 5.1 (Continued)

Fentanyl will be delivered by constant rate infusion and Equations (1) and (2) apply.

Fentanyl is often initially infused at 5 mcg/kg/h and it is readily available in 50 mcg/mL. We would like to infuse this drug for at least 12 h.

Volume to be infused per hour = 15 kg × 5 mcg/kg/h/50 mcg/mL = 1.5 mL/h

Volume of drug that should be drawn up = 1.5 mL/h × 12 h = 18 mL (additional drug can be drawn up to prime the infusion lines.)

The infusion rate will be 1.5 mL/h in this case. This drug is usually delivered by an electronic syringe driver set to 1.5 mL/h.

Propofol will be infused as a variable rate infusion and Equations (1) and (3) apply. Propofol has a wide infusion dose in dogs, and it is recommended to start at 0.3 mg/kg/min (18 mg/kg/h). For the procedure, a planned surgical time is two hours and this may be doubled to plan for events arising (surgical preparation time, potential intra-operative complications, etc.).

Planned infusion time = 2 h × 2 = 4 h

Drug concentration propofol = 10 mg/mL

Using Equations (1) and (3):

Volume to be infused per hour = 15 kg × 18 mg/kg/h/10 mg/mL = 27 mL/h

Volume of drug that should be drawn up = 27 mL/h × 4 h × 1.5 = 162 mL

Step 3: Deciding on an infusion technique.
Because the volumes are larger than commercial medical syringes, it would be easier to prepare this infusion in a (for example) 200 mL 0.9% saline bag using one of two techniques.

Technique 1: Discard the volume of 0.9% saline that is equivalent to the volume of drug being added to the 200 mL bag (i.e., a volume of 162 mL of 0.9% saline must be discarded, and then the drugs can be injected into the bag.

$$\begin{aligned}&\text{The starting infusion rate}\\&= \text{volume of bag / hours to be infused}\\&= 200\ \text{mL} / (4\ \text{h} \times 1.5)\\&= 200\ \text{mL} / 6\ \text{h} = 33\ \text{mL} / \text{h}.\end{aligned}$$

Upward and downward titration requires some more mathematics not covered in this example.

Technique 2: Aseptically empty the entire 200 mL from the 0.9% saline bag, and then inject the 162 mL of propofol into the bag.

$$\begin{aligned}&\text{The starting infusion rate} = \text{Propofol volume}\\&\text{of to be infused per hour} = 27\ \text{mL/h}.\end{aligned}$$

A tip, when starting out, is to calculate the propofol infusion rate for 0.2 and 0.4 mg/kg/min (12 and 24 mg/kg/h) and be ready to alter the infusion rate according to depth of anesthesia and response to surgical stimulation. If the animal is responding to surgical stimulation, then a 0.5 mg/kg IV bolus of propofol will help rapidly increase the plasma drug concentration (and therefore increase depth of anesthesia), allowing time for the increased infusion rate to take effect.

If electronic pumps are not available, then the drip rate can be calculated using the following equation:

$$\begin{aligned}&\text{Drip rate (drops/second)} = (\text{volume infused per hour}\\&\times \text{admins set drops per mL}) / 3600\ \text{s}\end{aligned}$$

If we use 60 drops/mL admin set in our hypothetic example, then

= (27 mL/h × 60 drops/mL)/3600 s

= 0.45 drops per second

[≈1 drop every 2 s].

Target-Controlled Infusion Technique

Target-controlled infusion is a common technique in human anesthesia, and many electronic pumps/syringe drivers are available programmed with drug and population pharmacokinetic data to facilitate TCI. There are two methodologies commonly used to define *target concentration*. The first is to target a desired plasma concentration and the second is to target an effect site concentration. Based on available pharmacokinetic and population data, a drug is administered at a variable rate controlled by the device to achieve the target concentration. This approach allows better control of anesthetic depth so that drug use (and adverse effects) is decreased. TCI approaches have been most commonly described for dogs, but this technique is not in mainstream use.

Pharmacogenomics and Pharmacovigilance

Pharmacogenomics describes how genetic variation influences drug pharmacokinetics and pharmacodynamics. Although this field of research is in its infancy in veterinary medicine, analgesic and anesthetic drugs have been investigated. Pharmacovigilance is the science and practice of detecting, understanding, and preventing adverse drug reactions. When a suspected reaction occurs, it should be reported to the relevant oversight organization and/or pharmaceutical company that produced the drug. Reporting plays an important role in collecting drug performance data under real-world conditions and in facilitating analysis to prevent future reactions.

Pharmacogenomics

In human medicine, pharmacogenomics has the ultimate goal of achieving individualized medical therapy. In veterinary medicine, this goal is not currently achievable because of the high cost to benefit ratio. However, veterinary pharmacogenomics has expanded understanding of differences in pharmacokinetic and pharmacodynamic effects between species and between individual breeds within a species.

Pharmacokinetic differences can arise because of different expressions of enzymes responsible for alterations in transporters that move drugs across membranes (e.g., blood–brain barrier) and those responsible for drug metabolism (biotransformation). For example, herding breeds of dog have variable inherited susceptibility to central nervous system depression after being given certain drugs (e.g., butorphanol, acepromazine, and ivermectin). This results from differences in the ABCB1 gene (also known as "MDR1 gene"), which expresses a variation in the P-glycoprotein drug transporter. While Collies are the prototypical example of ABCB1 gene variation, other herding breeds are also affected, including the Australian Shepherd, German Shepherd, Shetland Sheepdog, and long-haired Whippets.

Enzymes responsible for phase I biotransformation (i.e., the P450 system) have been implicated or known to cause poor metabolism of many drugs used in human medicine, but a few have been investigated in veterinary medicine. In dogs, the metabolism of the nonsteroidal anti-inflammatory celecoxib by the CYP-2D15 was investigated in Beagles and it was found that half of the dogs studied were classified as poor metabolizers. This is important because many other drugs act as substrates for this enzyme pathway. CYP-2B11 mutation has been implicated in Greyhounds for the delayed recovery observed from barbiturate drug administration. Similar mutations may explain delayed recovery (e.g., propofol) or poor metabolism of other drugs (e.g., celecoxib and ketoconazole) described in Greyhounds. Other examples of variable gene expression that alter biotransformation are esterase enzymes, as described in horses and rabbits. In horses, inefficient esterase activity has been implicated in adverse reactions to procaine penicillin. In some rabbits, esterases are very efficient, leading to rapid metabolism of atropine, rendering it less effective.

A well-recognized pharmacodynamic variation in both human and veterinary medicine is malignant hyperthermia. This adverse reaction, primarily triggered by inhalational anesthetics, has been described mainly in pigs (and humans) but also in dogs, cats, and horses. The prototypical gene responsible for this adverse reaction is that which encodes the type-1 ryanodine receptor located in skeletal muscle. This is an intracellular calcium transporter, with activation resulting in increased calcium concentration within the cytosol of muscle cells causing widespread muscle contractions, increased metabolism, and resultant heat production. Malignant hyperthermia has been bred out of commercial pig lines, so its occurrence is now rare. The incidence in dogs, cats, and horses is considered very rare.

Pharmacovigilance

In order for pharmacovigilance to be practiced, most authorities have made reporting of suspected adverse events straightforward. Reporting is not restricted to veterinarians and can be performed by veterinary technicians (nurses), farmers, and companion animal owners. An adverse event can be (1) a lack of efficacy, drug did not work as intended; (2) a hypersensitivity reaction; (3) an adverse reaction in people handling a drug or in untreated animals exposed to a drug; (4) drug residue detected despite observing an appropriate withdrawal period; or (5) an environmental incident where fauna or flora are affected. Reporting mechanisms vary by jurisdiction, with most offering confidentiality and varying levels of anonymity. Providing contact information is helpful with facilitating a proper investigation. Reporting suspected adverse drug reactions is an important part of practicing veterinary medicine.

Further Reading

Ainscough, L.P., Ford, J.L., Morecroft, C.W. et al. (2018). Accuracy of intravenous and enteral preparations involving small volumes for paediatric use: a review. *Euro J Hosp Pharma* 25: 66–71.

Aitken, M. (2016). Understanding the pharmaceutical value chain. *Pharmaceut Polic Law* 18: 55–66.

Duke, T. (2013). Partial intravenous anesthesia in cats and dogs. *Can Vet J* 54: 276–282.

Dutta, A., Malhotra, S.K., and Khoche, S. (2007). Tuberculin syringes: a convenient way to administer intravenous anesthetics in neonates and infants. *Pediac Anesth* 17: 501–502.

Jacques, E.R. and Alexandridis, P. (2019). Tablet scoring: current practice, fundamentals, and knowledge gaps. *Appl Sci* 9: 3066.

Petrie, K.W. and Wallace, S.L. (2015). The Care and Feeding of an IACUC: The Organization and Management of an Institutional Animal Care and Use Committee (IACUC). Florida: CRC Press.

Sampat, K.M., Wolfe, J.D., Shah, M.K. et al. (2013). Accuracy and reproducibility of seven brands of small-volume syringes used for intraocular drug delivery. *Ophthalmic Surg Lasers Imaging Retina* 44: 385–389.

Vallee, M., Barthelemy, I., Friciu, M. et al. (2021). Compatibility of lactated Ringer's injection with 94 selected intravenous drugs during simulated Y-site administration. *Hosp Pharma* 56: 288–234.

7

Injectable Drugs Used for Premedication, Induction, and Maintenance of General Anesthesia

Khursheed Mama and Gareth Zeiler

Introduction

The injectable drugs used in veterinary anesthesia are described in this chapter. Inhalational drugs are discussed in Chapter 8. Many of the drugs used by anesthetists are under government regulation (scheduled) and require some form of drug register and controlled access (kept under lock and key). Each country has its own drug schedule scheme, and it is the responsibility of the veterinarian to become familiar with the relevant legislation in the country in which they practice. Legislation typically describes requirements for drug purchasing, storage, and use. Failure to adhere to legislation could result in a suspension or loss of license to practice and possible criminal prosecution. Drugs will be presented following the peri-anesthetic pathway (see Chapter 2): premedication, induction, maintenance, and recovery phases. Species-specific chapters provide suitable drug combinations to use in healthy animals. Organ-system-focused chapters provide suitable drug combinations to use in patients with various diseases.

Drugs Used for Premedication

The premedication phase is an important step in preparing a patient for general anesthesia. There are critical outcomes that an anesthetist wants to achieve that will help guide which drug or combination of drugs to select. These outcomes are to reduce anxiety, provide sedation, provide analgesia, decrease drug dose requirements for induction and maintenance phases of anesthesia, reduce nausea and vomiting, and treat nonanesthetic processes related to the patient (e.g., insulin therapy for diabetes mellitus) or procedure (antihistamines and bronchodilators for bronchoalveolar lavage). Not every patient requires all of these key outcomes to be met. Ideally, following premedication, a patient should be calm, receptive to handling, and hemodynamically stable. Enough time must be allowed for the drug(s) used for premedication to have a clinical effect and this delineates how long the premedication period lasts. Typically, 30 min should be enough time to achieve the desired outcomes. A shorter timeframe is often achievable if drugs are given IV (versus IM or SC). Anxious patients may benefit from receiving an anxiolytic or sedative drug (e.g., trazodone; see Chapter 10) at home, before the animal is transported to the practice.

The most common drug combination in most species undergoing a surgical or invasive procedure is a sedative in combination with an analgesic (primarily opioids), such as (dex)medetomidine with methadone (dogs and cats) or xylazine and butorphanol (horses).

Phenothiazine and butyrophenone derivatives

Drug class summary	
Subclassification	None relevant to clinical anesthesia
Core drugs	Acepromazine, azaperone, and droperidol
Used for	Anxiolytic effects
Major receptor binding site(s)	Antagonist effects on dopamine (D2) receptors. Other important receptors that are antagonized (to a variable degree) include alpha-1 adrenergic receptors, histamine (H1), serotonin (5-HT2), and muscarinic cholinergic (M1) receptors
Used in	All species of healthy animals

(Continued)

Fundamental Principles of Veterinary Anesthesia, First Edition. Edited by Gareth E. Zeiler and Daniel S. J. Pang.

Companion Website: www.wiley.com/go/VeterinaryAnesthesiaZeiler

(*Continued*)

Drug class summary	
Cautioned use in	Hypovolemia, preexisting hypotension, expected peri-operative blood loss, or if packed cell volume is low (<25%) or total plasma proteins are low (<45 g/L; albumin <25 g/L). Very anxious or excited animals or those actively displaying aggressive behavior have a high circulating level of epinephrine (epinephrine causes beta-2 adrenergic-receptor-mediated vasodilation and acepromazine alpha-1 adrenergic receptor antagonism that can result in peripheral vasodilation and profound hypotension)
Dosing routes	IV, IM, SC, and oral for ACP
Treatment plans	Once, or repeated at 6–8 h intervals, or more frequently depending on the dose given, route of administration, and patient's response to the drug
Pharmacological antagonist	None
Species notes	Cautioned use in breeding stallions because treatment could result in paraphimosis (or more rarely, priapism) that could damage the penis. Cautioned when used alone in nervous or poorly socialized dogs, where aggression could be unmasked. Butyrophenone derivatives are reserved for use in pigs and wildlife because their clinical effect in other species is considered to be unpredictable

Drugs in these classes can cause anxiolysis and muscle relaxation, which can result in a reduction (approximately 20–50%) of the dose requirement for anesthetic induction and maintenance. These drugs also have anti-emetic, anti-spasmodic, and weak antihistaminic effects. They also impair the animal's ability to thermoregulate so that hypothermia and hyperthermia (depending on environmental temperature and temperature management interventions) can occur, thus regularly monitoring body temperature is recommended.

The most commonly used phenothiazine derivative in clinical use is *acepromazine* (acetylpromazine, ACP). Administration of acepromazine provides anxiolysis, anti-nausea, and anti-arrhythmic effects but does not provide analgesia. However, acepromazine does potentiate the beneficial effects of opioid agonists and thus they are frequently used in combination in dogs, cats, and horses.

The effects on the respiratory system following acepromazine alone are a decrease in respiratory rate, but tidal volume is minimally affected, which results in a minor decrease in minute volume.

The major effect on cardiovascular function is vasodilation, resulting from peripheral alpha-1 adrenergic receptor antagonism. Therefore, its use is avoided in hypovolemic or hypotensive patients. The alpha-1 adrenergic receptor antagonism also affords protection against catecholamine-induced cardiac arrhythmias.

Acepromazine can relax the gastroesophageal sphincter and may predispose animals to reflux and regurgitation during anesthesia. Other phenothiazine derivatives are reported to lower the seizure threshold, but there is no evidence that acepromazine does so and its use in animals with a history of seizures is at the discretion of the veterinarian. Weak antihistaminic effects support avoiding its use in patients undergoing skin testing for allergies. Repeated or large single doses (above the ranges recommended in this text) given to pediatric or geriatric patients could result in extrapyramidal symptoms (akathisia and tardive dyskinesia). A decrease in the packed cell volume (up to 10%), secondary to splenic sequestration, and mild inhibition of platelet function should be considered in patients with anemia or platelet-related bleeding disorders, respectively.

Azaperone is the most commonly used butyrophenone derivative in clinical use, whereas *droperidol* is used in some geographical regions in dogs and wildlife. Administration of azaperone results in similar effects to acepromazine; however, these effects can be unpredictable and unreliable in most domestic species and so its use has been mostly limited to pigs to combat stress during transport, introducing unfamiliar animals to a group, or farrowing. However, if azaperone is to be used in pigs for premedication or sedation, it should be administered in combination with other drugs to facilitate handling. Opioids, alpha-2 adrenergic receptor agonists, benzodiazepine agonists, and ketamine have been used in various combinations with azaperone to effectively sedate pigs (see Chapter 14). Azaperone has also been used in wildlife capture (chemical immobilization when used in combination with etorphine or thiafentanil, or as part of a butorphanol–azaperone–medetomidine drug combination and as an anxiolytic during transport or enclosed-confinement [boma] management).

Benzodiazepine agonists

Drug class summary	
Subclassification	None relevant to clinical anesthesia
Core drugs	Diazepam and midazolam
Used for	Sedative (not reliable in all species), anxiolytic, and muscle relaxation effects
Major receptor binding site(s)	$GABA_A$ receptor agonist, a specific benzodiazepine binding site has been identified

Drug class summary	
Used in	All species of animals
Cautioned use in	For sedation in respiratory compromised patients (especially brachycephalic animals) due to muscle relaxation causing upper airway obstructions. Unreliable in nervous, excited, or aggressive animals when used alone
Dosing routes	Both can be given IV, but midazolam can also be given IM or SC
Treatment plans	Single dose for premedication or constant rate infusion during general anesthesia
Pharmacological antagonist	Yes: flumazenil (or sarmazenil in some geographical regions)
Species notes	A good sedative drug in all ages of cattle, sheep, goats, camelids, and pigs. Good sedation in neonatal puppies, kittens and foals, geriatric dogs (in combination with an opioid), and sick (ASA IV+ cats and dogs). Limited (unpredictable) sedation in young or adult healthy dogs, cats, and horses when used alone; reserved for use as a co-induction drug

Diazepam and midazolam are two benzodiazepine agonists (commonly referred to as "benzodiazepines") available as injectable formulations for use in veterinary anesthesia. Midazolam is water soluble at an acidic pH (pH < 4.0), and once injected into an animal its molecular structure undergoes transformation making it highly lipid soluble when exposed to normal body pH (approximately 7.4). This unique quality allows for midazolam to be given SC or IM with a rapid, reliable onset of clinical signs. Diazepam, an older drug in this class, is not very soluble and commonly formulated with propylene glycol to improve solubility. Propylene glycol causes pain and potential muscle damage if given IM and is unreliably absorbed when administered via this or the SC route. Therefore, injections should be limited to the IV route.

Benzodiazepines mediate their clinical effects by their actions on the $GABA_A$ receptor. While dose-dependent ataxia, postural changes, and apparent sedation are observed in adult dogs, cats, and horses following administration, some animals may be difficult to restrain and become agitated or aroused ("paradoxical excitement"). As a result, sole administration of a benzodiazepine for premedicating adult, healthy dogs, cats, and horses is not generally recommended. However, its administration in combination with a potent opioid drug, especially in dogs, is still practiced because of the combination's "safety" profile (minimal cardiovascular depression), but the downside is variable, unpredictable sedation and limited dose-sparing effects of induction drugs, compared to other drug combinations routinely used for premedication. Alternatively, these drugs are commonly used following premedication as a co-induction drug in horses, dogs, and cats, mainly for their muscle relaxation properties, to reduce the dose of anesthetic induction drug and increase the duration of anesthesia following induction. Interestingly, in other species, notably sheep, goats, cattle, pigs, and potentially camelids, they tend to produce reliable sedation, even when administered alone and offer dose-sparing effects on induction drugs (approximately 20–30%). Concurrent administration with other drugs especially in older or debilitated patients offers many advantages as they enhance sedative properties of other drugs and reduce the dose of the primary anesthesia induction or maintenance drugs.

Minute ventilation is depressed for approximately 10 min following IV administration.

While benzodiazepines are generally considered to have insignificant cardiovascular effects, hypotension and arrhythmias are reported with rapid IV administration of diazepam. These effects are attributed to the propylene glycol vehicle.

Benzodiazepines can also be used to control seizures. It is not recommended to use these drugs in dogs and cats undergoing cesarean section as they undergo ion trapping in the neonate (due to lower pH environment) resulting in prolonged sedation and muscle relaxation in the neonate. These drugs are useful as sedatives in foals and crias (young camelids) where other medications (e.g., alpha-2 adrenergic receptor agonist drugs) result in undesirable cardiovascular effects. Note that benzodiazepines do not have any direct anti-nociceptive properties and should not be considered analgesic.

Alpha-2 adrenergic receptor agonists

Drug class summary	
Subclassification	Thiazine derivates and imidazoline derivatives. These subclasses are important to understand because the drugs within each class have different physiological effects
Core drugs	Thiazine derivates: xylazine Imidazoline derivatives: detomidine, romifidine, medetomidine, and dexmedetomidine
Used for	Sedative (reliable in all species), anxiolytic, muscle relaxation, analgesia, and anesthetic dose-sparing effects

(*Continued*)

(Continued)

Drug class summary	
Major receptor binding site(s)	Alpha-2 adrenergic receptors, alpha-1 adrenergic receptors, and imidazoline receptors
Used in	All species of healthy animals
Cautioned use in	Animals with organ dysfunction (cardiovascular, renal, hepatic, etc.). Sheep (and goats) because they can develop pulmonary hypertension and lung edema more readily compared to other species. Romifidine should be used cautiously in dogs because it can cause severe pulmonary derangements, including life-threatening pulmonary edema
Dosing routes	IV, IM, epidural (horses and cattle, and good analgesia with less risk of recumbency)
Treatment plans	Single dose for premedication or constant rate infusion during general anesthesia (or ICU sedation)
Pharmacological antagonist	Yes: Yohimbine, Tolazoline, and Atipamezole
Species notes	Species-specific and breed-specific range in drug sensitivity have been described (see the following text)

The alpha-2 adrenergic receptor agonists (commonly referred to as "alpha-2 agonists") have applications in a broad range of species: horses, ruminants, dogs, cats, non-human primates, small mammals, etc. These drugs may be administered by multiple routes including IV, IM, SC, epidural, spinal, oral transmucosal, and intra-articular. They are considered to be the most reliable sedatives in many species and excellent analgesics (albeit duration of analgesia is shorter than duration of sedation). When alpha-2 agonists are used for premedication, there is a significant reduction in dose required for anesthetic induction and maintenance (approximately 40–60% reduction), especially when used in combination with opioids (up to 80% reduction when deep sedation is achieved).

Recognizing differences may exist according to local availability, and drugs in this class commonly used in domesticated species are as follows: xylazine (horses, ruminants, dogs, and cats), romifidine (horses), medetomidine (dogs, cats, and horses), dexmedetomidine (dogs, cats, and horses), and detomidine (horses). Each drug has both alpha-2 and alpha-1 adrenergic receptor effects. *Xylazine*, the least specific member of this class (alpha-2:alpha-1 binding ratio of approximately 160:1), continues to be commonly used in many parts of the world. *Detomidine* and *romifidine* exhibit higher alpha-2:alpha-1 binding ratios than xylazine, 260:1 and 360:1, respectively. They can be used in the peri-anesthetic period and are commonly used for standing sedation (horses, ruminants, and pigs) due to their longer duration of action. In horses, romifidine is associated with less ataxia and head drop compared to detomidine and is thus preferred for procedures on the head. All three drugs are most commonly administered IV or IM and other routes include intra-articular, epidural, and oral transmucosal (Dormosedan Gel; see Chapter 10). *Medetomidine* has the highest degree of alpha-2 adrenergic receptor specificity of this class (alpha-2:alpha-1 binding ratio of approximately 1620:1). It is a racemic mixture of two optically active stereoisomers, levomedetomidine and dexmedetomidine, in equal quantities. *Dexmedetomidine*, the active dextro-isomer of medetomidine (same alpha-2:alpha-1 binding ratio as medetomidine), is also available commercially and, like medetomidine, is preferred over xylazine in dogs as reports indicate an increase in mortality following administration of xylazine during anesthesia. Recently, *Zenalpha*, a proprietary combination of medetomidine and peripheral alpha-2 adrenergic receptor antagonist vatinoxan (previously MK467), has become available. The intent in developing this combined product was to improve cardiovascular safety of medetomidine. Vatinoxan partially counters the peripheral vasoconstriction and resulting bradycardia and decrease in cardiac output observed with medetomidine without significantly influencing centrally mediated effects such as sedation and analgesia. Behavioral and cardiovascular effects of medetomidine and vatinoxan have been evaluated independently and administered simultaneously at different ratios; the current formulation provides a fixed ratio (20:1) of vatinoxan (10 mg/mL) and medetomidine (0.5 mg/mL). This combination is licensed in the United States of America and Europe for sedation in healthy dogs (ASA I-II/V) dogs (not recommended in cats). Clinical experience suggests a more rapid onset of sedation when compared to administration of an alpha-2 adrenergic receptor agonist alone. Zenalpha is licensed for short duration sedation, not for premedication before anesthesia. Bradycardia and occasional hypotension of a clinically relevant magnitude, which can be difficult to treat, have been observed in anesthetized patients premedicated with Zenalpha.

As mentioned, dose-dependent sedation and analgesia are features of these drugs in domestic species. Species differences are noteworthy: dose requirement for equivalent sedation with xylazine is lowest in goats and cattle (0.05–0.1 mg/kg IV) and highest in pigs (2 mg/kg IV). Sheep, camelids, horses, dogs, and cats span this gap from low to high dose requirements, respectively. This variation in dosing is not as notable for romifidine, detomidine, medetomidine, and dexmedetomidine. The duration of action (if drug effects are not reversed) does vary significantly between species. For example, the actions of (dex)medetomidine are of a significant duration in dogs and cats (hours) and of a very short duration (minutes) in horses. Some breeds within a species are more "sensitive" to these drugs regardless of drug subclass. This may reflect a metabolic scaling effect (e.g., draft breed horses more sensitive compared to warmbloods). Some breeds within a species are more sensitive to one drug (e.g., *Bos indicus* cattle breed appear more sensitive to xylazine compared to *Bos taurus* breeds).

Dosing depends on desired outcome (e.g., standing sedation versus anesthesia premedication). Higher doses provide muscle relaxation and, above a certain dose, prolong the duration rather than the intensity of sedation and analgesia. The reliability of sedation is improved with the concurrent administration of other drugs (e.g., opioids and acepromazine). The incidence of occasional aberrant behavior (e.g., increased sensitivity to tactile stimulation so that apparently sedated animals can react quickly and unexpectedly, such as with a kick or a bite) is also reduced.

While generally considered to cause minimal respiratory depression (decreased respiratory rate is compensated by an increase in tidal volume, to maintain minute ventilation), respiratory depression, stridor, and occasional cyanosis have been reported when alpha-2 agonists are given alone. Cyanosis is usually secondary to decreased cardiac output rather than arterial hypoxemia in healthy, normovolemic patients. The increased transit time of the erythrocyte through the capillary bed resulting from a decrease in cardiac output increases the amount of oxygen being extracted such that available hemoglobin is desaturated (and the tissue appears blue). Localized vasoconstriction may also play a role in observation of cyanosis. The incidence and severity of true respiratory effects is greater when these drugs are administered in combination with other drugs in most species. However, pulmonary hypertension with the possibility of lung edema has been described with sole use of alpha-2 agonists in many of the domesticated species, most notably sheep.

Importantly, this class of drugs is associated with significant cardiovascular adverse effects, and these can be divided into peripheral effects and central effects (these effects occur concurrently, with central effects more apparent as the peripheral effects wane). Peripheral effects include an increase in systemic vascular resistance (peripheral vasoconstriction), causing systemic hypertension and consequent baroreceptor-mediated decrease in heart rate, to approximately 40–50% of pre-injection values. This bradycardia is accompanied by a corresponding decrease in cardiac output. These peripheral effects occur at very low doses (e.g., 0.001 mg/kg of medetomidine in dogs), and higher doses increase the duration but not the magnitude of effect. Second-degree atrioventricular block and other bradyarrhythmias may also be observed. However, when administered alone, arterial hypoxemia rarely occurs. As peripheral effects wane, central effects become predominant and are caused by decreases in norepinephrine release. This results in decreased sympathetic outflow (sympatholytic effect) that result in a continuation of bradycardia and decreased cardiac output. Hypotension, when the central effects are dominant, can occur especially in hypovolemic animals or in animals maintained under inhalational anesthesia. The duration of these peripheral and central effects varies with drug, route of administration, and species. Despite the presence of bradycardia, concurrent use of an anticholinergic drug is not recommended due to the potential increase in myocardial work (in the face of peripheral vasoconstriction and increased afterload) and lack of efficacy in increasing cardiac output. However, anticholinergic drugs can be considered to treat bradycardia caused by central effects if an animal is also hypotensive.

Because of potential cardiovascular and respiratory complications, the routine use of alpha-2 agonists should be focused toward patients with good cardiovascular function (see Chapter 17). Close monitoring, even in healthy patients, is recommended to quickly identify problems, should they occur.

Other adverse effects are species dependent and include vomiting (which is especially common in cats receiving xylazine but may be seen with any alpha-2 agonist in dogs and cats), gastrointestinal stasis, diarrhea, hyperglycemia (anti-insulin effect), and diuresis (anti-ADH effect).

Opioids

Drug class summary	
Subclassification	Pure-*mu* agonists, partial-*mu* agonists, and *kappa* agonist–*mu* antagonist
Core drugs	Pure-*mu* agonists (morphine, fentanyl, remifentanil hydromorphone, methadone, and meperidine [pethidine]), partial-*mu* agonist (buprenorphine), *kappa* agonist, and *mu* antagonist (butorphanol and nalbuphine)
Used for	Analgesia and sedative effects (not reliable in all species)
Major receptor binding site(s)	*Mu*, *kappa*, and *delta* opioid receptors
Used in	All species of animals
Cautioned use in	High doses of pure-*mu* agonists in patients with respiratory compromise. Patients prone to histamine release (meperidine [pethidine] more of a concern than morphine)
Dosing routes	IV (not meperidine [pethidine]), IM, OTM (buprenorphine in horses and cats, and methadone in cats), epidurally, intra-articular, and topical (cornea)

(Continued)

(*Continued*)

Drug class summary	
Treatment plans	Single or repeated doses, or IV infusion during general anesthesia and recovery. Repeated dosing intervals have traditionally been based on pharmacokinetic recommendations where set time intervals are used for each drug. However, patients should be monitored regularly and dosed according to pain assessment
Pharmacological antagonist	Yes: Naloxone and in some cases butorphanol and nalbuphine have been used to antagonize pure-*mu* agonists
Species notes	There are species differences in opioid receptor densities and locations within the brain and spinal cord which results in variable clinical effects. Cattle, sheep, goats, pigs, and horses can demonstrate signs of hypermetria, vocalization, muscle twitching, and behavioral excitement (particularly horses) when opioids are administered alone or at high doses. Ileus and gastric stasis (or rumen statis) and constipation are common concern in all species. In dogs, body temperature tends to decrease slightly (<1 °C) whereas cats can develop hyperthermia (occasionally >40 °C). Effects on ocular pupil size also differ among species. Dogs often develop miosis whereas cats develop mydriasis

Opioids are commonly used for premedication and perioperative analgesia. In many species, the opioids cause variable sedation when given alone; however, when given in combination with a drug that causes anxiolysis or sedation, the resultant sedation is deeper and more reliable. This is especially the case when opioid drugs are combined with alpha-2 adrenergic receptor agonists in almost all species.

Pure-mu Opioid Receptor Agonists

Morphine is the prototypical pure-*mu* agonist but has agonist action on *mu*, *kappa*, and *delta* opioid receptors. It is often sold in vials of different concentrations and as either preservative-free or containing preservatives (usually multidose vials). It is efficacious for mild to severe pain and, when given alone, can cause mild-to-moderate sedation in some species (e.g., dogs). Histamine release is seen with rapid administration of IV morphine so slow administration (over five minutes) is recommended. IM or SC administration is unlikely to be of concern in animals without predisposing factors (e.g., known hypersensitivity reactions and mast cell tumor). Morphine is the most water soluble of the pure-*mu* opioids. Consequently, it is sequestered for a longer period of time within the epidural space and considered the opioid of choice for epidural administration. When given by this route, two potential adverse effects are urine retention and pruritis. For reasons that are not entirely clear, the incidence of urine retention appears to vary considerably among practices. One suggestion is that the practice of routinely emptying the bladder at the end of surgery masks retention as the bladder does not fill until effects on retention have waned. Following an epidural injection containing morphine, regularly checking bladder size (e.g., every four hours) is recommended until the animal begins urinating. Urinary retention has been reported in most species. Pruritis is a rare complication, reported in dogs and cats with mostly anecdotal reports in other species. When pruritis occurs, it can be severe and self-mutilation is common, warranting immediate treatment. Severe pruritis is often difficult to treat, unresponsive to antihistamines and systemic opioid receptor antagonists. Patients unresponsive to initial therapy could benefit from sedation with propofol or intralipid therapy (Gent et al. 2013). Morphine (use of preservative-free formulations is recommended) has also been used successfully as an analgesic when administered into joints (most commonly, dogs and horses) and topically on the cornea in most species. Intra-articular and topical administration limits systemic adverse effects, especially gastrointestinal ileus, that are commonly reported with systemic administration. *Hydromorphone* is an equally effective analgesic as morphine but does not cause histamine release following intravenous administration of clinically used doses. *Methadone* is unique among the pure-*mu* agonists in that it is also an N-methyl-D-aspartate (NMDA) receptor antagonist. Therefore, it may produce analgesia through both mechanisms and is an attractive choice in patients with central sensitization (see Chapter 3). In dogs, it does not tend to cause vomiting and causes panting less frequently than observed with either morphine or hydromorphone. Its limited adverse effect profile makes methadone an appealing alternative to morphine and hydromorphone. Methadone causes similar, or slightly less, sedation as compared to morphine and hydromorphone. The effect observed in cats can be best described as euphoria, creating a state in which this species is less perturbed by restraint and IV catheter placement. *Meperidine* (pethidine) is a short-acting, pure-*mu* agonist. Histamine release (and potentially associated hypotension) is a frequent observation that occurs when this drug is administered IV, so it is contraindicated by this route and given IM instead. Furthermore, meperidine is thought to have some anticholinergic effects because heart rate is usually maintained or increased, which contrasts with lower heart rates, even bradycardia, usually seen when administering other pure-*mu* agonists. However, the increased heart rate may not be related to anticholinergic effects but rather a baroreceptor-mediated response to histamine-induced vasodilation (and subsequent decrease in systemic vascular resistance). Unlike other opioids, meperidine causes some direct myocardial depression though this is of little consequence in healthy patients. Other pure-*mu* agonists such as fentanyl, alfentanil, sufentanil, and remifentanil are not typically used as premedication drugs in private practice but rather as either an induction drug or to provide analgesia during surgery and will be discussed later. However, if a patient is transferred from an ICU or critical care ward, then they may already be receiving a constant rate infusion (CRI) of one of these drugs and this should be considered when planning premedication.

Summary of drug effects is as follows:

Respiratory adverse effects are generally dose and route dependent and include respiratory depression (nonhuman primate species are most sensitive) and panting (dogs). Use of doses at the lower end of the recommended dose range is appropriate when treating severe trauma or in brachycephalic dogs to limit respiratory depression. Further doses can be provided, as necessary. When administered intravenously under general anesthesia, hypoventilation and apnea may occur.

The most common adverse effect is bradycardia, especially with high IV doses. Species differences in heart rate are anecdotally reported. Any associated decrease in cardiac output is usually well tolerated in healthy patients, but treatment may be required if hypotension develops (typically with an anticholinergic to increase heart rate).

Other adverse effects of the pure-*mu* agonists include hyperthermia (cats), mild hypothermia (dogs), vomiting (morphine/hydromorphone in dogs and cats), defecation, gastrointestinal ileus, and, with high doses, dysphoria. Vomiting is often undesirable in patients with esophageal or gastric foreign bodies and should be avoided in traumatic brain injury (especially if there is evidence of increased intracranial pressure, decreased level of consciousness, slow heart rate, high blood pressure, and possible erratic breathing pattern), deep corneal ulcers, and brachycephalic dogs. In these cases, these drugs can either be given once the animal is already anesthetized or, if included in premedication, select those that do not cause vomiting or administer anti-emetics (e.g., maropitant, ondansetron, and dolasetron) beforehand.

Partial-Mu Opioid Receptor Agonist

Buprenorphine is unique in that it is (currently) classified as a partial-*mu* agonist. Unlike the pure-*mu* opioid agonists, which are strictly regulated because they have a high potential for abuse, buprenorphine, in most countries, has fewer restrictions on its use and lower requirements for recordkeeping. It is most commonly given IV or IM, and sustained-release formulations are given SC. This drug has been studied mostly in dogs, cats, and horses. In cats and horses, OTM administration is effective but less so in dogs and can induce hypersalivation regardless of species. Its longer duration of action (6–8 h with recommended dosing) allows for less frequent dosing that has practical benefits. Its availability in high concentration and sustained-release preparations adds value in managing patients for up to three days from a single or once daily SC injection. Although buprenorphine is now considered a good analgesic, in cases in which pain may be severe, it is often better to manage pain initially with a pure-*mu* agonist. This is because buprenorphine is tightly bound to the *mu* receptor (displays high affinity) and cannot easily be displaced by a pure-*mu* agonist drug should additional analgesia be required. Likewise, if adverse effects are noted, it can be difficult to reverse buprenorphine with opioid antagonists.

Summary of drug effects is as follows:

Respiratory adverse effects are less pronounced compared to the pure-*mu* agonists and are often not clinically significant, with the exception of nonhuman primates.

None have been reported (or investigated specifically in animals) but appear to be limited to occasional reports of bradycardia that respond to anticholinergic treatment.

Buprenorphine can cause an increase in body temperature in cats. Gastrointestinal ileus is less of a concern than with the pure-*mu* agonists.

Kappa agonist–mu antagonist

Butorphanol is generally considered less effective than pure-*mu* and partial-*mu* agonist drugs for moderate-to-severe pain. Butorphanol has a short to intermediate duration of action in horses, and possibly ruminants (especially in patients suffering from gastrointestinal disorders). In dogs and cats, butorphanol is a reasonable sedative (similar or better efficacy compared to morphine and hydromorphone, especially in older or compromised patients) and is thought to causes less respiratory depression (and panting is infrequent) when compared to the pure-*mu* and partial-*mu* opioid agonists. However, its variable, and therefore, unpredictable duration of action and limited analgesic efficacy (compared with pure-*mu* and partial-*mu* agonists) limit clinical use to minimally invasive, short duration procedures. In some countries, it is a controlled substance.

Respiratory depression is of little clinical concern when administered alone.

Minimal cardiovascular adverse effects occur at recommended doses.

Other adverse effects include hypermetria, muscle twitching, and increased vocalization in horses and ruminants when given alone, and potentially other species when high doses are given alone. Occasionally, muscle and limb twitches are observed in horses and dogs.

Anticholinergics

Drug class summary	
Subclassification	None relevant
Core drugs	Atropine, glycopyrrolate, and butylscopolamine (N-butylscopolammonium bromide)
Used for	To reverse the clinical effects of increased parasympathetic autonomic nervous system activity
Major receptor binding site(s)	Muscarinic acetylcholine receptors
Used in	All species
Cautioned use in	Use of atropine and glycopyrrolate in horses is generally contraindicated and restricted to emergency use due to gastrointestinal ileus and risk of colic. Use in ruminants to decrease salivation is generally not indicated because it thickens saliva that can cause airway plugs
Dosing routes	IV, IM, and topical (eye drops)
Treatment plans	Single dose or repeated as required
Pharmacological antagonist	None
Species notes	Some rabbits have circulating atropinase (atropine esterase) that metabolizes atropine rapidly, making it less effective (shorter duration of action)

The anticholinergic drugs most commonly used in small animal practice are *atropine* and *glycopyrrolate*. They compete with the actions of acetylcholine at muscarinic postganglionic acetylcholine (cholinergic) receptor sites, and their predominant clinical effect is to increase heart rate in patients with vagally induced bradycardia. At therapeutic doses, the heart rate can increase to either the intrinsic sinoatrial (SA) node firing rate (80–100 beats per minute) or higher (>140 beats per minute) if circulating catecholamines are increasing sympathetic tone. Doses higher than recommended can cause centrally mediated tachycardia. These drugs also decrease bronchial and oral secretions, cause bronchodilation, cycloplegia, mydriasis, and increase stomach pH. In humans, and likely most species of animals, the onset of effect of atropine on heart rate is faster but with a shorter duration of action compared to glycopyrrolate, following IV administration. In extremely bradycardic patients, the onset maybe slowed for both drugs (due to a slowed circulation). Atropine crosses the blood–brain barrier and placental barrier, while glycopyrrolate does not. Atropine's distribution into the central nervous system is one of the reasons why it should be considered when treating a patient with a life-threatening bradyarrhythmia to treat both central and peripherally mediated causes. When low doses are given, bradycardia and bradyarrhythmias (primarily first- and second-degree AV block) may occur. This results from a direct, dose-dependent peripheral cholinergic effect. Treatment is to give a further dose. For this reason, higher doses are recommended during use in emergencies. An alternative drug that can be used to increase heart rate in horses (rather than atropine or glycopyrrolate) is N-butylscopolammonium bromide (hyoscine butylbromide). It is typically used to relieve spasmodic colic (hyoscine component is anti-spasmodic) but also elevates heart rate. An increase in heart rate lasts approximately 30 min. Tachyarrhythmias may be observed.

Respiratory effects are bronchodilation and cause a decrease in airway secretions. Both of these effects are desirable in brachycephalic dogs and patients with asthma or chronic bronchitis.

Anticholinergic drugs suppress parasympathetic tone to the SA node. Therefore, when given to animals with high parasympathetic (vagal) tone, heart rate will increase.

Other adverse effects: gastrointestinal ileus, mydriasis that, in humans and possibly animals, can cause photophobia. A central anticholinergic syndrome (dry mouth, constipation, urinary retention, mydriasis, and hyperactivity which includes confusion, restlessness, and delirium) is reported in humans with repeated and high doses.

Other Drugs Used for During the Premedication Period

On occasion, some patients who are not receptive to safe handling (fractious domestic animals) require the addition of drugs that can induce anesthesia as part of a premedication drug combination in order to achieve deep sedation (or anesthesia). The inclusion of these induction drugs is a form of chemical immobilization where the level of consciousness is decreased. This should not be confused with the administration of a peripheral muscle relaxant (succinylcholine, atracurium, etc.; see Further Reading) alone, which will cause chemical immobilization, but the animal remains aware of its surroundings but paralyzed.

Drugs Used for Induction of General Anesthesia

When given intravenously, these drugs will induce unconsciousness in a wide range of animal species. They are typically used to provide conditions favorable for endotracheal intubation and facilitate the transition to anesthesia maintenance. The clinical usefulness of these drugs for maintenance of anesthesia is determined by pharmacokinetic and pharmacodynamic properties in each species. Induction drugs are broadly classified into two groups: the hypnotic-sedatives and dissociative anesthetics. Hypnotic-sedatives provide dose-dependent effects ranging from sedation to unconsciousness. After an appropriate induction dose, patients are typically relaxed and appear asleep. By contrast, dissociative anesthetic drugs are associated with a cataleptic state where patients may look awake and maintain muscle tone and somatic reflex activity. This is described as a dissociated state. During induction, the induction drug is given alone or administered with other drugs to help reduce the dose or provide additional desirable properties (such as muscle relaxation). Some of the drugs described in the premedication section in this chapter may be used in this manner. Some additional adjunctive or co-induction drugs are discussed in this section.

Hypnotic-Sedatives

The major hypnotic-sedatives belong to the following drug classes: barbiturates (thiopental), alkyl phenols (propofol), neuroactive steroids (alfaxalone), and imidazoline derivatives (etomidate). These drugs are administered intravenously, with the exception of alfaxalone, which can also be given intramuscularly. The anesthetic activity of hypnotic-sedatives is mediated through the $GABA_A$ receptor. As a drug binds to its unique binding site on the receptor, an ion channel opens, allowing influx of chloride ions, resulting in neuronal hyperpolarization and a generalized depression of the central nervous system. None of these drugs have analgesic effects and thus, when required (i.e., noxious procedures or painful animals), drugs with analgesic properties should be included in the anesthetic plan.

Thiopental

Thiopental (also known as "thiopentone"), by virtue of a sulfur group substitution at position 2 of the barbituric acid ring, is classified as a thiobarbiturate. Thiopental is presented in powder form for reconstitution. Alkalinization (pH 10–11), which is necessary to render the compound water soluble, imparts a bacteriostatic property and also causes the drug to precipitate if reconstituted with an acidic solution (e.g., normal saline) or calcium-containing fluids (e.g., lactated Ringer's solution). Sterile water for injection is the preferred fluid for reconstitution. In part due to the alkalinity of the solution, perivascular administration can result in sloughing of the skin (within a day or two) especially at drug concentrations greater than 2%. Small animal formulations are generally reconstituted to 2.5–5.0%, but concentrations as high as 10% may be used in horses to facilitate faster delivery (smaller injectate volume). This weak acid ($pK_a \sim 7.6$) is approximately 61% unionized (i.e., lipid soluble and readily crosses the blood–brain barrier) at body pH; acidemia will increase the unionized drug proportion and may result in a relative overdose. The recommended clinical dose range in unsedated animals is broad (6–20 mg/kg; small animals, 4–10 mg/kg; horses) to account for individual variability and the effects of other drugs. For example, the dose necessary for intubation is reduced by up to 50% following premedication.

Thiopental produces dose-dependent hypnosis and central nervous system depression without compromise to cerebral perfusion. The onset of action is 15–30 s following IV administration, and the anesthetic duration after a single dose is determined by redistribution. Excitement is seen with slow administration (especially in unsedated animals); therefore, an initial bolus of approximately half of the calculated dose is recommended, followed by a quarter dose at 15 s intervals. In horses, the entire calculated dose is generally administered as a single bolus. Clearance from the body is dependent almost exclusively on hepatic metabolism; its use in animals with significant hepatic disease is not recommended. Greyhounds are known to have a reduced ability to metabolize thiopental so its use in this breed is discouraged (where other options are available) because of the risk of delayed recovery. In horses, especially when performing a field anesthetic, repeated doses are not recommended as recoveries are prolonged and associated with ataxia and stumbling. Thiopental has a duration of approximately 10–20 min before recovery starts.

Summary of relevant pharmacodynamic effects is as follows:

Respiratory rate may be decreased following administration, but the response varies with dose and speed of administration and is influenced by the patient's oxygenation status. At appropriate induction doses, transient, short-lasting apnea may be seen. However, if higher doses are given, then prolonged periods of apnea can occur, and ventilation should be assisted until spontaneous ventilation returns.

An increase in heart rate and a transient decrease in myocardial contractility are observed following administration. Changes in blood pressure, stroke volume, and cardiac output are more variable. Commonly, a decrease in stroke volume, reflecting decreased inotropy, is observed. Thiopental sensitizes the myocardium to the effects of circulating catecholamines, and animals can develop arrhythmias (such as ventricular bigeminy and trigeminy and sinus tachycardia) during induction. Cardiovascular adverse effects are magnified during acidemia and hypoxemia.

Both intracranial and intraocular pressures are decreased following administration. The drug has anticonvulsant properties. Phlebitis occurs when high concentrations (>5%) are administered via a peripheral catheter. If perivascular injection occurs, it is important to discuss the incident with owners and prepare them for the possibility of skin sloughing. Immediate treatment recommendations are to remove the catheter and treat the area of perivascular contamination. Injecting an isotonic crystalloid solution subcutaneously (10–20 mL) and administering 2% lidocaine (1–2 mg/kg) provides drug dilution, and lidocaine may help to neutralize the pH of the thiopental, cause vasodilation (increased removal of drug from perivascular contamination site), and provide analgesia.

Propofol

Propofol is an alkyl phenol. Propofol is commercially available in 1% (10 mg/mL) and 2% (20 mg/mL) formulations. Propofol is not very water soluble and solubilized as an oil-in-water emulsion consisting of various proprietary combinations of soybean oil, palm oil, coconut oil, long-chain or medium-chain triglycerides, glycerol, egg phosphatide, and egg lecithin. Some formulations may include a preservative (such as benzyl alcohol, disodium edetate, and sodium metabisulfite). Formulations that do not have a bacteriostatic preservative are prone to microbial growth. The unused drug of unpreserved formulations remaining in an opened vial or bottle should be discarded at the end of the day. Keeping the unpreserved drug in the fridge does not retard microbial growth. Unused drug from preserved formulations can usually be stored for up to 28 days following bottle penetration (depending on licensing). Perivascular injection does not cause inflammation or tissue damage. Propofol is commonly used for induction of anesthesia of dogs and cats but has been used in many other species for a wide range of clinical situations. The recommended clinical dose range in unsedated animals (3–8 mg/kg for small animals versus 2–4 mg/kg for horses) is broad to account for individual variability and the effects of other drugs. For example, the dose necessary for intubation is reduced 50–75% following premedication with some drugs, notably alpha-2 agonists.

Intravenous administration (generally over one minute) results in dose-dependent effects ranging from sedation to general anesthesia. Both sedation and the use of with benzodiazepine agonists with propofol (co-induction) will reduce the dose requirement (to as low as 1 mg/kg, even in healthy animals) and potentially reduce adverse effects and cost associated with propofol. Excitement can occur (but is uncommon in sedated animals) with administration of propofol in dogs and cats and tends to be more common when conservative initial doses are given too slowly to unsedated, anxious animals. Smooth induction of anesthesia is also typical in sheep, goats, and camelids with propofol alone or in combination with a benzodiazepine. Horses may exhibit tremors (muscle fasciculations) and paddle if propofol is used as the sole induction drug. However, this is less frequent following deep sedation achieved with an alpha-2 adrenergic receptor agonist ± opioid. Propofol can be combined with ketamine for induction, with the aim of providing muscle relaxation. This combination is known colloquially as "ketofol" or "propoket" but is not a commercially available preparation, and readers should be aware that there is no standard proportion of propofol and ketamine.

Unlike thiopental, which requires a large initial bolus given rapidly to achieve unconsciousness, propofol should be administered slowly, to effect (except in horses), resulting in use of a reduced overall dose (and fewer adverse effects). Propofol is rapidly redistributed and cleared from both hepatic and extrahepatic sites. Its short duration and clearance make it a suitable choice for patients with moderate-to-severe hepatic disease (if there is no significant concurrent cardiovascular compromise). The effective duration of general anesthesia is slightly less than 10 min with complete recovery to ambulation within 20 min in dogs and 30–40 min in cats. Clinically, this promotes the use of propofol as an anesthetic induction drug before maintenance with inhalational anesthesia or for short procedures.

Summary of relevant pharmacodynamic effects is as follows:

Respiratory depression and apnea are commonly observed following propofol administration, but these effects can be reduced by appropriate rates of drug administration (one-quarter of the calculated total dose injected every 15 s, taking 1 min to inject the full dose, if needed). Apnea can occur anytime within five minutes after administering a bolus, and delayed apnea can occur in dogs and cats that have been heavily sedated with a combination of an alpha-2 agonist and opioid. The decrease in cardiac output resulting from this premedication combination results in a slower onset of action for propofol, causing the delay in apnea.

A decrease in systemic arterial blood pressure, which can result in transient hypotension, is a common adverse effect following bolus administration of propofol in dogs and cats, even at recommended induction doses. This is secondary to a decrease in systemic vascular resistance (affecting both the venous and arterial circulation) and, to a lesser extent, negative inotropic effects. Animals that are hypovolemic may benefit from an intravenous fluid bolus before propofol administration.

Infrequently, propofol administration causes focal muscle twitches ("propofol twitches"), often affecting the face, limbs, or shoulders. These should not be mistaken for seizures but can be disruptive if exhibited at the surgical site. This effect is usually short-lived but infrequently lasts for >1 h. Uncommonly, some dogs and cats may withdraw their limb in response to propofol administration. The cause is unclear, but propofol injection is reported as painful in humans (as a warm burning sensation). Propofol reduces seizure activity and is considered appropriate for use in animals with raised intracranial pressure (as, for example, secondary to a brain tumor). There is conflicting evidence on the effect of propofol on intraocular pressure. This likely reflects the combined effect of propofol, different premedication drugs, and timing of pressure measurement. An increase in the incidence of infections in joints or wounds has been described with propofol use in septic or bacteremic human patients, and this may also be true in septic or bacteremic animals.

Alfaxalone

Alfaxalone is a neuroactive steroid. It is available as a clear, colorless, sterile, 1% (w/v) solution (10 mg/mL) in 2-alpha-hydroxypropyl-*b*-cyclodextrin. Cyclodextrin is inert, does not cause histamine release, and is excreted in its parent form through the kidney. In many pharmacokinetic and pharmacodynamic respects, alfaxalone is similar to propofol. It is recommended to administer alfaxalone IV over at least 60 s for a smooth transition to general anesthesia and good intubating conditions. The occasional animal may paddle, shake their head or have muscle fasciculations, and may be hypersensitive to environmental stimuli during induction. Premedication, especially with alpha-2 agonists, reduces the dose required for anesthesia induction. Recumbency lasts approximately 20 min following 2 mg/kg in dogs (longer in cats), but response to noxious stimulation returns in about half that time. This short duration of action is due to redistribution and rapid hepatic metabolism.

In addition to IV use of alfaxalone in small animals, alfaxalone has been used successfully in other species, including ruminants, camelids, and horses. It has also been evaluated for IM use in a wide range of species. While the large volume needed currently limits routine IM use of alfaxalone, this route may be considered in species where IV access is challenging because of anatomy (e.g., chelonians), size (e.g., small rodents), and/or behavior (e.g., marmoset and cats). IM injection does not cause tissue damage. It may also be used in combination with other premedication drugs to enhance sedation in domestic animals that are challenging to handle. Reports indicate peak sedation at 10–15 min following doses of 2.5–5.0 mg/kg IM when given alone. Peak sedation can, but not always, be shortened to 2–5 min if injected in combination with an opioid and alpha-2 agonist, but cyanosis can occur. When animals are anesthetized, or heavily sedated, oxygen should be provided because hypoventilation and hypoxemia are frequent clinical concerns. This is especially true when alfaxalone is used in combination with an opioid and alpha-2 agonist, mixed in a single syringe for IM injection.

Summary of relevant pharmacodynamic effects is as follows:

Respiratory depression, including post-induction apnea, is commonly observed in dogs and to a lesser extent in cats when IV doses at the higher end of the recommended range are administered. The incidence of post-induction apnea appears to be as common as with propofol.

At recommended induction doses, vasodilation occurs but is thought to be less pronounced than with propofol. Post-induction hypotension can occur at recommended doses secondary to a transient decrease in inotropy and cardiac output. Reductions in arterial blood pressure may be partly offset by an increase in heart rate, but this is not reliably present. This cardiovascular depression is likely to be magnified in compromised animals.

As with IV administration, hypersensitivity to stimuli may be observed following IM administration. Hyperactivity and increased sensitivity to sound may also be observed in recovery (following induction by either the IV or IM route in dogs and cats) especially when the anesthesia period is short or sedation from premedication is minimal. Hence, a quiet environment with dimmed lighting is suggested in animals recovering from alfaxalone. Excitement is self-limiting and short-lived and does not require treatment, with the exception of animals recovering from an orthopedic operation or at risk of becoming hyperthermic. Other clinical effects are muscle fasciculations and "jaw chattering." These tend to be seen more commonly when sedation is mild.

Etomidate

Etomidate is an imidazole compound. It is a weak base (pK_a 4.2) and is available in different formulations including a 2 mg/mL solution (pH 8.1) in 35% propylene glycol, which renders it hyperosmolar (4640 mOsm/L versus approximately 300 mOsm/L for plasma). In some countries, it is also available as an intralipid formulation that is white in color. The drug is approximately 75% protein bound and undergoes ester hydrolysis and glucuronide conjugation in the liver (recall that this enzyme system is rapidly saturated in cats; see Chapter 6). Etomidate has minimal adverse cardiopulmonary and central nervous system effects following administration. Consequently, it offers an attractive alternative for anesthesia induction in critically ill patients and cats with hypertrophic cardiomyopathy. It is also useful as an anesthetic induction drug in both dogs and cats with concurrent thoracic and head trauma. For induction of anesthesia, the drug should only be given IV. Premedication is highly recommended before etomidate administration to reduce the incidence of adverse effects during induction (e.g., myoclonus and vomiting). Alternatively, or in addition to premedication, etomidate may be co-administered with a benzodiazepine.

Summary of relevant pharmacodynamic effects is as follows:

Minor, self-limiting transient decrease respiratory rate of little clinical relevance.

Minor, self-limiting transient decrease in heart rate of little clinical relevance.

Etomidate interferes with cortisol synthesis for a period of 6–24 h. Administration of a physiologic dose of dexamethasone, or other short-acting glucocorticoid, before etomidate use is often suggested for hospitalized (and especially debilitated) patients if there is no relative contraindication (as, for example, in a diabetic animal). Usually, dexamethasone is used because it does not interfere with hypothalamic–pituitary–adrenal axis testing, which may be required in a debilitated animal. Pain on injection and hemolysis of red blood cells following administration are attributed to the hyperosmolar nature of the propylene glycol formulation. These effects can be minimized by diluting the drug significantly (using a 1:4 or 1:6 dilution with isotonic intravenous fluids) or co-administering it with intravenous fluids. Use of topical local anesthetic is recommended because increased airway reactivity following etomidate administration may make intubation difficult. Co-administration with a benzodiazepine agonist provides sufficient jaw muscle relaxation to facilitate tracheal intubation. Opisthotonos is sometimes observed in cats recovering from etomidate and this does not seem to be associated with any long-term consequences.

Dissociative Anesthetics

The dissociative anesthetics have unique central effects that include thalamocortical depression, and hippocampal and limbic activation. Clinically, these manifest as rigidity and muscle hypertonicity in the face of apparent absence of awareness, i.e., a dissociative state. Excessively high doses can cause a seizure-like appearance. The manifestation of a dissociative state is pronounced in dogs, cats, horses, and pigs, whereas cattle and small ruminants do not demonstrate muscle rigidity and hypertonicity. They are a versatile group of drugs and have been administered to many different species. In contrast to other anesthetic induction drugs, ketamine, and likely tiletamine, have some analgesic properties (see Chapters 3 and 9). However, any analgesia conferred must not be considered sufficient for surgical or invasive procedures and other analgesics should be provided. Intravenous and intramuscular administration routes are preferred to ensure a reliable effect. Unlike the hypnotic-sedatives, which act at $GABA_A$ receptors, the dissociative anesthetics act at many different receptors, the most important of which is NMDA receptor antagonism in the brain and spinal cord. This action blocks the influx of calcium (and other cations) into the nerve, which decreases the release of excitatory neurotransmitters and causes the dissociative state.

Ketamine Hydrochloride

Ketamine hydrochloride, a weak base (pK_a of 7.5), is a racemic mixture of two isomers formulated at various ready-mixed concentrations (most commonly as 100 mg/mL, but 50 mg/mL may be available) or in powder form ready for reconstitution. Sterile water for injection is the preferred fluid for reconstitution, and a concentration of less than 200 mg/mL is considered stable for clinical use. Reconstituted concentrations greater than 200 mg/mL are unstable (even when the solution is warmed) and are not recommended. It has been administered via IV, IM, oral, and rectal transmucosal routes at a wide range of doses, varying with species and route of administration. Ketamine has a very wide therapeutic index. The onset of action following IV administration is 45–60 s, slower than with propofol or alfaxalone. About 93% of the drug is absorbed within 20 min following IM administration, whereas only 16% is available to exert its effects 30 min after oral administration in the dog. Recovery from a single dose is determined by redistribution. Clearance from the body is through hepatic metabolism and renal excretion of both the parent drug and active metabolites (notably norketamine). Therefore, drug accumulation and associated effects are possible in all species with repeated dosing, infusions or single high-dose administration. In dogs, ketamine is metabolized by N-demethylation to norketamine (10–20% activity) and then to hydroxynorketamine (no activity), which is conjugated and excreted. In cats, only norketamine is formed due to their limited ability to conjugate with glucuronyl transferase. Hence, cats are more susceptible to prolonged effects with high or repeated dose administration. This is magnified if they also have a limited ability to excrete ketamine and norketamine as may occur in cats with significant renal dysfunction.

Respiratory effects include mild transient hypoventilation unless excitement is observed during induction, in which case an increased respiratory rate is observed. A transient apneustic breathing pattern (a long pause held for as long as 40 s after inspiration followed by 2–4 rapid breaths) is frequently observed in cats, dogs, and horses, especially when administered at high doses. Pharyngeal responses (swallowing) may be maintained following drug administration, but this swallowing reflex should not be considered as being protective and aspiration can still occur. It has been suggested that this, coupled with increases in tracheobronchial and salivary secretions, can make intubation more challenging, but experience suggests that at an appropriate depth of anesthesia this is not the case.

An increase in sympathetic tone, which clinically manifests as an increase in heart rate, myocardial contractility, and blood pressure is usually seen following ketamine administration. This increase in sympathetic tone is by indirect mechanisms, causing an increase in norepinephrine concentrations in the brain and peripheral nervous system. The consequent increase in myocardial work and oxygen consumption is undesirable in patients with restrictive or hypertrophic cardiac disease, where ketamine is contraindicated. It should also be avoided in the compromised patient or when sympathetic tone is reduced because myocardial contractility may be depressed following drug administration in patients with depleted sympathetic reserve.

Increased muscle tonicity, swallowing and maintained (albeit somewhat diminished) ocular reflexes, makes assessing depth of anesthesia during induction and maintenance a challenge. The anesthetist is therefore advised to assess the patient prior to administering more drug. The response to stimuli and return of limb withdrawal reflexes can indicate a lighter plane of anesthesia that may require additional doses. Recovery from ketamine-based anesthesia can be prolonged and associated with ataxia and dissociated behaviors, especially if high doses are used for induction and the anesthetic duration is short.

Tiletamine

Tiletamine is available in powder form as a 1:1 mixture with the benzodiazepine zolazepam. Like ketamine, it has been administered via many routes at a wide dose range in many different species. The reconstituted solution contains 50 mg/mL of each drug. Refrigeration extends the recommended shelf life to 56 days following reconstitution, but this drug may be stored for 7 days at room temperature. Some veterinarians do not use the provided fluid for reconstitution but rather use an alpha-2 adrenergic receptor agonist (typically medetomidine or dexmedetomidine) and an opioid (typically butorphanol) in various ratios to formulate a low-volume injectable dose. Zolazepam reduces the incidence of muscle rigidity and excitement that can occur with tiletamine immobilization, and the combination results in dose-dependent central nervous system depression. Like ketamine, IM tiletamine–zolazepam injection can elicit an avoidance response (believed to relate to stinging on injection). Recumbency is usually observed within 5–10 min of IM administration. Prolonged sedation and/or residual ataxia may last 2–4 h after administration of doses greater than 5–7.5 mg/kg. Hypothermia, hepatic or renal insufficiency, and hypoxemia may contribute to residual effects. Cardiovascular and respiratory considerations are similar to those listed for ketamine.

Similar to ketamine hydrochloride.

Similar to ketamine hydrochloride.

Similar to ketamine hydrochloride in many respects, but with the addition of zolazepam, recovery characteristics are dependent on which drug is eliminated first. Dogs tend to eliminate zolazepam faster than tiletamine and thus the recovery characteristics are similar to ketamine. Whereas felines (small and large) tend to eliminate tiletamine faster than zolazepam and generally have smoother but sometimes prolonged recoveries.

Other Drugs Used During Induction of General Anesthesia

Opioids

Due to the large margin of cardiovascular safety, some opioids are used for induction of anesthesia and/or as part of a balanced anesthetic induction technique in compromised patients. The use of opioids for induction of anesthesia is reserved primarily for critically sick dogs (ASA IV and V) or those with severe cardiac disease. Opioid induction in cats should generally be reserved for moribund (ASA V) patients. However, if an opioid induction is attempted in nonmoribund cats, then a hypnotic-sedative should be readily available to complete induction should increase in arousal or excitement occur. Of the available pure-*mu* agonists suitable for this approach, fentanyl and its analogs (alfentanil, sufentanil, and remifentanil) are most commonly used because they are rapid acting. However, the duration of action from a single bolus is short and, in most cases, less than 15 min. Other opioids that could be considered are methadone and hydromorphone; however, the time until tracheal intubation can be performed usually takes longer compared to fentanyl. If an opioid is used as the induction drug, then it is often administered with a benzodiazepine, or if this combination is insufficient to allow tracheal intubation, a small dose (about a quarter of the normal induction dose) of a hypnotic-sedative induction drug may be required.

Fentanyl is one of the more commonly used opioids for anesthesia induction. It is a synthetic phenylpiperdine derivative that is usually presented in vials or bottles at a 50 mcg/mL concentration. An example of an induction strategy in dogs (and cats) is to give an initial dose of 0.005 (5 mcg/kg) to 0.010 mg/kg (10 mcg/kg) IV followed 2 minutes later by a dose of a benzodiazepine (diazepam or midazolam at 0.2–0.3 mg/kg) and then additional boluses of fentanyl (0.005 mg/kg [5 mcg/kg]) or a very low dose of a hypnotic drug (propofol 0.5 mg/kg or alfaxalone at 0.25 mg/kg) to induce anesthesia and allow for tracheal intubation. Fentanyl is highly lipid soluble and readily crosses the blood–brain barrier resulting in its rapid action. Once fentanyl reaches the central nervous system, sedation occurs (more so in dogs than cats). Other effects seen in some dogs include panting, bradycardia, apnea, and excitement. These vary according to health status and presence of other drugs. Panting results from the effect of fentanyl to decrease the thermoregulatory set point so that the body attempts to lower core temperature. Of the analogs, remifentanil and sufentanil (both discussed later) are more prone to cause vagal mediated bradycardia during induction compared to fentanyl. The short duration of effect is largely because of rapid redistribution and hepatic metabolism. When fentanyl is used as an induction drug, then the short duration of action needs to be considered and a plan for intra- and post-operative analgesia instituted (see drugs used for maintenance of general anesthesia).

Central Muscle Relaxants

Drugs that have central muscle relaxant effects are often used for co-induction because they facilitate a reduction in the dose of primary agent required for tracheal intubation. They may also provide relaxation when used with drugs that do not provide muscle relaxation (e.g., ketamine). Benzodiazepines are a common choice and have been discussed in the previous section on premedication drugs.

Guaifenesin or GGE (abbreviation for glycerol guiacolate ether) is another central muscle relaxant that is routinely used as an IV co-induction drug in large, domesticated animals (horses and cattle). GGE acts at inhibitory interneurons at the level of the spinal cord and brainstem to cause muscle relaxation and mild sedation. The drug is presented in a powder form ready for reconstitution using an isotonic crystalloid fluid (like 0.9% sodium chloride). It is strongly advised to limit the reconstituted concentration to a 5% solution (e.g., by mixing the 50 g of powered drug to a 1 L intravenous fluid bag). The reconstituted drug is rapidly infused to effect (commonly under pressure) using an intravenous fluid administration set (e.g., 20, 15, or 10 drops/mL, except 60 drops/mL). Given the required dose (50–100 mg/kg for anesthesia co-induction in horses and cattle), a large volume of drug must be administered to achieve the desired effect. This and the potential to cause tissue necrosis with accidental perivascular administration (especially when the drug concentration exceeds 5%) result in the strong recommendation for IV catheter placement. When used as part of the anesthesia protocol, it is important to recognize that there is a lag between drug administration and effect. Toxicity initially manifests initially as rigidity, followed by respiratory depression or apnea. The latter can result in death if not treated and occurs at approximately 200 mg/kg.

Drugs Used for Maintenance of General Anesthesia

Injectable drugs are used during the maintenance period of general anesthesia to fulfill either the requirements of keeping the patient anesthetized or to decrease the amount of anesthetic (inhalational or injectable) required to maintain a surgical plane of anesthesia, or both. The technique of administering solely injectable drug(s) to maintain anesthesia is called "total intravenous anesthesia" (TIVA). The absolute requirement is to ensure that a drug that causes unconsciousness is incorporated into the TIVA protocol, thus drugs used for induction must be included. Injectable drugs that have analgesic and/or muscle relaxant properties are usually included as part of a balanced anesthetic and/or multimodal analgesic plan. These drugs decrease the amount of the anesthetic (injectable or inhalational) required to maintain anesthesia.

Primary Injectable Drugs Used for TIVA

While anesthesia is most commonly maintained with inhalational anesthetics and adjunct drugs, there are specific circumstances in which injectable-only maintenance protocols may be preferred. Examples include animals with neurological compromise and concerns for raised intracranial pressure. In this scenario, propofol or alfaxalone is often used in combination with fentanyl (or other opioid) and ventilatory support provided. Concurrent use of a benzodiazepine may also be considered. Other situations, where injectable drugs are needed or preferred, may also arise and additional drugs such as lidocaine and ketamine may be considered as appropriate for the species (e.g., small dog requiring bronchoscopy).

Propofol

Propofol (0.1–0.4 mg/kg/min) may be used for TIVA in dogs and to a limited extent in cats where it may accumulate due to their limited ability to glucuronidate. Its use is described in other species such as horses, but the technique has not gained widespread popularity. Target-controlled administration is described for propofol in dogs and may shorten recovery time, which seems both animal and dose dependent, but is not available to most veterinarians. Propofol provides dose-dependent effects ranging from sedation to unconsciousness. It is frequently used as a CRI to facilitate diagnostic procedures (e.g., MRI for patient with brain tumor), but its sole use is not recommended for noxious procedures as it does not provide analgesia. The use of analgesic drugs by bolus or CRI is strongly recommended and has the added benefit of reducing the dose of propofol needed. Cardiovascular parameters are usually well maintained with combinations of propofol and analgesic drugs, but ventilation may be necessary. Intubation and oxygen administration are strongly recommended when using propofol for anesthetic maintenance. A caution when using propofol in this manner is to recognize monitoring depth of anesthesia is different than observed for inhalational anesthetics. Most notably, the palpebral response is often present at an adequate anesthetic plane and to abolish it may result in an animal that is too deep.

Alfaxalone

As with propofol, use of alfaxalone (3–8 mg/kg/h) for maintenance of anesthesia in dogs and cats has been described. Similar to propofol, it too should be used with analgesic medications for noxious procedures. Support and monitoring considerations are also similar. While the drug is reported to be noncumulative in both dogs and cats, long-term use has not been evaluated and clinical experience suggests that recovery time can be variable and occasionally prolonged. Since glucuronidation is not required for its clearance, it is likely the better choice in cats requiring an injectable-only anesthetic protocol. As with single dose use, excitatory behaviors and tremoring may be seen during recovery and can be cause for concern where increased metabolic requirements and heat generation (from motor activity) are not desirable.

Ketamine

While ketamine may be used to maintain anesthesia alone as part of a short duration TIVA protocol in small animal, it tends to accumulate and result in a prolonged recovery with adverse behavioral effects. It is more commonly used for short-term anesthesia maintenance in horses (2–3 mg/kg/h) in combination with alpha-2 agonist drugs and either guaifenesin or a benzodiazepine. Recovery time may be prolonged, and ataxia is observed if the horse attempts to stand early. Horses maintained with these combinations generally maintain ocular reflexes and demonstrate good blood pressure and normal to low heart rates. Apneustic respiration is common at an appropriate anesthetic plane.

Drugs Used as Part of a Balanced Anesthetic and/or Provide Multimodal Analgesia

The concept of multimodal analgesia is described in Chapter 3.

Opioids

Fentanyl and its analogs are very effective at reducing the MAC (and MIR) during constant administration in both dogs and cats. In the dog, reduction in MAC of isoflurane is approximately 50% with the concurrent administration of a fentanyl infusion at a rate of 20 mcg/kg/h (0.33 mcg/kg/min). In cats, a ceiling effect at 10 mcg/kg/h in MAC reduction of around 25–30% is observed. A significant advantage of combining an inhalational anesthetic with an opioid such as fentanyl is that cardiovascular function is better maintained with a combination of opioid and inhalational anesthetic (providing bradycardia is treated) than an equivalent dose of inhalational anesthetic alone. However, respiratory depression is a significant concern and ventilation may need to be assisted or controlled. Lower doses (2–5 mcg/kg/h) may also be used during anesthesia, with some advantage in minimizing bradycardia and hypoventilation. This is the same dose range as that used for postoperative analgesia with fentanyl. If fentanyl is used at moderate to high doses (>7–10 mcg/kg/h), the infusion should be discontinued or reduced approximately 30 min before the end of the procedure to facilitate a timely return to spontaneous ventilation and avoid a delayed recovery.

Alfentanil is another opioid with a short half-life suited for administration by infusion during anesthesia. It has been evaluated for use in cats and is used in dogs. Isoflurane requirements are reduced by around 65% with an infusion rate targeting a plasma concentration of 500 ng/mL. Cardiovascular variables were also better maintained. As with at least some other opioids in cats, body temperature increased. Clinical use in the dogs supports a reduction in propofol dose with concurrent use of alfentanil when infused at 60 mcg/kg/h. In cats, alfentanil has been administered at 30 mcg/kg/h.

Sufentanil, like alfentanil, is a derivative of fentanyl. Similarly, as a consequence of its short duration of action, it is also administered as an IV infusion. Its pharmacodynamic properties are similar to alfentanil, fentanyl, and remifentanil, with its use associated with bradycardia (with potential to decrease cardiac output at higher infusion rates) and hypoventilation. If used to facilitate induction of general anesthesia in dogs (as described in the preceding text with fentanyl), a bolus of 0.5 mcg/kg can be delivered IV, followed by 0.5 mcg/kg/h. This infusion protocol produced similar cardiorespiratory changes to fentanyl delivered at 4 mcg/kg/h, reflecting its greater potency compared to fentanyl.

Remifentanil is unique among the opioids in that it is broken down in the plasma, which results in very high clearance and short duration of clinical effects, even in patients with significant hepatic disease. While analgesic effects also dissipate quickly, it is favored by some for its intra-operative titratability and lack of residual adverse effects. In cats, administered doses ranging from 0.25 to 1.0 mcg/kg/min (15–60 mcg/kg/h) reduces the isoflurane dose between 23 and 30%. There was no difference with increasing dose. In dogs, significant decreases in isoflurane dose requirements were seen with increasing doses of remifentanil. An infusion of 0.1 mcg/kg/min (6 mcg/kg/h) resulted in a dose reduction of round 30% with a 50% reduction when the infusion is increased to 0.25 mcg/kg/min (15 mcg/kg/h).

Morphine may be administered alone or as part of the combination colloquially known as "MLK," where morphine, lidocaine, and ketamine are mixed together as a single solution for CRI in dogs. Anesthetic dose reduction with minimum respiratory depression is reported at doses of 0.1–0.2 mg/kg/h as is commonly recommended. Other drugs with longer actions such as *methadone* and *hydromorphone* are also generally limited to use at the low end of their dose range when given as an infusion due to the potential to cause a prolonged recovery.

Benzodiazepine Agonists

Midazolam is more miscible than diazepam and less likely to bond to plastics; thus, it has commonly been used as the benzodiazepine of choice for intravenous infusion. Midazolam is incorporated for its muscle relaxant properties. The dose reduction of MAC and MIR is not as profound as with opioids and alpha-2 agonists, and administration causes a reduction of between 10 and 15%. However, additive effects of benzodiazepines with other drugs are likely. Typically, midazolam is infused at 0.1–0.3 mg/kg/h in most species. CRIs of longer than 60 min are cautioned in cats and horses because they can develop excitement and muscle weakness (horses) during recovery.

Alpha-2 Adrenergic Receptor Agonists

Medetomidine and dexmedetomidine CRIs have been used in dogs, cats, and horses with a substantial reduction in MAC (approximately 40–70%), especially when combined with an opioid. In addition to MAC reduction, they also provide good analgesia. Cardiovascular depression from these drugs is significant and should be considered; however, the effect of low doses administered by CRI may not have the same reduction in cardiac output as bolus dosing. In healthy dogs, cats, and horses, an infusion rate of 1–3 mcg/kg/h (medetomidine) is frequently used after a loading infusion to provide analgesia and anesthesia-sparing effects.

Ketamine

Ketamine, at sub-anesthetic doses, has been shown to mitigate or prevent central sensitization. At doses as low as 10–20 mcg/kg/min (0.6–1.2 mg/kg/h), after a loading dose of 0.5 mg/kg, ketamine will reduce anesthetic requirements up to 25%. Higher doses (up to 3 mg/kg/h) are reported to reduce inhalational anesthesia requirements further but exhibit a ceiling effect. Ketamine use in this manner has been reported in dogs, cats, and horses. While reported benefits are largely anecdotal, ketamine infusions may be continued into the post-operative period in conscious animals. Doses in the range of 1–3 mcg/kg/min (0.06–0.18 mg/kg/h) are suggested in awake animals to minimize behavior changes. In horses, prolonged infusions (>2 hours) during maintenance of anesthesia are avoided, and the infusion stopped 30 min before recovery to minimize the risk of excitement and incoordination during recovery.

Lidocaine

Lidocaine has grown in popularity since reports of its beneficial effects in ameliorating gastrointestinal stasis, especially in the horse. Lidocaine has anti-inflammatory and free-radical scavenging properties that have increased its popularity in small animal practice. Most veterinarians are comfortable with its use as it is often used to treat ventricular tachyarrhythmias in the dog. Adverse effects, which include seizures from overdose, are rare if appropriate doses are used. Anesthetic dose reduction was reported with a dose of 50 mcg/kg/min in dogs, but doses as low as 10–20 mcg/kg/min are used with perceived benefit in clinical patients. If used in the cat, a low dose (5–10 mcg/kg/min) must be used as the potential for toxicity is greater and many anesthetists avoid its use as an infusion in this species for this reason. Additionally, while a reduction in isoflurane dose was seen with lidocaine use in cats, cardiovascular depression was greater than with isoflurane alone, suggesting little benefit in this species. In horses, an infusion of 50 mcg/kg/min resulted in a 25% reduction in the sevoflurane dose requirement. In horses, the cardiovascular effects with equivalent doses of sevoflurane or a combination of sevoflurane and lidocaine did not differ, but there are potential analgesic effects, cost savings, and benefits to gastrointestinal motility. However, prolonged infusions of lidocaine during general anesthesia can cause a delayed, ataxic recovery and the infusion should be discontinued 30–45 min before recovery.

Questions and Answers

There are more practice questions and answers available for this chapter on the website. Please visit http://www.wiley.com/go/VeterinaryAnesthesiaZeiler.

Questions

1) Give three reasons justifying the use of ACP (acepromazine) as a premedication in dogs.
2) Give three reasons justifying the use of medetomidine as a premedication.
3) What is the likely behavioral effect of administering opioids to nonpainful horses?
4) Which drug can be used to treat central sensitization (windup pain)?
5) What condition do sheep or goats develop after administering xylazine?

Answers

1) Any three of anti-arrhythmic, anti-emetic, muscle relaxation, antihistamine effects, and anxiolysis.
2) Any three of sedation, analgesia, muscle relaxation, and anxiolysis.
3) Hypermetria, neighing, head bobbing, and sweating (excitement).
4) Ketamine.
5) Pulmonary edema and pulmonary hypertension.

Further Reading

Arnold, B.D.C. and Bilski, A.J.T. (1994). Drawing up propofol. *Anaesth* 49: 738–739.

Aydin, N., Aydin, N., Gultekin, B. et al. (2002). Bacterial contamination of propofol: the effects of temperature and lidocaine. *Eur J Anaesthesiol* 19: 455–458.

D'Aubioul, J., Van Gerven, W., Van de Water, A. et al. (1984). Cardiovascular and some respiratory effects of high doses of alfentanil in dogs. *Eur J Pharmacol* 100: 79–84.

Gent, T., Iff, I., Bettschart-Wolfensberger, R., and Mosing, M. (2013). Neuraxial morphine induced pruritus in two cats and treatment with sub anaesthetic doses of propofol. *Vet Anaesth Analg* 40: 517–520.

Hall, L.W. (1982). Relaxant drugs in small animal anaesthesia. *J Assoc Vet Anaesth Gr Brit Ire* 10: 144–155.

Hall, R.I., Szlam, F., and Hug, C.C. (1987). The enflurane-sparing effect of alfentanil in dogs. *Anesth Analg* 66: 1287–1291.

Haskins, S.C., Farver, T.B., and Patz, J.D. (1985). Ketamine in dogs. *Am J Vet Res* 46: 1855–1860.

Hayashi, Y., Sumikawa, K., Yamatodani, A. et al. (1989). Myocardial sensitization by thiopental to arrhythmogenic action of epinephrine in dogs. *Anesthes* 71: 929–935.

Hellyer, P.W., Mama, K.R., Shafford, H.L. et al. (2001). Effects of diazepam and flumazenil on minimum alveolar concentrations for dogs anesthetized with isoflurane or a combination of isoflurane and fentanyl. *Am J Vet Res* 62: 555–560.

Joerger, F.B., Wieser, M.L., Steblaj, B. et al. (2023) Evaluation of cardiovascular effects of intramuscular medetomidine and a medetomidine-vatinoxan combination in Beagle dogs: A randomized blinded crossover laboratory study. *Vet Anaesth Analg* 50: 397–407.

Jones, R.S., Auer, U., and Mosing, M. (2015). Reversal of neuromuscular block in companion animals. *Vet Anaesth Analg* 42: 455–471.

Kaartinen, J., Pang, D., Moreau, M. et al. (2010). Hemodynamic effects of an intravenous infusion of medetomidine at six different dose regimens in isoflurane-anesthetized dogs. *Vet Ther* 11: E1–E16.

Michelsen, L.G., Salmenpera, M., Hug, C.C. et al. (1996). Anesthetic potency of remifentanil in dogs. *Anesthes* 84: 865–872.

Muir, W.W., Wiese, A.J., and March, P.A. (2003). Effects of morphine, lidocaine, ketamine, and morphine-lidocaine-ketamine drug combination on minimum alveolar concentration in dogs anesthetized with isoflurane. *Am J Vet Res* 64: 1155–1160.

Murphy, M.R. and Hug, C.C. (1982). The anesthetic potency of fentanyl in terms of its reduction of enflurane MAC. *Anesthes* 57: 485–488.

Pascoe, P.J., Raekallio, M., Kuusela, E. et al. (2006). Changes in the minimum alveolar concentration of isoflurane and some cardiopulmonary measurements during three continuous infusion rates of dexmedetomidine in dogs. *Vet Anaesth Analg* 33: 97–103.

Pypendop, B.H. and Verstegen, J.P. (1998). Hemodynamic effects of medetomidine in the dog: a dose titration study. *Vet Surg* 27: 612–622.

Weaver, B.M. and Raptopoulos, D. (1990). Induction of anaesthesia in dogs and cats with propofol. *Vet Rec* 126: 617–620.

8

Inhalational Anesthetic Drugs

Nigel Caulkett and Daniel Pang

Mechanisms of Action

The use of inhalational (volatile) anesthetic drugs dates back to the 1840s with the introduction of ether by Dr. Crawford Long. This was soon followed by the introduction of nitrous oxide in the United States of America. Inhalational anesthetics have been in clinical practice for almost 200 years, but we still do not fully understand their mechanism of action. Early theories of anesthetic action focused on the ability of chemicals to disrupt the lipid bilayer of the cell membrane. Two investigators, Meyer and Overton, had independently observed that potency of anesthetics was increased in proportion to their lipid solubility.

For many years, research primarily focused on actions of anesthetics at the level of the cell membrane. In the 1970s and 1980s, some researchers began to question these theories and suggested that a protein target may be an alternate site of action for these drugs. Two researchers in particular, Nick Franks and Bill Lieb, performed some very elegant research to determine the effects of inhalational drugs on the firefly luciferase enzyme (Franks and Lieb 1984). In this work, they showed that a number of general anesthetics could inhibit the activity of this enzyme by binding with it. They also demonstrated that there was a good correlation between the concentrations required for enzyme inhibition and the concentrations required for anesthesia in animals. They further demonstrated that this binding was competitive in nature and appeared to occur at a common binding site. Taken together, this suggested that the action of the anesthetics was not via a disruption of the lipid bilayer but resulted from binding to a specific protein site.

Once it was determined that the mechanism of action of inhalational anesthetics resulted from binding to a specific protein site, the next step has been to determine which receptor(s) are involved. One of the more obvious sites is the gamma-aminobutyric acid A ($GABA_A$) receptor. A number of anesthetics, including propofol, thiopental, alfaxalone, and the benzodiazepines, have been shown to act on $GABA_A$ receptors. Inhalational anesthetics appear to have some of their activity at $GABA_A$ receptors, whereas gas anesthetics such as nitrous oxide and xenon do not appear to affect $GABA_A$ receptors. Glycine receptors and certain potassium channels are also potential targets for inhalational anesthetics. For example, sevoflurane has been shown to increase potassium conductance both pre- and post-synaptically resulting in hyperpolarization of neurons. These actions of sevoflurane are mediated by two specific potassium channels, TREK-1 and TASK-1. As with other anesthetics, such as ketamine, there is also evidence that inhalational anesthetics competitively bind to N-methyl-D-aspartate (NMDA) receptors with an antagonistic effect at this receptor. Ultimately, it is likely that the mechanism of action of inhalational anesthetics involves a number of different binding sites. Once these are determined, we will be better able to design drugs with more beneficial effects and fewer adverse effects. For more complete information on this subject please refer to the Further Reading section.

Even though we do not fully understand the mechanism of general anesthesia with inhalational drugs, there are many things that we do know concerning the pharmacokinetics and pharmacodynamics of these drugs. It is important to understand these concepts to use these drugs appropriately in a clinical setting. This chapter discusses some of the physical characteristics of these agents, factors that influence the onset and offset of these drugs, the important impact of delivery equipment, and the adverse effects that we should be aware of as anesthetists.

Fundamental Principles of Veterinary Anesthesia, First Edition. Edited by Gareth E. Zeiler and Daniel S. J. Pang.

Companion Website: www.wiley.com/go/VeterinaryAnesthesiaZeiler

Uptake and Excretion of Volatile Anesthetics

Inhalational anesthetics are unique in that they are delivered to the lungs and must transit the alveolar membrane to enter the circulation. In some cases, there is limited metabolism that occurs in the liver, but for the most part these drugs are not metabolized, and excretion occurs through exhalation from the lungs. These drugs are delivered as vapors or gases; therefore, we are unable to dose them in milligrams per kilogram as we would do with injectable drugs. Inhalational drugs are dosed as a percent of the inspired gas concentration. When we think about the pharmacokinetics of these drugs and the relative potencies of these drugs, it is important to always think in terms of inspired and expired concentrations. One of the unique things about inhalational anesthetics is that equipment is readily available to determine inspired and expired concentration of these drugs. With airway gas analysis, we can determine the uptake and excretion of these drugs in real time. There are a number of factors that will influence uptake and excretion of inhalational drugs, which are discussed in the following sections. In most of these discussions, we will provide examples based on the use of isoflurane and sevoflurane as they are the most commonly used inhalational anesthetics in North America and Europe. Halothane is an older drug that is still used in some countries, so it is included for completeness and provides a useful contrast to isoflurane and sevoflurane.

Saturated Vapor Pressure

The majority of inhalational drugs (excluding nitrous oxide) are delivered as vapors. They are in a liquid state at room temperature, but, being highly volatile, the resulting vapor is readily delivered to the patient via an anesthetic machine. Desflurane has a very high vapor pressure and is almost in a gaseous state at room temperature. It requires specialized equipment for delivery. In the early days of anesthesia, ether was delivered by a technique called the "open drop technique" (see Chapter 5). Liquid anesthetic was poured onto a sponge and placed into a device called a "Cox's mask." The mask would be placed over the animal's muzzle to induce and maintain general anesthesia as the animal inhaled the anesthetic vapor. Table 8.1 shows the open drop concentration for select inhalational anesthetics. These concentrations are considerably higher than necessary for maintaining general anesthesia (see the concept of minimum alveolar concentration (MAC) in the following text), explaining why an open drop approach is not generally considered appropriate for inhalational anesthetics in current use. In order to illustrate the danger of open drop administration, take the value from Table 8.1 for potential open drop isoflurane concentration (31.5%) and divide this by the MAC value in Table 8.2 (1.28%). It is apparent that the maximum open drop concentration is 25 times the MAC concentration. If we do the same for sevoflurane (open drop concentration of 21%/MAC value of 2.36%), the maximum open drop concentration is nine times the MAC concentration. Volatile anesthetics need to be delivered via *precision vaporizers* (Chapter 5) to avoid these dangerously high concentrations.

Table 8.1 Vapor pressure (mmHg) and open drop concentration for different inhalational anesthetic drugs. The potential open drop concentration is calculated when the vapor pressure is divided by atmospheric pressure (760 mmHg at sea level).

	Desflurane	Isoflurane	Halothane	Sevoflurane
Vapor pressure at 20 °C	700	240	243	160
Potential open drop concentration at sea level	92.1%	31.5%	31.9%	21%

Table 8.2 The minimum alveolar concentration of selected inhalational anesthetic drugs in dogs. Values of MAC are similar among mammalian species.

Inhalational anesthetic	MAC	Reference
Halothane	0.89%	Kazama and Ikeda (1988)
Isoflurane	1.28%	Steffey and Howland (1977)
Sevoflurane	2.36%	Kazama and Ikeda (1988)
Desflurane	7.2%	Doorley et al. (1988)

In clinical practice, isoflurane is typically delivered at a maximum concentration of 5% for mask induction of anesthesia and is delivered at 1–2% for maintenance of anesthesia. The open drop concentration of 31.5% would represent a large overdose of the drug. It is for this reason that these anesthetics are typically delivered via a precision vaporizer. The liquid anesthetic is contained within the vaporizer, and it is used to deliver an accurate concentration of the drug. An isoflurane vaporizer is calibrated to precisely deliver isoflurane at increments between 0 and 5%, a concentration range relevant to clinical practice. From Table 8.1 it is also apparent that these drugs should only be used in a vaporizer that is labeled and calibrated for the individual drug as their different volatilities will impact the concentration of the drug delivered from the vaporizer. A similar saturated vapor pressure of isoflurane and halothane means that they could theoretically be delivered safely from the same vaporizer. This practice is not recommended as vaporizers are specifically calibrated and labeled for the individual drug.

Wash-in and Wash-out of Anesthetics

To illustrate the uptake and excretion of volatile anesthetic drugs, it is helpful to consider an animal (e.g., dog) having general anesthesia induced by mask ("mask induction"). Note: Mask (or chamber) induction is no longer a commonly used technique in many species. It can be distressing to the animal, it is difficult to accurately titrate anesthetic depth, and causes workplace pollution with anesthetic drug (a concern for human health). The concept of uptake and excretion of volatile drugs described in the following text equally applies after induction of general anesthesia by intravenous injection.

Typically, we can administer a higher concentration of inhalation anesthetic during the induction period in order to rapidly *wash-in* the anesthetic, and we may even use close to the maximum concentration on the vaporizer. We would never maintain our dog with this concentration, but during mask induction there is no anesthetic in the dog's system and we need to maximize the concentration during the induction period. This concept of using a high drug concentration early in the anesthetic is called "overpressure." The use of overpressure is particularly important when a *rebreathing circuit*, such as circle system, is used as it takes time to maximize inspired anesthetic concentration when exhaled gases are rebreathed as these gases often have a lower anesthetic concentration than the gas being delivered into the circuit from the vaporizer (see Chapter 5 for a complete description of breathing circuits). The overpressure technique must be used more cautiously with a *nonrebreathing circuit*, such as a Bain system, as the concentration delivered from the circuit is the same as the vaporizer concentration. Therefore, it is easier to overdose an animal with a nonrebreathing circuit. Another factor that influences wash-in of the anesthetic with a rebreathing system is the *fresh gas flow*. The fresh gas flow is the mixture of gases flowing into the breathing circuit from the flowmeter(s) and the anesthetic vaporizer. In veterinary medicine, this is typically a mixture of oxygen and the inhalational anesthetic. Rebreathing circuits allow for rebreathing of exhaled gases for economic reasons (reduction of oxygen and inhalational anesthetic administered), and rebreathing helps preserve heat and moisture of the inhaled gas. As stated in the preceding text, rebreathing of gases during the wash-in period will slow induction of anesthesia as the rebreathed gas is low in anesthetic drug when compared to the fresh gas mixture. In addition to the use of overpressure, it is important to use high fresh gas flows during induction of anesthesia (typically 2–3 times the maintenance flow) when using a rebreathing circuit as this will flush the expired gas out of the pop-off valve and into the scavenging system. This results in a relatively greater proportion of fresh gas being delivered, helping to speed the induction of anesthesia. It is typical to deliver higher fresh gas flows for the first 15–20 min of the anesthetic procedure. The impact of increased fresh gas flow and overpressure are illustrated in Figures 8.1 and 8.2. Following the induction period, we hope to maintain our dog at a relatively steady plane of anesthesia, adjusting the vaporizer as needed to maintain an adequate depth of anesthesia for the procedure being performed. Once the procedure is completed, we will need to *wash-out* the inhalational anesthetic for the dog to wake up. The anesthetic is excreted from the lungs and follows a concentration gradient from the alveoli to the anesthetic machine. In order to speed the wash-out of anesthetic, the concentration in the breathing circuit should be as close to zero as possible. If a nonrebreathing circuit is being used, simply adjusting the vaporizer setting to zero or "off" will quickly eliminate the inhalational anesthetic from the circuit and facilitate wash-out from the dog. With a rebreathing circuit, the vaporizer should be turned off, but it is also important to increase the fresh gas flow to minimize rebreathing of exhaled gases (which contain anesthetic drug from the lungs). If the fresh gas flow is not increased, the dog will continue to inhale exhaled anesthetic and recovery will be slower. The timing of when to do this will vary according to circumstances. For instance, if post-operative radiographs are to be taken after surgery, care should be taken to not reduce the anesthetic concentration immediately following surgery to avoid an animal waking up unexpectedly during transfer for radiographs.

Blood/Gas Partition Coefficient

The movement of inhalational anesthetic from the alveolus to the blood and into the brain (site of action to cause general anesthesia) is dependent on the partial pressure of the inhalational anesthetic and ultimately concentration gradients. As the pressure of the gas builds in the alveolus, it will move into the bloodstream until equilibration occurs between the alveolus and the blood. When we think of speed of induction, one of the most important factors is the solubility of the anesthetic in the blood. The development of a high partial pressure of inhalational anesthetic occurs when the anesthetic molecules do not easily go into solution (blood). Therefore, as induction is dependent on a high partial pressure of the drug, induction times with poorly soluble drugs are rapid. By contrast, inhalational anesthetics that are more soluble in blood take a longer time to develop a high partial pressure; consequently, onset of action is slow. We can compare solubility of inhalational

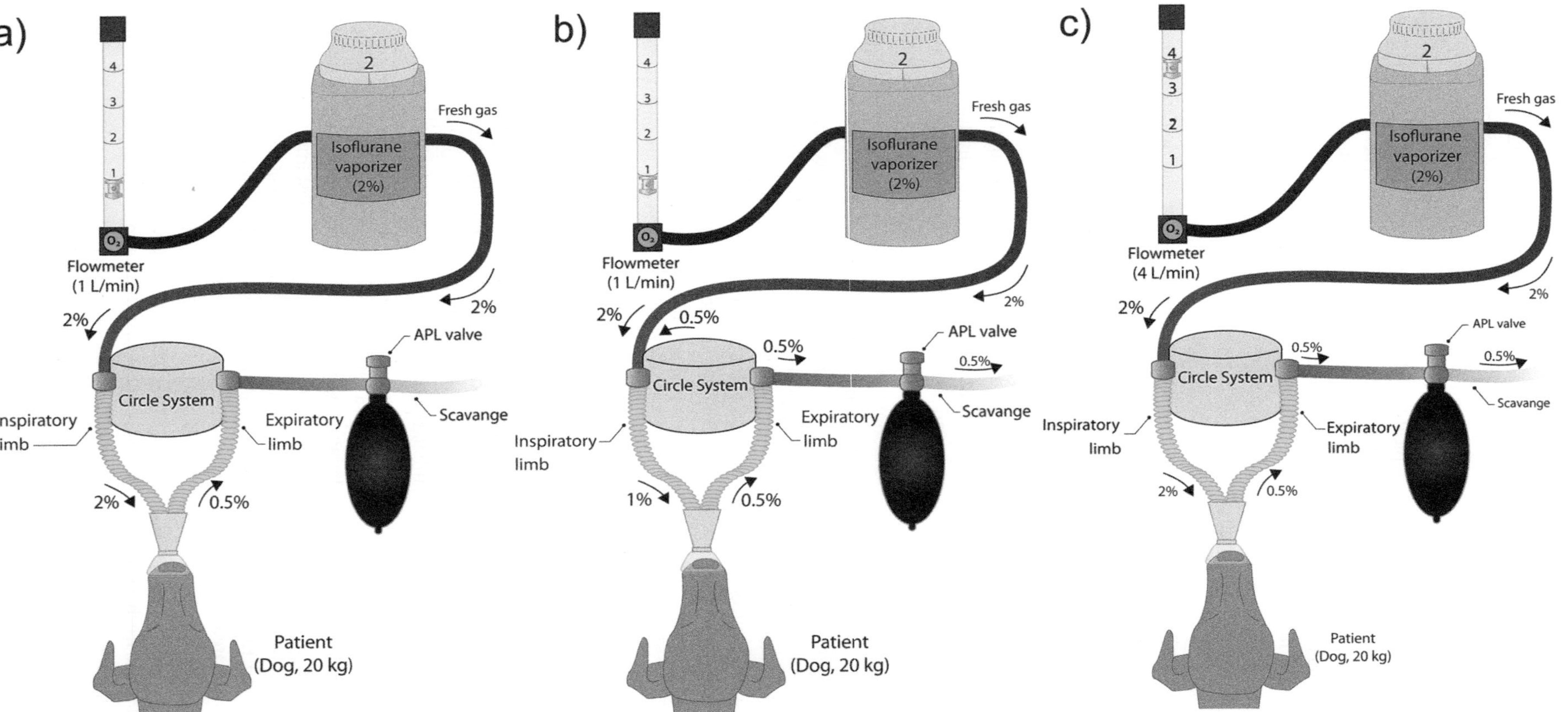

Figure 8.1 Impact of fresh gas flow on inspired anesthetic concentration with a circle rebreathing system. In the following example, isoflurane anesthesia is initiated in a 20 kg dog. The minute ventilation of this dog is 20 kg × 200 mL/kg/min (4 L/min). The accompanying panels illustrate the impact of providing a maintenance flow on a circle system (50 mL/kg/min) versus a flow of 200 mL/kg/min (high enough to minimize rebreathing) on inspired isoflurane concentration. In (a), the oxygen flow rate is set at 50 mL/kg/min for a total flow of 1 L/min and the vaporizer setting is 2% isoflurane. At the start of anesthesia, there is a significant uptake of isoflurane and the dog exhales 0.5% isoflurane. In (b), the exhaled isoflurane is soon rebreathed. As the flow meter is set to 1 L/min, 50 mL/kg/min of the dog's minute ventilation (one-quarter of 200 mL/kg/min) is provided by the fresh gas flow at a concentration of 2% isoflurane. The remaining 150 mL/kg/min of the dog's minute ventilation is provided by the rebreathed gas (with an isoflurane concentration of 0.5%). When the fresh gas and the rebreathed gas mix in the inspiratory limb of the circuit, the resulting inspired concentration of the gas will be approximately 1% isoflurane. As we are ultimately trying to achieve an alveolar concentration of approximately 1.5% isoflurane, it is apparent that this low fresh gas flow will slow the increase in isoflurane concentration. In (c), the oxygen flow rate is increased to 200 mL/kg/min (4 L/min) and the vaporizer is still set at 2%. As this flow rate matches the dog's minute ventilation, the breathing system is now functioning as a nonrebreathing system. The exhaled gas (200 mL/kg/min of 0.5% isoflurane) is all expelled from the circuit via the APL valve and the dog only inhales the fresh gas delivered into the inspiratory limb of the circuit. This gas contains isoflurane at a concentration of 2%. It is apparent that the use of this higher flow, to prevent rebreathing, will maximize the inspired concentration of isoflurane.

anesthetics by looking at the blood/gas partition coefficient. Drugs with greater solubility in blood have a greater blood/gas partition coefficient. The drugs that have been used in the dog are listed in the following text, from the most rapid to the slowest onset, with their blood/gas partition coefficient in parentheses (see Further Reading). It is also apparent from this list that more recent advances in the development of inhalational drugs have focused on developing anesthetics with a rapid onset and offset of effect (i.e., desflurane and sevoflurane):

desflurane (0.63); sevoflurane (0.66); isoflurane (1.40); halothane (3.51)

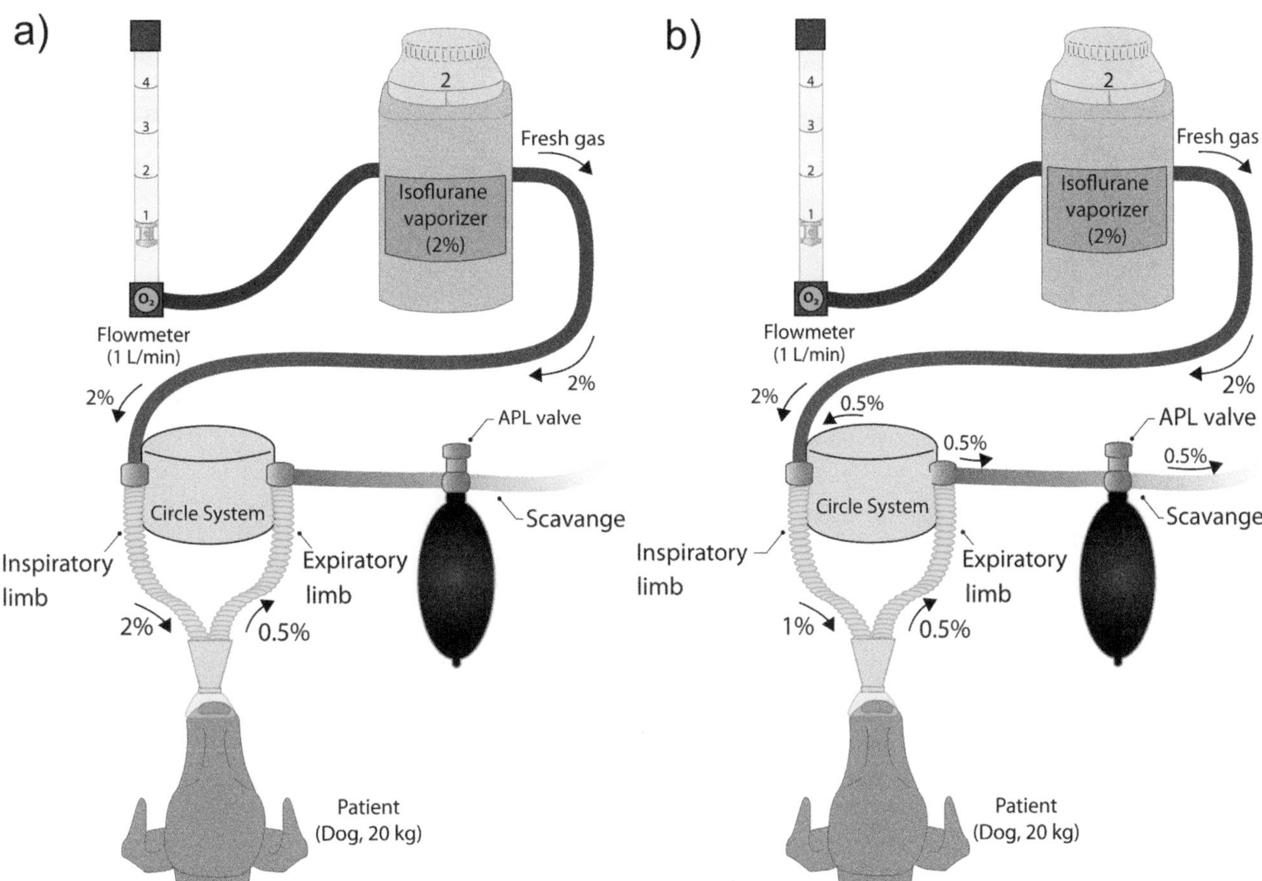

Figure 8.2 The impact of overpressure on inspired concentration of isoflurane in a circle system. Overpressure is often used early in the anesthetic period to maximize inspired concentration of the anesthetic gas. When using isoflurane in the dog, we can anticipate a necessary maintenance concentration of approximately 1.5–2%. It takes time to achieve this concentration in the alveoli and the brain. Early in the anesthetic period, the vaporizer is often set higher than the anticipated maintenance concentration in order to maximize the inspired concentration. In the following example, isoflurane anesthesia is initiated in a 20 kg dog using a fresh gas flow of 50 mL/kg/min (1 L/min). The initial vaporizer concentration is 2% isoflurane. The figure illustrates the impact of increasing the vaporizer concentration to 5% on inspired concentration. In (a), as in Figure 8.1a, the oxygen flow rate is set at 50 mL/kg/min for a total flow of 1 L/min and the vaporizer setting is 2% isoflurane. There is significant uptake of isoflurane and the dog exhales 0.5% isoflurane. In (b), as in Figure 8.1b, the exhaled isoflurane is soon rebreathed. As the flowmeter is set to 1 L/min, 50 mL/kg/min of the dog's minute ventilation is provided by the fresh gas at a concentration of 2% isoflurane. The remaining 150 mL/kg/min of the dog's minute ventilation is provided by the rebreathed gas at an isoflurane concentration of 0.5%. When the fresh gas and the rebreathed gas mix in the inspiratory limb of the circuit, the resulting inspired concentration of the gas will be approximately 1% isoflurane. In (c), the vaporizer setting is now increased to 5% isoflurane. The fresh gas flow of 1 L/min provides 50 mL/kg/min of the dog's minute ventilation. The remaining 150 mL/kg/min of the dog's minute ventilation is provided by the rebreathed gas at an isoflurane concentration 0.5%. When the fresh gas and the rebreathed gas mix in the inspiratory limb of the circuit, the resulting inspired concentration of the gas will be approximately 1.6% isoflurane. The increase in vaporizer setting has an almost instantaneous effect of increasing the inspired concentration of isoflurane from 1 to 1.6%. In (d), very soon after the increase in vaporizer setting, the expired concentration of isoflurane will also increase. Here, it has increased to 3%. When this exhaled gas mixes with the 5% isoflurane in the fresh gas flow, a concentration of 3.5% results in the inspired gas. When overpressure is used, it is important to monitor our patient closely and only use these high vaporizer settings for the shortest time necessary. In this example, a maintenance flow of oxygen was used to illustrate the concept of overpressure, but typically overpressure and high fresh gas flows are used in combination to maximize the inspired inhalational anesthetic concentration and speed uptake of the anesthetic.

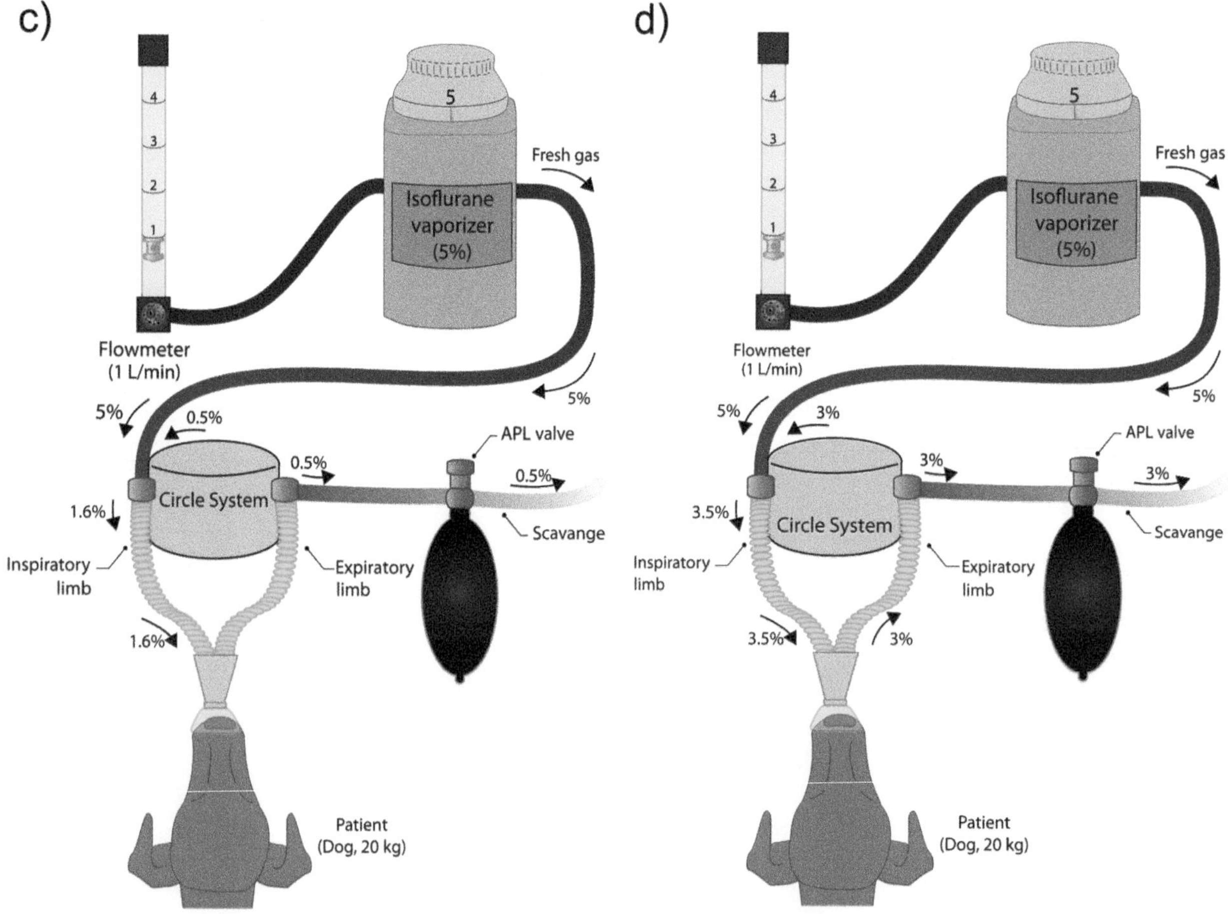

Figure 8.2 (Continued)

In order to fully understand the relationship between solubility, partial pressure, and concentration, it is important to remember Henry's law: "The amount of gas dissolved in a liquid is directly proportional to the partial pressure of the gas in equilibrium with the liquid." Refer to Figure 8.3 to view this concept using the canine blood/gas partition coefficients (abbreviated as λ) listed in the preceding text. Remember that onset of anesthesia is dependent on the *partial pressure* of the drug in the alveolus. In Figure 8.3, we have achieved an equal alveolar drug *concentration* of 2% (2 mL of drug in 100 mL of gas) at atmospheric pressure. This results in a *partial pressure* of 15 mmHg (2% of 760 mmHg). At equilibrium, the partial pressure of the drug in the blood is equivalent to the partial pressure in the alveolus (15 mmHg). In order to achieve this partial pressure with halothane, 7.02 mL of halothane must be dissolved in 100 mL of blood [2 mL $\times \lambda$ (3.51)]. With isoflurane, 2.8 mL of the drug must be dissolved in 100 mL of blood [2 $\times \lambda$ (1.4)]. Finally, with sevoflurane only 1.32 mL of drug must be dissolved in the blood [2 $\times \lambda$ (0.66)]. When the three drugs are compared, the onset of anesthesia is most rapid with sevoflurane and slowest with halothane.

Patient Factors That Influence Uptake of Anesthetics

Much of the discussion in the preceding text has focused on the effect of inspired concentration and alveolar partial pressure on uptake of inhalational anesthetics and speed of induction. Another major factor influencing anesthetic uptake is alveolar ventilation. Uptake increases with increased ventilation and, conversely, uptake is reduced with hypoventilation. In clinical practice, we typically use an injectable drug such as propofol or alfaxalone to induce general anesthesia. Both of these drugs are respiratory depressants, which induce hypoventilation. This will impact the uptake of inhalational anesthetics, and some assisted ventilation is often required during the induction period to facilitate uptake of the inhalational anesthetic and ensure a smooth transition from the induction to the maintenance period. Inhalational drugs are also respiratory

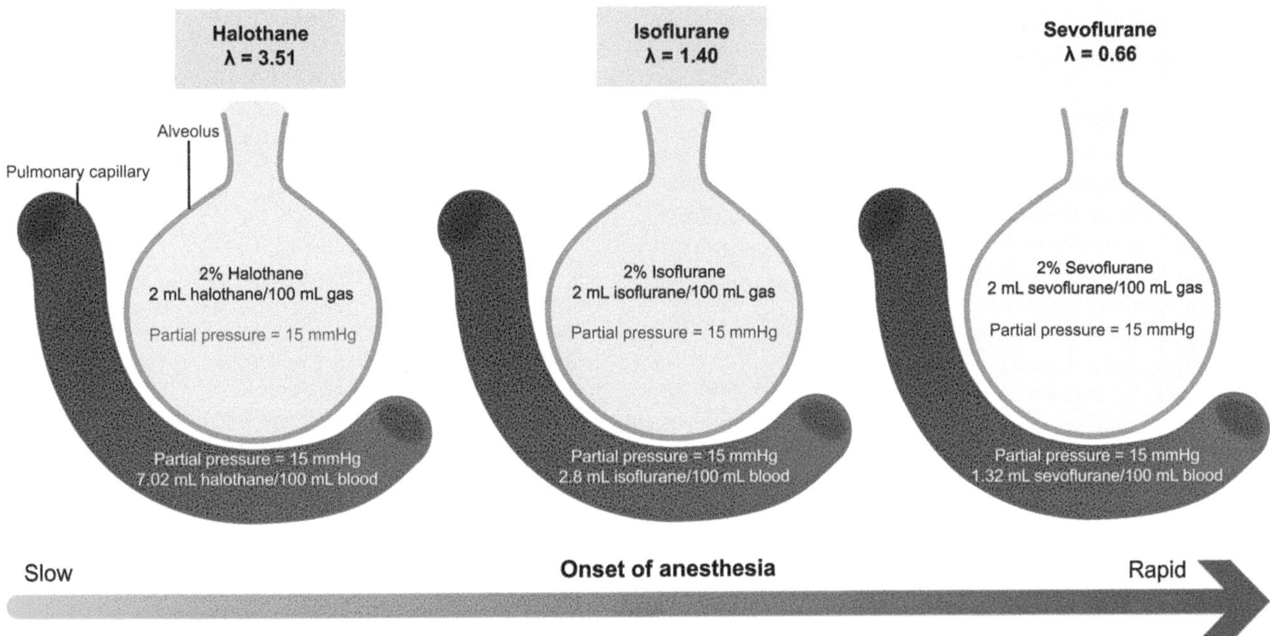

Figure 8.3 Relationship between drug concentration, partial pressure, and blood/gas partition coefficient (λ) in alveolar gas and pulmonary capillary blood at equilibrium. Refer to the text for a complete explanation.

depressants, and hypoventilation induced by these drugs results in a feedback loop that results in reduced uptake during spontaneous ventilation as the plane of anesthesia deepens. It is also important to note that initiation of controlled ventilation can make uptake more efficient and deepen the plane of anesthesia. Cardiac output also has an influence on uptake of inhalational anesthetics. Increased cardiac output increases blood flow to the lungs and slows the rate of rise in alveolar partial pressure, whereas reduced cardiac output will have the opposite effect, partial pressure of anesthetic in the alveolus increases and uptake is more rapid. The impact of cardiac output is particularly important in patients with shock as a deep plane of anesthesia can be quickly induced with adverse cardiovascular consequences that may lead to decompensation. Inhalational drugs should be used cautiously and sparingly in patients in shock, with appropriate pre-anesthetic stabilization whenever possible (Chapter 16).

Concept of Minimum Alveolar Concentration and Potency of Inhalational Anesthetics

Whenever we deliver an anesthetic drug, it is important to know the appropriate dose to achieve the desired effect. With injectable anesthetic drugs, we will often determine the mean dose required in a population to induce general anesthesia and allow tracheal intubation. This dose is often expressed in mg/kg and provides a good starting point to determine what dose will be required in an individual patient. For example, for two commonly used injectable drugs, alfaxalone and propofol, the alfaxalone dose required for anesthetic induction of lightly premedicated dogs is around 1.7 mg/kg (O'Hagan et al., 2012), whereas the propofol dose required in premedicated dogs is around 2.8 mg/kg (Watney and Pablo 1992). Knowing these doses provides a good starting point for administration in a clinical setting under similar circumstances (premedicated animals). Dosing of inhalational anesthetics is slightly more challenging as they are delivered as a vapor, so rather than dosing in mg/kg we dose inhalational drugs as a concentration; they are delivered as a percentage of the inspired gas. Since many factors will influence the actual delivered concentration, we focus on the expired concentration of the gas when we are trying to determine an effective concentration. This expired (end-tidal) concentration reflects the alveolar concentration. An airway gas analyzer can be used to determine these end-tidal concentrations. In essence, we can determine the pharmacokinetics of inhalational anesthetics in real time. In order to determine the effective concentration of an inhaled anesthetic, the concentration of drug that will prevent skeletal muscle movement in response to a noxious stimulus (traditionally, skin incision) in 50% of patients is determined (at sea level). This concentration is known as the "minimum alveolar concentration" (Merkel and Eger 1963). Obviously, in a clinical situation we would like to prevent response in all of our patients, and we either deliver the anesthetic at a slightly higher concentration than the MAC value or we use our knowledge of other drugs that reduce MAC to allow delivery of inhalational anesthetics at a lower concentration. Reducing the inhalational anesthetic concentration delivered has the important additional advantage of reducing adverse effects associated with this drug class (described in the following text). The MAC value of isoflurane in the dog is 1.28%, whereas the MAC of sevoflurane in the dog is 2.36% (see Further Reading). The lower MAC value of isoflurane reflects that isoflurane is the more potent drug (less isoflurane is required to prevent response to a surgical stimulus). MAC is *additive*, meaning that it would be possible to combine isoflurane and sevoflurane to anesthetize a dog (for example, though this is not performed under normal clinical situations). For example, if half the MAC value of isoflurane (0.64%) was combined with half the MAC value of sevoflurane (1.18%), the mixture would be equipotent to one MAC of isoflurane or sevoflurane (*MAC equivalent*). MAC tends to be relatively constant among species (Table 8.2). Slight differences are commonly seen with different study designs within and between species. A useful practical application of MAC is the concept of a *MAC multiplier*: this is an estimate, based on MAC, to achieve different end points. For example, *MAC* is defined based upon preventing a response in 50% of a patient population. In order to reduce the likelihood of a response in a given individual patient, it is common to initially set a vaporizer concentration of 1.3 × MAC. For isoflurane, this is approximately 1.7%, which is the concentration required to prevent a response in 95% of patients. The same concept can be applied to recovery, where the alveolar (end-tidal) concentration of most inhalational anesthetics must fall to approximately 40% of MAC for recovery to occur (e.g., 0.9% for sevoflurane). Note: The MAC multiplier required to prevent autonomic responses to noxious stimuli is approximately 1.5–2 MAC. At this concentration, there is a greater likelihood of encountering multiple adverse effects from the inhalational anesthetic (i.e., hypotension and hypoventilation), hence the advantages of balanced anesthesia (described in the following text) in allowing a reduction in inhalational drug requirement.

Factors That Influence MAC

There are a few factors that will increase MAC and more factors that will decrease MAC. A list of these factors is included in Table 8.3. The most clinically relevant are discussed in the following text.

Table 8.3 Factors that increase or decrease minimum alveolar concentration (MAC) in veterinary anesthesia.

Factors that increase MAC
Drugs that induce CNS stimulation (ephedrine)
Morphine in horses
Hyperthermia
Hypernatremia
Factors that decrease MAC
Drugs that induce CNS depression: injectable anesthetics and lidocaine
Sedatives and tranquilizers: acepromazine, alpha-2 adrenergic receptor agonists, and benzodiazepines
Opioids (most species)
Hypothermia
Hyponatremia
Pregnancy
Increasing age
$PaO_2 < 40$ mmHg
$PaCO_2 > 95$mmHg
Mean arterial blood pressure < 40 mmHg

Some of these factors are important considerations in pre-operative assessment, such as the impact of pregnancy and age on MAC. A number of these factors are controlled by provision of appropriate supportive care including maintenance of normoxemia, normocarbia, normotension, and normothermia. The recognition that ephedrine can increase MAC is important since, if it is administered to an animal in a light plane of anesthesia, it can result in arousal. This is particularly important in equine patients as moving limbs can cause damage to equipment or personnel.

One of the most important considerations in reference to factors that will reduce MAC is the impact of tranquilizers, sedatives, analgesics, and injectable anesthetics. As described below, inhalational anesthetics have some significant adverse effects, the most notable of these are hypotension and hypoventilation. In general, it is not advisable to use them as the sole drug for maintenance of anesthesia as the concentration rquired is likely to result in these adverse effects. The concept of *balanced anesthesia* uses the inhalational anesthetic to maintain unconsciousness but utilizes appropriate doses of other drugs to enhance sedation, analgesia, and muscle relaxation in order to reduce the patient requirement for the inhalational anesthetic. For example, premedication of a dog with acepromazine or dexmedetomidine, combined with an opioid, such as methadone or hydromorphone, will significantly reduce inhalational anesthetic requirements. If even greater reductions are desired intra-operatively, such as in hemodynamically unstable patients, an intravenous constant rate infusion (CRI) of a potent opioid such as fentanyl or remifentanil can significantly reduce volatile anesthetic requirements, resulting in greater hemodynamic stability (Chapters 16 and 17). Horses and cats can prove slightly more challenging as opioids induce CNS stimulation, and while they provide analgesia, which is certainly beneficial, they may not induce a MAC-sparing effect due to CNS excitation (see Further Reading). Another technique to reduce inhalational drug requirements is to deliver an injectable anesthetic in combination with the inhalational anesthetic to maintain general anesthesia. This may be as simple as delivering a bolus of alfaxalone or propofol to a lightly anesthetized dog or ketamine to a horse to acutely deepen the plane of anesthesia when it is demonstrating signs of arousal. Or, it may be the concurrent administration of a CRI of an anesthetic such as alfaxalone, propofol, or ketamine to reduce inhalational anesthetic requirements. This technique is termed "partial intravenous anesthesia" (PIVA). A CRI of an alpha-2 adrenergic receptor agonist can be particularly useful in horses as it will result in significant MAC reduction when opioids may not. Medetomidine, at a dose of 3.5 mcg/kg/h, reduced desflurane MAC in ponies by 28% (see Further Reading). The quality of anesthesia and recovery may also be enhanced with these techniques.

One of the best ways to reduce MAC in veterinary patients is with the concurrent use of a local anesthetic technique. An effective local anesthetic technique will provide profound analgesia to the surgical site and prevent intra-operative nociception (Chapter 3). In these situations, animals can often be maintained anesthetized with a concentration of inhalational anesthetic that is less than the MAC value (e.g., close to 1% isoflurane in dogs). Interestingly, systemic administration of the local anesthetic lidocaine can also induce a significant reduction in MAC. Again, this can be particularly useful in horses. A bolus dose of 2.5 mg/kg administered over 10 min followed by a CRI of 50 mcg/kg/min produced an average MAC reduction of 25% (see Further Reading). Minimal cardiovascular impairment is noted with lidocaine. This can be an important technique for colic surgery as horses can demonstrate significant cardiovascular instability with high doses of volatile anesthetic, with additional potential benefits from lidocaine of a prokinetic effect on the gastrointestinal tract and anti-inflammatory effect.

Operating the Anesthetic Vaporizer

Currently, the majority of anesthetic machines utilize a precision variable-bypass vaporizer located out of circuit (Chapter 5). An isoflurane vaporizer can deliver between 0 and 5%, whereas a sevoflurane vaporizer delivers between 0 and 8%. The higher percentage for sevoflurane reflects that it is less potent (Table 8.2). The dial of the vaporizer is adjusted to deliver the desired inspired concentration. Maintenance of anesthesia with isoflurane is typically achieved with a vaporizer setting of 1.5–2% (this relates to the MAC multiplier concept described in the preceding text). If the plane of anesthesia suddenly lightens and the animal shows signs of arousal, the setting may be increased to 3–5% for a short period of time to deepen the plane of anesthesia. The setting should be decreased as soon as an appropriate plane of anesthesia is achieved. This may be done in combination with an intravenous bolus of an anesthetic or analgesic.

Integrating the Fresh Gas Flow Rate and the Vaporizer Setting

If we recall from the discussion regarding wash-in of anesthetics, rebreathing can have a major impact on inspired gas concentration. In the preceding example of an unacceptably light plane of anesthesia, if a rebreathing circuit is used, in addition to increasing the vaporizer concentration, it is equally important to increase the fresh gas flow to decrease rebreathing or the animal will rebreathe a higher proportion of gas that contains less anesthetic. This is important for all patients anesthetized with a nonrebreathing circuit, but especially large patients, such as horses, as rebreathing tends to be more profound due to limitations in how much the fresh gas flow can be increased as a result of the limited maximum output of commercially available flowmeters. In equine and large ruminant anesthesia, rapid increases in depth of anesthesia are not achievable with inhalational anesthetics alone and an injectable anesthetic, such as ketamine or thiopental, is needed to acutely deepen the plane of anesthesia when needed.

Pharmacodynamics

Respiratory System

All inhalational anesthetics produce a dose-dependent depression of central ventilatory drive, characterized by an increase in arterial partial pressure of carbon dioxide ($PaCO_2$). This may be more pronounced in some species, particularly diving animals. Inhalational anesthetics also depress hypoxic respiratory drive, even at low doses. This depresses an important rescue mechanism as hyperventilation in the face of hypoxemia is profoundly depressed or absent during inhalational anesthesia. Surgical stimulation can result in an increase in minute ventilation, but it is not always accompanied by a significant reduction in $PaCO_2$. The odor of most volatile anesthetics has been shown to be aversive in a number of species and may result in bradycardia and apnea (see Further Reading). Mask (face mask) induction is not advised without deep sedation and, in most species, induction with an injectable drug is preferred. All volatile anesthetics will induce bronchodilation. This can be useful in the prevention and treatment of bronchospasm during anesthesia.

Cardiovascular System

All inhalational anesthetic drugs induce a decrease in arterial blood pressure. Some of this effect is due to a reduction in cardiac output. This is most predominant with halothane. Modern drugs tend to induce a decrease in blood pressure via vasodilation with a lesser, but not negligible, reduction in myocaridal contractility. This reduction in blood pressure may be further compounded by the use of positive pressure ventilation, which decreases venous return during the inspiratory phase (positive intrathoracic pressure causes venous compression). Effects on heart rate are variable between species but, in general, a slight increase in heart rate may be observed with isoflurane, sevoflurane, and desflurane (effect varies according to the presence of other drugs, e.g., opioids that promote bradycardia). Arrhythmias, particularly ventricular arrhythmias, are relatively common with halothane and often induced by catecholamines. These arrhythmias are much less frequent with newer inhalational drugs. In general, hypotension is the most clinically relevant adverse cardiovascular effect. As it is dose dependent, steps should be taken to reduce the concentration of volatile anesthetic administered (such as with provision of balanced anesthesia).

Renal and Hepatic Systems

All of the inhalational anesthetics will induce a decrease in renal blood flow, with a concurrent decrease in glomerular filtration rate and urine production. These effects are typically resolved following recovery and can be minimized by appropriate pre-operative and intra-operative fluid therapy. All of the inhalational drugs have been implicated in post-operative liver dysfunction. With isoflurane and desflurane it is mild and self-limiting, whereas more severe hepatic impairment has been seen with halothane, particularly in humans. Reduced hepatic blood flow during anesthesia and other intrinsic factors can lead to increased plasma concentrations of concurrently administered drugs. This can be particularly pronounced in animals that present with significant pre-operative liver dysfunction.

Malignant Hyperthermia

This is a very rare condition that has been observed predominantly in pigs but also reported in dogs and horses. The condition is triggered by administration of an inhalational anesthetic. It is characterized by severe muscle contraction and a hypermetabolic state. Hypercarbia, hyperthermia, and acidosis are characteristic of the condition. Tachycardia may also be observed. Animals will rapidly decompensate and die unless they are quickly treated with dantrolene and delivery of the inhalational anesthetic is stopped (need to convert to a total intravenous anesthesia protocol). Unfortunately, most clinics do not stock dantrolene.

Inhalational Anesthetics

Halothane

Halothane is a halogenated ethane molecule. It is the oldest inhalational anesthetic still in use in veterinary patients but is no longer available in most parts of the world. It has largely been replaced by isoflurane and sevoflurane. Halothane has a less irritating odor than isoflurane and is the most potent of the current inhalational drugs, but, as it is the most soluble of these drugs (high blood/gas partition coefficient), induction and recovery are slower. Halothane undergoes more extensive metabolism than the other inhalational anesthetics (approximately 20–45% in humans). Ventricular arrhythmias are not uncommon with halothane, particularly under light planes of anesthesia. As with all inhalational anesthetics, respiratory depression and hypotension are the predominant adverse effects.

Isoflurane

Isoflurane is a halogenated methyl-ethyl ether. Currently, it is probably the most commonly used inhalational anesthetic in veterinary medicine. Its lower blood/gas partition coefficient, when compared to halothane, confers a quicker onset and offset than halothane. The odor is irritating and can cause breath-holding in some patients should mask or chamber induction be attempted. It is slightly less potent than halothane and is minimally metabolized (0.2% in humans). It is less arrhythmogenic than halothane. The major adverse effects are hypotension, primarily the result of vasodilation, and respiratory depression.

Sevoflurane

Sevoflurane is a halogenated methyl-isopropyl ether molecule. It has a lower blood/gas partition coefficient than isoflurane resulting in a more rapid onset and offset of anesthesia. It is less potent than halothane or isoflurane but has a slightly less irritating odor than isoflurane. Elimination is primarily via respiratory excretion, but there is some hepatic metabolism (2–5% in humans). Major adverse effects are similar to isoflurane (hypotension and respiratory depression) though there is some evidence to suggest that respiratory depression is less profound. Currently, the cost of sevoflurane when compared to isoflurane is probably the major limitation to it being adopted in routine veterinary practice.

Desflurane

Desflurane is a halogenated methyl-ethyl ether molecule with the lowest blood/gas partition coefficient of inhalational drugs in current use, conferring the most rapid onset and offset of anesthesia. It is the least potent of the inhalational anesthetics. As the vapor pressure of desflurane is close to atmospheric pressure (Table 8.1), it is near its boiling point and requires a specially designed vaporizer (gas–vapor blender). Desflurane undergoes very minimal hepatic metabolism (0.02% in humans). Respiratory and cardiovascular adverse effects are similar to isoflurane and sevoflurane. As with sevoflurane, the cost of the drug, when compared to isoflurane, is a limitation to widespread use in veterinary practice. The requirement for a specialized vaporizer and contribution to climate change are further limitations.

Linking MAC, Potency, and Onset of Action

To summarize the preceding text, MAC is simply a measure of potency, which allows us to effectively dose our inhalational anesthetics by providing a good starting point for the vaporizer setting. It is apparent that all of the inhalational anesthetics have significant dose-dependent adverse effects, particularly respiratory depression and hypotension. Our knowledge of MAC reducing drugs and techniques will help us pick appropriate premedications, PIVA techniques, and local anesthetic blocks to reduce the required inhalational anesthetic concentration and produce a more stable plane of anesthesia. The blood/gas partition coefficient provides a good indication of onset and offset of action, acknowledging that there are several other factors to consider including concentration of the anesthetic administered, impact of rebreathing, hemodynamic status, and ventilation. The final section discusses some unique situations where we use inhalational anesthetics and how to protect ourselves and our planet from the adverse effects of these drugs.

Delivery of Inhalational Anesthetics in Unique Settings

Considerations for Delivery of Inhalational Anesthetics in the Field

In general, we deliver inhalational anesthetics in a very controlled clinical environment. One of the most important aspects of this controlled environment is ambient temperature. Modern variable-bypass vaporizers are temperature compensated to deliver reliable, predictable concentrations over a range of around 20–35 °C. Anesthesia performed outside a clinical setting may be required for anesthesia of some challenging wildlife species (Figure 8.4), when surgery is performed in remote locations or in disaster situations. In these settings, one of the major challenges is vaporization of the anesthetic at low ambient temperatures. Hot water bottles or warm fluid bags have been used to warm vaporizers in order to maintain a predictable output. Another challenge in remote settings is the availability of cylinder oxygen. If a power supply or generator can be accessed, portable oxygen concentrators can be used to effectively deliver oxygen to an anesthetic machine in remote locations (see Further Reading).

Use in Euthanasia

Inhalational drugs have been used as the sole method of euthanasia with the open drop technique described in the preceding text (see the section on saturated vapor pressure). It is important to remember that studies in animals have shown that these techniques can be aversive, and the American Veterinary Medical Association guidelines on euthanasia recommend that this technique is only used "In

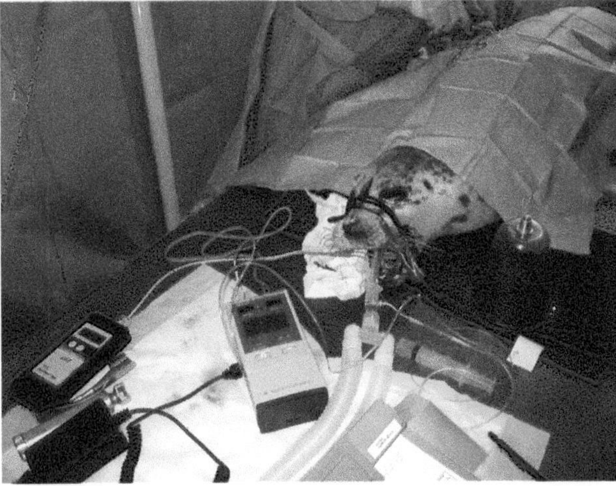

Figure 8.4 Harbor seal anesthetized with isoflurane on the deck of a ship.

those species where aversion or overt escape behaviors have not been noted, exposure to high concentrations resulting in rapid loss of consciousness is preferred" (AVMA Guidelines for the Euthanasia of Animals: 2020 Edition). It is difficult to euthanize animals with anesthetic delivered via a precision vaporizer as lethal concentrations are not rapidly obtained. In these situations, the animal is anesthetized with inhalational anesthetic, and a secondary euthanasia technique (such as intravenous potassium chloride) is used to complete euthanasia in the anesthetized animal.

Environmental Impact of Inhalational Anesthetics

When we consider the environmental impact of inhalational anesthetics, it is important to consider the impact on individuals exposed to low concentrations of these drugs over a prolonged period and the impact on the atmosphere of our planet. Appropriate scavenging of waste gases (see Chapter 5) must be in place wherever these drugs are used and exposure avoided as much as possible. We are still learning about the long-term effects of inhalational anesthetics through occupational exposure, but there is some evidence that they may be pro-inflammatory, promote genomic instability, and possibly impact hepatic and renal function with prolonged exposure. Appropriate scavenging should always be used, and face mask or chamber induction should be avoided as much as possible. Anesthetic machines should be serviced and checked for leaks regularly (see Further Reading), and facility concentrations should be checked for potential occupational exposure on a regular basis.

Climate change is probably the greatest challenge we face in this century. The inhalational anesthetics are greenhouse gases and significantly contribute to this problem. Of these, nitrous oxide and desflurane have the greatest impact. Current scavenging methods vent these drugs unchanged into the atmosphere. Unless we can significantly improve scavenging techniques, we must seriously consider other mitigation methods. Recent suggestions include eliminating the use of desflurane and nitrous oxide, and using total intravenous anesthesia whenever possible (see Further Reading).

Questions and Answers

There are more practice questions and answers available for this chapter on the website. Please visit http://www.wiley.com/go/VeterinaryAnesthesiaZeiler.

Questions

1) Excretion of modern volatile anesthetics occurs predominantly at the level of the:
   a) Lungs
   b) Liver
   c) Kidneys
   d) Combination of hepatic and renal excretion
2) In order to appropriately dose volatile anesthetics, we need to know the:
   a) Dose in mg/kg/min
   b) Dose in mg/kg/h
   c) Minimum alveolar concentration as a percent of inspired gas
   d) Dose in milliliters
3) Early in the course of an anesthetic procedure, the major impact of rebreathing exhaled volatile anesthetic delivered via a circle system is to:
   a) Dilute the inspired concentration of the anesthetic gas
   b) Augment the inspired concentration of the anesthetic gas
   c) Have no impact on inspired concentration of the anesthetic gas
   d) Increase the level of CO_2 in the circuit via rebreathing
4) "Newflurane" is a theoretic volatile anesthetic with a blood/gas partition coefficient of 0.8 in the dog. When compared to isoflurane and sevoflurane, we would predict the following regarding onset of action:
   a) Newflurane has a more rapid onset of action than either isoflurane or sevoflurane
   b) Newflurane has a less rapid onset of action than either isoflurane or sevoflurane
   c) Newflurane has an intermediate onset of action: slower than sevoflurane or more rapid than isoflurane
   d) Newflurane has an intermediate onset of action: slower than isoflurane or more rapid than sevoflurane
5) Newflurane has a MAC of 0.82% in the dog. Based on our knowledge of MAC, we would expect that the potency of newflurane is:
   a) More potent than isoflurane and sevoflurane
   b) Less potent than isoflurane and sevoflurane
   c) Intermediate potency between isoflurane and sevoflurane
   d) We cannot predict potency based on MAC, and we would need to know the blood/gas partition coefficient

Answers

1) a
2) c
3) a
4) c
5) a

Further Reading

Bettschart-Wolfensberger, R., Jäggin-Schmucker, N., Lendl, C. et al. (2001). Minimal alveolar concentration of desflurane in combination with an infusion of medetomidine for the anaesthesia of ponies. *Vet Rec* 148: 264–267.

Burn, J., Caulkett, N.A., Gunn, M. et al. (2016). Evaluation of a portable oxygen concentrator to provide fresh gas flow to dogs undergoing anesthesia. *Can Vet J* 57: 614–618.

Doorley, M.B., Waters, S.J., Terrell, R.C., and Robinson, J.L. (1988). MAC of I-653 in beagle dogs and New Zealand white rabbits. *Anesthes* 69: 89–92.

Dzikiti, T.B., Hellebrekers, L.J., and Dijk, P. (2003). Effects of intravenous lidocaine on isoflurane concentration, physiological parameters, metabolic parameters and stress-related hormones in horses undergoing surgery. *J Vet Med Assoc* 50: 190–195.

Flecknell, P., Roughan, J., and Hedenqvist, P. (1999). Induction of anaesthesia with sevoflurane and isoflurane in the rabbit. *Lab Anim* 33: 41–46.

Franks, N. (2006). Molecular targets underlying general anaesthesia. *Br J Pharmacol* 147: S72–S81.

Franks, N. and Lieb, W. (1984). Do general anaesthetics act by competitive binding to specific receptors? *Nature* 310: 599–601.

Gaya da Costa, M., Kalmar, A., and Struys, M. (2021). Inhaled anesthetics: environmental role, occupational risk, and clinical use. *J Clin Med* 10: 1306. https://doi.org/10.3390/jcm10061306.

Iqbal, F., Thompson, A., Riaz, S. et al. (2019). Anesthetics: from modes of action to unconsciousness and neurotoxicity. *J Neurophysiol* 122: 760–787.

Kazama, T. and Ikeda, K. (1988). Comparison of MAC and the rate of rise of alveolar concentration of sevoflurane with halothane and isoflurane in the dog. *Anesthes* 68: 435–438.

Marchiori, J.M.M., Prebble, M.J., and Pang, D.S.J. (2023). A prospective survey of veterinary anesthesia equipment in Alberta, Canada, using a standardized checkout procedure. *Can Vet J* 64: 159–166.

Merkel, G. and Eger, E.I., II (1963). A comparative study of halothane and halopropane anesthesia: including method to determine equipotency. *Anesthes* 24: 346–357.

O'Hagan, B., Pasloske, K., McKinnon, C. et al. (2012). Clinical evaluation of alfaxalone as an anaesthetic induction agent in dogs less than 12 weeks of age. *Aust Vet J* 90: 346–350.

Steffey, E.P., Eisele, J.H., and Baggot, J.D. (2003). Interactions of morphine and isoflurane in horses. *Am J Vet Res* 64: 166–175.

Steffey, E.P. and Howland, D. Jr (1977). Isoflurane potency in the dog and cat. *Am J Vet Res* 38: 1833–1886.

Watney, G. and Pablo, L. (1992). Median effective dosage of propofol for induction of anesthesia in dogs. *Am J Vet Res* 53: 2320–2322.

9

Nonsteroidal Anti-inflammatory Drugs, Local Anesthetic Drugs, and Adjunct Drugs Used for Pain Management

H. Nicole Trenholme, Gareth Zeiler, and Daniel Pang

Nonsteroidal Anti-inflammatory Drugs

Metabolic Pathways of Arachidonic Acid

In order to understand the mechanism of action of nonsteroidal anti-inflammatory drugs (NSAIDs) and their effects, the biosynthesis and metabolism of arachidonic acid requires explanation. Arachidonic acid (AA) is an omega-6 polyunsaturated fatty acid that is naturally found bound in structural phospholipids of cell membranes and proteins (e.g., albumin) or stored in lipid bodies of immune cells. Free AA can either be sourced exogenously from diet, synthesized from linoleic acid, or produced endogenously by enzymatic release from phospholipids by phospholipases, usually during injury or inflammation. Free AA undergoes oxidation via one of three pathways, resulting in bioactive metabolites essential for immune system function. This function includes the inflammatory response to pathogens and trauma, anti-inflammatory response, wound healing, modulation of mood, and energy balance (Table 9.1). Pathways of enzymatic oxidation reactions are catalyzed by (1) cyclooxygenases (COX), (2) lipoxygenases (LOX), and (3) cytochrome P450 enzymes (Figure 9.1). The bioactive metabolites act as local hormones or participate in lipid signaling by binding to their respective receptors, which are distributed all over the body.

The mechanism of action of NSAIDs is through the drug binding to COX (and LOX, in the case of dual inhibitors) enzymes to inhibit their function as catalysts. This inhibition hinders the production of prostaglandins and thromboxane (and leukotrienes). Inhibiting one of the metabolic pathways of free AA can increase metabolism via the uninhibited pathways. The clinical consequences of free AA being metabolized via uninhibited pathways are largely unknown and an area of active investigation.

Classification of NSAIDs

The first-generation NSAIDs (e.g., aspirin, phenylbutazone, and meclofenamic acid) have good anti-inflammatory and antipyretic effects through their effect in inhibiting COX. However, patients administered this generation of NSAIDs were prone to gastrointestinal and renal adverse effects, even when administered at recommended therapeutic doses. On further investigation, it was discovered that the COX enzyme was, in fact, a group of isoenzymes. There is strong evidence that two isoenzymes exist, namely COX-1 and COX-2, with a third being described (no current consensus on nomenclature but often described as splice variant COX-1.2 or COX-3). This chapter focuses on COX-1 and COX-2, being the more important. The discovery of these isoenzymes brought about the often oversimplified, classic COX theory that COX-1 produces "housekeeping" prostaglandins (essential for normal physiologic function in many organ systems but notably the gastrointestinal tract and renal system) and COX-2 is induced during inflammation or trauma, producing pro-inflammatory prostaglandins. This theory spurred the discovery of the second-generation of NSAIDs (e.g., carprofen, meloxicam, ketoprofen, etc.) which preferentially inhibited COX-2 over COX-1, maintaining desirable anti-inflammatory analgesic and antipyretic effects. However, although less frequent, gastrointestinal adverse effects are still reported when these NSAIDs are administered at therapeutic doses. Renal adverse effects are mostly limited to overdosing of these drugs or prescribing them to patients at risk of renal injury (see later). This drug development approach continued, with the theory that producing selective COX-2 inhibitors would eliminate the gastrointestinal adverse effects, and resulted in the third-generation of NSAIDs (tepoxalin, deracoxib, fibrocoxib, mavacoxib, cimicoxib, robenacoxib, etc.). However,

Fundamental Principles of Veterinary Anesthesia, First Edition. Edited by Gareth E. Zeiler and Daniel S. J. Pang.

Companion Website: www.wiley.com/go/VeterinaryAnesthesiaZeiler

Table 9.1 Physiologic effect of bioactive metabolites of free arachidonic acid metabolism via the cyclo-oxygenase, lipoxygenase, and cytochrome P450 pathways.

Ligand	Site of production	Target receptor	Physiologic effect
Cyclo-oxygenase pathway			
PGD2	Mast cells and central nervous system	DP1 and CRTH2	Vasodilation, edema, and inhibition of platelet function. Also recruits basophils and eosinophils during allergic responses
PGE2	Kidney and inflamed or injured tissue	EP1, EP2, EP3, and EP4	Decreased tumor necrosis factor alpha production, increased anti-inflammatory cytokines expression in macrophages, uterine contraction, vasodilation, and pyrexia
PGI2	Vascular endothelium and cardiac tissue	IP	Inhibit, platelet aggregation, downregulates tumor necrosis factor alpha, and upregulates anti-inflammatory cytokines
PGF2alpha	Reproductive system	FP	Vasoconstriction, bronchoconstriction, smooth muscle, and uterine contraction
Thromboxane A2 and B2	Platelets	TP alpha TP beta	Regulates platelet aggregation Vasoconstriction and bronchoconstriction
Lipoxygenase pathway			
Many	Mast cells and alveolar macrophages	Many	Collectively, the major effects include increase in vascular permeability, neutrophil chemotaxis to site of infection or inflammation, T-cell lymphocyte proliferation, stimulation of bronchoconstriction, trigger for asthma and anaphylaxis, increase mucous secretion in airways and gastrointestinal tract, promote wound healing by macrophages, and regulate cholesterol levels in the liver
Cytochrome P450 pathway			
EETs	Kidney	PPAR alpha and gamma	Vasodilation, anti-inflammatory and angiogenic function, and inhibition of sodium transport
HETE	Kidney	–	Vasoconstriction

PG: prostaglandin; EETs: epoxyeicosatrienoic acids; HETE: 20-hydroxyeicosatetraenoic acids.

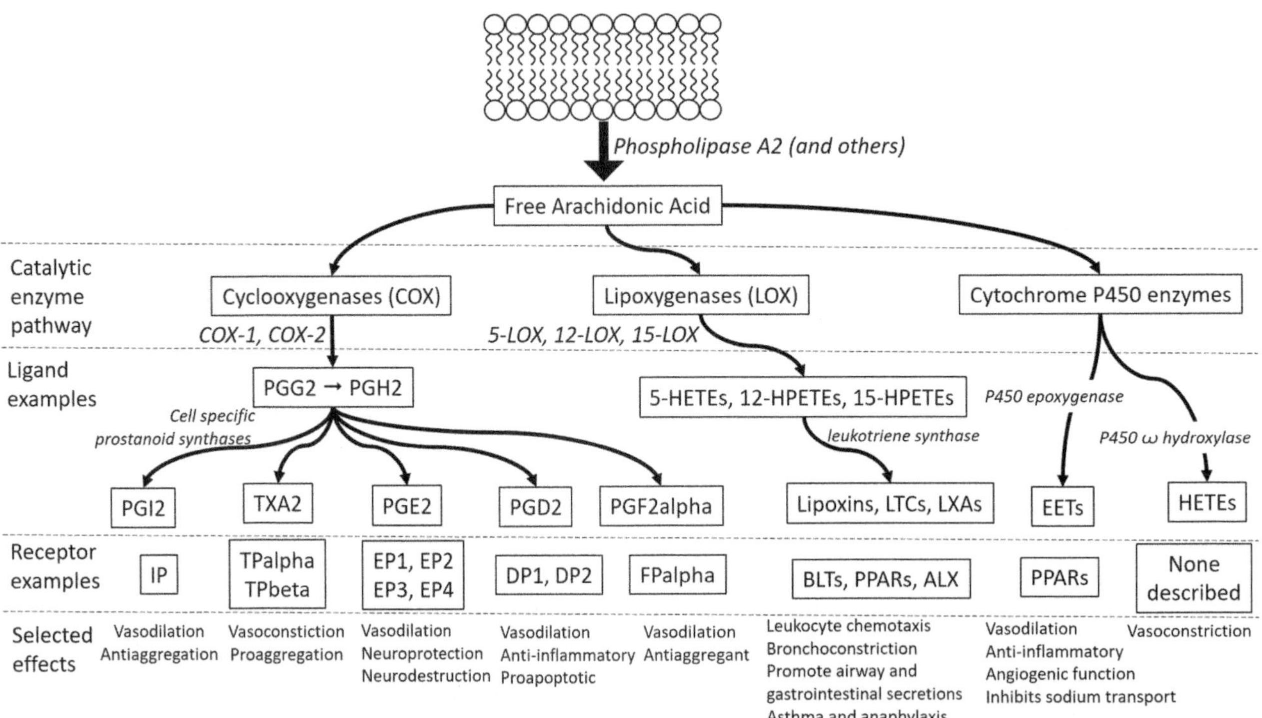

Figure 9.1 A flow diagram depicting the metabolism of free arachidonic acid. There are three enzyme pathways that arachidonic acid can be metabolized, and these are catalyzed by cyclooxygenases, lipoxygenases, and cytochrome P450 enzymes to produce a plethora of bioactive metabolites (ligands) responsible for local hormonal and lipid signaling effects. Examples of ligands, their receptors, and physiologic effects are summarized.

gastrointestinal adverse effects still occur, an indication that the classic COX theory is simplistic, with the function of the two isoenzymes overlapping, or that other, yet undiscovered isoenzymes exist and are also inhibited. Regardless of the factors mentioned in the preceding text, it is now known that for gastrointestinal wall maintenance and healing, both COX-1 and COX-2 functions are necessary.

While most NSAIDs will inhibit COX and LOX, the duration of binding and inhibition of LOX are very short (minutes) for most drugs and they are therefore classified as COX-inhibitors only. However, some NSAIDs (e.g., tepoxalin and ketoprofen) block LOX activity for a sufficient amount of time (hours) to be considered a dual inhibitors (i.e., inhibiting both COX and LOX). These dual inhibitors are recommended for use in species of animals that are prone to bronchoconstriction. When these species are given a COX-inhibitor, free AA is metabolized by the LOX pathway that biosynthesizes metabolites that can cause bronchoconstriction (see Chapter 18).

The latest generation of NSAIDs does not inhibit COX (or LOX) catalytic function in prostaglandin and thromboxane (and leukotriene) biosynthesis but rather targets their receptors. The prostaglandin E2 receptor blocker (antagonists) grapiprant (a member of the novel piprant class of drugs) is the first of its type to be licensed to treat osteoarthritis in dogs in many countries. Grapiprant blocks the EP4 receptor. Current evidence suggests that this drug has a low risk of gastrointestinal (no gastric or intestinal ulceration or perforation reported) and renal (no acute kidney injury reported) adverse effects when used appropriately.

Indications for Use

NSAIDs have been prescribed for acute and chronic use to treat pain states associated with tissue inflammation. They are either prescribed as a sole analgesic or in combination with adjuvant drugs, especially in patients with chronic pain. When they are prescribed for chronic use, the lowest effective dose should be determined by asking the owner to steadily decrease the dose (or increasing the dose interval, from daily to every second day, for example) with the purpose of limiting their adverse effects. When treating food-producing animals with NSAIDs, it is important to follow recommendations for meat, milk, and egg withdrawals, even if it is being given to a "pet" and not a production animal. The best resource for this is the Food Animal Residue Avoidance Databank (FARAD; www.farad.org). In the United States of America, the only drug that is Food and Drug Administration (FDA) approved for treatment of inflammation and fever in food-producing animals is flunixin meglumine. Under the Animal Medicinal Drug Use Clarification Act (AMDUCA; https://www.fda.gov/animal-veterinary/guidance-regulations/animal-medicinal-drug-use-clarification-act-1994-amduca), NSAIDs can be used extra-label (i.e., in a manner that differs from the drug's approved license) and requires a valid veterinary–client–patient relationship as well as following FDA rules and regulations. A full list of drugs that are prohibited for use, even extra-label (off-label), in food animals is available through resources citing AMDUCA. The anesthetist should also refer to FARAD (if a local resource is not available in the country in which they practice) to determine appropriate withdrawal times to inform clients of these stipulations.

When choosing a particular NSAID, it is important to consider drug availability, species being treated, therapeutic indication, and potential adverse effects and/or risk of toxicity. A summary of some of these is listed in Table 9.2 for dogs and cats. See Chapter 13 for NSAID use in equids and Chapter 14 for use in exotic mammals, pigs, and ruminants.

Contraindications and Cautions of Use

NSAIDs are contraindicated for use in patients with gastrointestinal tract illnesses that include vomiting, diarrhea and anorexia, or those undergoing gastrointestinal surgery. They are also generally contraindicated in patients that are hypovolemic, hypotensive, or azotemic. Cats with stable chronic kidney disease may be administered meloxicam chronically (at the lowest effective dose), but this is not recommended in dogs (see Chapter 19). NSAIDs are commonly used in horses with colic, a population that is often hypovolemic and may undergo gastrointestinal surgery. NSAID use is generally avoided in patients with hepatopathies or coagulopathies. The liver is the major site of NSAID metabolism where most will undergo phase I and phase II biotransformation. Hepatopathies that decrease the metabolic functional capacity of the liver can result in higher plasma concentrations of NSAIDs that can increase the risk of adverse drug effects. In cases with hepatopathies that are not life-threatening or severe, administering an NSAID that only undergoes phase I biotransformation (i.e., meloxicam) can be considered. Idiosyncratic hepatopathies have been reported but most have been limited to a single breed of dog (e.g., carprofen in Labrador retrievers) but are of limited clinical concern. The first-generation NSAIDs, most notably aspirin, bind irreversibly to COX-1, preventing the production of thromboxane A2 and thus platelet aggregation. This effect persists for the lifespan of the platelet and therefore caution is advised if elective surgery is undertaken because of decreased hemostasis. In patients treated with aspirin (alone or in combination

Table 9.2 Nonsteroidal anti-inflammatory drugs utilized frequently in small animal patients.

Drug	Dogs	Cats	COX-inhibitor generation	Chemical group	Use
Phenylbutazone	X		First	Pyrazolone	Musculoskeletal disease, antipyretic
Meclofamic acid	X		First	Anthranilic acid (fenemates)	Musculoskeletal disease
Aspirin	X	X	First	acetylated salicylates	Antiplatelet therapy, osteoarthritis, inflammatory pain
Tolfenamic acid	X	X	Second	Anthranilic acid (fenemates)	Acute and chronic pain
Carprofen	X	X	Second	Propanoic acid	Osteoarthritis pain, peri-operative period, and neoplasia with COX-2 expression
Piroxicam	X		Second	Enolic acid (oxicams)	Certain neoplasia conditions and osteoarthritis pain
Meloxicam	X	X	Second	Enolic acid (oxicams)	Osteoarthritis pain and peri-operative period
Etodolac	X		Second	Indol acetic acid	Osteoarthritis pain
Ketoprofen[a]	X	X	Second	Heteroaryl acetic acid	Musculoskeletal disease and pain, and short-term analgesia cats
Deracoxib	X		Third	Coxibs	Peri-operative pain and osteoarthritis pain
Robenacoxib	X	X	Third	Coxibs	Osteoarthritis pain (dogs) and musculoskeletal disease (cats)
Mavacoxib	X		Third	Coxibs	Osteoarthritis pain
Firocoxib	X		Third	Coxibs	Osteoarthritis pain and peri-operative pain
Tepoxalin[a]	X		Third	Hydroxamic acid	Osteoarthritis pain in dogs
Galliprant		X	Not applicable	Pipirant	Osteoarthritis pain dogs

a) Considered dual blockers, see text for details.

with clopidogrel), treatment should be discontinued for a 7–9-day period before surgery.

Adverse Effects of NSAIDs

The major adverse effects, at recommended therapeutic doses, are related to the gastrointestinal tract and include anorexia, vomiting, and diarrhea. These result from both the direct irritation of the mucosa due to the acidic nature of NSAIDs causing mucosal and villus injury, as well as from reduced cytoprotection and blood flow secondary to decreased prostaglandin synthesis. These adverse effects can occur in patients given an NSAID alone but are more frequently encountered in dogs given both NSAIDs and steroids. In some cases, gastrointestinal signs can be transient (2–4 days) due to development of tolerance. This occurs due to enhanced production of growth factors, increased cell proliferation, and mucosal regeneration over time. Less commonly, in some patients, gastrointestinal ulceration can occur. If unrecognized, these ulcers can perforate if NSAID therapy is continued. Gastric or duodenal perforation can be life-threatening. It is important to note that these gastrointestinal adverse effects can occur with the use of any NSAID from any generation of drugs, i.e., the risk remains present with the newer generations. When adverse effects (at therapeutic doses or overdose) are encountered, supportive care includes stopping drug administration, administering gastroprotectant medications (e.g., omeprazole/pantoprozole), and a synthetic prostaglandin analog (e.g., misoprostol) to promote healing of the gastrointestinal tract.

Tips for Switching One NSAID to Another

Different NSAID classes represent different chemical groups. It is important to take this into consideration when selecting an alternative NSAID. Ideally, an NSAID from a different chemical group should be selected. The two major reasons for switching from one NSAID to another are lack of efficacy or because of adverse effects. Both reasons recognize that each individual will respond differently to an NSAID, so the ideal choice that provides efficacy without adverse effects is based on an individual's response. In general, it is recommended to observe a wash-out period of a few days (e.g., six half-lives of the drug, which is 5–7 days for most) before administering a different NSAID; however, there is no evidence to support this common recommendation. During the transition, when no NSAID is given, adjunct drugs (such as paracetamol [not to cats]) may be given to continue provision of analgesia. Switching from a COX-inhibiting NSAID to a receptor antagonist NSAID (i.e., grapiprant) does not seem to require a wash-out period. The practice of using an injectable NSAID during the peri-operative period and then a different NSAID for oral administration post-operatively and for at-home administration is known to occur. However, there is no evidence to recommend this practice and it is probably best avoided. Ideally, the same NSAID should be given during the peri-operative period and continued following discharge from the hospital.

Local Anesthetic Drugs

There are two main groups of local anesthetic (LA) drugs, namely the *esters* and *amides*. These are differentiated by the presence of an oxygen–carbon bond (esters) or nitrogen–carbon bond (amides) in the intermediate chain (Figure 9.2). These intermediate chains link an aromatic ring (improves lipid solubility) to a terminal amine. The terminal amine can exist in either a tertiary form (three bonds) that makes it lipid soluble, or as a quaternary form (4 bonds) that is positively charged and makes the drug molecule polar and thus water soluble. There are differences in the pharmacokinetics and pharmacodynamics between these two groups that are highlighted in this chapter. Most LAs are racemic mixtures of two different enantiomers. In some cases, one of the enantiomers is removed, so the final product for use contains a single enantiomer. This may be performed when one of the enantiomers is more effective and/or has fewer adverse effects. For a racemic mixture to exist, these drugs need to have a chiral center. Naming the different enantiomers is where atoms can be differentiated into left-hand (S-; counterclockwise) and right-hand (R-; clockwise) orientations around the chiral center, according to Cahn–Ingold–Prelog rules of nomenclature. Furthermore, some of the enantiomers are optically active and rotate plane polarized light in opposite directions and are indicated as *levo* (rotates light to the left; counterclockwise) or *dextro* (rotates light to the right; clockwise). In general, the R-enantiomers are associated with greater toxicity with the exception of levobupivacaine and ropivacaine that are both pure S-enantiomers.

Indications of Use

The use of locoregional anesthesia techniques provides an efficient means of reducing pain sensation and, whenever

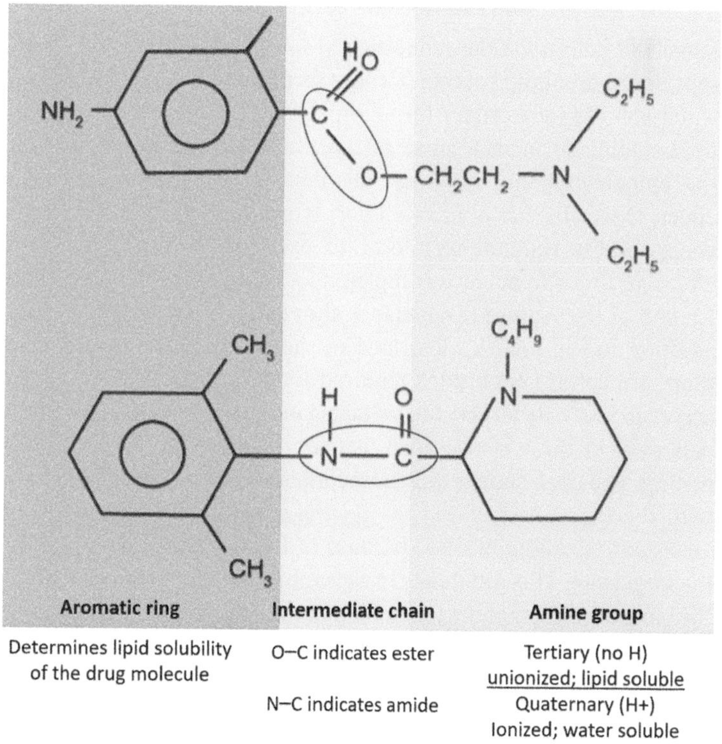

Figure 9.2 The chemical structure of prilocaine (an ester; top) and bupivacaine (an amide; bottom) local anesthetic drugs. There are three major regions of interest: the aromatic ring, the intermediate chain, and the terminal amine group. The significance of these regions is summarized.

Aromatic ring	Intermediate chain	Amine group
Determines lipid solubility of the drug molecule	O–C indicates ester	Tertiary (no H) unionized; lipid soluble
	N–C indicates amide	Quaternary (H+) Ionized; water soluble

possible, plays an important part of a balanced anesthetic plan, allowing for reduction of systemic opioid administration and inhalational anesthetic. This helps reduce adverse effects from these drugs. Furthermore, locoregional anesthetic techniques have an important role in Enhanced Recovery After Surgery (ERAS) protocols, an approach that takes a holistic view of patient care to optimize the numerous factors that influence recovery (e.g., surgical technique, anesthetic technique, nutrition and fluid management, and physical rehabilitation). LA drugs are used in locoregional anesthesia. Typically, LA are deposited perineurally, intrathecally, and epidurally to provide locoregional anesthesia. However, lidocaine can also be administered systemically for reasons other than locoregional anesthesia, such as for its anti-arrhythmic properties, as a systemic (visceral) analgesic to reduce minimum alveolar concentration requirement in anesthetized patients, as a free-radical scavenger, and as a gastrointestinal prokinetic.

Mechanism of Action

These drugs block voltage-gated sodium channels by binding at the *intracellular* DIV-S6 site. This means that the LA must be able to enter the axoplasm (inside the cytosol of the neuronal axon) to exert it blocking effect. The aromatic ring of the LA determines lipid solubility (see later) and the terminal amide determines the water solubility (alters between the tertiary or quaternary form according to tissue pH). When the LA is deposited around a nerve, the tissue pH in relation to the drug's pK_a (see later) will determine the proportion of LA molecules present in either a lipid soluble (tertiary form; unionized) or water-soluble (quaternary form; ionized) form. Only the lipid-soluble form can move intracellularly (traversing the epineurium and neuronal membrane) to exert its effect. Once the LA is intracellular, it transforms to its water-soluble (quaternary) form to exert its blocking effect. In order to achieve complete blockade of a nerve, 75–80% of the sodium conductance should be blocked. In addition to the LA pK_a described in the preceding text, there are certain conditions required for the LA to gain access to block its target site. Voltage-gated sodium channels exist in three states: open (active), inactivated, and resting. The open state is most susceptible to LA blocking, with the inactive state and the resting states somewhat "resistant" to being blocked because of limited access to the target site. This difference in accessibility of the site to the blocking effects of the LA can explain the phenomenon of "use-dependent onset" where, as more action potentials are traveling through the axon, the higher the chance of the receptor being blocked because the sodium channel is in an open state during action potential propagation. Other factors influencing LA access to the nerve are fiber thickness, amount of myelination, and nerve bundle size. Perhaps the consideration with the most clinical relevance is nerve bundle size and the "mantle effect." If a large nerve bundle is blocked, analgesia will be more reliable proximally than distally. Taking the ischiatic nerve as an example: if blocked at the level of the pelvis, analgesia will be more reliable in the proximal regions of the pelvic limb compared to the distal regions. This results in good analgesia to the mid to distal femur but not to the phalanges. This is because the outer parts of the nerve are blocked while the center of the nerve bundle is less reliably blocked. Proximal nerve branches emanate from the outer parts (i.e., the mantle), while distal nerves emanate from the central parts. For nerve fibers that are myelinated, at least three nodes of Ranvier are blocked (i.e., approximately 1 cm of nerve fiber exposed to LA). Although voltage-gated sodium channels are the primary target of LAs, other receptors on potassium and calcium channels and G-protein-coupled receptors have been identified. Nerve fiber size (thickness and diameter) can influence the onset of the block where thinner nerve fibers will block quicker compared to thicker ones. This longer onset is because it takes time for the LA to penetrate thicker nerves.

Pharmacokinetics of LAs

As with all drugs, pharmacokinetics (absorption, distribution, metabolism, and elimination) must be considered. The site of drug administration also alters the pharmacokinetics of LAs. In general, those tissues with greater perfusion (i.e., more vascular) will have greater drug absorption form than the site of injection into the circulation. The order from most vascular to least vascular, for common locoregional techniques, is as follows:

Intercostal > epidural > brachial plexus > femoral/sciatic

LA pharmacokinetics vary according to factors specific to individual members, including lipid solubility, protein binding, and dissociation constant (see the following text and Table 9.3).

In pregnant animals, placental transfer of LAs occurs. This is most relevant to amides, which exhibit *ion trapping*. Here, the nonionized base of the LA crosses the placenta rapidly. As fetal tissue is more acidic than maternal blood and tissue, a greater proportion of drug exists in its ionized (free/active) form and is trapped in the fetal circulation. The degree to which this occurs depends on the drug. Bupivacaine ($pK_a = 8.1$), for example, will transfer back to the mother, whereas lidocaine ($pK_a = 7.8$) does not.

Table 9.3 Physiochemical properties of various local anesthetics.

Drug	pK_a	% ionized	Lipid solubility	% Protein binding	Potency	Duration	Maximum dose (mg/kg)	CNS toxicity (mg/kg)	Miscellaneous
Esters									
Procaine	8.9	97	100	6	1	Short			Fast onset 30–60 min DOA CNS stimulant PABA
Chloroprocaine	9	95	810	7	1	Short			Highest pK_a Fastest onset 30 min DOA
Tetracaine	8.3	93	5822	94	8	Long			Slow onset unless intrathecal Highest toxicity potential
Benzocaine	2.51		1310	3–7.5		Short			Topical only – fast onset 5–10 min DOA PABA/MetHb Fish anesthesia
Amides									
Lidocaine	7.8	76	366	64	2	Medium	Dogs: 6 Cats: 6 Sheep: 6	Dogs: 21–22 Cats: 12 Sheep: 6.8	Fast onset of action 1 h DOA Multiple uses EMLA cream (eutectic)
Mepivacaine	7.7	61	130	77	2	Medium	Dogs: 5–6 Cats 2–3 Sheep: 5–6		Fast onset 1–2 h DOA Poor topical efficacy Drug of choice for diagnostic blocks in horses – less neurotoxicity Slow metabolism in fetus and newborn
Prilocaine	8	76	130	55	2	Medium			
Ropivacaine	8.1	83	775	94	6	Long	Dogs: 3 Cats: 1.5	Dogs: 5 Sheep: 3.5	S enantiomer only → less CV toxicity Slow onset (20–30 min) Biphasic effect on vasculature *>1% → vasodilation* *<0.5% → vasoconstriction*
Bupivacaine	8.1	83	3420	95	8	Long	Dogs: 2 Sheep: 2 Cats: 2	Dogs: 4–5 Cats: 5 Sheep: 1.6	Slow onset (20–30 min) Long DOA (3–10 h) Poor topical efficacy Cardiotoxic
Levobupivacaine	8.1	83	3480	>97	8	Long			S enantiomer only Less cardiotoxic Can cause vasoconstriction
Etidocaine	7.8	66	7317	94	6	Long			

DOA: duration of action; CNS: central nervous system; CV: cardiovascular; PABA: para-aminobenzoic acid; MetHb: methemoglobin; EMLA: eutectic mixture of local anesthetics.

However, the fetus is able to metabolize and eliminate lidocaine better than bupivacaine, so lidocaine may be a better option for epidurals in small animal Cesarean sections compared to bupivacaine. This is in addition to lidocaine having a shorter half-life and allowing for the mother to ambulate sooner and potentially be returned to the owner earlier.

The pharmacodynamics of LAs are altered by several factors, including age, comorbidities, and body temperature (Table 9.4).

When a combination of substances melts at a different temperature than each substance alone, this is known as a "eutectic mixture." An example of a eutectic mixture is EMLA cream, a combination of lidocaine and prilocaine intended for topical application, such as desensitizing skin before IV catheter placement.

Table 9.4 Patient factors that alter pharmacodynamics of local anesthetics.

Factor	Affect
Age	*Neonates*: Increased absorption Increased volume of distribution Increased plasma esterase activity *Geriatrics*: Decreased hepatic clearance Increased half-life
Pregnancy	Increased nerve sensitivity Increased hepatic blood flow → faster clearance lidocaine Decreased hepatic enzyme activity → slower bupivacaine/ropivacaine clearance
Liver disease	Decreased metabolism Decreases plasma esterases Decreased clearance
Anesthesia	Decreased hepatic blood flow → slower lidocaine clearance
Renal failure	Decreased plasma pseudocholinesterease activity Decreased amide metabolite excretion Increased amide metabolites
Diabetes mellitus	Increased hepatic clearance of lidocaine but decreased amide metabolites excretion
Drugs	Any that alters plasma esterase activity Decreased hepatic blood flow
Temperature	Cooling → increase pK_a → increased in ionized/active form
Baricity	*Isobaric (= 1)* most local anesthetic at room temperature *Hypobaric (<1)* → goes to independent site (e.g., local anesthetic warmed to body temperature) *Hyperbaric (>1)* → goes to dependent site (e.g., decreased temperature or diluted with hypertonic solution or dextrose)

Characteristics of LAs and Clinical Correlations

Lipid Solubility

Lipid solubility correlates to LA *potency*. The greater the lipid solubility the greater the diffusion of the drug through the epineurium and neuronal membrane. Thus, the greater the lipid solubility the lower the dose of drug required to block the nerve (increased potency).

Dissociation Constant (pK_a)

pK_a of an LA correlates to *time of onset*. Drugs with a lower pK_a (closer to healthy tissue pH) will have a higher concentration of the tertiary form (lipid-soluble and non-ionized), resulting in a shorter time to onset compared to LAs with a higher pK_a. However, in inflamed or infected tissues, the tissue pH is more acidic and less of the LA will be in its tertiary form, reducing entry into the nerve and block efficacy.

Intermediate Chain

The *intermediate chain* of LAs correlates to *metabolism*. Esters are primarily hydrolyzed by plasma cholinesterase enzymes while amides are biotransformed by hepatic metabolism (and excreted in bile). Clearance of amides varies, with the order from most to least rapidly cleared as follows:

Lidocaine > mepivacaine > ropivacaine > bupivacaine

Protein Binding

Protein binding of LAs correlates with *duration of action* (Table 9.5). The affinity of an LA to plasma proteins corresponds to its affinity at the target site (which is a protein). The higher the protein binding, the longer the LA will be present at the target site, thereby extending its duration.

Table 9.5 Typical duration of action of commonly used local anesthetics when administered alone. Variability of onset and duration is influenced by the concentration of the drug (and dose), volume injected, and nerve proximity.

Drug	Onset of effect	Duration of action
Lidocaine 2%	5 min	1–2 h
Mepivacaine 2%	5–10 min	1–3 h
Bupivacaine 0.5%	15–25 min	4–12 h
Ropivacaine 0.75%	10–20 min	4–12 h

Adverse Effects and Toxicity

Adverse effects of LAs are associated with their intermediate chain group. Esters, such as benzocaine and procaine, can cause allergic reactions due to the metabolite para-aminobenzoic acid (PABA). Amides can be associated with methemoglobinemia (metHb) through various mechanisms. Prilocaine causes metHb through production of the O-toluidine metabolite. Benzocaine causes metHb through direct oxidation of the iron in heme in humans, dogs, and cats. Lidocaine can cause metHb through production of the metabolite monoethylglycinexylidine (MEGX), leading to renal failure. When metHb occurs, the occurrence of clinical signs is dependent on percentage. 10–20% metHb is generally tolerated without clinical consequence. Patients become hypoxemic at concentrations >30% and cardiac arrest occurs at concentrations >70%. Treatment of metHb is with slow intravenous administration of injectable methylene blue: 4 mg/kg in dogs and 1–2 mg/kg in cats. This reduces ferric iron to ferrous so that oxygen can again be carried.

In addition to group-specific toxicity described in the preceding text, amide LAs have the potential for generalized systemic toxicity. The potential for toxicity increases with increasing solubility. Additionally, S-enantiomers are generally less toxic, so LAs presented as S-enantiomers have a better safety profile. Risk and signs of toxicity depend on the route and speed of administration, species (cats are more sensitive than other species), the acid–base balance of a patient, and concurrent therapies. In humans in the early stages of LA toxicity, several signs are reported, including numbness of the tongue, lightheadedness, and visual/auditory disturbances. As toxicity increases, muscle twitching, unconsciousness, seizures, and coma occur.

The most severe effects of LA toxicity are respiratory depression and cardiac arrest. In the cardiovascular system, sodium channel blockade leads to a reduction of phase 0 depolarization. This causes prolongation of the PR and QRS intervals, lengthening the refractory period. If a patient is hyperkalemic, these effects will be more severe. The ECG changes observed are dependent on the dose administered. At subconvulsant doses, an increased heart rate with widening of the QRS complexes occurs. At convulsive doses, there is an increase in sympathetic nervous system stimulation that leads to tachycardia, hypertension, and arrhythmias, such as ventricular tachycardia and ventricular fibrillation. At supraconvulsive doses, bradycardia, hypotension, decreased cardiac contractility, and asystole are seen. Bupivacaine is considered more toxic than other LAs because it exhibits greater cardiovascular toxicity. Unlike other LAs, in addition to the effects described in the preceding text, bupivacaine also causes direct myocardial depression at toxic doses. Consequently, it is usually avoided in blocks with a high rate of absorption into the systemic circulation, e.g., intratesticular blocks. Unfortunately, under general anesthesia, early signs of toxicity may not be apparent due to the combined effect of other drugs and their impact on the cardiovascular and respiratory systems. Intermittent positive pressure ventilation will mask respiratory depression. Therefore, care must be taken to carefully administer LA and monitor for complications. If a nonlethal toxicity occurs, administration of the LA should be discontinued and supportive care should be initiated. This includes oxygen supplementation, treatment of seizures, and treatment of arrhythmias. Fatal toxicities should also include cardiopulmonary resuscitation. As toxicity severity increases, intralipid emulsion therapy should be included. As LA are lipid soluble, they will solubilize in intralipid, lowering the plasma concentration and risk of toxicity. Intralipid is given as a 1–2 mL/kg bolus IV, followed by 0.25–0.5 mL/kg/min IV for 30–60 min, and then 0.5 mL/kg/h until serum is lipemic. Concurrent use of lidocaine, vasopressin, calcium, and beta-blockers should be avoided when treating LA toxicity.

General Notes on Performing Locoregional Anesthesia

Aside from the occurrence of adverse effects, there may be other contraindications for performing locoregional procedures, including coagulopathy, peripheral neuropathy, cutaneous infections or tumor at the site of needle entry, and unstable fractures, due to the risk of inadvertent vascular damage, transient worsening of neurological signs, risk of spreading infection/ tumor cells, and inability to identify anatomical landmarks for performing a block, respectively. When administering LA, we can also mix in additives to prolong the effects of the primary drug. These are summarized in Table 9.6.

Adjunct Drugs Used for Pain Management

Adjunctive analgesics are commonly used in outpatient treatment for owners to administer at home. Additionally, these medications serve as alternative therapies to add on to traditional analgesic options for hospitalized patients or those with both acute and chronic pain. The goals with multimodal therapy are to adequately treat pain while reducing adverse effects, such as activation of sympathoneuroadrenal pathways, behavior changes, and ileus.

Table 9.6 Additives for local anesthetics that may improve duration of action.

Drug	Effects on local anesthetics	Most useful	Dose	Notes
Epinephrine	Decreased absorption, decreased plasma concentration, and increased duration	Short-acting local anesthetics	2.5–5 mcg/mL (0.1 mg epi:20 mL LA)	May enhance analgesia due to alpha-2 adrenergic receptor agonist effects
Hyaluronidase	Increase tissue penetration, shorten onset of action, and increase local tissue pH, which increases unionized form			May increase toxicity by increasing plasma concentration
Sodium bicarbonate (controversial use)	Increase pH, which increases unionized form that results in quicker onset	Decrease pain with injection		Leads to ion trapping and increased intensity and duration of action
Alpha-2 adrenergic receptor agonists	Hyperpolarization of C fibers causes LA blockade of shorter onset, increased duration of action, and improved quality of block			Reversal of alpha-2 adrenergic receptor agonists not reverse blockade Xylazine – large animal epidural [Dex]medetomidine – small animal

Opioids are frequently used in the management of acute pain; however, some pain can be refractory to classic analgesic options (i.e., opioids, NSAIDs, and locoregional anesthesia), or there may be contraindications to administration of a particular type of pain medication. Although there are innumerable drugs included within this sector, the most common in current use are presented in the following text.

Amantadine

Amantadine has the potential to provide analgesia through its antagonist action at the N-methyl-D-aspartate (NMDA) receptor. As this receptor is principally active in central sensitization (see Chapter 3), the use of NMDA antagonists, such as amantadine, can be valuable in reducing chronic pain, including neuropathic pain, where there is a reduced response to opioids. Amantadine also increases dopamine in the circulation, which may provide an additional analgesic mechanism. Although this drug does not relieve acute pain, it is an anti-hyperalgesic in chronic pain conditions. It is also neuroprotective, enhancing the efficacy of other analgesic drugs as well as reducing glial activation (implicated in chronic pain states) and, in human medicine, decreasing opioid tolerance. When treating pain, amantadine should not be used alone but instead given as an adjunct to work synergistically with other therapies. In dogs and cats, it has high bioavailability with a short half-life (5 h). Typically, amantadine is administered at a dose of 3–5 mg/kg every 12–24 h, taking three weeks to reach maximum efficacy. It has a lower safety margin than other analgesics used in veterinary medicine: a 10 times overdose has been associated with arrhythmias and death in humans. The most common adverse effects seen in dogs include gastrointestinal distress, agitation, and the potential for lowering of seizure thresholds. Dose reductions are recommended in patients with renal and/or hepatic insufficiency. Although amantadine has been used as an antiviral in horses, its efficacy as an analgesic has not been thoroughly investigated in any species. It is available as liquid oral suspensions, as well as tablet and capsule forms.

Cannabinoids

The endocannabinoid system is present in nearly every vertebrate, with receptors in both the central and peripheral nervous system. The density of receptors greatly varies between species, leading to different levels of sensitivity. There are two types of receptors: CB1 are located in the central nervous system and CB2 are located on monocytes and microglia. The latter is important for regulation of inflammatory processes and suppression of activation of glial cells through G-protein-coupled action. Both the CB1 and CB2 receptors are important in pain pathways and are involved with anxiety, neuroinflammation, immune function, and many other physiologic functions. Current understanding of the cannabinoid pathway physiology, thought to be similar among species, involves two neurotransmitters: arachidonoyl ethanolamide (AEA) and 2-arachidonoyl glycerol (2-AG). These are endogenously released from the post-synaptic membrane and interact with CB1 and CB2. This leads to intracellular influx of calcium and subsequent inhibition of neurotransmitter release. When injury occurs to neurons or neurons are excessively firing, the production of AEA and 2-AG increases transiently, with subsequent rapid intracellular uptake and degradation. The endocannabinoid system also interacts with numerous other receptors, including *mu* and *delta* opioid receptors as well as serotonin (5HT2A) and dopaminergic (D2) receptors.

When used therapeutically, there is suppression of neurons in the spinothalamic tracts, leading to the alteration of pain processing. Additionally, cannabinoids have peripheral sites of action as well, especially in regions of acute tissue injury and nerve injury. The role of cannabinoids in veterinary medicine, including efficacy, routes of administration, and dosing regimens, is currently unclear. Pharmacokinetic studies have been performed for different routes of administration, including transmucosal, oral, and transdermal administration. The results of investigations into their analgesic potential have been mixed, with canine studies showing both no analgesic effect and measurable analgesia. Interpretation of these data is difficult due to differences in study populations and the concurrent use of other analgesics. Dogs are sensitive to cannabinoids, making them prone to toxicities from exposure to tetrahydrocannabinol (THC). At doses up to 100 mg/kg in dogs, adverse effects include mild, transient gastrointestinal distress and increases in alkaline phosphatase. However, at higher doses, hypothermia, urinary incontinence, ataxia, and seizures can develop. Presently, medical marijuana cannot be prescribed, dispensed, or recommended for use in veterinary patients. Cannabinoid use is further complicated by the variability between concentrations and formulations of available over the counter products. Some of these contain THC concentrations as low as 0.3%. At this time, the veterinary profession is still early in the process of determining if cannabinoids can be used in practice and, if so, the best methods for their use. This is an active area of research. As this class of drugs is controlled in many countries, anesthetists must be aware of local regulations and restrictions. In some countries, products with low THC concentrations may be legally available, sold as cannabidiol-based products, the ideal dose, route, and dosing interval, with evidence to support their use as analgesics remain to be determined.

Gabapentin and Pregabalin

These drugs are structurally similar to gamma-aminobutyric acid (GABA) but do not bind to GABA receptors. Although the mechanism of action is not well understood, their antihyperalgesic effects are thought to be mediated by binding to the alpha-2-delta subunit of voltage-gated calcium channels, leading to decreased frequency of neuronal firing. They also inhibit presynaptic release of GABA and induce glutamate release in the locus coeruleus of the brainstem. Together, these effects induce central nervous system depression, hence their potential use in epilepsy management and management of neuropathic pain. As for amantadine, these drugs are not generally used as sole analgesics but rather given for their synergistic effects with other medications. While they appear to have a wide safety margin in veterinary species, target therapeutic plasma concentrations, effective dosing regimens, and risk of adverse effects (aside from sedation and ataxia, which improve over time) are unknown. In dogs and cats, gabapentin has been shown to have high oral bioavailability, at 80% and 90–95%, respectively, with peak plasma concentrations in 1–2 h after dosing. A common dose of gabapentin to achieve anxiolysis before a veterinary visit in cats is 100 mg/cat, given several hours before beginning transport. It may be helpful to give a first dose the evening before, followed by a second dose on the morning of the visit. For management of chronic pain, typical dosing is approximately 8 mg/kg every 6 h in cats and 10–30 mg/kg every 8 h in dogs. In dogs, 30% of administered drug is metabolized into N-methyl-gabapentin by the liver, with a renal elimination half-life of 4 h. Consequently, dosing intervals are short in order to maintain a useful plasma concentration. As the administered dose is increased in small animal veterinary patients, the percentage of absorption decreases (e.g., at 20 mg/kg, <50% absorbed enterally). Clinical trials are ongoing to evaluate efficacy in other species, such as horses. Gabapentin has gained popularity as an adjunctive treatment in acute pain in dogs and cats but should not be used as a sole analgesic to manage post-operative pain. Overall, gabapentin is fairly inexpensive and available as capsules (50, 100, 300, and 600 mg) and liquid formulations. If smaller patients are being treated with a liquid oral formulation, it is important that the clinician ensure that it is a nonxylitol containing liquid, as these formulations can cause hypoglycemia and liver failure, especially in dogs and cats.

Pregabalin, which is similar to gabapentin, has been used predominantly as adjunctive therapy for dogs, and is well absorbed orally. It has a longer half-life than gabapentin. It is typically dosed at 4 mg/kg orally twice daily, which may improve compliance. Unfortunately, the cost of pregabalin is often prohibitive (around 2–3 times greater than the cost of gabapentin).

Tramadol

Tramadol acts at numerous receptors, including opioid, noradrenergic, and serotonergic receptors. Tramadol is a *mu* opioid receptor agonist and serotonin and noradrenaline reuptake inhibitor, providing effective analgesia in people. It is available in injectable and tablet forms and has been frequently recommended in the past as an at-home oral treatment for pain management in dogs. However, tramadol has been found to be minimally effective in providing pain relief in many veterinary species. This is thought to be mainly due to the low ability of some species (i.e., dogs and horses) to metabolize tramadol into its active form, the metabolite O-desmethyltramadol, which is primarily a *mu* opioid receptor agonist. Cats can metabolize tramadol more readily than dogs and horses and it may therefore have an analgesic role in this species. In horses, tramadol has also not been associated with improvement of lameness. Overdoses of tramadol can theoretically induce a serotonin syndrome although this has not been reported in veterinary species. Clinical signs of toxicity include excitability, tachyarrhythmias, gastrointestinal distress, dyspnea, and death. The risk of developing serotonin syndrome is higher when other drugs that block serotonin reuptake are co-administered with tramadol (e.g., serotonin reuptake inhibitor antidepressants, and trazodone). Therefore, appropriate dose reduction should be applied in the event that these drugs are co-administered. Given the questionable analgesic efficacy, the use of tramadol for pain management in dogs and horses is not recommended. Its use in cats requires further investigation and should not replace proven therapies (e.g., buprenorphine), where available.

Central Endogenous Neuromodulators

Medications that affect this system have the potential to provide intense analgesia. There are multiple binding sites within the spinal cord that can be targeted for pain management, including serotonin (5HT) and norepinephrine (NE) receptors, which are involved with the descending inhibitory pathway from the brainstem (see Chapter 3). However, response to these drugs is highly individual – what may work well in one patient, may have little effect in another, or even amplify the pain signal some patients (though it is rare to have drug-associated hyperalgesia). Consequently, when using these drugs, it is usually necessary to conduct a drug trial, adjusting doses based on individual response. Some of this inter-individual variation reflects differences in mood and behavior, which have a large influence on descending inhibition pathways. Drugs in this group include serotonin or norepinephrine reuptake inhibitors, such as tapentadol, amitriptyline, and trazodone.

Tapentadol is a centrally acting oral analgesic that not only acts as a direct *mu* opioid receptor agonist but also inhibits reuptake of NE. There are a handful of studies within veterinary medicine describing the use of tapentadol. Although it has a limited bioavailability (4.4% when administered orally), studies have shown promise as an analgesic in dogs and cats, e.g., antinociception in beagles undergoing thermal stimulation, and improvement of lameness scores in dogs following orthopedic surgery. Intravenous dosing has been associated with hypersalivation and nausea, and caution should be exercised when given in combination with other central endogenous neuromodulators, such as tricyclic antidepressants, or serotonin/norepinephrine reuptake inhibitors. Tapentadol is typically administered orally at 10–30 mg/kg in dogs and 5.7–11.4 mg/kg in cats.

Amitriptyline is a tricyclic antidepressant drug (TCA), which is considered first-line therapy for neuropathic pain in humans. It primarily works by nonselectively inhibiting reuptake of serotonin and norepinephrine. It is also an antagonist at the NMDA receptor, blocks voltage-gated sodium channels, enhances activity of adenosine and GABA receptors, and has anti-inflammatory effects. Amitriptyline has been used in the treatment of multiple behavior disorders in veterinary medicine, such as separation anxiety in dogs, barbering and urine spraying in cats, and feather plucking in birds. When treating dogs for neuropathic pain and associated itchiness, it can be dosed orally once daily at 3–4 mg/kg. Unfortunately, studies of its efficacy as an analgesic are sparse, so dosing of other species is mostly empirical. Negative sequelae have been reported due to muscarinic and alpha-1 adrenergic receptor antagonism, as well as antihistamine effects. These have been shown to lead to xerostomia (dry mouth), polyuria, polydipsia, urinary retention, blurred vision, sedation, and hypotension. In human patients, weight gain, seizures, agitation, cardiac arrhythmias, and bone marrow suppression have all been reported. There are also a large number of potential drug interactions, so concurrent medications being administered should be carefully evaluated before beginning TCA use.

Another popular treatment for behavioral problems that may alter pain perception includes selective serotonin or norepinephrine reuptake inhibitors (SSRI or SSNRI). These drugs, such as fluoxetine and duloxetine, are typically more costly than TCAs. They also act within the complex descending inhibitory systems and can reduce pain (in addition to their behavioral modification effects) though their effects on enhancing descending inhibition is unpredictable. However, they may be an option when traditional means of analgesia have been exhausted. In humans, SSRIs are one of the first drugs chosen for treatment of neuropathic pain and may be useful in somatosensory disease. However, due to the high cost, lack of evidence, and potential adverse effects, these drugs are not typically used as a first- or second-line analgesic in veterinary patients. As described in the preceding text, there is a risk of serotonin syndrome with these drugs, especially when combined with TCAs, SSRIs, or SSNRIs.

Trazodone, a serotonin-2A receptor antagonist and mild reuptake inhibitor, is frequently used in veterinary medicine to manage anxiety. In human medicine, it causes sedation and is often used as a sleep aid. Although canine studies of analgesic benefit are lacking, in rodent models it shows promise through its effects on the endogenous opioid system as well as via serotonin receptors. Typical doses to provide anxiolysis in dogs and cats are 2–10 mg/kg (oral tablet), 2–3 times daily. The wide dose range reflects inter-individual variability.

Polysulfonated Glycosamino-Glycans (PSGAGs)

Injectable PSGAGs can be administered by intramuscular or intra-articular injection with the intention of reducing inflammation within joints though the exact mechanism of action is not fully understood. Their use can improve range of motion and orthopedic lameness scores in treated patients. Injectable PSGAGs have been used in horses, dogs, and cats. Adverse effects of PSGAGs include vomiting, diarrhea, inappetence, and sedation. When patients are concurrently treated with NSAIDs or platelet inhibitors, it is recommended to proceed cautiously, as there may be additive effects, such as enhanced platelet inhibition.

Immunotherapy

This is a rapidly growing area of pain management, with several monoclonal antibody treatments licensed in the past few years. Frunevetmab works by binding to nerve growth factor, which modulates pain signals and is elevated in joints affected by osteoarthritis. Its use leads to significant improvements in pain, mobility, and activity. Administration is a once monthly subcutaneous injection dosed according to body weight (1 mL for 2.5–7 kg cats; 2 mL for 7.1–14 kg cats), with improvements observed after 2–3 injections. The most common adverse effects noted with therapeutic dosing include injection site discomfort, vomiting, diarrhea, and anorexia. At five times the licensed dose, azotemia and hyperbilirubinemia can occur. Frunevetmab is presented in a single-use vial that requires refrigeration and is light sensitive. Its use in the presence of chronic conditions, such as cardiac disease or chronic kidney disease, has not studied but no immediate contraindication to its use in this patient cohort has been identified. Frunevetmab is minimally immunogenic, but chronic studies following drug use over the course of years would be necessary to determine the likelihood of immune effects.

Similar to frunevetmab, bedinvetmab is a monoclonal antibody licensed in some countries for the treatment of osteoarthritis in dogs. Two studies have been completed with client-owned dogs, administering 0.5 mg/kg subcutaneously every 28 days. In these studies, it was found that compared to placebo, bedinvetmab was effective at improving pain related to osteoarthritis. Adverse events at therapeutic doses have included azotemia, pain at the site of injection, vomiting, and weight loss. As described in the preceding text, further studies are needed evaluating chronic use and use in patients with coexisting diseases.

Question and Answers

There are more practice questions and answers available for this chapter on the website. Please visit http://www.wiley.com/go/VeterinaryAnesthesiaZeiler.

Questions

1) Although originally marketed as an antiviral agent, amantadine is now frequently used as an analgesic agent, with activity at what receptor?
   a) NMDA
   b) AMPA
   c) KAI
   d) Adrenergic
2) What is the target of frunevetmab, drug used to treat osteoarthritic pain in cats?
   a) Nerve growth factor
   b) Nuclear factor *kappa* B
   c) Natural killer cells
   d) Neuronal NK cells
3) The amide local anesthetics are metabolized through the cytochrome P450 system. Which of the following drugs is safer to use in a dog with liver failure?
   a) Bupivacaine
   b) Mepivacaine
   c) Procaine
   d) Prilocaine
4) Which nonsteroidal anti-inflammatory drug irreversibly blocks platelet aggregation and therefore increases the risk of intra-operative bleeding?
   a) Etodolac
   b) Aspirin
   c) Tepoxalin
   d) Carprofen
5) Which receptor does gabapentin act upon?
   a) $GABA_A$
   b) $GABA_B$
   c) Calcium channels
   d) Sodium channels

Answers

1) a
2) a
3) c
4) b
5) c

Further Reading

Becker, D.E. and Reed, K.L. (2006). Essentials of local anesthetic pharmacology. *Anesth Prog* 53: 98–109.

Budsberg, S.C., Kleine, S.A., Norton, M.M., and Sandberg, G.S. (2019). Comparison of two inhibitors of E-type prostanoid receptor four and carprofen in dogs with experimentally induced acute synovitis. *Am J Vet Res* 80: 1001–1006.

Corral, M.J., Moyaert, H., Fernandes, T. et al. (2021). A prospective, randomized, blinded, placebo-controlled multisite clinical study of bedinvetmab, a canine monoclonal antibody targeting nerve growth factor, in dogs with osteoarthritis. *Vet Anaesth Analg* 48: 943–955.

Dewey, C.W. and Xie, H. (2021). The scientific basis of acupuncture for veterinary pain management: a review based on relevant literature from the last two decades. *Open Vet J* 11: 203–209.

Domínguez-Oliva, A., Casas-Alvarado, A., Miranda-Cortés, A.E., and Hernández-Avalos, I. (2021). Clinical pharmacology of tramadol and tapentadol, and their therapeutic efficacy in different models of acute and chronic pain in dogs and cats. *J Adv Vet Anim Res* 19: 404–422.

Donati, P.A., Tarragona, L., Franco, J.V.A. et al. (2021). Efficacy of tramadol for postoperative pain management in dogs: systematic review and meta-analysis. *Vet Anaesth Analg* 48: 283–296.

Ferreira da Cruz, F.S., Natalini, C.C., Pellin de Molnar, B.F. et al. (2020). Tramadol effects on lameness score after inhibition of P-GP by ivermectin administration in horses: preliminary results. *J Equine Vet Sci* 92: 103163.

Gamble, L.J., Boesch, J.M., Frye, C.W. et al. (2018). Pharmacokinetics, safety, and clinical efficacy of cannabidiol treatment in osteoarthritic dogs. *Front Vet Sci* 23: 165.

Hanna, V.S. and Hafez, E.A.A. (2018). Synopsis of arachidonic acid metabolism: a review. *J Adv Res* 11: 23–32.

Indrawirawan, Y. and McAlees, T. (2014). Tramadol toxicity in a cat: case report and literature review of serotonin syndrome. *J Feline Med Surg* 16: 572–578.

Kieves, N.R., Howard, J., Lerche, P. et al. (2020). Effectiveness of tapentadol hydrochloride for treatment of orthopedic pain in dogs: a pilot study. *Can Vet J* 61: 289–293.

Lamont, L.A. (2008). Adjunctive analgesic therapy in veterinary medicine. *Vet Clin North Am Small Anim Pract* 38: 1187–1203.

Luna, S.P.L., Basilio, A.C., Steagall, P.V.M. et al. (2007). Evaluation of adverse effects of long-term oral administration of carprofen, etodolac, flunixin meglumine, ketoprofen, and meloxicam in dogs. *Am J Vet Res* 68: 258–264.

Mathews, K., Kronen, P.W., Lascelles, D. et al. (2014). Guidelines for recognition, assessment and treatment of pain: WSAVA Global Pain Council members and co-authors of this document. *J Small Anim Pract* 55: E10–68.

Monteiro, B.P., Lascelles, B.D.X., Murrell, J. et al. (2022). 2022 WSAVA guidelines for the recognition, assessment and treatment of pain. *J Small Anim Prac* 64: 177–254.

Sanderson, R.O., Beata, C., Flipo, R.M. et al. (2009). Systematic review of the management of canine osteoarthritis. *Vet Rec* 164: 418–424.

Taylor, A. and McLeod, G. (2020). Basic pharmacology of local anaesthetics. *Br J Anaesth Edu* 20: 34–41.

Ukai, M., McGrath, S., and Wakshlag, J. (2023). The clinical use of cannabidiol and cannabidiolic acid-rich hemp in veterinary medicine and lessons from human medicine. *J Am Vet Med Assoc* 261: 623–631.

Varcoe, G., Tomlinson, J., and Manfredi, J. (2021). Owner perceptions of long-term systemic use of subcutaneous administration of polysulfated glycosaminoglycan. *J Am Anim Hosp Assoc* 57: 205–211.

Walters, R.R., Boucher, J.F., and De Toni, F. (2021). Pharmacokinetics and immunogenicity of frunevetmab in osteoarthritic cats following intravenous and subcutaneous administration. *Front Vet Sci* 8: 687448.

10

Other Drugs Used During the Peri-anesthetic Period

Abdur Kadwa, Keagan Boustead, Justin Grace, Daniel Pang, and Gareth Zeiler

Oral Drugs

Some injectable drugs used during the peri-anesthetic period can be purchased in an oral formulation. This chapter covers information relevant to oral administration only and a complete discussion of injectable formulations can be found in Chapter 7. Drugs that are given orally are intended to be delivered through the oral transmucosal (OTM) or oral administration route. In the former, a drug deposited within the oral cavity (or sublingually) is absorbed through the oral mucosa. With oral administration, the drug reaches the stomach, where it is dissolved, with most absorption occurring within the proximal small intestines. The advantage of OTM administration is that the drugs are absorbed into the bloodstream via the sublingual vein, with blood containing drug returning to the heart via the jugular vein and cranial vena cava. This direct pathway to the heart means that absorbed drug is available for distribution to target sites (e.g., receptors) via the systemic circulation. Minimal drug metabolism occurs via this route of absorption as the liver is initially bypassed. By contrast, drugs given by oral administration are absorbed by the small intestines into the bloodstream via the portal blood vessels. Blood carried by these vessels drain into the liver. The liver is a major organ for drug metabolism, and this metabolism can result in a decrease in the amount of drug present in the bloodstream for distribution. Drug bioavailability (see Chapter 6) is decreased if liver metabolism of a particular drug is high. Metabolism by the liver before a drug reaches the systemic circulation is known as the "first pass effect" (also known as "pre-systemic metabolism"). Many oral drugs used during the peri-anesthetic period are prone to a high first pass effect (i.e., a low oral bioavailability). This explains why high doses may be necessary when using this route of administration and why other administration routes are generally preferred. If oral delivery is desired, OTM administration is preferred, but the efficacy of this route greatly varies according to drug pharmacokinetics (not all drugs are readily absorbed via an intact oral mucosa).

Anxiolytic and Sedative Drugs

Anxiolytic drugs are used to calm an excitable patient. They do not reliably result in a change in level of consciousness so that animals are calm but not sedated. Sedative drugs have anxiolytic effects but also result in dose-dependent sedation, whereby the greater the dose the more profound the sedation. Both anxiolytic and sedative drugs have been used in hospitalized patients to promote a calm and quiet environment. Anxious or aggressive patients may benefit from applying a "Chill Protocol" whereby a combination of drugs is given before being transport to a veterinary facility. The Chill Protocol was first described by veterinarians at the Cummings School of Veterinary Medicine (Tufts University) and includes a combination of gabapentin, melatonin and acepromazine. This is given the evening and a few hours before transportation. Drug efficacy is generally improved when these drugs are given before the arousal phase of distress, fear, and anxiety occurs.

Acepromazine (ACP) is a phenothiazine derivative. It is also discussed in the injectable drug chapter and only information relevant to oral formulations is discussed here. Acepromazine is available in many different oral formulations, including pastes, syrups, and tablets. These are often prepared by compounding pharmacies. Acepromazine has been given to a wide range of species but is most commonly prescribed for use in dogs, cats, and horses. In general, oral bioavailability ranges from 20% to 55% depending on the dose and species; therefore, a higher oral dose is required

Fundamental Principles of Veterinary Anesthesia, First Edition. Edited by Gareth E. Zeiler and Daniel S. J. Pang.

Companion Website: www.wiley.com/go/VeterinaryAnesthesiaZeiler

compared to injectable doses. Following oral administration, the elimination half-life is 2–3 times longer than IV injection (i.e., clinical effects last longer, up to 15 h). Furthermore, adverse effects (decreased blood pressure, decreased hematocrit, paraphimosis, etc.) are less prominent. Use of this drug is cautioned in dogs with an ABCB1 (MRD1) gene mutation because the clinical effects can be profound (greater level of anxiolysis and adverse effects). In dogs suspected or confirmed to have this gene mutation, a quarter of the recommended oral dose should be administered first to determine the response before further doses are given. An alternative approach is to reduce the dose by 25–50%. Use in Boxer dogs is controversial. Early, largely anecdotal, reports indicated a greater than expected cardiovascular effect, resulting in marked hypotension. However, anecdotal evidence suggests that the risk of boxer dogs developing severe hypotension is no different to other dog breeds and acepromazine may be used cautiously when indicated. This may reflect early reports being associated with a specific genetic line of these dogs. Acepromazine is either given alone or in combination with other drugs, such as a benzodiazepine or gabapentin. Dogs and cats that develop motion sickness during ground transport benefit from being treated with acepromazine because it has anti-emetic and mild antihistaminic effects. Use for air transport is controversial because of concerns of drug-induced poikilothermia (body temperature varies with environmental temperature, which may lead to hypothermia or hyperthermia). Use of acepromazine alone to treat noise phobias is controversial because this drug does not decrease an animal's cerebral response to noise, but it is effective when given with a benzodiazepine. However, in cats, oral benzodiazepine use has been associated with hepatopathy (see later).

Trazodone (a triazolopyridine derivative serotonin antagonist and reuptake inhibitor) has a range of effects that resemble benzodiazepines, phenothiazine derivatives, and tricyclic antidepressants in humans. The mechanism of action is not well understood, especially in animals. Despite this lack of information, its off-label use in animals is popular, especially for management of anxiety at home and before transport to the clinic, and in hospitalized animals. Adverse effects include gagging, vomiting, diarrhea, colitis, increased appetite, paradoxical excitement, and, in dogs, panting and hypersalivation. The incidence of adverse effects is low and the drug is generally well tolerated in dogs and cats. This drug is frequently prescribed to reduce anxiety and may be given alone or in combination (e.g., as part of the Chill Protocol) before transport to a veterinary clinic. Its sedative effects are somewhat variable in dogs and more predictable in cats. Trazodone has mild cardiovascular effects, including a dose-dependent decrease in systemic arterial blood pressure, heart rate, and myocardial contractility in dogs. Overall, the effect is comparable to that of an acepromazine–opioid combination used for premedication. This effect suggests that its use in hypovolemic animals, or animals with significant cardiovascular disease, should be cautioned.

Clonidine and *dexmedetomidine* are alpha-2 adrenergic receptor agonists (alpha-2 agonists) and are available in various formulations (pastes, liquids, syrups, tablets, etc.) commercially or by compounding pharmacies, for oral use. Alpha-2 agonists are widely available as injectable formulations and are discussed in detail in the injectable drug chapter. Information about oral and OTM dosing is provided here.

Clonidine is a human antihypertensive drug that is presented in tablet form and has traditionally been used off-label alone or in combination with other drugs for behavioral issues, mainly in dogs but also in cats. Examples of use include noise phobias (e.g., thunderstorms and fireworks), fear-related aggression, separation anxiety, and to treat diarrhea in patients with stress-induced inflammatory bowel disease. Doses in use span a wide range because they have been extrapolated from doses used in humans and based on clinical experience. Pharmacokinetic data in dogs and other species is lacking. In some countries, clonidine is used for sedating hospitalized patients. Reported adverse effects include ataxia, constipation, and sedation. Caution is advised when prescribing this drug in patients with cardiovascular disease because of the cardiovascular changes induced by this drug class (see Chapter 7 for more details). Treatment should not be abruptly discontinued in patients on long-term treatment because hypertension is likely to occur. If this drug is used intermittently to treat fear-related behavioral issues, then it should be given 90–120 min before an event.

The injectable formulation of dexmedetomidine has been used (off-label) for OTM application in situations where the commercially available gel or compounded formulations is not available. Compounded formulations do not appear as reliable or effective as the commercially available gel formulation, probably because of poorer OTM absorption and lower bioavailability. Note: Other alpha-2 agonists have been used by OTM route, with similar effects to those described here. Dexmedetomidine gel, when given by the OTM route at least 20 min before an event that can cause acute anxiety, is effective in dogs and cats (off-label use). It has been used to treat distress, fear and anxiety resulting from veterinary visits, noise phobias (e.g., thunderstorms, fireworks, etc.), and exposure to novel environments or situations. Reported adverse effects include vomiting, hypersalivation, and excessive sedation (can be undesirable if the intention is to provide anxiolysis).

Cardiovascular adverse effects are not as profound as when injected (IV and IM). At doses sufficient to cause sedation, effects are longer lasting after OTM administration compared to by injection.

Gabapentin and *pregabalin* (grouped together as gabapentinoids) are classified as anticonvulsant and analgesic drugs (antihyperalgesic and antiallodynic, but not antinociceptive; see Chapter 3). These drugs have been successfully used in the treatment of neuropathic pain and are increasingly used as anxiolytics, especially in cats (administering a dose before a stressful event, e.g., veterinary clinic visit). Both drugs are analogs of gamma(γ)-aminobutyric acid (GABA, an inhibitory neurotransmitter); however, neither drug acts directly on the $GABA_A$ receptor (as an agonist or antagonist). The mechanism of action is not fully understood but evidence of multiple receptor interactions exists (i.e., antagonism at voltage-dependent neuronal calcium channels and interaction with voltage-sensitive potassium channels), as well as an increase in GABA synthesis. Inhibition of N-type voltage-dependent neuronal calcium channels decreases calcium influx, which results in a reduced release of predominantly excitatory, but also inhibitory neurotransmitters from the presynaptic neurons. There is little effect from this inhibition of these calcium channels on healthy neurons, but during a stimulated state (epilepsy and hyperalgesia) these calcium channels are upregulated and thus these drugs suppress function of these neurons.

Gabapentinoids are administered per *os* either as a capsule, tablet, or oral solution (liquid formulation). However, the oral solution contains xylitol as a sweetener that can lead to profound insulin secretion, resulting in severe hypoglycemia and hypokalemia, and even death. Gabapentin is absorbed more slowly and variably compared to pregabalin, which is absorbed approximately three times faster. It is theorized that any condition causing a decreased gastrointestinal motility will result in increased gabapentin absorption but not with limited effects on pregabalin due to its ready absorption. In humans, gabapentin has resulted in false positive urine protein on urine dipstick.

Pregabalin has demonstrated various pharmacokinetic (stronger affinity for its receptors and is more potent) and pharmacodynamic advantages over gabapentin, and switching between the drugs is well tolerated in dogs, and likely other animals as well. The relatively high cost of treatment with pregabalin, compared to gabapentin, may limit its use to animals weighing less than 10 kg. Gabapentinoids are not recommended during gestation (because of a lack of safety data) but is safe during lactation. The most common reported adverse effects of gabapentinoids are sedation and ataxia though these are viewed as benefits when used for anxiolysis. It has been recommended to taper the dose downward when discontinuing these drugs after prolonged use (>30 days) to minimize the risk of seizures resulting from acute withdrawal. Gabapentinoids are administered off-label in veterinary medicine and no withdrawal times are available for food-producing animals (Table 10.1).

Melatonin is an endogenous amine hormone produced primarily in the pineal gland from tryptophan via serotonin. Melatonin synthesis is controlled by circadian rhythm (light–dark cycle), where the highest concentration of melatonin is present during the nocturnal period. This is due to increased release of noradrenaline, during the period where light is absent, from sympathetic nerve terminals. Noradrenaline binds to beta-adrenergic receptors leading to synthesis of melatonin. Melatonin then binds melatonin receptors and inhibits neuronal activity in the suprachiasmatic nucleus of the mammalian brain which is the circadian pacemaker.

Melatonin is well known for its use in human medicine, for the treatment of insomnia and jet lag, and has become popular as a calming drug for dogs (though high-quality supporting evidence is limited). It has been used in combination with amitriptyline for the management of thunderstorm phobia. Clinical data on the efficacy, safety, and appropriate dosage regimen for melatonin is lacking and further research is warranted. However, current dosage recommendations range from 0.1 mg/kg (every 8–24 h) to 3–6 mg/dog (every 8 h) and 1.5–6 mg/cat (every 12 h).

Benzodiazepines are positive allosteric modulators on $GABA_A$ receptors. These are ligand-gated anion channels that allow influx of chloride ions and result in hyperpolarization of the neuron. This modulation causes its anxiolytic

Table 10.1 Summary of current dose (mg/kg) recommendations for gabapentin and pregabalin in dogs, cats, and horses, usually dosed twice daily.

Use	Dog	Cat	Horse
Gabapentin			
Anticonvulsant	10–20	5–10	–
Neuropathic pain	5–15	5–10	2.5
Behavioral disorder	5–30	–	–
Anxiolysis*	10–15	100 mg/cat (20–30 mg/kg)	–
Laminitis	–	–	2.5
Pregabalin			
Anticonvulsant	2–4	2–4	–
Neuropathic pain	4–5	2–4	4

*90 min prior to stressful event.

and sedative (in some species; see Chapter 7) drug effects for which they are often prescribed. Drug effects on behavior occur in the hypothalamus and limbic system of the brain. There are many benzodiazepine drugs available for oral use and they have been prescribed to treat fear, anxiety, phobias, and stimulate appetite in many species. However, fear-related aggression is not reliably inhibited. Benzodiazepines are often combined with tricyclic antidepressants to reduce the panic-like states associated with fears and phobias (e.g., thunderstorms and fireworks). This drug group is prone to tachyphylaxis, where repeated daily dosing results in decreased drug efficacy and clinical effect. In dogs, the decreased clinical effect may prompt an increase in dose. This is not recommended because of the development of physical dependency (a withdrawal abstinence syndrome: weight loss, increased anxiety, limb tremors, muscle pain, and seizures) in this species and possibly others.

Oral formulations of benzodiazepines are well absorbed via the gastrointestinal tract. Injectable formulations can be used for oral administration but have a bitter taste and are therefore commonly mixed with fruit juice. These drugs undergo a high first pass effect, but hepatic biotransformation results in the formation of active metabolites that contribute to the desired clinical effect. Benzodiazepines are excreted in urine and feces; therefore, they should be used with care in patients with hepatic and renal dysfunction.

Adverse effects of benzodiazepines include sedation, myorelaxation, ataxia, increased appetite, disinhibition (paradoxical excitation), and idiopathic hepatic necrosis (reported in cats given oral diazepam). Clinical signs of benzodiazepine toxicity include ataxia, lethargy, emesis, nausea, nystagmus, disinhibition, sedation, and cardiopulmonary depression (at very high doses). Flumazenil and sarmazenil are administered to antagonize the effects of benzodiazepines, as indicated. Oral benzodiazepines are not recommended during gestation period due to an increased risk of congenital malformation of the fetus. However, a once off dose of an injectable drug has been used in equines undergoing general anesthesia for cesarian section.

The use of oral formulations of benzodiazepines is off-label dogs, cats, and horses (Table 10.2). Benzodiazepines are controlled substances in many countries with the potential for human abuse.

Imepitoin is a centrally acting drug that acts as a low affinity, partial agonist at its benzodiazepine binding site on the $GABA_A$ receptor. It is classified as an imidazolone and not a benzodiazepine. It was originally developed for idiopathic canine epilepsy but has also been approved in some countries for noise aversion. The anxiolytic effect of imepitoin is similar to that of benzodiazepines, with fewer adverse effects, such as sedation. However, emesis, ataxia, and lethargy are still observed.

Information on other oral medications for analgesia (opioids, nonsteroidal anti-inflammatory drugs, etc.) and appetite stimulation (mirtazapine) can be found in other chapters and in Further Reading.

Table 10.2 Summary of suggested doses (mg/kg) of oral benzodiazepines used in dogs, cats, and horses. A dose can, generally, be repeated 4 h later to prolong clinical effect. Daily dosing is not recommended.

Drug	Dog	Cat	Horse
Alprazolam	0.02–0.1	0.0125–0.25	0.1 once
Chlordiazepoxide	2.0–6.5	0.2–1.0	–
Clonazepam	0.1–1.0	0.015–0.2 mg/kg q8h	–
Clorazepate	0.5–2.0	0.5–2.0 mg/kg q12h	–
Diazepam	0.5–2.0	0.1–1.0 or 1.0–4.0 mg/cat*	10–30
Flurazepam	0.1–0.5	0.1–0.4	–
Lorazepam	0.02–0.5	0.03–0.08	–
Midazolam	0.5–2.0	0.1–1.0	0.05–0.1
Oxazepam	0.2–1.0	0.2–1.0	–

*Acute fulminant hepatic necrosis has been reported in cats given diazepam per os, thus caution is advised, especially with repeated dosing (see Further Reading).

Cardiovascular Support Drugs

The cardiovascular support drugs are used when there are concerns with the heart (e.g., inadequate contractility, an arrythmia negatively affecting arterial blood pressure) or blood vessels (to cause vasoconstriction or vasodilation).

Positive Inotropes

Positive inotropes increase contractility of the ventricles, thereby promoting ventricular emptying and an increase in stroke volume and cardiac output. Commonly used drugs include dobutamine, dopamine, ephedrine, and pimobendan. Other examples are epinephrine (adrenaline) and norepinephrine (noradrenaline). Dopamine, norepinephrine, and epinephrine are naturally occurring monoamine neurotransmitters synthesized in the adrenal glands (chromaffin cells of the adrenal medulla) and postganglionic fibers of the sympathetic nervous system. They are classed as catecholamines. As with all catecholamines, the blood pH and electrolyte concentrations, if outside of the normal physiologic range, can alter the pharmacodynamic effect of these drugs.

Dobutamine is a synthetic catecholamine drug that primarily acts as an agonist at beta-adrenergic receptors, with limited alpha-adrenergic receptor agonist effects. It has a very short half-life (approximately 2 min), reflecting its clinical use as an intravenous infusion. Dobutamine is used for its positive inotropic effects which increases arterial blood pressure (but increases in blood pressure can potentially be offset by vasodilation in skeletal muscles). As the dose increases (generally greater than 10 mcg/kg/min), a positive chronotropic effect (increased heart rate) can occur. Inhalation drugs used to maintain general anesthesia commonly cause a decrease in cardiac output because of their negative inotropic effects. Therefore, dobutamine is a common choice, especially in equine anesthesia, to maintain a mean arterial blood pressure above 70 mmHg. Dobutamine is contraindicated in animals with tachycardia or thickened ventricular walls (i.e., hypertrophic cardiomyopathy).

Dopamine is a naturally occurring catecholamine, the effects of which are dose dependent. It has a short half-life of approximately 3 min and, as for dobutamine, is delivered via intravenous infusion. In humans, at low doses (1–2.5 mcg/kg/min) the drug is an agonist primarily at the dopamine (D1 and D2) receptors, mediating splanchnic and renal vasodilation. These low-dose effects have been questioned in animals, especially cats. In humans and in animals, at moderate doses (up to 10 mcg/kg/min), beta-adrenergic effects predominate, resulting in increased cardiac output as a result of positive inotropy. As the dose increases, an undesirable positive chronotropic effect may occur. At higher doses, alpha-adrenergic effects predominate, leading to an increase in systemic (and pulmonary) vascular resistance. Some anesthesiologists prefer dopamine to dobutamine (in cats and dogs) because of its ability to increase blood pressure through vasoconstriction at higher doses. In addition to its direct sympathetic effects, dopamine also stimulates the release of noradrenaline from preganglionic neurons, stimulating an endogenous sympathomimetic effect.

Ephedrine is a synthetic, substituted amphetamine that has primarily indirect sympathomimetic activity. It exerts its effects by stimulating the release of norepinephrine from sympathetic neurons as well as delaying the catabolism of norepinephrine by inhibiting monoamine oxidase (MAO) activity. At lower doses, it stimulates beta-adrenergic activity (positive inotropic effect). Alpha-adrenergic activity (vasoconstriction) appears at higher doses. Ephedrine is usually administered as an intravenous bolus (0.05–0.15 mg/kg in most species) due to its longer duration of action compared to other catecholamines but can be administered as an intravenous infusion. The duration of action is species dependent, up to 30 min in cats and dogs and 60 min in horses (following intravenous bolus). Repeated administration may have diminished efficacy (tachyphylaxis) due to the incomplete replenishment of norepinephrine within sympathetic nerve terminals.

Pimobendan (a benzimidazole–pyridazinone derivative) is a synthetic drug that is a selective inhibitor of a hydrolytic enzyme called "cyclic nucleotide phosphodiesterase 3" (PDE3). Pimobendan causes a positive inotropic effect and vasodilation (it is classified as an inodilator drug). A secondary effect of this drug is that it sensitizes the cardiac myocyte troponin C to the binding of calcium, which further contributes to its inotropic effects. Oral doses are effective within an hour or two in cats and 2–4 h in dogs. When an injectable formulation is used, these effects occur within 5 min of injection. Dogs and cats presenting with stage B2 cardiac disease (see Chapter 17) that require urgent surgery can benefit from starting pimobendan therapy with an injectable formulation, if available, before continuing with the oral formulation. While most often used in dogs, pimobendan use is also reported in cats and horses.

Epinephrine (adrenaline) is a naturally occurring catecholamine with dose-dependent cardiovascular effects. It has a short half-life of approximately 3 min and is administered either by frequent dosing (e.g., during cardiopulmonary resuscitation) or via an intravenous infusion. It is most frequently used during cardiopulmonary resuscitation (see Chapter 20). An intravenous dose of 0.01 mg/kg or an infusion of less than 0.5 mcg/kg/min will predominantly have beta-adrenergic effects, typified by a positive inotropic effect and vasodilation. Intravenous doses of 0.1 mg/kg or infusions exceeding 0.5 mcg/kg/min will cause alpha-adrenergic effects to predominate, characterized by an increase in systemic vascular resistance. Therefore, epinephrine, depending on the dose, can be utilized as both a positive inotrope drug and a vasopressor drug. However, some animals may develop cardiac arrythmias (usually tachyarrhythmias) that may necessitate discontinuation of an intravenous infusion. In addition to its cardiovascular effects, epinephrine is a bronchodilator. This combination of cardiovascular and pulmonary effects makes it the recommended treatment for hypersensitivity reactions and anaphylaxis.

Anti-arrhythmic Drugs

Adequate cardiac output depends upon coordinated function of the atria and ventricles. Excitation–contraction coupling refers to the electrical signals of the heart being converted into contraction of the cardiomyocytes. Electrical signals normally originate in the sinoatrial (SA) node, traverse the internodal tract and Bachmann's bundle (a branch of the internodal tract that innervates the inner wall of the left atrium), enter the atrioventricular (AV) node, are conducted through the bundle of His, and onto the left and right bundle branches, finally terminating in the Purkinje fibers. Normal functioning of this electrical system is dependent upon normal plasma pH and electrolyte concentration, input from the autonomic nervous system appropriate for the current mental and physical status of the animal, and no physical disruptions. The decision to treat arrythmias is complex and relates to the impact of the arrhythmia on the cardiovascular status of the animal and the stability of the arrhythmia.

Anti-arrhythmic drugs are classically grouped according to their mechanism of action (the Vaughn–Williams classification; Table 10.3). These drugs have also been classified according to their indication and drug action on the pathophysiologic cause of the arrhythmia (the Sicilian Gambit) or a combination of the Sicilian Gambit and Vaughn–Williams classification (the Oxford Classification).

Vasopressors

Vasopressors are indicated during hypotension typified by vasodilation. They induce vasoconstriction, raising mean arterial blood pressure (MAP), and therefore increase organ perfusion. Situations that may warrant the use of vasopressors include, but not limited to, septic shock, neuraxial local anesthesia-induced vasodilation, or general anesthetic-induced vasodilation. Vasopressors should be used cautiously, at the lowest effective dose, as the induced arteriolar vasoconstriction may compromise tissue perfusion. Furthermore, due to the increased afterload (secondary to vasoconstriction), cardiac output is decreased and myocardial workload and oxygen consumption are increased. Cardiac output may be further decreased by the activation of a baroreceptor-reflex-induced reduction in heart rate. Thus, vasopressors should be titrated to achieve a MAP not exceeding 60–65 mmHg and administered for the shortest possible duration. Both natural (noradrenaline and vasopressin) and synthetic (phenylephrine) vasopressors exist and are catabolized by catechol-O-methyltransferase (COMT) and MAO (except vasopressin, which is broken down by vasopressinases in the liver). Like positive inotropes, the pharmacodynamics of catecholamine vasopressors may be altered by aberrations in blood pH and plasma electrolyte derangements.

Norepinephrine is a naturally occurring catecholamine with dose-dependent receptor interactions. It has a short half-life of approximately 2 min and is administered by intravenous infusion. It is both an alpha- and beta-adrenergic agonist, with its beta effects predominating at lower infusion rates (less than 0.025 mcg/kg/min). The dose range commonly used clinically is 0.1–2 mcg/kg/min. At the lower end of this range, alpha-adrenergic effects become apparent alongside beta-adrenergic activity so that both cardiac output and systemic vascular resistance increase. At the upper end of this range, the alpha-adrenergic effects override the beta-adrenergic effects with a decrease in cardiac output.

Table 10.3 The Vaughn–Williams classification of anti-arrhythmic drugs.

Class	Pharmacodynamics	Indications	Examples
Class I	Sodium channel blockers and decreases the rate of initial depolarization of cardiac myocytes (Phase 0 of the cardiac action potential)	Ventricular arrythmias and atrial fibrillation	Lidocaine Quinidine Mexiletine
Class II	Beta-blockers, negative chronotropy, and reduces automaticity of nodal tissue	Tachyarrhythmias	Propanalol Esmolol Sotalol*
Class III	Potassium channel blockers and reduces the rate of repolarization of cardiac myocytes (Phase 3 of the cardiac action potential) prolonging refractory period	Supraventricular and ventricular arrythmias	Amiodarone** Dronedarone
Class IV	Calcium channel blocker, negative chrono- and dromotropy, and positive lusitropy	Supraventricular arrythmias	Diltiazem Verapamil
Class V	Multiple and depends on individual drug	Supraventricular and ventricular arrythmias	Magnesium sulfate Digoxin

*Sotalol has both beta-blocking and potassium channel blocking effects.
**Amiodarone, although classed as a potassium channel blocker, also has blocking effects at sodium channels, beta receptors, and calcium channels.

Phenylephrine is a synthetic catecholamine with alpha-adrenergic activity. Its short half-life of 5 min results in it being delivered primarily by intravenous infusion. It decreases cardiac output in a dose-dependent manner by causing both an increase in afterload and a baroreceptor-mediated decrease in heart rate. Furthermore, the alpha-adrenergic activity also decreases perfusion of the splanchnic organs (and skeletal muscles) in a dose-dependent fashion. In equine practice, phenylephrine may be administered systemically or injected directly into the spleen to reduce its size. Reduction of splenic size is used during management of entrapment of the left dorsal ascending colon over the nephrosplenic ligament. Phenylephrine topically applied to mucosa mediates vasoconstriction. A dilute solution is commonly instilled into the nares of horses recovering from general anesthesia to reduce nasal congestion and facilitate airflow.

Vasopressin (arginine-vasopressin [AVP]) is a naturally occurring propeptide hormone released from the paraventricular nucleus of the hypothalamus. In addition to its role in free water conservation, it also mediates vasoconstriction by interacting with the AVP 1 receptor. This contrasts with the action of the catecholamine vasopressors (described in the preceding text), which act through adrenergic receptors. Compared to the catecholamines, it has a relatively long half-life of approximately 20 min and can therefore be administered as either an intravenous bolus or intravenous infusion. Unlike the catecholamines, it is unique in that its pharmacodynamics are minimally affected by aberrations in blood pH and electrolyte derangements. As a result of these differences, it serves as a good alternative in cases of hypotension refractory to other vasopressors, such as in patients in septic shock.

Vasodilators

Sustained hypertension is damaging to tissues. This damage is referred to as "target organ damage" or "end-organ damage." Hypertension results in histological damage to the kidneys and has been associated with proteinuria. Proteinuria is associated with accelerated progression of kidney disease and an increased risk of mortality. Sustained hypertension also results in hypertensive choroidopathy and retinopathy, hypertensive encephalopathy and cerebrovascular accidents, as well as hypertensive cardiomyopathy (with associated ventricular hypertrophy).

Hypertension can be classified as situational, secondary hypertension and primary (idiopathic and essential) hypertension. Situational hypertension occurs in an otherwise normotensive animals as a result of autonomic nervous system input due to anxiety or fear (e.g., the so-called "white coat phenomenon"). Secondary hypertension occurs as a result of underlying conditions such as kidney disease or endocrinopathies. Primary hypertension is a diagnosis of exclusion where no underlying cause for hypertension can be elucidated.

The American College of Veterinary Internal Medicine (ACVIM) defines hypertension in conscious patients as a systolic arterial blood pressure of greater than 160 mmHg in cats and dogs. Hypertension should be treated if there is evidence of end-organ damage and the systolic blood pressure remains above 160 mmHg over eight weeks or above 180 mmHg over two weeks. The primary mechanism by which antihypertensive drugs mediate their action is vasodilation.

Vasodilatory drugs can be grouped according to their mechanism of action.

Angiotensin-converting enzyme inhibitors (ACEi) exert their action by inhibiting the downstream production of angiotensin II and aldosterone, both of which mediate vasoconstriction. These drugs also dilate the afferent arterioles of the glomerulus, thereby decreasing pressure within the glomerulus and ultimately the degree of proteinuria. Due to their effects on intraglomerular pressure, ACEi should be used with caution in dehydrated and hypovolemic patients as they can cause a significant reduction in glomerular filtration rate. Angiotensin-converting enzyme inhibitors are the preferred first-line antihypertensives in dogs, but not cats. These drugs are administered orally, usually twice daily. Examples of drugs within this class are *enalapril, benazepril, and captopril.* Intravenous formulations of ACEi exist; however, these have been minimally investigated for use in veterinary species.

Calcium channel blockers bind to calcium channels of vascular smooth muscle, inhibiting calcium influx, thereby causing vasodilation. This drug class is preferred as a first-line antihypertensive in cats. There are two classes of calcium channel blockers: dihydropyridines and nondihydropyridines, which comprise phenylalkylamines and benzothiazepines. The dihydropyridines are most selective for vascular smooth muscle and therefore primarily used as vasodilators. The nondihydropyridines are more selective for cardiac calcium channels. The dihydropyridine *amlodipine* is administered orally, once daily.

Phosphodiesterase 5 inhibitors (PDE5i) increase the concentration of cyclic guanosine monophosphate (cGMP) within the corpus cavernosum and pulmonary vascular smooth muscle. An increased concentration of cGMP inhibits calcium entry into pulmonary vascular smooth muscle thereby mediating vasodilation of the pulmonary vasculature. *Sildenafil* is an example of a PDE5i that is commonly used to treat pulmonary hypertension in dogs. It is dosed orally, twice daily.

Alpha-adrenergic receptor antagonists function by inhibiting the binding of norepinephrine to alpha-adrenergic receptors on vascular smooth muscle cells. These drugs are commonly used to stabilize patients before phaeochromocytoma excision surgery. Examples of drugs in this group include *prazosin, phentolamine, doxazosin, and phenoxybenzamine.* All of these drugs can be administered orally. It must be noted that phenoxybenzamine has a half-life of 24 h; therefore, it is dosed for at least two weeks to achieve hemodynamic control.

Nitrodilator drugs mediate vasodilation by producing nitric oxide. Nitric oxide (NO) is a potent endogenous vasodilator. *Nitroglycerine* may be used in acute exacerbations of left heart failure. It primarily acts as a venodilator, reducing cardiac work by decreasing cardiac preload. It is available as a transdermal patch or ointment, to be applied to the hairless inner surface of the pinna. Its onset time is unpredictable due to variable absorption; it is reported to produce vasodilation between 15 min to an hour after application. Personnel must wear gloves during application as it will be absorbed through the skin, potentially causing dizziness and migraines. *Sodium nitroprusside* is primarily an arteriodilator. It acts rapidly after administration and has a short half-life of 2 min so that it is primarily delivered by intravenous infusion. Its pharmacokinetic profile makes it suitable for use in acute hypertensive crises and acute heart failure (to reduce cardiac afterload). A common adverse effect of nitroprusside infusion is cyanide toxicity, especially in patients receiving high doses, those with hepatic or renal impairment, or with vitamin B12 deficiency.

Corticosteroids

The term "corticosteroids" generally refers to the synthetic analogs of hormones produced by the adrenal cortex; it is an all-encompassing term for both glucocorticoids and mineralocorticoids, which are produced by the *zona fasciculata* and *zona glomerulosa* of the adrenal cortex, respectively. Synthetic versions of these hormones have varying glucocorticoid and mineralocorticoid activity. These drugs interact virtually with every organ system. In general, glucocorticoids have primarily anti-inflammatory (prevent formation of arachidonic acid by inhibiting the enzyme phospholipase A2-alpha; arachidonic acid is required for prostaglandin synthesis), immunomodulating, and metabolism-altering effects. Mineralocorticoids primarily act on the distal convoluted tubules of the nephrons within the kidneys to regulate serum sodium and potassium concentrations and water balance. Corticosteroids therefore have a wide range of applications, including treatment of allergic and inflammatory conditions, autoimmune diseases, and the diagnosis and management of hypo- and hyperadrenocorticism (Addison's and Cushing's disease, respectively).

Corticosteroid drugs can be classified according to their onset and duration of action as well as their glucocorticoid or mineralocorticoid activity (Table 10.4). Multiple corticosteroid formulations exist for administration by numerous routes, including oral syrups and tables, inhalational delivery, topical ointments and sprays, and injectables.

Antimicrobials

Antimicrobials are a group of drugs used routinely by veterinary anesthetists. As with the selection and administration of other peri-anesthetic drugs, there should be a rational approach to their use. The increasing development of antimicrobial resistance is a major concern in both humans and animals. The responsible and rationale use of antimicrobials to limit antimicrobial resistance is termed "antimicrobial stewardship." The ACVIM has issued a consensus statement on therapeutic antimicrobial

Table 10.4 Commonly used corticosteroids in veterinary practice classified according to activity, speed of onset, and duration of action.

Corticosteroid	Glucocorticoid activity	Mineralocorticoid activity	Onset of action	Duration of action
Cortisol*	+	+	Immediate	6 h
Hydrocortisone	+	+	Immediate	6 h (S)
Prednisolone	++	+	6 h	36 h (I)
Triamcinolone	++	–	12 h	36 h (I)
Dexamethasone	+++	–	1 h	72 h (L)
Aldosterone*	–	+	Immediate	1 h
Fludrocortisone	–	+++++	24 h	48 h (L)

S: short acting; I: intermediate acting; L: long acting.
*Cortisol and aldosterone are included as physiologic references.

use in animals, which also covers aspects of antimicrobial resistance (see Further Reading). Furthermore, the American Veterinary Medical Association has provided a checklist of criteria to be met before a practice can state that they are conforming to antimicrobial stewardship (https://www.avma.org/sites/default/files/2020-06/Veterinary-Checklist-Antimicrobial-Stewardship.pdf). Administering an antimicrobial creates a selection pressure on pathogens or commensal microbes to develop resistance. Therefore, preventing infection rather than treating it should be a key objective. With evidence that antimicrobial resistant bacteria may be passed from animals to humans, all persons involved with antimicrobial use have an obligation to practice infection prevention and antimicrobial stewardship. The World Health Organization has published a list of antimicrobials of critical importance for human medicine. Veterinarians should be conscious of this list when selecting antimicrobials for animal use. The use of antimicrobials classified as critically important should be limited to select veterinary cases. This is especially true for antimicrobials that meet the "highest priority" classification. The WHO document can be found here https://www.who.int/publications/i/item/9789241515528.

In the peri-anesthetic and critical care setting, antimicrobials may be used for two reasons: prevention of surgical site infections and the treatment of a bacterial infection. When developing an antimicrobial plan, one should consider the bacterial species being targeted, its antimicrobial susceptibilities, the type of tissue infected, and the pharmacodynamic and pharmacokinetic profile of the antimicrobial of choice. In order to be effective, an antimicrobial must achieve a concentration above its minimum inhibitory concentration (MIC) in the target tissue. When a sample is sent for bacterial culture, some laboratories report an MIC along with the species of bacterium and its susceptibility profile. This MIC should be used as the therapeutic target (Figure 10.1). Achieving a drug concentration above the MIC requires knowledge of the pharmacokinetic profile of the selected antimicrobial, that is, its absorption, volume of distribution, and clearance. Antimicrobials killing/inhibiting activity can be considered *time dependent* or *concentration dependent*. With time-dependent killing, tissue concentrations of the antimicrobial must remain above the MIC for the entire treatment duration. In this group of antimicrobials, dosing interval determines efficacy. The dosing interval varies according to the initial dose, the volume of distribution, and drug clearance. These antimicrobials are usually dosed every 6, 8, or 12 h. With concentration-dependent killing, drug efficacy is determined by the maximum tissue concentration (Cmax) above MIC. Furthermore, the concentration-dependent antimicrobials have a

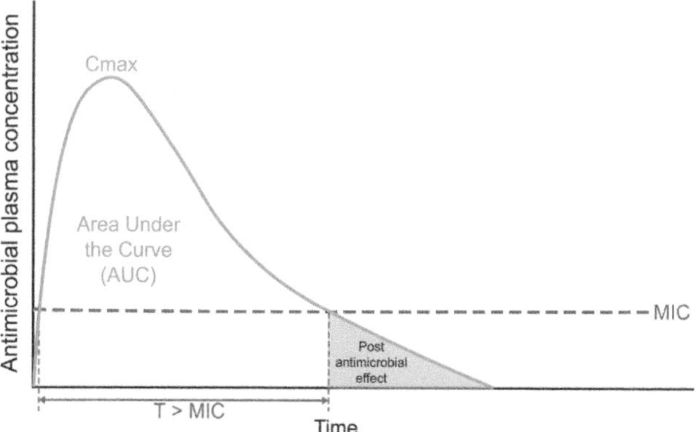

Figure 10.1 Antimicrobial plasma concentration (or effect site or tissue concentration) change over time following a single bolus of drug. Key pharmacokinetic parameters are illustrated. MIC: minimum inhibitory concentration; Cmax: maximum drug concentration (see text: concentration-dependent antimicrobials); T > MIC; time above MIC (see text: time-dependent antimicrobials).

post-antibiotic effect whereby the inhibitory or killing effect of these drugs lasts longer than the time they are above the MIC. Usually, these antimicrobials are dosed once daily. Some antimicrobials exhibit a combination of concentration- and time-dependent efficacy. In this group, the area under the concentration–time curve to MIC ratio (AUC/MIC ratio) is what determines the efficacy. The AUC/MIC ratio for antimicrobials has been established for some companion animals and can be readily found using an online search.

In the peri-anesthetic and critical care setting, it is common to begin antimicrobial therapy without a bacterial culture and susceptibility analysis. This is because it takes a few days to culture a sample. This approach to antimicrobial therapy is called "empiric antimicrobial therapy." In this situation, an antimicrobial is selected based on the pathogens most likely to be encountered, the site of infection/trauma/surgery, and patient species. Bacterial culture of the local clinic environment can help with drug selection. Cytology and Gram staining helps broadly identify bacterium into rods or cocci, and Gram positive or Gram negative. These characteristics can help choose the appropriate antimicrobial. When infection is present, a sample for culture should always be taken as soon as possible (before beginning empirical therapy) so that an evidence-based decision can be made following the results of culture and susceptibility testing. Empirical therapy is usually considered escalating or de-escalating. Escalating therapy is where a first-line antimicrobial is used empirically but is proven to be ineffective because, for example, a resistant microbe is cultured. In this scenario, the therapy will be "escalated" by changing the antimicrobial therapy (e.g., adding another antimicrobial or changing to a second-line antimicrobial the microbe is sensitive to). A de-escalating therapy is where a second-line (or third-line) antimicrobial is initially used in at-risk patients (e.g., with sepsis or severe trauma, etc.), but after receiving the culture and sensitivity results, it becomes apparent that a first-line antimicrobial could have been effective. In this case, the antimicrobial therapy is "de-escalated" to a first-line antimicrobial. First-line, second-line, etc., grouping of antimicrobials differs from geographical region; however, the logic of their grouping is similar. For example, a first-line antimicrobial may be grouped as those that are frequently prescribed but require prudent use. Whereas the second- and third-line antibiotics should have restricted use (or use should be avoided) and only included once culture and sensitivity reports are available. Combining two or more antimicrobials can either result in synergy or antagonism. It was proposed that using a bacteriostatic and bactericidal antimicrobial promoted antagonism and decreased efficacy of therapy. Also, combining two antibiotics with the same mechanism of action (such as using two beta-lactams) is not more effective than using them alone. However, emerging evidence suggests that antimicrobial combinations are far more complex than previously thought. An expert (e.g., specialist veterinarian in medicine) or medical journal articles should be consulted before routinely combining antimicrobials. In addition to selecting an appropriate antimicrobial, the adverse effect and toxicity profile should be known. Considering this may exclude the use of a particular antimicrobial in our patient even though it has a suspectable bacterial infection. Table 10.5 summarizes the antimicrobial classes most frequently encountered in veterinary medicine.

Table 10.5 Summary of different antimicrobial classes used in veterinary medicine.

Drug class	Examples	Mechanism of action	PK/PD	Bacteriostatic or bactericidal	Side effects and toxicity
Aminoglycosides	Gentamicin Amikacin	Inhibition of protein synthesis at 30 s ribosomal subunit	Concentration dependent	Bactericidal	Renal tubal dysfunction, neuromuscular blockade, and ototoxicity
Beta-lactams (penicillins, cephalosporins, and carbapenems)	Ampicillin Amoxicillin Cefazolin Cephalexin Cefuroxime Cefotetan Meropenam	Inhibition of cell wall synthesis	Time dependent	Bactericidal	Immune mediate disease, allergic reactions (hypersensitivity and anaphylaxis), acute renal tubular necrosis, and hypotension (especially Amoxycillin–Clavulanate)
Quinolones and fluoroquinolones	Enrofloxacin Ciproflaxacin Marbofloxacin	Stops DNA synthesis by inhibiting DNA gyrase function	Concentration dependent (or AUC/MIC ratio)	Bactericidal	Cartilage damage in growing animals, retinal toxicity in cats, reduced seizure threshold, and QT prolongation
Phenicols	Chloramphenicol	Inhibition of protein synthesis at 50 s ribosomal subunit	Time dependent	Bacteriostatic	Bone marrow suppression, CYP450 inhibitor, peripheral neuropathy, gastrointestinal upset, and prolonged half-life in cats as relies heavily on glucuronidation
Macrolides	Erythromycin Tylosin	Inhibition of protein synthesis at 50 s ribosomal subunit	AUC/MIC ratio	Bacteriostatic	Injection site irritation, nausea, intestinal hypermotility, vomiting and diarrhea, CYP450 inhibition, QT prolongation, hepatotoxicity, colitis in horses and rabbits, and anhidrosis in foals
Lincosamides	Clindamycin Lincomycin	Inhibition of protein synthesis at 50 s ribosomal subunit	AUC/MIC ratio	Bacteriostatic	Diarrhea, esophagitis after oral administration in cats, neuromuscular blockade, and pseudomembranous enterocolitis in hind gut fermenters

Table 10.5 (Continued)

Drug class	Examples	Mechanism of action	PK/PD	Bacteriostatic or bactericidal	Side effects and toxicity
Nitroimidazoles	Metronidazole	Inhibition of DNA synthesis	Concentration dependent	Bactericidal	CNS toxicity and bone marrow suppression
Sulphonamides	Trimethoprim–sulfadiazine Trimethoprim–sufamethoxazole	Inhibition of folic acid metabolism	Time dependent	Bacteriostatic	Hypersensitivity, cholestasis, acute hepatic necrosis, macrocytic anemia, thrombocytopenia, nonseptic arthritis, keratoconjunctivitis sicca, hyperkalemia, and functional hypothyroidism
Tetracyclines	Tetracycline Doxycycline	Inhibition of protein synthesis at 30 s ribosomal subunit	AUC/MIC ratio	Bacteriostatic	Hypotension with IV injection, calcium chelation, nephrotoxicity, hepatotoxicity, teeth discoloration, esophagitis in cats after oral dosing, neuromuscular blockade, immunosuppression, hypersensitivity, propylene glycol carrier can cause hemolysis, CNS signs, and hypotension
Rifamycin	Rifampicin	Inhibition of RNA polymerase	Concentration dependent (or AUC/MIC ratio)	Bactericidal	Hepatotoxicity, CNS symptoms, and CYP450 inducer
Polymixin	Polymixin B Colistin	Destabilize phospholipids and lipopolysaccharides of Gram-negative bacteria	AUC/MIC ratio	Bactericidal	Nephrotoxicity and neurotoxicity: neuromuscular blockade, ataxia, paresthesia, and histamine release
Glycopeptides	Vancomycin	Inhibition of cell wall synthesis	Time dependent	Bactericidal	Nephrotoxicity, hypersensitivity, hypotension, and ototoxicity

PK/PD: pharmacokinetic and pharmacodynamic characteristics of the drug that determine if their killing or inhibitory effects are time or concentration dependent; AUC/MIC: area under concentration–time curve to minimum inhibitory concentration ratio (see text for details); CYP450: cytochrome P450 gene; CNS: central nervous system; IV: intravenous; QT: Q and T waves of an electrocardiogram tracing; prolonged QT means ventricular repolarization is prolonged.

The use of peri-anesthetic antimicrobials should be based on the risk for surgical site infections and the possible consequence to the patient should an infection develops. Peri-anesthetic antimicrobial therapy is the delivery of an antimicrobial intravenously 30–60 min before skin incision, with appropriate redosing until wound closure. The ASA classification of the patient undergoing a surgical procedure can help guide peri-anesthetic antibiotic use (Table 10.6). There is growing evidence that in the absence of a bacterial infection the continuation of antimicrobial therapy into the post-anesthetic period is not required. It must be remembered that there are multiple factors that may influence the development of surgical site infections, such as hypothermia, hypotension, anesthetic drug selection, anesthesia duration, surgical duration, operating room conditions, and atraumatic tissue handling. The anesthetist should optimize factors under their control.

Table 10.6 Recommendations for peri-operative antimicrobial use.

Should not receive peri-operative antimicrobials	Should receive peri-operative antimicrobials
• ASA I–II undergoing a clean procedure • Apyrexia ASA III undergoing a clean or clean-contaminated procedure	• ASA III with contaminated or infected wounds • Pyretic ASA I–V patients • ASA IV–V patients • Patients where surgical site infections would be catastrophic (e.g., orthopedic implantation and neurosurgery)

Nutraceutical or Herbal Remedies

"Nutraceutical" is a portmanteau of "nutrition" and "pharmaceutical." A working definition has been suggested to eliminate confusion and to better define the concept of "nutraceuticals," which could allow for effective regulation of these products. The North American Veterinary Nutraceutical Council (now defunct) defined *veterinary nutraceuticals* as "a substance which is produced in a purified or extracted form and administered orally to patients to provide agents for normal body structure and function and administered with the intent of improving the health and well-being of animals."

Nutraceuticals encompass isolated nutrients (Table 10.7), phytochemicals (Table 10.8), herbal products, functional foods, and engineered foods, when these are specifically used to treat or prevent diseases.

Herbal remedies or herbal medicine are plants or parts of a plant (roots, leaves, stems, seeds, etc.) which contain active compounds and are used as medicinal products

Table 10.7 Nutraceuticals prepared as isolated nutrients (amino acids, vitamins, minerals, and fatty acids) that owners may be administering to their companion animal.

Drug Description	Proposed effect	Toxicity	Adverse drug–drug interactions
L-Arginine • Precursor for NO and proteins	• Antihypertensive • Growth promoter	• Abdominal discomfort • Asthma • Diarrhea • Nausea • Bloat	• Anticoagulants • Antihypertensive drugs • Diuretics • Insulin • Nitrates
Glutamic acid • Excitatory neurotransmitter • Precursor to GABA	• GI lining health • Muscle anabolism	• Excitotoxicity	• Anticonvulsants
L-Lysine • Competes with arginine • Promotes calcium uptake • Protein synthesis	• Anti-inflammatory • Herpes viral particle inhibition • Limiting amino acid	• Abdominal discomfort • Diarrhea • Cholelithiasis • Nephrotoxicity	• No reported interaction
L-Tryptophan • Precursor to melatonin and serotonin • Protein synthesis	• Anxiolytic • Calming • Limiting amino acid	• Diarrhea • Emesis • Lethargy • Serotonin syndrome	• MAOI • SSRIs • TCAs
Methionine • Precursor compound • Protein synthesis • Acidifies urine	• Antioxidant • Limiting amino acid	• Anorexia • Ataxia • Diarrhea • Emesis • Nausea • Seizures	• Charcoal • Ephedrine (decreased plasma concentration) • Mexiletine (decreased plasma concentration) • Pseudoephedrine (decreased plasma concentration)
Vitamin A (Retinol) • Fat-soluble	• Antioxidant • Bone growth • Cellular division • Embryo development • Immunity • Reproduction • Vision	• Abdominal discomfort • Emesis • Hemorrhagic diathesis • Hepatotoxicity • Irritability • Nausea • Skin sloughing	• Tetracycline • Warfarin
Vitamin B3 (Niacin) • Water-soluble	• Antioxidant • Energy production • Homeostasis	• Anorexia • Diarrhea • Nausea	• CBD products • Insulin (decreased efficacy)

Table 10.7 (Continued)

Drug Description	Proposed effect	Toxicity	Adverse drug–drug interactions
Vitamin B6 (Pyridoxine) • Water-soluble • CNS homeostasis • Metabolism	• Antidepressant • Immunity	• Neurotoxicity • Photosensitivity • Seizures	• Barbiturate (decreased plasma concentration) • Phenytoin (decreased plasma concentration)
Vitamin B9 (folic acid) • Water-soluble • DNA synthesis • Erythrocyte production	• Homeostasis	• No reported toxicities	• Barbiturates (impair folic acid absorption) • Sulfonamides (folic acid antagonists) • Trimethoprim (folic acid antagonists)
Vitamin C (ascorbic acid) • Water-soluble • Collagen synthesis	• Antioxidant • Immunity	• Acidic urine • Diarrhea	• Ephedrine (decreased plasma concentration) • Propranolol (decreased plasma concentration) • Pseudoephedrine (decreased plasma concentration)
Vitamin D • Fat-soluble • Calcium and phosphorus homeostasis	• Antidepressant • Bone homeostasis	• Anorexia • Emesis • Hypersalivation • Polyuric/polydipsic • Renal damage	• Cimetidine (interfere with Vitamin D metabolism) • Digoxin (arrhythmia) • Magnesium (hypermagnesemia) • CYP450 isoenzymes inducers (decreased drug plasma concentration)
Vitamin E • Fat-soluble	• Antioxidant • Immunity	• Asthenia • Diarrhea • Fatigue • Hemorrhagic diathesis • Nausea	• Anticoagulants (potentiated) • Immunosuppressants
Vitamin K • Fat-soluble	• Coagulation	• No reported toxicities	• Anticoagulants
Calcium • Coagulation • Muscle contraction • Cardiac rhythm • Nerve function	• Homeostasis	• Anorexia • Diarrhea • Emesis • Kidney failure • Lethargy • Nausea	• Levothyroxine (decreased absorption) • Quinolones (decreased absorption) • Tetracyclines (decreased absorption)
Iron • Component of hemoglobin	• Erythrocyte production • Anemia prevention • Homeostasis	• Abdominal discomfort • Emesis • Hematochezia • Hemodynamic disturbances • Lethargy • Tremors	• Vitamin E (diminishes response to iron) • Quinolones (decreased absorption) • St. John's wort (tannins decreases iron absorption)
Selenium • DNA synthesis • Protection against cell damage	• Antioxidant	• Alopecia • Anemia • Anorexia • Depression • Emesis • Nausea • Stunted growth	• Anticoagulants • Quinolones (decreased absorption)

(Continued)

Table 10.7 (Continued)

Drug Description	Proposed effect	Toxicity	Adverse drug–drug interactions
Zinc • DNA synthesis • Immunity • Metabolism • Protein synthesis	• Anti-inflammatory • Antioxidant • Improve immunity • Wound healing	• Anorexia • Depression • Diarrhea • Emesis • Hemolysis • Hepatic damage • Lethargy	• Quinolones (decreased absorption) • Tetracyclines (decreased absorption)
Omega fatty acid • Sources: fish, algae, nuts, seeds, and plant oils Omega-3 • Anti-inflammatory • NB in neurological and retinal development Omega-6 • Pro-inflammatory Omega-9 • Anti-inflammatory • Reduces insulin resistance	• Aggression • Analgesic – OA • Anti-arrhythmic (VPC) • Anti-inflammatory (IBD, COPD) • Antineoplastic • Immunoinhibitory • Improves anorexia • Hypercholesterolemia • Hypertriglyceridemia • Neurological and retinal development • Nephroprotective • Pruritus/atopy • Reduces cachexia • Reduce preterm labor • Wound healing	Omega-3 • Immunodeficiency • Platelet dysfunction • Altered lipid and glucose metabolism Omega-6 • Retinopathy • Worsens glomerular hypertension and hypertrophy in CKD Cautionary use in patients with thrombocytopenic conditions	• NSAID (hemorrhagic diathesis) • Anticoagulants (hemorrhagic diathesis)
SAMe • S-adenosyl-L-methionine • Precursor to cysteine	• Increases serotonin, noradrenaline and dopamine • Maintenance of cell membranes • Regulate hormones • Restores glutathione deposits	• Diarrhea • Nausea	• MAOI (serotonin syndrome) • SSRIs

CBD: cannabidiol; CKD: chronic kidney disease; COPD: chronic obstructive pulmonary disease; CYP450: cytochrome P450 gene; GABA: gamma-aminobutyric acid; IBD: inflammatory bowel disease; MAOI: monoamine oxidase inhibitors; NO: nitric oxide; NSAID: nonsteroidal anti-inflammatory drug; OA: osteoarthritis; SSRIs: selective serotonin reuptake inhibitors; TCAs: tricyclic antidepressants; VPC: ventricular premature contractions.

Table 10.8 Nutraceuticals prepared as phytochemicals that owners may be administering to their companion animal.

Drug Description	Proposed effect	Toxicity	Adverse drug–drug interactions
Berberine • Isoquinoline alkaloid • Obtained from various plants, i.e., *Berberis* spp., *Argemone* sp., *Hydrastis* sp., and *Coptis* spp. • Poor oral bioavailability • Crosses blood–placenta and blood–mammary barrier Caution in pregnant and lactating animals	• Antibiotic • Antidiabetic (Type II) • Antifungal • Anti-inflammatory • Antineoplastic • Antioxidant • Antiprotozoal • Antipyretic • Congestive heart failure • Hepatoprotective • Hyperlipidemia • Hypertension • Nephroprotective • Neuroprotective • Obesity	• Low toxicity and adverse effects • Hypotension • Dyspnea • GI disturbances • Cardiac damage	• Antihypertensive drugs (hypotension) • Insulin (hypoglycemia) • CYP450 inhibitors

Table 10.8 (Continued)

Drug Description	Proposed effect	Toxicity	Adverse drug–drug interactions
Glucosinolates • Commonly found in plants of the *Brassicaceae* family • Concentration higher in roots • NB glucosinolates: glucobrassicin, glucoraphanin, progoitrin, and sinigrin • Metabolites are bioactive	• Antioxidant • Antimicrobial • Anti-inflammatory • Regulates Phase I hepatic metabolism	• Carcinogenic • High sulfur content in brassicas leads to trace mineral deficiencies and polioencephalomalacia • Goiter/thyromegaly (iodine metabolism disrupted) • Decreased T_4 • Genotoxic • Heinz body anemia • Hepatotoxic (nitriles) • Nephrotoxic	• CYP450 inhibitors
Polyphenols • Commonly found in cereals, chocolates, beverages, fruits, vegetables, etc. • >8000 polyphenols; divided into four main chemical configurations: 1. Flavonoids Anthocyanins Anthocyanidins Flavonols Flavanols Flavones Chalcones 2. Phenolic acid Hydroxybenzoic acid Hydroxycinnamic acid 3. Lignans Secoisolariciresinol Matairesinol 4. Stilbenes Resveratrol	Flavonoids (mostly) • Analgesic • Anti-inflammatory • Antimicrobial • Antineoplastic • Antioxidant • Cardioprotective • Chemopreventive • Immunomodulatory • Neuroprotective	• Carcinogenesis (phytoestrogens and genistein) • Kidney damage • Mutagenic (quercetin) • Pro-oxidant • Thyrotoxicity	• CYP450 inhibitors

CYP450: cytochrome P450 gene; GI: gastrointestinal.

(Table 10.9). Some classifications put herbal remedies as a subcategory of nutraceuticals. Animal-derived nutraceuticals are frequently used and include substances such as chondroitin sulfate, glycosaminoglycans, etc. (Table 10.10). Essential oils are classified as phytonutrients (Table 10.11). They contain natural volatile aromatic compounds and are used as aromatherapy. Essential oils are inhaled either directly from the bottle or from a diffuser or humidifier. They can also be applied topically; however, ingestion of these oils can cause toxicity even in small amounts. Essential oils can be mixed with food and water for ingestion but only following dilution. Generally, these oils are avoided in puppies and kittens less than 10 weeks of age.

In recent decades, nutraceutical and herbal remedies have gained popularity among pet owners. Not only are they believed to provide health benefits, but they are also readily available. The relative lack (variable by country) of regulatory oversight and approval processes (safety, efficacy, and labeling) promotes ease of access. Unfortunately, the use of nutraceuticals or herbal remedies is often not disclosed by owners unless specific questions are asked by veterinarians. Their use can be associated with deleterious effects due to possible drug–drug interaction *in vivo*.

Tables 10.7–10.11 highlight the common nutraceuticals administered by pet owners and includes their toxicities and possible drug–drug interactions. The clinical relevance of drug–drug interactions remains to be established with most nutraceuticals. The majority of the information presented is derived from human literature and extrapolated to the veterinary medicine. More research is needed in this area. For more in-depth information, reader is referred to Further Reading.

Table 10.9 Nutraceuticals prepared as herbal remedies that owners may be administering to their companion animal.

Drug Description	Proposed effect	Toxicity	Adverse drug–drug interactions
Aloe vera • *Aloe vera* belonging to *Asphodelaceae* family • Phytochemical constituents: amino acids, anthraquinones, saponins, minerals, vitamins, etc.	• Analgesic • Angiogenesis • Antibacterial • Antidiabetic • Antifungal • Anti-inflammatory • Antineoplastic • Antioxidant • Antiviral • Immunostimulatory • Laxative • Periodontal disease • Prebiotic • Wound healing	• Diarrhea • Emesis • Hypoglycemia	• Anticoagulants • Insulin (hypoglycemia) • Laxatives
Babool • *Acacia nilotica* belonging to *Fabaceae* family • Root extract appears safer than rest of plant • Phytochemical constituents: alkaloids, flavonoids, glucosides, polyphenols, saponins, tannins, terpenes, and fatty acids • Mature seeds contain: copper, iron, zinc, manganese, potassium, and zinc	• AChE inhibitor • Analgesic • Antidiabetic • Antidiarrheal • Antifungal • Anthelminthic • Antihypertensive • Anti-inflammatory • Antimicrobial • Antimutagenic • Antineoplastic • Antioxidant • Antiplasmodial • Antiplatelet aggregation • Antipyretic • Diuretic • Gastroprotective • Hepatoprotective • Immunostimulatory • Metal chelation • Spasmolytic	• Hepatotoxicity	• Amoxicillin (decreased absorption)
Black seed • *Nigella sativa* belonging to *Ranunculaceae family* • Phytochemical constituents: alkaloids, anthraquinones, coumarins, flavonoids, glucosinolates, phenolics, saponins, tannins, and terpenoids	• Analgesic • Anticonvulsant • Antidiabetic • Antihistaminic • Anti-inflammatory • Antimicrobial • Antineoplastic • Bronchodilation (asthma) • Cardioprotective • Hepatoprotective • Gastroprotective • Immunomodulatory • Increase reproductive responses • Spasmolytic	• Dyspnea • Lethargy • Decreased GSH	• Anticoagulants (hemorrhagic diathesis) • Antihypertensive drugs (hypotension) • Calcium channel antagonists (amlodipine and diltiazem) • Immunosuppressants • Insulin (hypoglycemia) • Potassium sparing drugs (i.e., spironolactone) • SSRIs (increase serotonin levels)

Table 10.9 (Continued)

Drug Description	Proposed effect	Toxicity	Adverse drug–drug interactions
Chamomile Contains coumarin, apigenin, etc. Look at chamomile oil	• Anti-inflammatory • Anxiolytic • Spasmolytic	• Anorexia • Dermatitis • Diarrhea • Emesis • Hemorrhagic diathesis	• Anticoagulants • Benzodiazepines
Cannabis • *Cannabis sativa* belonging to *Cannabaceae* family • Hemp has <0.3% THC cf. marijuana • 113 phytocannabinoids and 140 terpenes • THC: main psychoactive cannabinoid • CBD: main medicinal cannabinoid	• Analgesic (OA) • Anticonvulsant • Antidepressant • Anti-inflammatory • Antimicrobial • Antineoplastic • Antioxidant • Anxiolytic • Chemopreventive	• Agitation • Ataxia • Decreased heart rate • Depression • Diarrhea • Dyspnea • Emesis • Hyperesthesia • Hypotension • Lethargy • Mydriasis • Poikilothermia • Sedation • Tremors • Urine dribbling	• Antihypertensive drugs • α_2-Adrenoceptor agonists • Benzodiazepines • CYP450 inhibitors • Gabapentin/pregabalin • Injectable anesthetics (additive) • Levetiracetam (somnolence) • Metoclopramide (additive) • Monoamine inhibitors (selegiline) • Opioids • Promethazine (additive) • SSRIs (e.g., fluoxetine) • Theophylline clearance increased • TCAs (amitriptyline) • Warfarin (increase in hypoprothrombinemic effect)
Fenugreek • *Trigonella foenum-graecum* belonging to *Fabaceae* family • Phytochemical constituents: flavonoids, saponins, pyridine alkaloids, and steroidal sapogenins; high vitamin, protein, amino acid, and minerals content • Contains coumarin constituents	• Analgesic • Antibacterial • Antifungal • Antidepressant • Antidiabetic • Anti-inflammatory • Antineoplastic • Antipyretic • Antiulcerogenic • Hepatoprotective (antioxidant, antiradical, and iron metabolism normalizing effect) • Hypercholesterolemia • Hypotension	• No significant toxicity • Avoid in pregnancy and lactation (may have neurodevelopmental, neurobehavioral, and neuropathological adverse effects)	• No severe interaction • Possibly with aspirin and other antiplatelet and anticoagulant drugs
Ginger • Root/rhizome from *Zingiber officinale* belonging to *Zingiberaceae* family • Phytochemical constituents: gingerol, shogaols, curcumene, zingerone, zingiberol, zingibain, and paradols	• Analgesic • Antidiabetic • Anti-emetic • Anti-inflammatory • Antineoplastic • Antioxidant • Cardioprotective • Chemopreventive • Gastroprotective • Immunomodulatory • Neuroprotective • Motion sickness	• GI disturbances • CNS depression • Cardiac arrhythmias • Hemorrhagic diathesis	• Anticoagulants (aspirin, clopidogrel, and heparin) • Morphine (increased plasma concentration due intestinal P-glycoprotein inhibition – enhanced oral absorption) • Tramadol (increased plasma concentration due to CYP450 isoenzyme inhibition)

(Continued)

Table 10.9 (Continued)

Drug Description	Proposed effect	Toxicity	Adverse drug–drug interactions
Ginkgo biloba extract • *Ginkgo biloba* belonging to *Ginkgoaceae* • Phytochemical constituents: ginkgolides, flavonoids, glycosides, etc.	• Antioxidant • Anxiolytic • Age-related behavioral disturbances • Mental performance • Quality of life	• Diarrhea • Nausea • Restlessness • Ginkgotoxin in seed: emesis, irritability, and seizures	• Anticoagulants (hemorrhagic diathesis) • CYP450 inhibitor • MAOI • SSRIs • TCAs
Ginseng • *Panax ginseng* belonging to *Araliaceae* family • Phytochemical constituents: ginsenosides	• Antioxidant • Anxiolytic • Immunomodulatory • Mental performance	• Anxiety • Diarrhea • Hypertension	• Anticoagulants (hemorrhagic diathesis) • CYP450 inhibitors • Insulin (hypoglycemia)
Hawthorn • *Crataegus* spp. belonging to *Rosaceae* family • Phytochemical constituents: flavonoids, glycosides, phenols, procyanidins, saponins, tannins, triterpenoids, etc.	• Antidepressant • Anti-inflammatory • Antimicrobial • Antioxidant • Anxiolytic • Cardioprotective • Gastroprotective	• Diarrhea • Emesis	• Anticoagulants • Antihypertensive drugs • Cardiotonic • Nitrates • Theophylline
Indian frankincense • *Boswellia serrata* belonging to *Burseraceae* family	• Anti-inflammatory • Antitussive • Antiulcerogenic (colon) • Arthritis • Asthma • Wound healing	• Diarrhea • Flatulence • Nausea	• Immunosuppressants • CYP450 inhibitor
Kava • *Piper methysticum* belonging to *Piperaceae* family • Phytochemical constituents: kavalactones	• Anti-inflammatory • Antineoplastic • Anxiolytic • Neurological benefit	• Anorexia • Ataxia • Hepatoxicity • Nausea	• Barbiturates • Benzodiazepines • Diuretics • Hepatotoxic drugs • Opioids • Cyclohexamines • NSAID • Trazodone
Milk thistle or Silymarin • *Silybum marianum* belonging to *Asteraceae* family • Phytochemical constituents: Silymarin (principle), glycosides, flavonoids, terpenoids, etc. • Accumulates nitrates	• Antidiabetic • Antifungal • Anti-inflammatory • Antineoplastic • Antioxidant • Hepatoprotective • Immunomodulatory	• Diarrhea • Emesis • Nitrate poisoning in sheep and cattle	• CYP450 inhibitor • Insulin (hypoglycemia)
Neem extract • *Azadirachta indica* belonging to *Meliaceae* family • Nonleguminous evergreen tree • Phytochemical constituents: bioactive triterpenoids (azadirachtin, nimbin, nimbinin, nimbidin, and salannin)	• Antibacterial • Antifungal • Anti-inflammatory • Antimalarial • Antimutagenic • Antineoplastic • Antioxidant • Antiulcerogenic • Antiviral • Contraceptive • Diabetes • Immunomodulatory	Side effects from leaf extract were more pronounced than with the seed oil • Lethargy • Weakness • Loss of body condition • Depression • Decreased T_3 • Increased T_4 • Increased lipid peroxidation • Decreased testosterone • Diuresis	• Immunosuppressants (azathioprine, cyclosporine, and corticosteroids) • Insulin (hypoglycemia)

Table 10.9 (Continued)

Drug Description	Proposed effect	Toxicity	Adverse drug–drug interactions
Sea Buckthorn • *Hippophae rhamnoides* belonging to *Elaeagnaceae* family • High in antioxidants • Phytochemical constituents: carotenoids, flavonoids, polyphenols, proanthocyanins, organic acids, amino acids, vitamins, and PUFA	• Antineoplastic • Antioxidant • Anxiolytic • Hepatoprotective • Immunomodulatory • Radioprotective	• No significant toxicities reported • Nontoxic carotenodermia from hypercarotenemia (prolonged ingestion)	• Anticoagulants (hemorrhagic diathesis)
St. John's Wort • *Hypericum perforatum* belonging to *Hypericaceae* family • MOA similar to TCA and SSRIs • Phytochemical constituents: hypericin, anthraquinones, mucilage saponins, and tannins; fats, proteins, and oils	• Antidepressant • Anxiolytic	• Photosensitivity	• CYP450 inducers • SSRIs • TCA • Trazodone
Turmeric and Curcumin • Dried rhizome from three *Curcuma* spp. belonging to *Zingiberaceae* family • Turmeric contains curcuminoids (i.e., curcumin, demethocurcumin, bismethoxycurcumin) • MOA: unknown but multiple pathways involved	• Immunomodulatory and anti-inflammatory in GIT, joints, eyes, and brain • Chronic disease states: inflammatory bowel disease, chronic pain, and Alzheimer's disease • Preventive potential in age-related disease • Analgesic: TRPV-1 receptor antagonist • *Morphine tolerance attenuated by low-dose curcumin but aggravated by high dose*	• Nausea • Diarrhea • Emesis • Hemorrhagic diathesis • Anemia	• Antithrombin (hemorrhagic diathesis) • Aspirin (hemorrhagic diathesis) • Clopidogrel (hemorrhagic diathesis) • Duloxetine (stomach ulceration, kidney stones, and hemorrhagic diatheses) • Fluoxetine (hemorrhagic diathesis) • Heparin (hemorrhagic diathesis) • Insulin (hypoglycemia) • NSAID (hemorrhagic diathesis) • Sertraline (hemorrhagic diathesis) • Urokinase (hemorrhagic diathesis) • Warfarin (hemorrhagic diathesis) • Inhibits drug-metabolizing enzymes (CYP450, GST, and UDP-glucuronosyltransferase) • Active iron chelator (anemia induced in mice)

AChE: acetylcholine esterase; CBD: cannabidiol; CKD: chronic kidney disease; COPD: chronic obstructive pulmonary disease; CYP450: cytochrome P450 gene; GABA: gamma-aminobutyric acid; GIT: gastrointestinal tract; GSH: glutathione; GST: glutathione S-transferases; IBD: inflammatory bowel disease; MAOI: monoamine oxidase inhibitors; NO: nitric oxide; NSAID: nonsteroidal anti-inflammatory drug; OA: osteoarthritis; SSRIs: selective serotonin reuptake inhibitors; TCAs: tricyclic antidepressants; THC: tetrahydrocannabinol; TRPV-1: transient receptor potential vanilloid 1; VPC: ventricular premature contractions.

Table 10.10 Animal-based nutraceuticals that owners may be administering to their companion animal.

Drug Description	Proposed effect	Toxicity	Adverse drug–drug interactions
Glucosamine • Compound in cartilage	• Joint health	• Diarrhea • Emesis	• Anticoagulants • Doxorubicin
Green lipped mussel • Rich in glycosaminoglycans, zinc, iron, selenium and vitamin B	• Analgesic • Anti-inflammatory • Improves quality of life	• GIT discomfort • Nausea	• Anticoagulant • NSAID
Honey • *Apis mellifera* • *Lactobacillus* and *Bifidobacterium* have evolved synergistically with *Apis mellifera*	• Antibacterial • Anticonvulsant • Antidepressant • Antifungal • Antimicrobial • Antioxidants • Anxiolytic • Laxative • Wound healing	• Bradycardia • Diaphoresis • Emesis • Hyperglycemia • Hypotension • Nausea	• No reported interactions

GIT: gastrointestinal tract; NSAID: nonsteroidal anti-inflammatory drug.

Table 10.11 Nutraceuticals prepared as essential oils that owners may be administering to their companion animal.

Drug Description	Proposed effect	Toxicity	Adverse drug–drug interactions
Chamomile oil • *Matricaria chamomilla* (German chamomile) • *Chamaemelum nobile* (Roman chamomile) • 28 terpenoids (α-bisabolol), 36 flavonoids, and 120 secondary metabolites • Not as frequently used in veterinary medicine cf. humans	• Antidiabetic • Anti-inflammatory • Antioxidant • Antiseptic • Anxiolytic • Eczema • GI disturbances • Neuralgia • Spasmolytic • Increased wound healing	• Anorexia • Diarrhea • Emesis • Hemorrhagic diathesis	• Anticoagulants • Benzodiazepines
Eucalyptus oil • *Eucalyptus* spp. • Phytochemical class: oxygenated monoterpenes, oxygenated sesquiterpenes, and monoterpene hydrocarbons • Major constituents: α-phellandrene, α-pinene, c-terpinene, *p*-cymene, and limonene	• Antibacterial • Antifungal • Anti-inflammatory • Antioxidant • Antipyretic • Antiradical • Asthma	• Toxic to dogs and cats • Anorexia • Diarrhea • Dysphagia • Emesis • Mydriasis • Lethargy • Salivation • Seizures	• CYP450 isoenzyme inducers
Hemp/CBD oil • Look at Cannabis • Phytochemical constituents: CBD, THC, β-caryophyllene, limonene, humulene, α-pinene, terpinolene, etc.	• Analgesic • Anticonvulsant • Antidiabetic • Antihypertension • Antineoplastic • Atopic dermatitis • Obesity • Osteoarthritis	• Abdominal discomfort • Diarrhea • Emesis	• Anticoagulants • Antidepressants • Anti-epileptic drugs

Table 10.11 (Continued)

Drug Description	Proposed effect	Toxicity	Adverse drug–drug interactions
Peppermint oil • *Mentha piperita* • Phytochemical constituents: menthol, menthone, menthyl acetate, limonene, flavonoids, and β-pinene	• Allergies • Analgesic • Antiulcerogenic • Burns • Cytoprotective • Digestion • Immunodeficiency • Lice and flea treatment	• Toxic to dogs and cats • Death • Diarrhea • Emesis • Lethargy • Asthenia	• CYP450 isoenzyme inhibitor (increase in drug plasma concentration)

CBD: cannabidiol; CYP450: cytochrome P450 gene; THC: tetrahydrocannabinol.

Further Reading

Agnew, W. and Korman, R. (2014). Pharmacological appetite stimulation rational choices in the inappetent cat. *J Fel Med Surg* 16: 749–756.

Center, S.A., Elston, T.H., Rowland, P.H. et al. (1996). Fulminant hepatic failure associated with oral administration of diazepam in 11 cats. *J Am Vet Med Assoc* 209: 618–625.

De Souza Dantas, L.M. and Crowell-Davis, S.L. (2019). Benzodiazepines. In: *Veterinary Psychopharmacology*, 2e (ed. S.L. Crowell-Davis, T.F. Murray, and L.M. De Souza Dantas), 67–102. New Jersey, USA: Wiley-Blackwell.

Engel, O., Masic, A., Landsberg, G. et al. (2018). Imepitoin shows benzodiazepine-like effects in models of anxiety. *Front Pharmacol* 9: 1–11.

Gruen, M.E., Sherman, B.L., and Papich, M.G. (2018). Drugs affecting animal behavior. In: *Veterinary Pharmacology and Therapeutics*, 10e (ed. J.E. Riviere and M.G. Papich), 416–448. New Jersey, USA: Wiley-Blackwell.

Gupta, R.C., Srivastava, A., and Lall, R. (2019). *Nutraceuticals in Veterinary Medicine*, 1e. Gewerbestrasse, Switzerland: Springer.

Jessen, L.R., Damborg, P.P., Spohr, A. et al. (2019). *Antibiotic Use Guidelines for Companion Animal Practice*, 2e. The Danish Small Animal Veterinary Association, SvHKS. https://www.ddd.dk/sektioner/familiedyr/antibiotikavejledning/Documents/AB_uk_2019.pdf.

McNicholas, L.F., Martin, W.R., and Cherian, S. (1983). Physical dependence on diazepam and lorazepam in the dog. *J Pharmacol Exp Ther* 226: 783–789.

Papich, M.G. (2021). *Papich Handbook of Veterinary Medicine*, 5e. Missouri, USA: Elsevier.

Quimby, J.M. and Lunn, K.F. (2013). Mirtazapine as an appetite stimulant and anti-emetic in cats with chronic kidney disease: a masked placebo-controlled crossover clinical trial. *Vet J* 197: 651–655.

Repova, K., Baka, T., Krajcirovicova, K. et al. (2022). Melatonin as a potential approach to anxiety treatment. *Int J Mol Sci* 23: 16187.

Ruiz-Cano, D., Sanchez-Carrasco, G., El-Mihyaoui, A. et al. (2022). Essential oils and melatonin as functional ingredients in dogs. *Anim* 12: 2089.

Sloan, J.W., Martin, W.R., and Wala, E.P. (1990). Dependence-producing properties of alprazolam in the dog. *Pharmacol Biochen Behav* 35: 651–657.

Weese, J.S., Giguere, S., Guardabassi, L. et al. (2015). ACVIM consensus statement on therapeutic antimicrobial use in animals and antimicrobial resistance. *J Vet Intern Med* 29: 487–498.

Weeth, L.P. (2015). Chapter 13: appetite stimulants in dogs and cats. In: *Nutritional Management of Hospitalized Small Animals*, 1e (ed. D.L. Chan), 128–135. USA: John Wiley & Sons, Ltd.

Section 2

Fundamental Aspects of Clinical Anesthesia

11

Standards of Practice for Performing Veterinary Anesthesia

Matthew Gurney, Robert Meyer, Stijn Schauvliege, and Daniel Pang

Overview of the Concept of Standards of Practice

In the European Union and United Kingdom, each country has its own Code of Professional Conduct (CPC), which defines the standards to which veterinarians should, or must, comply. The aim of a veterinary CPC is to ensure high standards of practice in veterinary medicine, thus optimizing not only animal and public health but also animal welfare. In general, most CPCs address eight overarching themes: definitions and framing concepts, duties to animals, duties to clients, duties to other professionals, duties to competent authorities, duties to society, and professionalism and practice-related issues (Magalhães-Sant'Ana et al. 2015). Typical examples of specific recommendations or requirements are (1) the duty for veterinarians to keep their knowledge on animal health and welfare legislation up to date; (2) the need to show respect for animals and avoid harm in handling, diagnosis, and treatment; (3) guidelines for animal euthanasia; (4) the obligation to obtain informed owner consent before carrying out a procedure; (5) responsible use of medicines (e.g. with regard to microbial resistance); and (6) the duty to report animal welfare violations to legal authorities.

The United States of America has 50 individual state boards of veterinary medicine, each with its own laws and regulations. Some states, such as Mississippi, have adopted the American Veterinary Medical Association Code of Veterinary Medical Ethics. Each state Veterinary Licensing Board sets minimum standards for granting a license to practice and adjudicates practice-related issues. While some states grant veterinary license portability (reciprocity) to individuals licensed in other states, this is currently not uniformly applied across all 50 states. Individuals seeking specific information regarding the practice of veterinary medicine at the state level must contact the relevant state veterinary licensing board.

In Canada, individual Provinces and Territories are responsible for legislating the practice of veterinary medicine, including requirements for registration as a veterinarian, regulations and bylaws, and professional conduct. For example, in Alberta, the relevant legislation is the Veterinary Profession Act (2000), which grants the Alberta Veterinary Medical Association (ABVMA) the authority to govern veterinary medical practice within Alberta.

Elsewhere in the world, the practice of veterinary medicine is generally regulated at a state (or equivalent) or national level by a legislative body that determines and upholds minimum standards of practice. The frameworks in place to achieve this are similar to those described in this chapter. Registered (licensed) veterinarians, veterinary nurses, or technicians/technologists must be familiar with, and adhere to, these standards of practice.

Regulatory Bodies That Set Minimum Standards of Practice

In the European Union, each country has its own CPC that sets minimum standards of practice. In 2009, the Federation of Veterinarians of Europe (FVE) published the European Veterinary Code of Conduct. This Code of Conduct is regularly updated by the FVE and is meant to serve as a framework for European countries when developing or updating their national CPCs. Although no specific guidelines are included with regard to anesthesia and analgesia, it is stated that veterinarians shall respect animals as sentient beings, should use the least stressful techniques necessary for sound diagnosis and treatment, and should attempt to relieve animals' pain and suffering. If their condition is untreatable, the option of euthanasia should be discussed

Fundamental Principles of Veterinary Anesthesia, First Edition. Edited by Gareth E. Zeiler and Daniel S. J. Pang.

Companion Website: www.wiley.com/go/VeterinaryAnesthesiaZeiler

with the owner and must be practiced with as little pain, distress, and fear as possible.

The Royal College of Veterinary Surgeons (RCVS) regulates standards of practice in the United Kingdom. The RCVS code of professional conduct states:

- "Inducing anaesthesia by administration of a specific quantity of medicine directed by a veterinary surgeon may be carried out by a Listed veterinary nurse or, with supervision, a student veterinary nurse, but *not* any other suitably trained person."
  - Note: "Listed" refers to a registered veterinary nurse.
- "Administering medicine to effect, to induce and maintain anaesthesia may be carried out *only* by a veterinary surgeon."
- "Maintaining anaesthesia is the responsibility of a veterinary surgeon, but a suitably trained person may assist by acting as the veterinary surgeon's hands (to provide assistance which does not involve practising veterinary surgery), for example, moving dials."
- Monitoring a patient both during anesthesia (and monitoring a patient at any other time) is the responsibility of the veterinary surgeon, but may be carried out on his or her behalf by a suitably trained person.
- The most suitable person to assist a veterinary surgeon to monitor and maintain a patient during anesthesia is a Listed veterinary nurse or, under supervision, a student veterinary nurse.

The RCVS officially recognizes vets with either particular or specialized knowledge and skills in a designated field of veterinary practice as Advanced Practitioners or RCVS Specialists. The RCVS maintains a list of each category to provide a clear indication to the profession and the public of those veterinary surgeons who have demonstrated knowledge and experience in a particular area of veterinary practice beyond their initial primary veterinary degree. Currently, there are 13 Advanced Practitioners and 71 Specialists of anesthesia listed. Diplomates of the European College of Veterinary Anaesthesia and Analgesia (ECVAA) practicing in the United Kingdom can gain automatic recognition.

In the United States of America and Canada, any licensed veterinarian can administer anesthesia to veterinary patients. Qualification is conferred by graduation from an American Veterinary Medical Association (AVMA) recognized school or college of veterinary medicine, a passing score on the North American Veterinary Licensing Examination (NAVLE), and a valid license issued by the State Veterinary Board or the provincial veterinary regulatory organization.

The AVMA Model Veterinary Practice Act (MVPA) is intended to serve as a set of guiding principles for those who are now, or will be in the future, preparing or revising a practice act under the codes and laws of an individual state (https://www.avma.org/sites/default/files/2021-01/model-veterinary-practice-act.pdf, accessed 31 May 2021). Similarly, the American Association of Veterinary State Boards (AASVB) Model Practice Act contains language that defines the procedures of the state regulatory board and provides Member Boards with current regulatory language covering a host of issues facing veterinary medicine regulatory boards (https://www.aavsb.org/board-services/member-board-resources/practice-act-model, accessed 31 May 2021).

The AAVSB recommends individual State Boards of Veterinary Medicine consider identifying minimum standards for delineating the various specific Veterinary Facilities within its rules (e.g., clinic, hospital, specialty or referral hospital, etc.). "Differing facilities can be defined within rules that can identify minimum standards and the allowable practices to insure public protection" (Veterinary Medicine and Veterinary Technology Practice Act Model with Commentary, p. 11, Section 104(bb). Veterinary Facility, available at https://www.aavsb.org/board-services/member-board-resources/practice-act-model, accessed 31 May 2021).

The American College of Veterinary Anesthesia and Analgesia (ACVAA) has taken the position to restrict veterinary technicians from performing certain anesthesia-related procedures (see Position Statement on the Supervision of Veterinary Technicians Performing Anesthetic and Analgesic Procedures, https://acvaa.org/wp-content/uploads/2020/10/ACVAA-2020-Position-Statement-on-Supervision-of-Technicians.final_.pdf, accessed 31 May 2021). This position statement represents an opinion of that Recognized Veterinary Specialty Organization™ (RSVO) and does not necessarily reflect current state veterinary board interpretation as reflected in the AVMA-MVPA and the AASVB Model Practice Act.

The AVMA-MVPA definitions of direct and indirect technician supervision are similar to those of the AASVB Model Practice Act. Immediate Supervision means the supervising veterinarian is in the immediate area and within audible and visual range of the patient and the individual treating the patient. *Direct Supervision* is defined as the supervising veterinarian is readily available on the premises where the patient is located. Indirect Supervision means a supervising veterinarian need not be physically on the premises but has given either written or verbal instructions for the treatment of the patient and is readily available for communication either in person or through use of electronic information and communication technology. Veterinary technicians may perform a wide range of procedures under conditions of immediate, direct, and indirect supervision of a licensed veterinarian as summarized in Table 11.1.

In Alberta (Canada), many tasks associated with anesthesia can be performed by a Registered Veterinary Technologist (Technician) under direct (supervising veterinarian is on the premises and is quickly and easily available, but not necessarily within sight or hearing range) or immediate (supervising veterinarian is in immediate area, within audible and visual range) veterinary supervision. An unregistered person (not a registered veterinary technologist or veterinarian) who works in the clinic may perform limited tasks under immediate veterinary supervision (e.g., adjust vaporizer setting and record monitoring data).

Associations and Committees That Publish Guidelines and Standards of Practice with Regard to Anesthesia and Analgesia

The Association of Veterinary Anaesthetists (AVA) published a set of guidelines for safer anesthesia (https://ava.eu.com/resources/anaesthesia-guidelines) (Table 11.2). This includes advice on anesthetic case planning, analgesia, monitoring, patient support, training of staff, etc. In addition, the AVA also provides example anesthetic records and checklists, which can be downloaded from their website.

The European College of Veterinary Anaesthesia and Analgesia (ECVAA) is part of the European Board of Veterinary Specialization (EBVS®), an organization that recognizes specialists in different areas of veterinary

Table 11.1 Allowable Animal Healthcare Tasks (from AAVSB Model Regulations Veterinary Technician Scope of Practice) (selected examples, from https://www.aavsb.org/board-services/member-board-resources/practice-act-model, accessed 31 May 2021).

Section 1. Immediate Supervision:
- (1) Assisting the veterinarian with surgical procedures
- (2) Placement of abdominal, thoracic, or percutaneous endoscopic gastrostomy (PEG) tubes

Section 2. Direct Supervision:
- (1) General anesthesia and sedation, maintenance, and recovery
- (2) Nonemergency endotracheal intubation
- (3) Regional anesthesia, including paravertebral blocks, epidurals, and local blocks
- (4) Dental procedures including, but not limited to, (a) the removal of calculus, soft deposits, plaque, and stains; (b) the smoothing, filing, and polishing of teeth; and (c) single root extractions not requiring sectioning of the tooth or sectioning of the bone
- (5) Euthanasia
- (7) Placement of tubes including, but not limited to, gastric, nasogastric, and nasoesophageal
- (10) Fluid aspiration from a body cavity or organ (i.e., cystocentesis, thoracocentesis, and abdominocentesis)
- (13) Placement of epidural, intraosseous, and nasal catheters

Section 3. Indirect Supervision:
- (1) Administration, preparation, and application of treatments including, but not limited to, drugs, medications, controlled substances, enemas, and biological and immunological agents unless prohibited by government regulation
- (2) Intravenous catheterizations and maintenance of intra-arterial catheterizations
- (4) Collection of blood except when in conflict with government regulations (i.e., Coggins Equine Infectious Anemia testing)
- (7) Monitoring including, but not limited to, electrocardiogram (ECG), blood pressure, carbon dioxide (CO_2), and blood oxygen saturation
- (8) Clinical laboratory test procedures
- (11) Laser therapy
- (12) Animal rehabilitation therapies
- (16) Emergency animal patient care including, but not limited to
  - (a) Application of tourniquets and/or pressure procedures to control hemorrhage, application of appropriate wound dressings in severe burn cases, resuscitative oxygen procedures, anti-seizure treatment, and supportive treatment in heat prostration cases
  - (b) Administration of a drug or controlled substance to manage and control pain, to prevent further injury, and prevent or control shock, including parenteral fluids, under direct communication with a veterinarian or in accordance with written guidelines consistent with accepted standards of veterinary medical practice
  - (c) Administration of a drug or controlled substance to prevent suffering of an animal, up to and including euthanasia, under direct communication with a veterinarian
  - (d) Initiate and perform CPR, including administration of medication and defibrillation, and provide immediate post-resuscitation care according to established protocols

Note: It is recommended that readers access the listed website to view the current task list.

Table 11.2 AVA guidelines for safer anesthesia (https://ava.eu.com/resources/anaesthesia-guidelines).

AVA guidelines for safer anesthesia

1. Patient safety
   - "AVA recommended procedures and safety checklist" incorporated into every case.
2. Anesthetic case planning
   - Anesthesia plan considered for each individual patient, covering patient risk factors, procedure risk factors, suitable anesthesia drugs, fluids, and monitoring aids.
   - Consideration given to the limits of anesthesia care that can be provided, and outside assistance sought or case referral to specialist anesthesia facilities arranged when required.
3. Analgesia
   - Analgesia should be a top priority of care.
   - A range of analgesic therapies should be available and utilised, including full opioid agonists, local anesthetics, NSAIDs, adjunctive drug therapies, and nondrug therapies
   - An analgesic plan should be made for each case recognising the expected level and modality of pain.
   - Patients should be actively assessed using validated pain scores and results responded to appropriately.
   - Patients with known or expected pain should be prescribed ongoing analgesia at discharge and the owners should be informed of pain-related behavioral signs.
4. Staff
   - Qualified veterinary staff, who have received anesthesia training, to monitor every anesthetic.
   - Veterinary students to be supervised by a qualified member of veterinary staff when monitoring an anesthetic.
   - Use of advanced anesthesia trained staff whenever available or required.
5. Monitoring
   - Dedicated anesthetist monitoring each case.
   - Additional monitoring equipment of pulse oximetry, capnography, and blood pressure monitors available and utilised.
6. Patient support
   - Active temperature monitoring and temperature support, including preventive measures and active warming devices available and utilised.
   - Fluid therapy considered for every anesthetic and goal-directed administration provided where indicated. Availability of fluid pumps and/or syringe drivers to ensure accuracy.
   - Blood pressure support considered from outset and managed where appropriate through anesthetic drug selection, fluid therapy, and appropriate drug administration.
   - Requirement of ventilation support considered from outset. Availability of manual or mechanical means of positive pressure ventilation utilised when necessary.
7. Emergency ready
   - All staff to have received CPR training and CPR simulations, to be practiced in-house during each year.
   - All patients to have IV access during anesthesia via an IV catheter.
   - Emergency equipment to be available at all times.
8. Recovery
   - Patient recovery from anesthesia to be adequately monitored and recorded.
   - Recovery to take place in a suitable location.
9. Training
   - All clinical staff involved with anesthesia to receive regular CPD on anesthesia and analgesia.
   - A dedicated member of staff to oversee practice policies and standards of care.
10. Records
    - Professional records of anesthesia kept, including patient details, procedure details, staff involved, drugs, monitoring, and recovery.
    - Records should be reviewed for morbidity and mortality issues.

Note: It is recommended that readers access the listed website to view the current version of the guidelines.

medicine. The ECVAA aims to advance veterinary anesthesia, analgesia, and peri-operative care in Europe. To become an EBVS® Specialist in Veterinary Anaesthesia and Analgesia, a veterinarian must complete additional training over a period of 3–5 years and pass the examination of the ECVAA. Diplomates of the ECVAA advance the subject of veterinary anesthesia, analgesia, and peri-operative care by high-quality practice, by research and by contributing to training of residents and veterinarians, the latter, e.g., in the form of Continuing Professional Development (CPD) or educational articles and in the provision of consultancy services to the pharmaceutical industry.

In the United Kingdom, the RCVS Practice Standards Scheme (PSS) is a voluntary initiative to accredit veterinary practices and approximately two-thirds of veterinary clinics are members of the scheme. Through setting standards and carrying out regular assessments, the scheme aims to promote and maintain the highest standards of veterinary care including, for example, conducting clinical audit and morbidity and mortality rounds. Guidance on these and other quality-improvement tools is available through the RCVS Knowledge website (https://knowledge.rcvs.org.uk/quality-improvement).

The ACVAA is an RSVO that certifies veterinary specialists in the practice of veterinary anesthesiology through an approved postgraduate residency training program and a multiday certifying examination. By virtue of their training, Diplomates of the ACVAA can provide the highest levels of peri-operative patient care and are experts in pain management as well as assessment and mitigation of anesthetic risks, delivery of anesthetic and analgesic drugs, and maintaining and monitoring the physiologic well-being of the anesthetized patient (https://acvaa.org/about/about-the-acvaa, accessed 31 May 2021). Diplomates of the ACVAA are permitted to present themselves as Board

Certified Specialists® in Veterinary Anesthesia and Analgesia.

A board-certified veterinary specialist is a veterinarian who has completed additional training in a specific area of veterinary medicine and has passed an examination that evaluates their knowledge and skills in that specialty area. Annotation 3.6 of the AVMA Principles of Veterinary Medical Ethics provides general guidance on who can present themselves to the public as a specialist and the difference between earning a certificate and the process of becoming board-certified by an AVMA-recognized specialty organization (https://www.avma.org/resources-tools/avma-policies/principles-veterinary-medical-ethics-avma, accessed 31 May 2021). Currently, there are 22 AVMA-Recognized Veterinary Specialty Organizations™ or RVSOs comprising 41 distinct specialties. The RVSOs are referred to as "colleges," but they are not schools or universities (https://www.avma.org/education/veterinary-specialties/what-board-certified-veterinary-specialists-do, accessed 31 May 2021).

The ACVAA and the American Animal Hospital Association (AAHA) have published position statements and guidelines for various aspects of veterinary anesthesia practice. The ACVAA position statements on anesthesia guidelines for horses, small animal monitoring, treatment of pain in animals, opioid sparing pain therapy in animals, and control of waste anesthetic gas can be found at https://acvaa.org/veterinarians/guidelines (accessed 31 May 2021). The AAHA guidelines on anesthesia for dogs and cats, fluid therapy, and referrals can be found at https://www.aaha.org/aaha-guidelines/what-are-aaha-guidelines (accessed 31 May 2021). While exemplifying good practices, these guidelines and position statements are not codified into the individual states' practice acts. While not legally enforceable on their own, these documents could be cited as standard of care in legal proceedings.

Handling Situations Where the Minimum Standards of Practice Are Not Met

Awareness of one's own limitations is considered an important aspect of the FVE's European Veterinary Code of Conduct. This means that veterinarians are expected to refer cases to colleagues or specialists when they do not have sufficient knowledge, experience, or appropriate equipment to establish a diagnosis, provide appropriate care, or carry out certain procedures. This also applies to the fields of anesthesia and analgesia, e.g., when treating patients with chronic pain and when performing advanced surgical procedures or treating severely compromised patients, with the need for extensive peri-operative monitoring, mechanical ventilation, one lung intubation, etc. In such cases, it may be indicated to refer the patient to a well-equipped hospital with specialized anesthetic personnel. The European Veterinary Code of Conduct indeed states that veterinarians, when unable to provide a service, should help their client find another veterinarian who is capable of providing the service concerned.

The RCVS expects veterinary surgeons to seek to ensure the health and welfare of animals committed to their care and to fulfill their professional responsibilities by maintaining five principles of practice:

1) Professional competence
2) Honesty and integrity
3) Independence and impartiality
4) Client confidentiality and trust
5) Professional accountability

Section 1.2 of the code of professional conducts states that veterinary surgeons must keep within their own area of competence and refer cases responsibly, and Section 3.5 states that veterinary surgeons must not hold out themselves or others as specialists or advanced practitioners unless appropriately listed with the RCVS, or as veterinary nurses unless appropriately registered with the RCVS.

The AVMA, in annotation 7.4 of the Principles of Veterinary Medical Ethics, provides a position statement recommending referrals when a case is outside a practitioner's level of experience: "Veterinarians who believe that they haven't the experience or equipment to manage and treat certain emergencies in the best manner, should advise the client that more qualified or specialized services are available elsewhere and offer to expedite referral to those services" (https://www.avma.org/resources-tools/avma-policies/principles-veterinary-medical-ethics-avma, accessed 31 May 2021).

Recordkeeping

The RCVS mandates that veterinary surgeons must keep clear, accurate, and detailed clinical and client records. These should include details of examination, treatment administered, procedures undertaken, medication prescribed and/or supplied, and the results of any diagnostic or laboratory tests. There is, however, no requirement for anesthetic records to be used although this is a requirement for practices in the PSS.

The AVA guidelines for safer anesthesia recommend that professional records of anesthesia are kept, including patient details, procedure details, staff involved, drugs, monitoring and recovery, and that records should be reviewed for morbidity and mortality issues.

The ACVAA Small Animal Monitoring guidelines make similar recommendations for contemporaneous record-keeping for legal purposes during both sedation and cases undergoing general anesthesia. The AAHA 2020 Anesthesia and Monitoring Guidelines recommend the use of patient safety checklists and documentation of patient parameters during anesthesia and recovery.

Further Reading

Grubb, T., Sager, J., Gaynor, J.S. et al. (2020). AAHA Anesthesia and monitoring guidelines for dogs and cats. *J Am Anim Hosp Assoc* 56: 59–82.

Magalhães-Sant'Ana, M., More, S.J., Morton, D.B. et al. (2015). What do European veterinary codes of conduct actually say and mean? A case study approach. *Vet Rec* 176: 654. https://doi.org/10.1136/vr.103005.

12

Approach to Healthy Dog and Cat Anesthesia and Analgesia, and Selected Disease Processes and Procedures

Pamela Murison and Gareth Zeiler

Risk of Anesthetic Mortality

Veterinary reports of anesthetic mortality show some variation, dependent on location and types of practices. According to the largest multicenter study (UK based, across referral and primary care practices), the Confidential Enquiry into Perioperative Small Animal Fatalities (CEPSAF; Brodbelt et al. 2008), anesthetic risk of death in dogs is around 0.17% (1 in 601) overall, with a risk of 0.05% in healthy animals and 1.33% in sicker animals (≥ASA III). In cats, the risk is 0.24% (1 in 419) with 0.11% in healthy animals and 1.40% in sick ones (≥ASA III). Although this study showed an improvement in mortality from previous large multicenter studies, the death rates are still greater than those reported in people of 0.003% (see Further Reading). It is important to note, however, that veterinary studies may show much higher survival rates in individual center studies and also that methodological differences prevent precise comparisons. Studies of primary care practice have shown a death rate of 0.01% within 48 h for dogs in the United Kingdom and 0.05% within seven days for the United States of America, with a higher mortality rate demonstrated in referral practices, e.g., 0.65% (see Further Reading). This difference is likely to be related to the different population of animals and range of procedures performed in referral practice.

There is a notable difference in mortality rates between healthy cats and dogs, which has been consistently observed across studies. Dog and cat mortality rates are much closer in sicker animals. It should be noted that time of anesthetic associated death is also rather different, with 61% of deaths reported in cats occurring in recovery, compared to only 47% of dogs (Brodbelt et al. 2008).

Breeds of Dog and Cat

Dogs are an incredibly diverse species, having been selectively bred for so many practical and impractical purposes over the centuries. It is inevitable therefore that we can have some very specific breed-related differences in dogs.

Size differences can be dramatic in dogs, with different breeds ranging in weight from 1.5 to 130 kg. The size impacts on equipment requirements, tendency toward heat loss and hypothermia, and many management factors that can be more difficult at both extremes. Care should be taken in the dosing of giant-breed dogs in particular, related to the allometric scaling of dose requirements.

Anatomical differences are particularly important. Brachycephalic animals are very popular in many countries and their conformation and associated risk factors can have a significant impact on anesthesia. Brachycephalic breeds include French and English bulldogs, Pugs, Boston terriers, etc. In these animals, the foreshortened muzzle creates less space in the nasal cavity. Many dogs suffer from what is known as "brachycephalic obstructive airway syndrome" (BOAS), with a variable degree of upper airway obstruction present at any time. The components of airway obstruction are produced by narrow nares, a long soft palate, and in some breeds a hypoplastic trachea (narrower). The tendency for sub-atmospheric pressures generated in the thorax to fail to cause adequate air admittance creates negative pressure effects elsewhere, for example, eversion of laryngeal ventricles or even laryngeal collapse in severely affected animals. The negative pressure may also have effects on the gastrointestinal tract with a high incidence of regurgitation in these breeds, possibly associated with hiatal hernia in some cases.

A mutation of the ABCB1-1Δ gene in dogs (formally known as "MDR1") has been noted with particular

Fundamental Principles of Veterinary Anesthesia, First Edition. Edited by Gareth E. Zeiler and Daniel S. J. Pang.

Companion Website: www.wiley.com/go/VeterinaryAnesthesiaZeiler

frequency in Collie type dogs. This gene controls production of P-glycoprotein. When mutations are present, this may affect the ability of drugs to cross the blood–brain barrier (which is relevant for anesthetics) and also bioavailability of orally administered drugs. The effect of these mutations is to cause increased sedation with a longer effect, for example, with acepromazine. Several opioid drugs are reported to be substrates for P-glycoprotein, which may imply a longer duration of action and more marked sedation in affected dogs; however, differing responses to opioids are related to many clinical factors in dogs.

Dachshunds have been observed to exhibit a significantly lower heart rate under anesthesia than other small breeds undergoing the same procedure (Harrison et al. 2012). The authors of this study also noted a small difference in body temperature, but this is unlikely to have completely explained the effect on heart rate.

Chondrodystrophic breeds (i.e., those with shortened and distorted legs, such as Bassett Hounds) may have considerable loose skin on the limbs which can result in surprisingly challenging intravenous access, a difficulty compounded with variable and somewhat tortuous venous pathways. It may also be noted that a dog breed with such limbs may have a larger trachea than expected for their weight (a large dog on short legs).

An idiosyncratic hepatotoxic reaction to carprofen has been reported, with Labrador retrievers being overrepresented. It should be noted that this was a report from the United States of America, and the same problem has not been reported with the same frequency in other countries, suggesting a possible relation to a genetic strain.

The Greyhound and other sight hounds will have a slower recovery after thiopental administration than other breeds. Although demonstrated to have a larger total body fluid volume (and hence lower proportion of fat, important in drug redistribution), the Greyhound has also been shown to have a slower metabolism associated with cytochrome P450 (CYP enzyme expression) activity, and both are probably contributory to the slower drug elimination seen. Although best known to be related to thiopental administration, this difference should also be acknowledged if administering other drugs that rely on the same CYP subtype for phase I biotransformation. Omeprazole, for example, relies on the CYP3A12 subtype and metabolism appears to be similar in Greyhounds to other breeds. Propofol, however, has a slower elimination via CYP2B11 though clinically this may not be significant due to the short duration of this drugs.

Some breed differences are very much related to their physical features. Breeds with dense coats, such as Newfoundland or Pyrenean Mountain dogs, may be more likely to retain heat during anesthesia and be more likely to become hyperthermic. It may also be more difficult to estimate weight. On the other hand, breeds with a larger surface-area-to-volume ratio (e.g., Yorkshire Terrier or Chihuahua) and/or poor coat (e.g., hairless Chinese Crested) will lose heat dramatically during anesthesia without careful measures to prevent this. Some breeds will have a higher incidence of certain diseases, which may be relevant for anesthesia.

In cats, breed variation is less marked than that of dogs; however, there are still some breed differences for the anesthetist to be aware of. Anatomical and size variation is less marked than in dogs. Brachycephaly is less common in cats than dogs,; however, Persian and some other cat breeds will have a foreshortened skull and reduced nasal airflow, but this should not be mistaken for BOAS, which is a syndrome exclusively described in dogs (see Chapter 18). Rex and hairless breeds of cats can have a significantly greater heat loss during anesthesia. Familial and genetic associations with hypertrophic cardiomyopathy (HCM) have been reported in several breeds of cats (e.g., Norwegian Forest) with a specific genetic mutation identified in Maine Coon and Ragdoll cats. In these animals, HCM may be asymptomatic. Importantly, the effects of anesthesia may cause decompensation in these animals (Chapter 17).

Principles of Intravenous Access Sites and Procedures

For dogs and cats, the most common routine intravenous access is a cephalic vein. The medial branch of this vein may also be cannulated. A note about terminology: Although a "catheter" may technically be termed a device entering a bladder or other organ to drain fluid, and a "cannula" is a tube inserted, e.g., into a blood vessel to administer fluids/drugs, the terms are often used interchangeably with regard to intravenous access. In the context of this chapter, "cannula" is used.

The procedure of inserting an IV cannula is described in Table 12.1.

Other Vascular Access Sites

A lateral saphenous vein is useful in dogs especially when thoracic limbs are not accessible (e.g., bilateral elbow arthroscopy). Some nervous animals may respond better to saphenous cannula placement.

These veins are usually more mobile than a cephalic vein. Using a thumb alongside the vein for stability may be helpful but do not compromise aseptic technique. In larger animals or those who are quite active, it may be helpful to

Table 12.1 Procedural steps of placing an over-the-needle intravascular cannula in dogs and cats. The principles are the same for all peripheral vein cannula placements.

Step	Procedure	Figure
1	Prepare all required materials and then engage an assistant to securely restrain the animal. Even a calm animal may jump as a cannula is inserted. It is common practice to provide sedation before placing an IV cannula in most animals, to reduce stress and facilitate restraint.	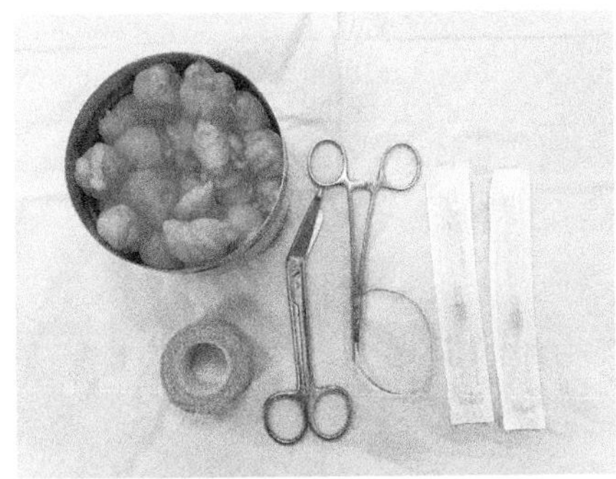
2	Operator clips and cleans area – Ensure a large enough clip distal to insertion site to prevent a sterile cannula contacting with hair – The operator should also ensure suitable hand hygiene (wash hands or apply alcohol rub) or nonsterile gloves (healthy patients) or sterile gloves (immunocompromised patients).	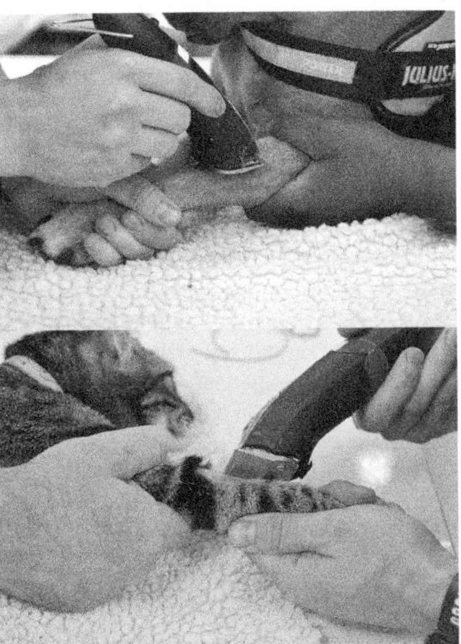
3	Assistant holds dog or cat in sternal recumbency and raise vein, by holding a hand around the elbow. ● Hooking the fingers above the elbow reduces the chance for the assistant's hand to slide downward. ● A tourniquet (e.g., rubber band and hemostat) can be used and may be helpful in larger animals in particular but can be more uncomfortable for the animal. In loose skinned animals, ensure skin held taut by both assistant and operator but do not flatten vein. In thick skinned or loose skinned animals, the skin may be broken with ● the tip of a no. 11 scalpel blade, or ● a hypodermic needle (18/21 Ga). ● Note: This is not a "cutdown" that is a surgical exposure of a vessel.	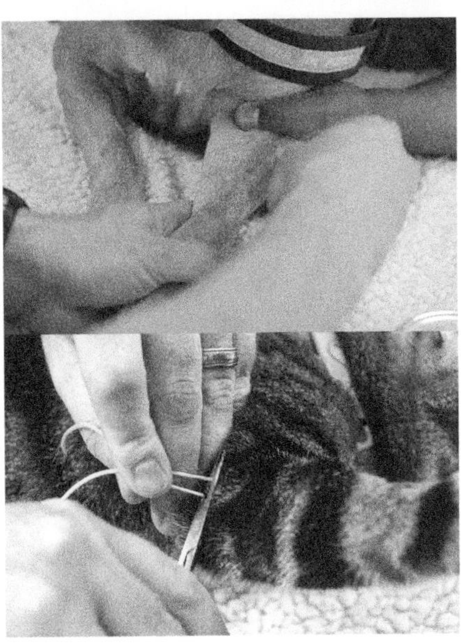

(Continued)

Table 12.1 (Continued)

Step	Procedure	Figure
4.1	Hold the cannula securely and in a way that flashback of blood can be seen. Ensure fingers do not touch the cannula itself. Insert at slight angle to skin (approximately 30° above the plane of the vein), over the top of the vessel. • The vessel is more palpable than visible in some animals.	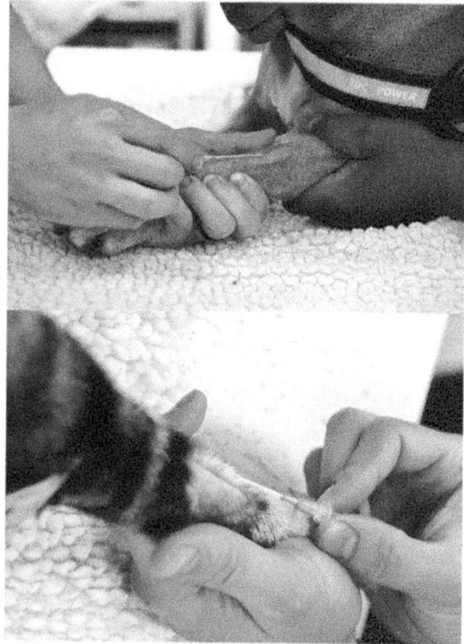
4.2	As the vein is entered, flashback of blood is seen (blue arrow). Stop inserting at this point. Flatten the angle of the cannula (more flat to the skin) and insert catheter a few millimeters with stylet. • The stylet will protrude from the catheter about 3 mm or so; therefore, if this step is omitted, there is a risk that the stylet is in the vein but the catheter is not, so it fails to thread.	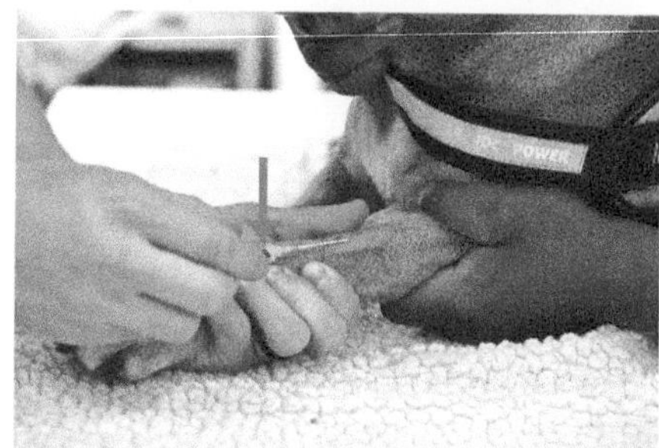
4.3	Then, thread catheter off stylet. • Importantly, advance the catheter off the stylet rather than withdrawing the stylet from the catheter.	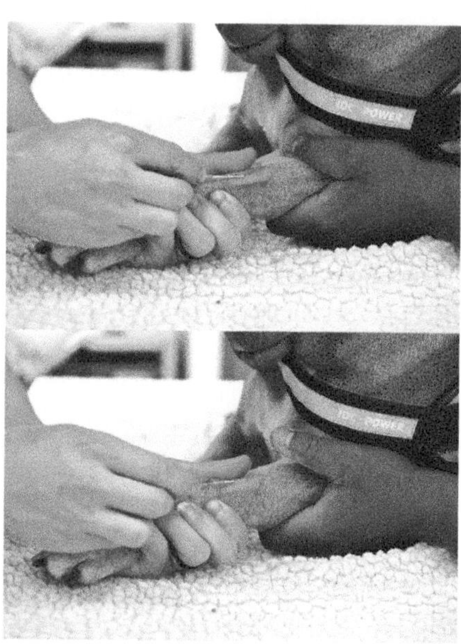

Table 12.1 (Continued)

<table>
<tr><th>Step</th><th>Procedure</th><th>Figure</th></tr>
<tr><td>4.4</td><td>Remove stylet
• It is not recommended to reinsert a stylet – this may cut off the tip of the cannula which may be released into the circulation
Once the catheter is inserted, the assistant can stop raising the vein, and if able to do so safely can move the hand to obstruct the flow of blood via the cannula by pressure.
Cap the cannula
• It may be easier to cap initially and add connectors later after securing.
• The operator's nondominant thumb can hold the cannula in place by pushing the cap inward to the leg or pressing down on a wing (if the variety of cannula has them).
Do not touch the insertion point into the skin.</td><td>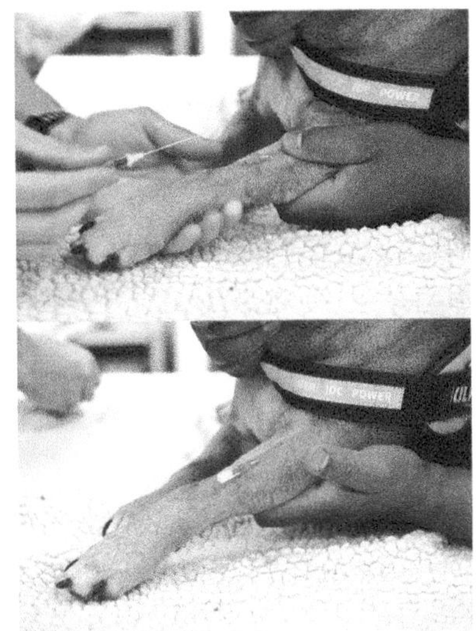</td></tr>
<tr><td>5</td><td>Secure in position, e.g., using adhesive tape
• Using tape that is relatively easy to remove will make this easier later
• Using tape that adheres well to the plastic of the cannula helps stop inadvertent removal.
• Pinch the tape down well over the plastic to ensure it grips.
• There is no benefit to wrapping many times around the leg, which may increase rigidity. Tightly wrapped tape may cause distal migration of the cannula or kinking.</td><td>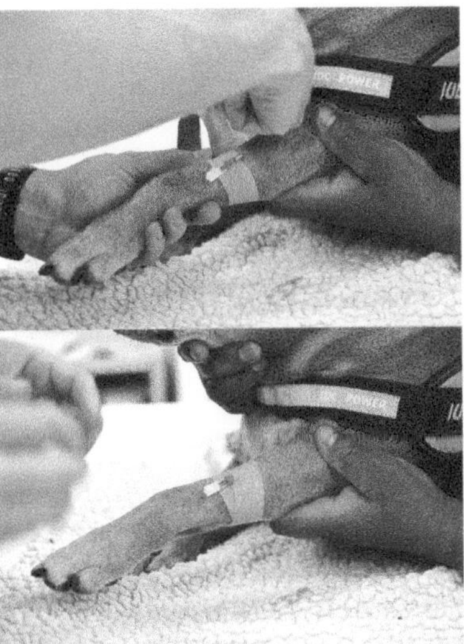</td></tr>
<tr><td>6</td><td>There are benefits to using an injectable port (pictured) or a T-port or Y-connector. Although not essential, this is very helpful when giving fluids and also for ease of drug administration.</td><td>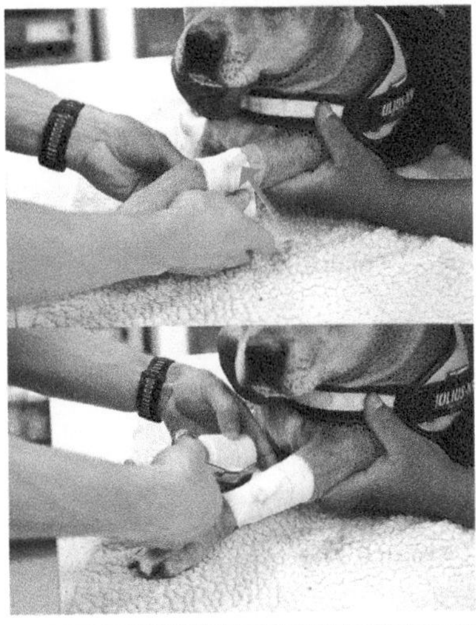</td></tr>
</table>

have a second assistant to raise the vein while the first is restraining the animal. Lateral recumbency is easier for cannulation, if tolerated. Raising the vein can be more difficult in larger animals especially for a small-handed assistant. If the animal is small enough, hold a hand above the stifle, and this has the advantage that it can also reduce the ability of the dog to withdraw the limb (which might happen in response to the stimulus of insertion). In larger dogs, pressure on the caudal aspect of the limb is sufficient to raise the vessel. The principle of placement is exactly the same as described in the preceding text for cannulating a cephalic vein.

On securing the cannula *in situ*, be aware that tight tapes proximal to the hock can restrict venous blood flow and can be uncomfortable for the animal. A tip is to flex the hock slightly when taping because this increases the width of the limb compared to the extended hock (Figure 12.1). If taped in this position, the tape will not be too tight. Be careful also about the angle; keep the cannula aligned with the vessel during the taping process.

In cats, the lateral saphenous veins are small. The medial saphenous veins are better developed, and also have the advantage of being a straight vessel for cannulation (Figure 12.2). It is best to position the cat in lateral recumbency. An

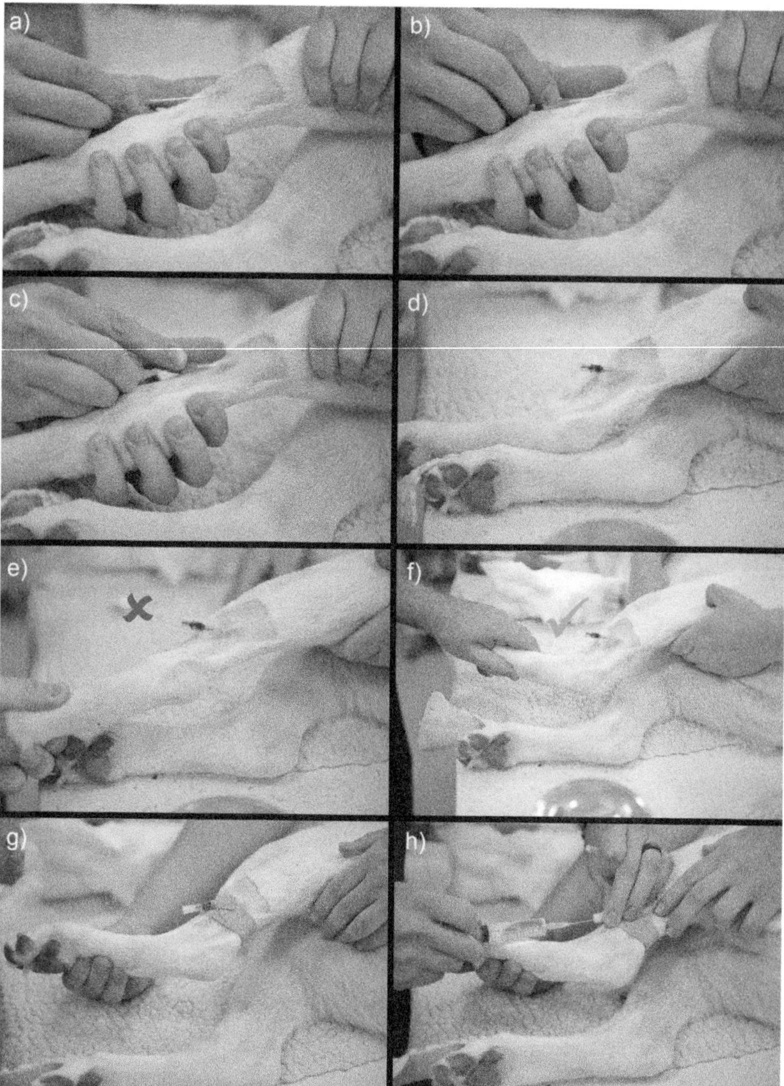

Figure 12.1 Intravenous cannulation of a lateral saphenous vein in a dog. After aseptic preparation, the vein can be raised by applying pressure behind the stifle (a), once blood enters the flash chamber, then the angle of insertion can be decreased to the level of the skin and the cannula, and stylet is advanced 0.5 mm as a unit to ensure that the cannula tip is within the vein (b). Then, the cannula is advanced into the vein while keeping the stylet stationary (c). Once the cannula is in the vein, it can initially be capped using the pre-packaged cap. Before securing the cannula using adhesive tape (25 mm), the leg should not be extended (e) but rather slight flexed (f) to prevent overtight wrapping of the tape. Once the cannula is taped (g), then an injection port stopper (or any other type of IV connector) can be attached to make IV injection easier without causing bleeding (h).

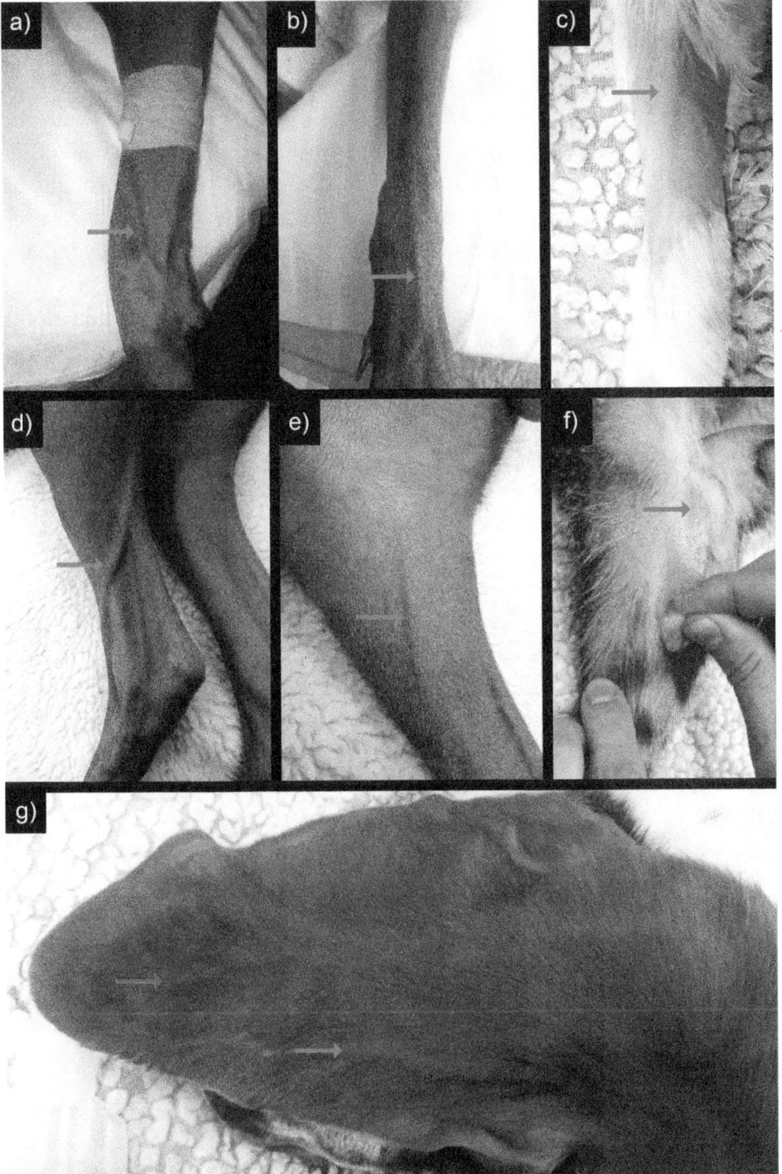

Figure 12.2 Other sites of venous access include: the accessory (medial) branch of the cephalic vein of a dog (a), the dorsal metacarpal III vein of a dog, cephalic vein in a cat (c), lateral saphenous vein in a dog (d), medial saphenous vein in a dog (e) and cat (f), and the marginal auricular veins (blue arrow) in a large ear dog (g). The auricular artery (red arrow, usually in the middle of the ear) should not be cannulated for IV access purposes.

additional assistant may help to hold the upper pelvic limb out of the way if required but may not be needed in more sedated animals. Be careful to not tape too tightly (as for dogs).

The marginal ear vein is also suitable for use, especially in animals with larger ears (Figure 12.2). It can be a useful site in animals with considerable loose skin and chondrodystrophy, such as Dachshunds and Basset hounds. The ear is mobile and should be held taut with an assistant raising the vessel. Be careful not to cannulate the artery inadvertently. The vessel is very superficial over the surface of the cartilage, and it is easy to go too deep and traverse the vein. Rolling the edge of the ear under when holding the ear with the nondominant hand ensures a straight line access. Keep the cannula very flat to the ear and, if very mobile, and ask an assistant to thread the cannula off the stylet.

When taping, secure the cannula flat to the ear. Some support (e.g., a few rolled gauzes) on the inside of the ear can be useful (and can assist in stabilizing the ear during cannulation), but if this cannula is to be left in a conscious animal, try to not allow dressings to become too heavy, unwieldy, and uncomfortable.

Jugular veins are not usually used for cannula placement in healthy animals. However, the jugular can be catheterized (usually using a long-stay central venous catheter) in situations such as, when placed and left in place for numerous days, to facilitate daily blood sampling, to administer large fluid volumes in larger patients, or if peripheral venous access is limited (e.g., damaged veins from previous cannula placement).

Principles of Airway Management

Options for airway management and supply of inhalational anesthetics during anesthesia include the use of facemasks, endotracheal intubation using an endotracheal tube (Figure 12.3 and Table 12.2), and supraglottic airway devices. In certain circumstances, alternative airways such as tracheostomies are used; however, this is beyond the scope of this chapter. Endotracheal tubes come in a wide range of sizes. The size of an endotracheal tube is the internal diameter (ID). There are size charts for dogs and

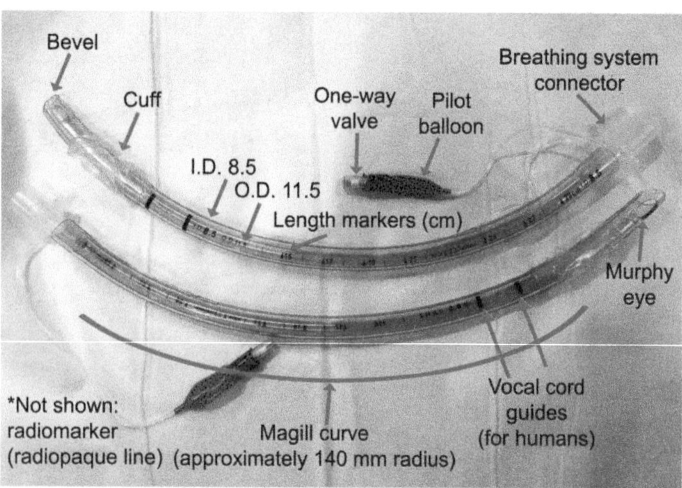

Figure 12.3 The anatomy of an endotracheal tube.

Table 12.2 Common types of endotracheal tubes used in small animal practice.

Composition	Endotracheal tube type	Advantages	Disadvantages	Photos
Polyvinyl chloride	Cuffed Uncuffed Armored Cole (reinforced) Shielded (for laser surgery)	Very affordable and can be cut to the correct length Usually, high-volume low-pressure cuffs that are less likely to cause trauma of perfusion concerns of the tracheal mucosa Transparent tubes that facilitate cleaning Preformed with a gentle curve (Magill curve) that follows the normal resting position of the mouth and neck	Smaller sized tubes often have relatively large cuffs that are difficult to pass through the *rima glottidis* Manufactured as a single-use item but can be used until the cuff is nonfunctional Can only use cold liquid sterilant to sterilize tubes In humans, plastic allergies have been described If bent too far, this tube will kink causing an airway obstruction Very small tubes can twist on themselves, especially when warmed to body temperature; therefore monitoring for obstruction is encouraged	

Table 12.2 (Continued)

Composition	Endotracheal tube type	Advantages	Disadvantages	Photos
Silicon	Cuffed	Available in any size and length Transparent tubes that facilitate cleaning Multiuse tube that can be sterilized using cold liquid sterilant or steam autoclave Silicon is inert and no hypersensitivity reaction has been reported in humans or animals	Very expensive Very easy for the animals to bite a section off and aspirate the distal tip Pilot balloon attachment site often tears causing cuff leaks Straight tubes and in certain breeds (bull terriers) intubation might be challenging Usually has low-volume high-pressure cuffs Rather rigid and if bent too much, it is prone to kinking and cracking the wall of the tube	
Siliconized polyvinyl chloride	Cuffed Uncuffed Armored (reinforced)	Flexible and soft material less prone to causing airway trauma	Generally sold as single use Prone to accidental occlusion when securing the tube May require a stylet to allow intubation, especially in small-sized tubes	
Red rubber	Cuffed	Multiuse tube that can be sterilized using cold liquid sterilant Midrange in price Manufactured with a Magill curve	Exposure to excessive heat make the tubes prone to cracking Opaque, resulting in difficulty visualizing any plugs or material not removed in the cleaning process which can lead to a partial or complete obstruction Wall of tube is often thicker than other materials and thus more rigid which can cause airway trauma Cuff is usually a low-volume high-pressure cuff and requires a tube clamp to ensure cuffs remain inflated	

cats to help prepare for tracheal intubation and a version of a chart can be found in Table 12.3.

The most common airway management technique is orotracheal intubation.

Benefits

- Ensuring a patent airway
- Protection against aspiration of material (e.g., regurgitated stomach contents, hemorrhage, etc.)
- Permits delivery of oxygen and inhalational anesthetics
- Facilitates assisted or controlled ventilation (e.g., manual breath or intermittent positive pressure ventilation [IPPV]).

Table 12.3 Size chart to estimate endotracheal tube size for different weights (kg) in dogs and cats (assumes normal anatomy).

Lean weight (lbs)	Endotracheal tube size (internal diameter: ID) in mm	
	Dogs	Cats
1 (2.2)	3.5–4.0	3.0
2 (4.4)	4.0–5.0	3.5
3.5 (7.7)	5.5	4.0
4.5 (9.9)	6.0	4.5
6 (13.2)	6.5	5.5
8 (17.6)	7.0	–
10 (22.0)	8.0	–
12 (26.5)	8.5	–
14 (30.9)	9.0	–
16 (35.3)	9.5	–
20 (44.1)	10.0	–
25 (55.1)	11.0	–
30 (66.1)	12.0	–
>35 (77.2)	14–16	–

Disadvantages

- In cats, a higher anesthetic risk associated with endotracheal intubation
- Takes time (varies with experience and may be affected by some breeds, e.g., brachycephalic dogs)
- Risk of trauma
  - Laryngeal swelling
  - Irritation to the tracheal mucosa and tracheitis
  - Rupture of the trachea: usually related to cuff overinflation (e.g., cats and small dogs)
  - Stricture (created by scar tissue formation after mucosal damage, can be slow, taking months, to become evident)
  - Laryngospasm (mostly cats)

Procedure for Orotracheal Intubation

Dogs

A laryngoscope may be useful but is not essential in most animals. However, laryngoscopy may be very helpful for difficult intubation, e.g., due to pathology or brachycephalic anatomy. Familiarization with the technique of using a laryngoscope on healthy animals can greatly facilitate its use in difficult cases. When using a laryngoscope, always use the longest blade that will comfortably fit in the oropharynx. Doing so optimizes illumination of the *rima glottidis*. The procedure of orotracheal intubation with an ET tube of a dog is outlined in Table 12.4.

If not using a laryngoscope, ensure the mouth is well open. A directable, bright light can be useful. In most healthy dogs with normal anatomy, the larynx will be visible. The tip of the ET tube can be used to displace the soft palate if required.

Cat

In cats, many veterinarians will use an uncuffed ET tube. Cats are, in general, less likely to regurgitate under anesthesia, so protection of the airway may be less important. However, bear in mind the potential for leakage of anesthetic gases. Use of IPPV could increase leaks and environmental contamination; therefore, the largest uncuffed ET tube that is possible should be used. This will be larger than a passable cuffed ET tube, partly as many cuffed ET tubes have a thicker wall but mainly due to the presence of a cuff making it more difficult to pass through the *rima glottidis* of the larynx (Figure 12.4). ET tube sizes of 4.0–5.5 mm uncuffed or 3.5–5.0 mm cuffed are likely to be suitable depending on cat size.

Cats are more susceptible to laryngospasm than other domestic species (except perhaps rabbits). In the authors' experience, the risk of laryngospasm is greatly increased if intubation is attempted at an insufficient depth of anesthesia (i.e., when a cough reflex is still present) or with a traumatic intubation. Similarly, late extubation, performed after return of the cough reflex, is more likely to precipitate laryngospasm. Most veterinarians will use local anesthetic to desensitize the larynx during intubation. In various countries, specifically designed local anesthetic spray (lidocaine) is available. This is safe to use in cats. However, there are two major caveats to using commercially available local anesthetic sprays: (1) there have been reports of swelling and damage to the cats' larynx when some human throat spay preparations were used (they often have flavoring or different excipients). If a licensed spray is not available, a safer option than using a human product is to use injectable lidocaine (some practices prefer stocking a preservative-free formulation); (2) care with doses of sprays, the dose of a spray can be rather variable (e.g., 2–10 mg per actuation). Be particularly careful with small cats that the drug is deposited onto the *rima glottidis* of the larynx and cords and not into the trachea (as the fluid can lead to increased upper respiratory sounds and coughing post-anesthetic). If there is a risk of local anesthetic toxicity in smaller cats, or a commercial spray formulation is not available, 0.1 mL of lidocaine 2%, onto the *rima glottidis* (half the volume on each side), is effective in desensitizing the area (Figure 12.5).

Table 12.4 Procedure of orotracheal intubation of a dog.

Step	Procedure	Figure
1	Prepare all materials Have a selection of tubes prepared ● Table 12.3 shows a size chart, and this is probably the largest you would be able to use so have two smaller sizes. It is generally recommended to prepare three different ET tube sizes for each patient (more for brachycephalic dog breeds). ● Other ways to estimate tube size include using the nasal planum or digital palpation, although these estimates may not be very accurate. Using the cube root of body weight ($\sqrt[3]{Body\ weight}$) in kg or one-third of the nasal width has been suggested to be more suitable (Tong & Pang 2019).	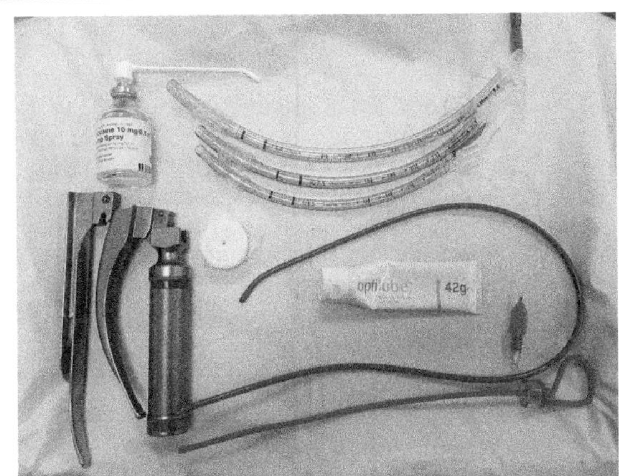
2	Check tubes ● Cleanliness. ● Length (from the end of the muzzle to the thoracic inlet [estimated as the point of the shoulder]) (red arrows indicate ET tube too long [left] and was cut to size [right]). ● Connector should be present and firmly attached. ● Cuffs should be inflated (not overdistended, which can cause cuff damage) and checked after about five minutes to ensure no loss of cuff pressure (yellow arrow). ● Lubrication can both aid in positioning and may help improve the seal around the cuff (Blunt et al. 2001). A water-based lubricant gel is suitable. ● If an ET tube stylet (blue arrow; used to either bend tip of ET tube or add strength in very flexible tubes) or intubating stylet (green arrow; tip of stylet inserted into the trachea and the ET tube is advanced over the stylet as a guide ["railroad-ing"]) is used, then they should be checked to see if they fit within the ET tube.	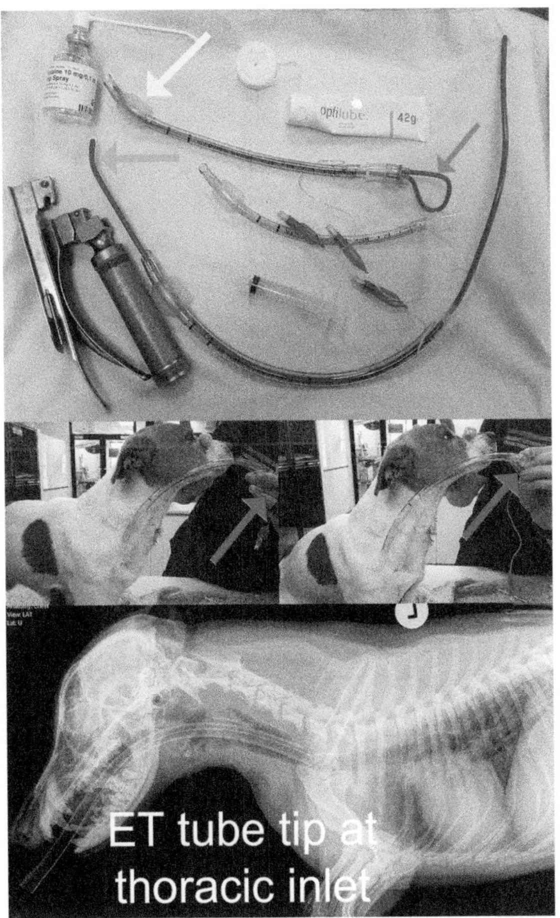

(Continued)

Table 12.4 (Continued)

Step	Procedure	Figure
3	Ensure depth of anesthesia is adequate before attempting to intubate the trachea (usually ventrally rotated eye, reduced or absent medial palpebral reflex, and relaxed jaw tone). • *Beware different anesthetic agents will give slightly different clinical signs (e.g., a central eye and retention of palpebral reflexes with ketamine or a tendency for less globe rotation with alfaxalone [Herbert & Murison 2013]). • Performing intubation with the patient in either sternal recumbency or lateral recumbency is feasible. It is a useful skill to be proficient at intubating in both positions. • In most animals, elevation of the head will facilitate intubation; however, care should be taken to avoid extension in animals with neck instability. • A bandage behind the upper canines may facilitate the assistant holding. • The assistant's other hand should be lifting the skull of the dog (Note: Scruffing gives less security and stability in positioning. Avoid any pressure on soft tissues around the neck area which will affect intubation). • Ensure neck is straight (not flexed or overextended). • Good head positioning makes intubation much easier.	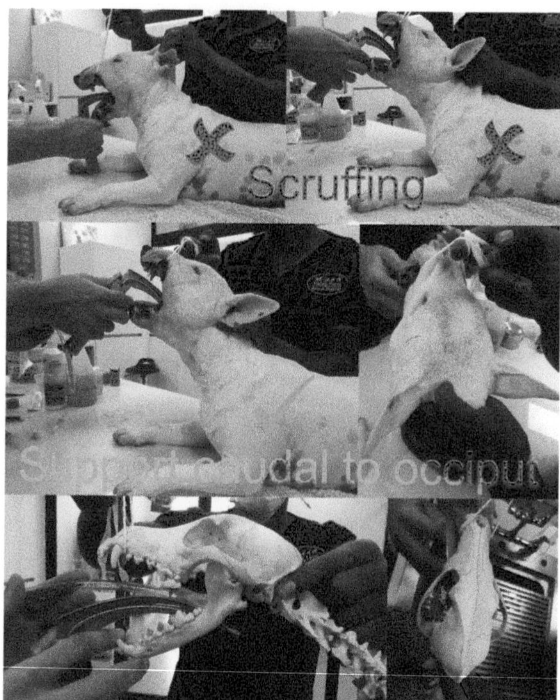
4	Position the laryngoscope blade • Gently but firmly pull the tongue forward. If using a laryngoscope, flicking the tongue out of the mouth with the blade of the laryngoscope can reduce the risk of an inadvertent bite. • Ensure the mouth is sufficiently open to permit visualization of the glottis. • Hold the tongue between fingers (usually of the nondominant hand) ± with the aid of a dry gauze. • Insert the laryngoscope to the base of the tongue just rostral to the epiglottis. Some practitioners place the laryngoscope on the epiglottis; this is not necessary in most animals in the authors' opinion and can cause an increased risk of post-anesthetic swelling but is useful in some difficult intubations. Once positioned, transfer the laryngoscope handle to the nondominant hand (also grasping the tongue) and use the dominant hand to manipulate the ET tube. Alternatively, practice keeping the laryngoscope in your right hand and always manipulate the ET tube with your left hand. See step 5 how the glottis is always clearly visible when your hands are not crossed while inserting the ET tube. • A straight (e.g., Miller) or curved blade (e.g., Mackintosh) may be used depending on preference of the anesthetist and anatomy of the dog. • If epiglottal tip is dorsal to the soft palate, it may be released by using the tip of the endotracheal tube to dislodge it. • A clear view of the whole glottis should be achievable in most healthy animals.	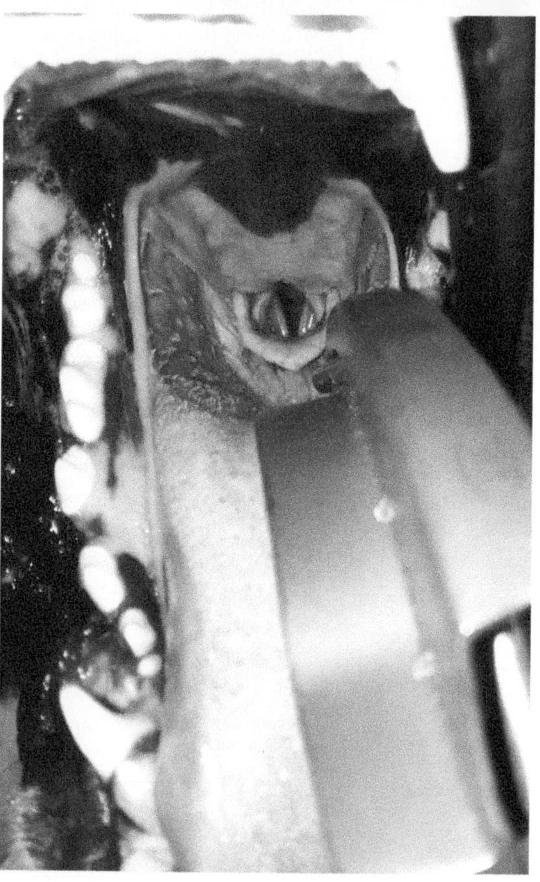

Step	Procedure	Figure
5	Insert the ET tube ● Insert the ET tube with bevel aligned to glottis. ● Do not push on the cords. ● The tip of the tube should be seen to pass through the cords. Trauma to the cords should be avoided. ● A gentle rotation while advancing may aid movement through the larynx. ● Ensure the curve of the ET tube follows the curve of the neck (this is less likely to create bevel occlusion in the trachea).	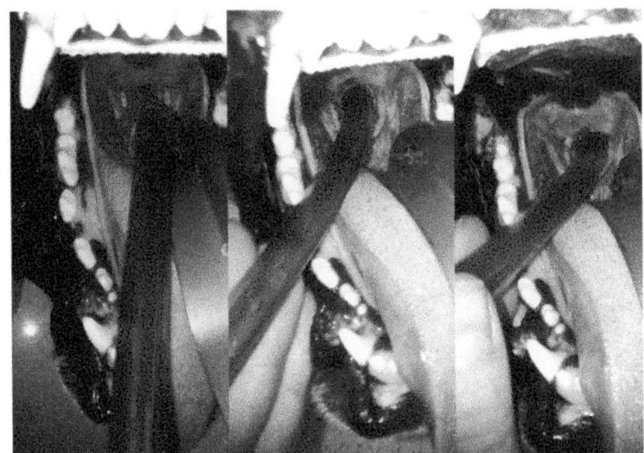
6	Secure the tube ● Specific tube ties are available, but narrow bandage (e.g., white open weave) is suitable. ● Be aware that tying tightly around the tube is quite likely to cause some restriction of the tube lumen (or if not tight enough tube can still move). ● If connector has wings, an overhand knot with one side in front and one side behind the wing secures and ensures but cannot move forward or backward (but *must* have secure connector). ● Can tie around back of head and upper or lower jaw (may depend on procedure) – be careful not to catch tongue and not be too tight (facial swelling rostral to tie can occur).	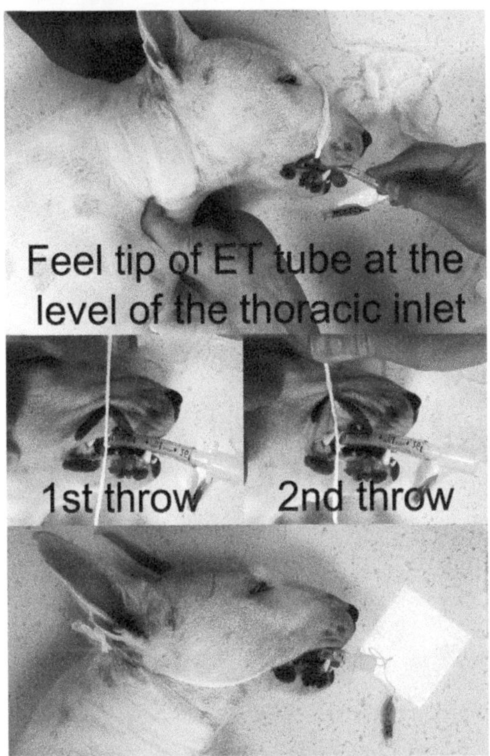
7	● Inflate cuff – Ideally inflate to 20–30 mmHg. – Specific pressure measuring syringes are available (e.g., AGCuffil; Hung et al. 2020). – Alternatively can inflate just enough to stop a leak when a pressure of 20 cmH_2O is applied to inflate the lungs; however, there are risks and some very high cuff pressures have been generated using this technique. It is important that the syringe used is proportional to the size of the cuff, and the smaller the animal, the smaller and slower incremental inflation should be performed to avoid overinflation. – Some practitioners will just inflate the pilot balloon to a pressure that they judge to be correct, which is relatively effective for experienced anesthetists. ● Be careful, silicon tubes in particular may be easy to overinflate and produce high cuff pressures (Briganti et al. 2012).	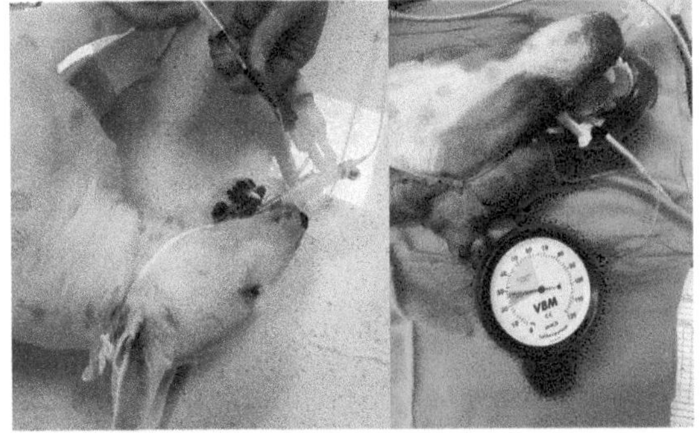

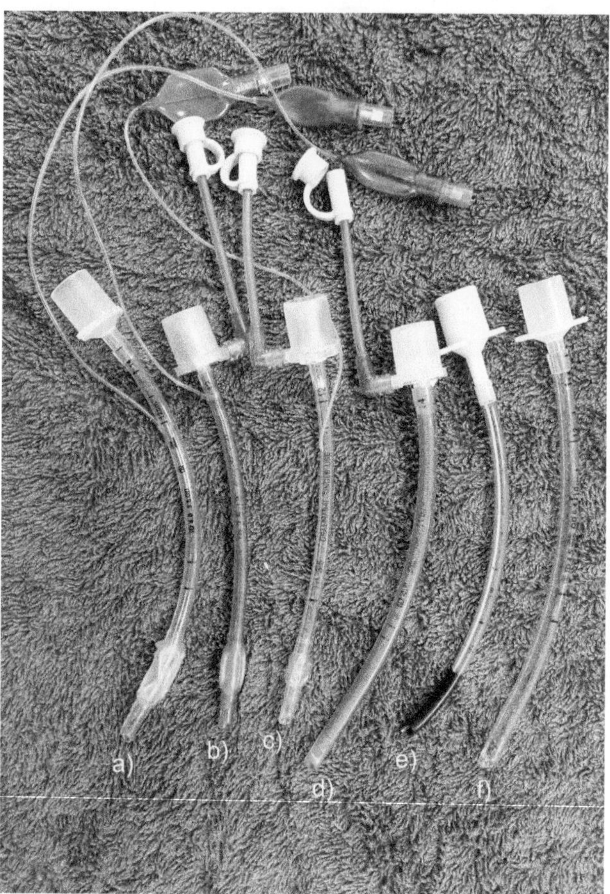

Figure 12.4 Endotracheal tubes that can be used in cats. They can be cuffed (a–c) or uncuffed (d–f). Generally, the largest uncuffed endotracheal tube is preferred for cats except in cats undergoing thoracotomy or dental procedures. Note that endotracheal tubes (b–d) have sidestream gas sampling ports incorporated into the breathing circuit connector.

The procedure of orotracheal intubation in cats is similar to dogs but with some notable considerations. The equipment and consumables need to be prepared before general anesthesia is induced. In many aspects, they are the same as for dogs but with the possible exception of including a local anesthetic and a different type of lubricant (lubrication is very important in cats and can really make a difference to the procedure). The authors' favor a medical grade silicon spray in cats. If using gel, ensure there is no occlusion of the tip of the tube, which can occur easily. Also, do not apply too much gel to the tube because this can result in increased upper airway sounds and coughing. Once all equipment is prepared and ready, then general anesthesia can be induced. Checking the depth of anesthesia is very important in cats and generally orotracheal intubation should only be performed if they are in a surgical plane of anesthesia. If ketamine is used, a swallowing reflex can still be present but there must be no head avoidance movements (turning the head away when the mouth is opened). If there are head movements, then additional induction drug(s) should be administered to deepen the plane of anesthesia before any further attempts to intubation. The steps of orotracheal intubation are summarized in Figure 12.6.

Avoid using a spring-loaded gag (sometimes used for orotracheal intubation, dental procedures, etc.), as opening of the jaws can be extreme and may cause reduction in maxillary artery blood flow in some cats (which can be related to post-anesthetic blindness). During orotracheal intubation, once the local anesthetic is applied to the *rima glottidis*, the operator should wait for a brief period (30–45 s) to allow the drug to work. The laryngoscope should be

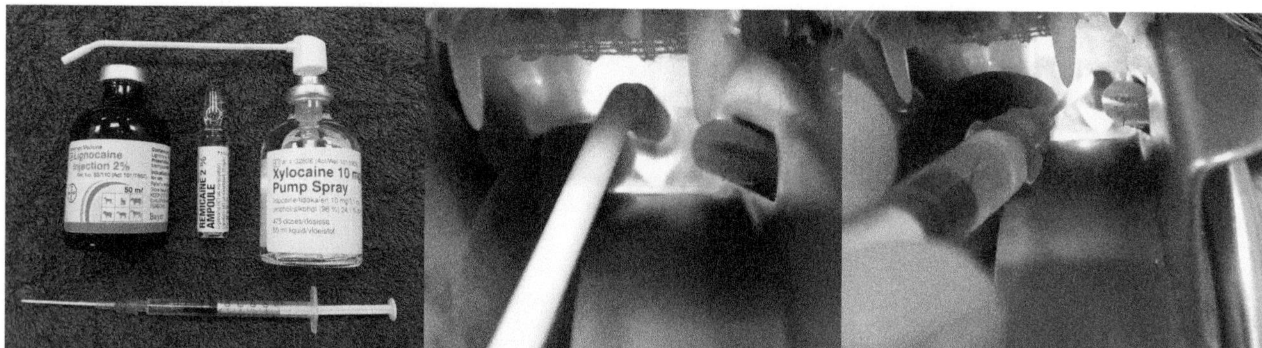

Figure 12.5 Various lignocaine products can be used to desensitize the *rima glottidis* in cats (left). An oral spray product (usually products for human use) can be used by placing the nozzle of the spray in the middle of the mouth to ensure a good single actuation is used to cover the entire *rima glottidis* (middle). Alternatively, an injectable product could be used by dripping the local anesthetic on the arytenoids (right).

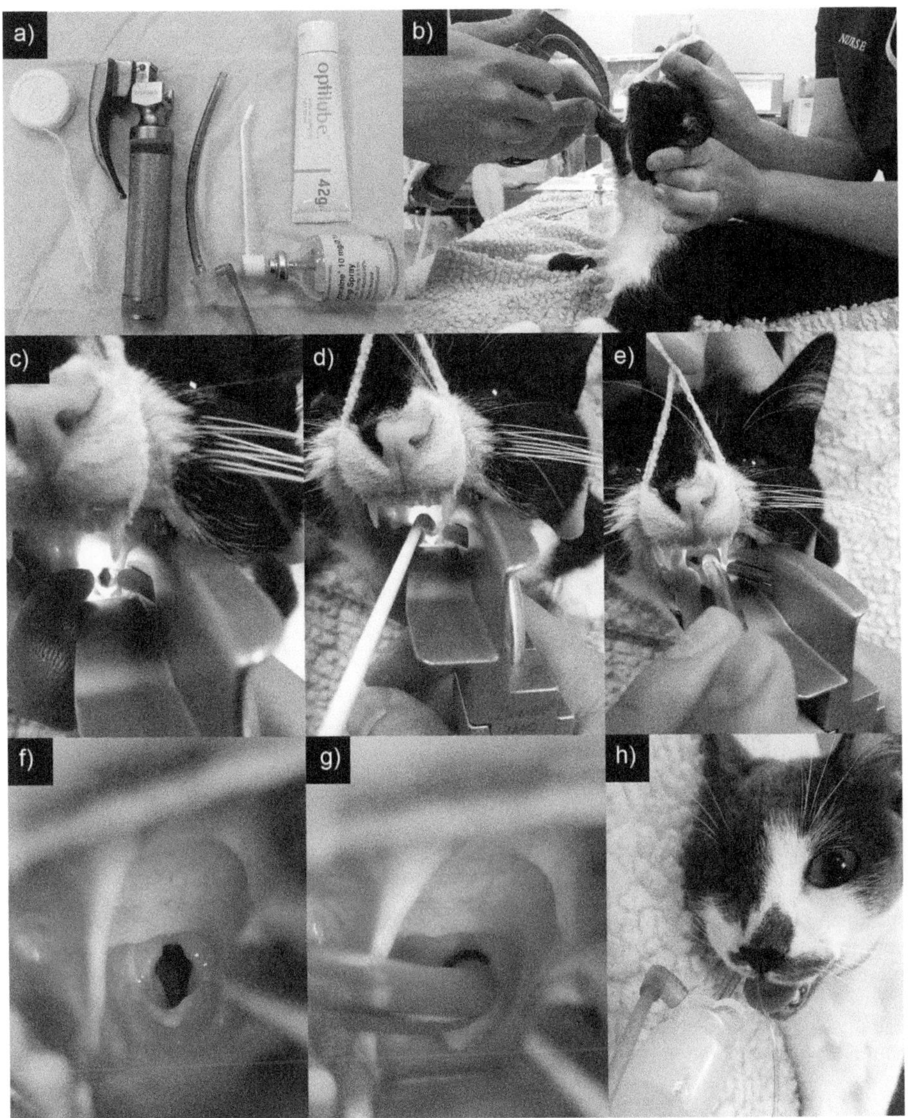

Figure 12.6 The procedure of orotracheal intubation in a cat starts with preparing all the materials and equipment required to swiftly secure the airways (a). After inducing general anesthesia, the depth of anesthesia is assessed, and if adequate, the mouth can be opened and the tongue pulled forward (b) and the blade of the laryngoscope positioned (c). Then, lignocaine can be applied (d) and then 10–30 s later the depth of anesthesia should be evaluated before attempting tracheal intubation (e). The endotracheal tube should only be advanced if the arytenoids are abducted (f) and then the endotracheal tube should be advanced in the center of the *rima glottidis* (g). Then, the tip of the endotracheal tube should be felt at the level of the thoracic inlet before securing and then connecting to a breathing circuit (h).

removed during this period. Cats can respond to the spray, and if they are lightly anesthetized the laryngoscope should be removed and an additional "top-up" dose of the induction drug should be given to deepen the plane of anesthesia. Furthermore, try not to wait too long before intubation either, as this can decrease quality of intubation conditions and require top-up induction drug. Once the laryngoscope is repositioned, it is helpful to watch a couple of breaths to note movement of the arytenoids (they should move freely without "vibrating" or being partially closed because this could indicate an impending complete laryngospasm; Figure 12.7). As much as possible, avoid contact with the vocal cords and attempt to slide the ET tube through the *rima glottidis* when it is open during inspiration. Pressure on the vocal cords is likely to produce laryngospasm. Once the ET tube is in the trachea, then it needs to be positioned so that the patient end is at the level of the thoracic inlet and the breathing system connector is at the level of the incisors. Then, the ET tube can be secured in place by using a 25 mm gauze ribbon (Figure 12.8).

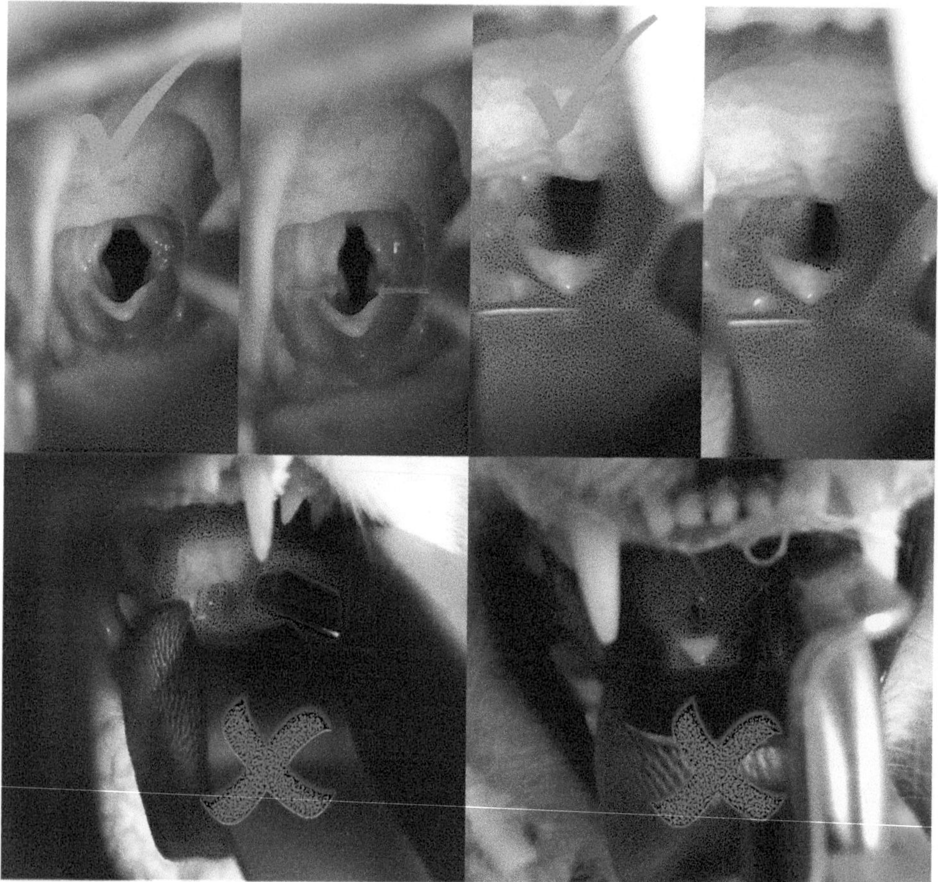

Figure 12.7 Cats are prone to laryngospasm and thus the endotracheal tube should never be advanced into the trachea if there is any suggestion that the arytenoids are not moving freely during the respiratory cycle. The top row of images are close-up views of arytenoids moving freely during the respiratory cycle, and the ideal time to perform tracheal intubation is during peak inhalation (green ticks). Note the vocal folds (blue arrows) seen behind the arytenoids and epiglottis cartilage of the larynx, and the bevel of the endotracheal tube should not be advanced into the vocal folds. The bottom row of images are of cats with partial laryngospasm (red crosses), and endotracheal intubation should not be attempted in these cats.

Techniques of Inflating an Endotracheal Tube Cuff

A cuffed endotracheal tube (ET tube) can be used in dogs and cats, and in most cases the cuff needs to be inflated. Cats are more prone to tracheal injury as a result of cuff (over)inflation compared to dogs. The major cause of damage is related to occlusion of the venous and lymphatic vessels in the tracheal mucosa. Average venous and lymphatic vessel pressures in the trachea of dogs are 16 cmH_2O (12 mmHg) and 4–7 cmH_2O (3–5 mmHg), respectively, and these pressures are thought to be similar in the cat. If the pressure exerted by the inflated cuff on the trachea mucosa exceed these values, it can result in edema and congestion of the tissues that ultimately result in a decreased perfusion or ischemia. Therefore, the amount of pressure that has been advocated to be applied to the trachea ranges between 20 and 25 cmH_2O. Dogs and cats that are hypotensive are at a higher risk of trauma due to cuff overinflation. Overinflation of the cuff has the risk of trauma to the tracheal mucosa that can result in scarring and stricture. A stricture may not be identified for many years after the anesthetic. In some cases, overinflation of the cuff has resulted in tracheal rupture. The benefit of inflating a cuff always outweighs the risk of trauma to the trachea. Therefore, learning how to properly inflate and test a cuff pressure is an important skill to master.

The methods that have been described to assess cuff inflation are for polyvinyl chloride (and siliconized polyvinyl chloride) endotracheal tubes with a high-volume, low-pressure cuff. These ET tubes are the most commonly used in dog and cat during anesthesia. These methods are not reliable for inflating cuffs of other types of ET tubes made from other compositions (i.e., silicon or red rubber). The preferred methods make use of either a commercial syringe device with a built-in pressure gauge

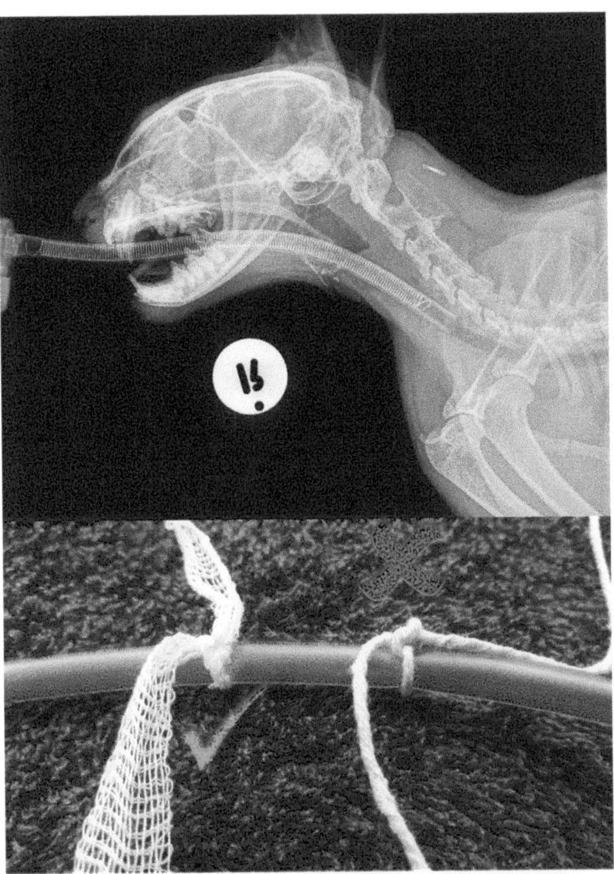

Figure 12.8 The tip (bevel) of the endotracheal tube should advance until the level of the thoracic inlet and the length of the endotracheal tube should be at the level of the incisor teeth (top). Note that this is a reinforced (armored) endotracheal tube with a metal coil in the wall of the endotracheal tube, and these tubes cannot be cut to size. Cats (and dogs) where small-sized endotracheal tubes are used (<5.0 mm), they should not be secured using string because of the risk of overtightening the knot (red cross) rather a gauze ribbon should be used (green tick).

or a purpose-built cuff inflation manometer (see Chapter 4). In these methods, the device is used to inflate the cuff, which simply involves connecting the device to the one-way valve and inflating the cuff to pressure not exceeding 25 cmH_2O. The advantage is that they are quick and easy to use and reliable. However, the disadvantage is that they are expensive devices and cannot be used in silicon and red rubber ET tubes. A less accurate method that often result in cuff pressures higher than intended is the minimum occlusive volume (MOV) method. This method is where the cuff is inflated until a leak around the cuff within the trachea is no longer heard, when a pressure of 20–25 cmH_2O is applied to the patient's respiratory system. This airway pressure is measured using a breathing circuit pressure gauge (see Chapter 5). The limitation to this method is that it becomes more unreliable in a loud environment where it can be difficult to hear the sound of leaking air. A variation of MOV method that has been described in human anesthesia and sometimes used in veterinary anesthesia is to inflate the cuff until the pilot balloon is fully inflated, apply the desired target pressure to the airways (close the pop-off valve, decrease the fresh gas flow rate to 150 mL/min, and squeeze the bag while observing the airway pressure gauge), and then to deflate the cuff until a leak can be heard. Once the cuff is inflated to the desired pressure, then the pop-off valve must be opened and the fresh gas flow rate can be returned to its planned rate. This variation of MOV is the least preferred method to use in dogs and cats because of the risk of tracheal rupture, especially if applied when inflating a low-volume high-pressure cuff in smaller animals. Other methods that have been described include digital palpation of the ET tube pilot balloon or inflating the cuff based on reproducing a previously learned cuff pressure through experience. However, these methods are not reliable or accurate and can potentially result in cuff overinflation and tracheal injury. Caution is advised when using these less preferred techniques, and they should only be used in scenarios where availability of equipment is limited.

Other Methods of Managing the Airway

If orotracheal intubation using an ET tube is not possible for whatever reason, then alternative techniques can be considered such as using a facemask or a supraglottic (laryngeal mask) airway device. A facemask (with a diaphragm) is adequate for short procedures to supplement oxygen. Hold the facemask securely and push the corner of mandibles forward into the facemask (which straightens the airway). This technique is suitable for cats undergoing short duration procedures such as sterilization (i.e., neutering, castration, etc.). Supraglottic airway devices are a compromise between a facemask and endotracheal intubation, and the *supraglottic airway* is defined as the region rostral (over) to the *rima glottidis* of the larynx and these devices are placed over this region without entering the larynx or trachea. Specifically designed devices for cats (and dogs) are available. However, it is also possible to use small human laryngeal masks (e.g., size 1–2), which have an inflatable cushion to improve pharyngeal fit. Supraglottic airway devices do not create such a good seal as a cuffed endotracheal tube and so are less reliable for intermittent positive pressure ventilation or manual ventilation or if there is a risk of aspiration (e.g., during a dental procedure). The technique is less popular in dogs than cats due to the relative ease and low complication rate associated with endotracheal intubation in dogs; however, supraglottic airway devices may be considered particularly in situations where repeated frequent intubation may increase risk of trauma (e.g., daily radiotherapy or dressing changes requiring general anesthesia).

Placing a supraglottic airway device:

- Check depth of anesthesia is adequate
- An assistant should hold the head as for intubation of the trachea
- Open the mouth and gently pull tongue forward (some veterinarians will use topical lidocaine in cats to reduce reactions)
- Advance the supraglottic airway device into the oropharynx until resistance is felt
- Secure and inflate cushioned seal (if present)
- Ensure correct location

Capnography is very useful (considered mandatory when using supraglottic airway devices by some anesthetists) to ensure a lack of obstructive ventilatory pattern (which may also produce paradoxical breathing) either due to the epiglottis being folded back into the larynx during device insertion or, more commonly, migration (e.g., twisting) of the device during use.

Principles of Local Anesthesia

Regional anesthesia is the depositing of a local anesthetic drug, using various techniques, to cause anesthesia of an anatomical region (e.g., a pelvic limb before stifle surgery). In contracts, *local anesthesia* is defined as the topical (e.g., spraying the *rima glottidis* before tracheal intubation) or local infiltration (e.g., ring-block around a cutaneous mass) of a local anesthetic drug. The techniques of regional anesthesia include locoregional blocks (peripheral nerve or ganglion or plexus blocks), epidural, spinal, and intravenous regional blocks. The common techniques used in dogs and cats are local and locoregional blocks and epidurals, which are described further.

Local and Regional Blocks

Local anesthetic drugs are cost-effective ways to provide additional analgesia or even complete desensitization of an area. Simple ways to use include infiltration (e.g., a "line" block, administered before or after surgery) or instilling into a wound before surgical closure (a so-called "splash block"). The authors usually avoid doses above 4 mg/kg lidocaine or 1.5 mg/kg bupivacaine or ropivacaine. Using a more dilute solution can assist spread in smaller individuals by allowing a larger volume to be used.

Testicular (sometimes called intratesticular blocks) injection of local anesthetic can provide additional analgesia for castration. Systemic uptake is high from this technique, so lidocaine is a better choice than bupivacaine. Many anesthetists will retain a small amount of the desired dose of local anesthetic to infiltrate around the spermatic cord.

Locoregional anesthesia in the form of peripheral or plexus nerve blocks requires a very good understanding of anatomy. Some of the techniques used to block the pelvic limb are easy to master compared to the thoracic limb. Ideally, an ultrasound machine and a nerve stimulator (used alone or together) should be used to improve the safety of performing these blocks. However, in the authors' experience, performing a "blind" (no ultrasound or nerve stimulator) block of the ischiatic nerve and saphenous branch of the femoral nerve is easy to master, with a very low complication rate (Figure 12.9). There is a growing body of evidence showing peripheral or plexus nerve blocks to be highly effective. Readers are encouraged to refer to readily available resources (reference texts, online materials, and training courses) before undertaking more advance locoregional techniques.

Epidural

Administration of analgesic drugs into the epidural space (extradural anesthesia/analgesia, commonly called an "epidural") can easily be performed in practice without any specialist equipment. It is important to maintain aseptic technique, however. Small plastic drapes are economical to purchase and can reduce the risk of contamination of the site. Sterile gloves should be worn.

An epidural with local anesthetic will cause desensitization of the pelvic limbs and abdomen (depending on volume administered). Use of an opioid in the epidural space can result in longer lasting analgesia than the drug administered systemically. Morphine is particularly useful in this scenario, as its relatively low lipid solubility increases retention, providing a long duration of action (18–24 h).

Contraindications to performing epidural injections are localized infection at the needle insertion site, clotting disorders, abnormal anatomy (landmarks cannot be identified), sepsis, and unresolved hypotension. Relative contraindications are bacteremia and peripheral neuropathy. Local anesthetic drugs administered epidurally will block sympathetic outflow from the spinal cord, producing vasodilation. For this reason, caution should be employed should hypotension be deemed a risk in a particular animal. A fluid bolus (10 mL/kg of an isotonic crystalloid such as lactated Ringer's solution, for example, administered over 15–30 min) may be appropriate to counteract the relative hypovolemia.

Most veterinarians find it easier to position the dog or cat in sternal recumbency; however, the procedure can also be

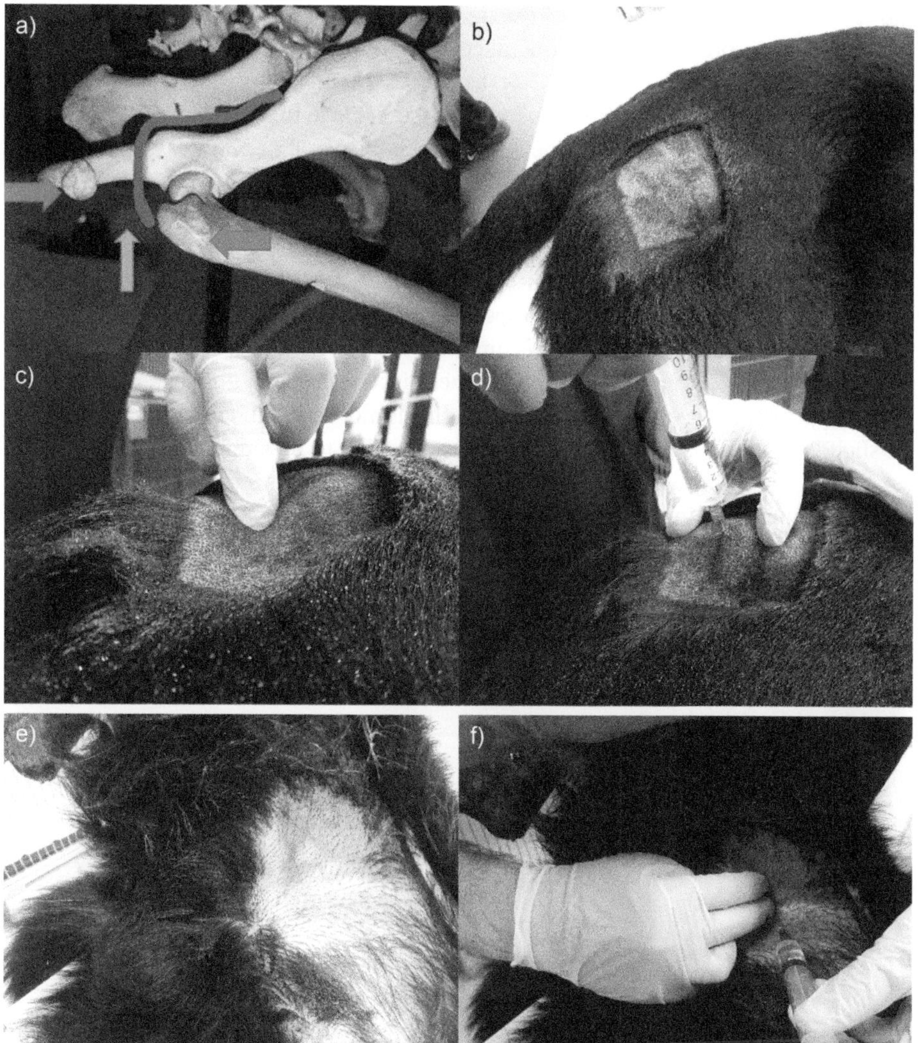

Figure 12.9 The ischiatic (sciatic) and saphenous (branch off the femoral) nerves can be blocked by administering a local anesthetic around these nerves. There are anatomical landmarks that are easy to palpate and can be used to block these nerves. The ischiatic nerve courses along the "sciatic notch" and body of the ischium caudal to the coxofemoral joint ((a) blue line). The ischiatic tuberosity ((a) left blue arrow) and trochanter major ((a) right blue arrow) of the femur are palpated. The needle is advanced between these two bone landmarks ((a) green arrow). First the region is aseptically prepared (b), then using sterile gloves, the gap between the two bone landmarks is felt (c), then a needle is advanced until it makes contact with the ischium (d), and finally once the bone is felt, the needle is retracted 1–2 mm and the syringe is aspirated before administering the local anesthetic (0.1–0.2 mL/kg). The medial aspect of the proximal pelvic limb is aseptically prepared over the "femoral triangle" (e). Then, the pulse of the femoral artery if felt (f), the needle is advanced subcutaneously immediately cranial to the femoral artery and after aspirating, and the local anesthetic is injected (0.1 mL/kg).

performed in lateral recumbency. Pulling the pelvic limbs cranially helps to "open up" the lumbosacral space. However, be mindful of displacing fractured bone fragments, especially of the pelvis or femur. Ensure that the animal is positioned with the spine straight (i.e., no twisting or bending of the thoracolumbar vertebral column).

The spread of the drug is related to the volume and speed of injection. Be aware that older or obese animals may have greater fat deposition in the epidural space and this may increase cranial spread. As a general rule, most anesthetists will suggest a maximum of 1 mL injectate per 5 kg but not exceeding a total volume of 6 mL. This volume should, if a local anesthetic is injected, cause anesthesia of the pelvic limbs and most of the abdomen. A larger volume has a risk of spreading further cranially and may affect intercostal muscle function.

Lidocaine (45 min to 1 h duration) or bupivacaine (a 3–6 h duration is often cited but, in the authors' experience, duration can exceed 6 h and last up to 12–18 h) are suitable local anesthetics. Avoid preparations that contain preservative. A spinal needle with central stylet is recommended (22–20 g, 1.5"–3"). A Tuohy needle may provide a better "feel" (loss of tissue resistance to advancement and "pop" sensation; see later) during the procedure (Figure 12.10).

After clipping and aseptic preparation of the area, skeletal landmarks can be identified (Figure 12.11). A thumb and middle finger on the wings of the ilium will usually present the palpable "dip" of the lumbosacral space to the forefinger. The needle should be inserted with the bevel facing cranially, at an angle perpendicular to the skin. In dogs, the placement should be approximately in the middle of this space; for cats, a slightly more caudal placement is usually more effective.

Advance the needle slowly and carefully, appreciating the feeling of the needle tip advancing though the tissue layers. Once through the skin and subcutaneous tissue, the stylet may be removed and a bleb of saline placed on the hub of the needle (the "hanging drop" technique). If the needle contacts bone, the tip of the needle may be "walked" forward or backward slightly, but moving too far away from a perpendicular angle to the skin may make insertion into the space impossible so, if necessary, withdraw most of the needle length and redirect. A slight "pop" is felt as the needle penetrates the ligamentum flavum. The saline drop may be aspirated into the needle upon entry to the epidural space (however, this sign is not seen in every animal, especially smaller patients and those positioned in lateral recumbency).

Observe to check if cerebrospinal fluid emerges from the needle. This finding is more common in cats or small-breed dogs than larger ones due to the spinal cord ending more caudally. If this happens, the authors prefer to adjust doses and continue with a "spinal" (intrathecal) injection rather than attempt to reposition into the epidural space. Use approximately one-third to half of the planned epidural dose if administering intrathecally. If blood emerges from

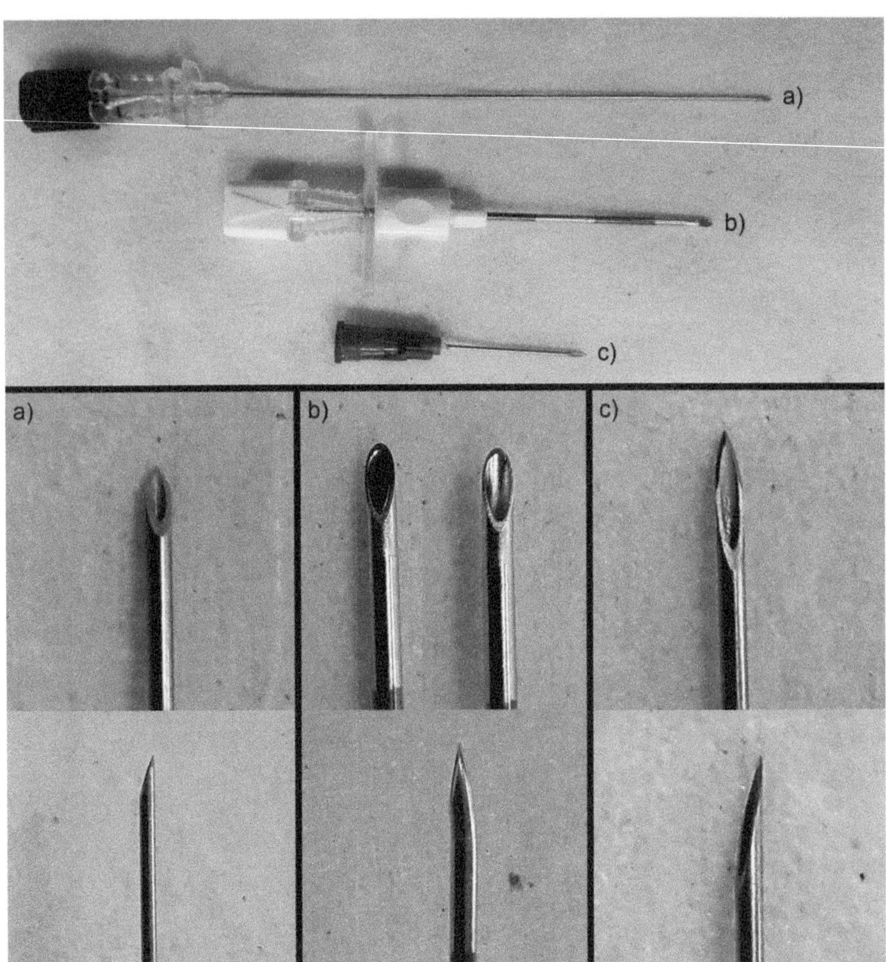

Figure 12.10 Epidural injections can be performed using an spinal needle (a) or a Tuohy needle (b) but not a hypodermic needle (c). The spinal (short bevel) and Tuohy (Huber point) needles have blunter points compared to the cutting-type needles such as the hypodermic needles (long bevel).

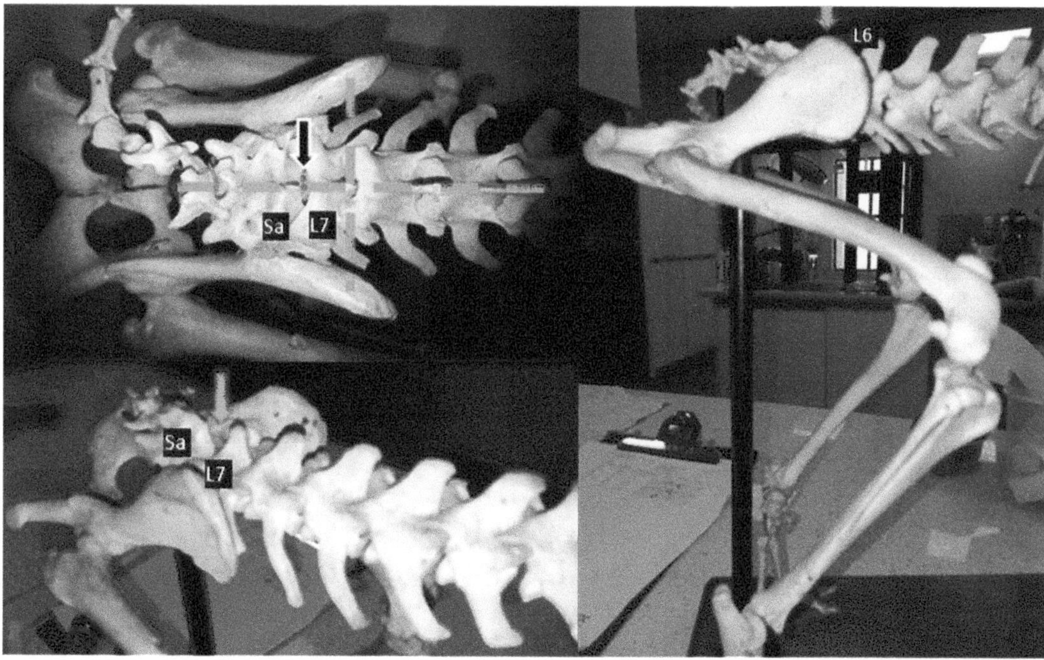

Figure 12.11 The epidural space in dogs and cats is usually entered using the lumbosacral puncture site (black and white arrow and green arrow of skeletal images). This puncture site can be identified by palpating boney landmarks. In these species, it is caudal to the seventh lumbar vertebra (L7) and cranial to the first sacral vertebra (Sa). Note that L7 is between the most dorsal arches of the ileums and that its dorsal spinal process is shorter compared to L6.

the needle, then it should be removed and the entire procedure restarted with a new needle.

When the needle is in position, it is very important that the needle does not move. Use the nondominant hand to hold the needle securely. Many anesthetists will inject a test volume of saline, which should be easily injected, with minimal resistance to flow of the injectate. Attach the syringe containing the drugs to be administered carefully, ensuring that the needle is not inadvertently pushed in (or rotated). An air bubble in the syringe can be used to identify resistance to injection. As the injection is performed, release the finger from the plunger. The air bubble should not compress (i.e., it should maintain its size) if the needle is correctly located in the epidural space. Injecting drugs into the epidural space should be done over 1–2 min. Fast injections can cause excessive cranial spread of injectate (risk of adverse cardiorespiratory effects) and an incomplete ("patchy") block.

Potential complications of performing an epidural injection are neural damage from the needle, neurotoxicity from injectate, spinal trauma, infection (abscess or meningitis), inadvertent spinal injection, inadvertent IV injection (venous sinus puncture), hypotension, bradycardia, Horner's syndrome, respiratory depression, total spinal anesthesia (cranial migration of local anesthetics), urinary retention (opioids), allergic reaction (recommended to use preservative-free drugs), pruritus (opioids), and accidental wrong drug administration.

Sedation and General Anesthesia

Additional information about sedation and induction drug protocols can be found on the American Animal Hospital Association website (https://www.aaha.org/aaha-guidelines/2020-aaha-anesthesia-and-monitoring-guidelines-for-dogs-and-cats/resource-center) and the Association of Veterinary Anaesthetists website (https://ava.eu.com/resources/checklists).

Sedation

The concept of sedation is explained in Chapter 2. Sedating dogs and cats are very common procedures in veterinary practice because it facilitates, for example, safe handling for animal and handler, allows for noninvasive (e.g., diagnostic imaging) and minor-invasive (e.g., cannulating veins, placing nasogastric tubes, etc.) procedures to be performed, and as premedication before inducing general anesthesia. The purpose of sedating a dog or cat needs to be established before selecting the drug(s) to be used and the route of administration (oral, oral transmucosal, SC, IM, and IV).

The purpose of sedation will determine the required depth of sedation, which ranges from mild to heavy (profound) sedation. In other words, the planned procedure influences both the choice of drugs and dosing. For example, for radiography with multiple positioning, and a requirement to be perfectly still, higher doses may be required than for other procedures, such as ultrasound. The animal's temperament will also affect dosing. A calm, quiet animal may require low doses. Regardless of the purpose of sedation, the overall goals are to cause anxiolysis (Chapters 2 and 6). A common misconception is that sedation is safer than general anesthesia. However, the deeper the level of sedation the higher the risk of an adverse event occurring (e.g., aspiration of refluxed gastric content), especially if the patient is moved to different location or restrained in various recumbencies. Any patient that is sedated should have their cardiovascular and respiratory systems monitored (see Chapter 4), and the deeper the level of sedation the more frequently these systems should be monitored (i.e., at 5–10 min intervals) until the animals are aware of their surroundings, can protect their airway, and raise their head.

With regard to drug selection (see Chapters 7 and 10), the alpha-2 adrenergic receptor agonists (alpha-2 agonists) are probably the most commonly used drug class in healthy dogs and cats. They are usually given IM or IV and are often combined with opioids. Even for a nonpainful animal, using an opioid can improve the quality of sedation and reduce doses of other drugs required. Butorphanol is popular for this purpose.

Ketamine combinations (e.g., with a benzodiazepine or an alpha-2 agonist) are popular in cats.

Alfaxalone, administered IM, is gaining popularity, especially in cats. However, the volume of injection is high. In the authors' opinion, sedation produced by alfaxalone, especially when given alone, is less reliable in healthy animals than those that are older or less stable.

Health screening programs in some countries may result in a requirement to sedate a dog for cardiac echocardiography. In these cases, drugs such as alpha-2 agonists are undesirable due to their cardiac effects. If examination is not possible without sedation, butorphanol may be chosen, perhaps with a low dose of acepromazine.

Benzodiazepines produce very little effect on the cardiovascular system; however, in healthy animals they can cause some excitement (reduced inhibition) and so are generally not administered alone. Benzodiazepines are much more useful for sicker animals (ASA IV or V) or in combination with ketamine or alfaxalone. Combining a benzodiazepine with an opioid (such as butorphanol) is very commonly used, perhaps due to perceived safety; however, this combination in healthy dogs and cats is not particularly effective in causing sedation.

Examples of drugs and doses are provided in Table 12.5.

General Anesthesia

General anesthesia is presented in detail in Chapter 2. For general anesthesia, most dogs and cats will be sedated (premedicated) either before or after placement of an intravenous cannula. Lighter sedation may be adequate to facilitate handling and a smooth induction compared to the deeper levels of sedation needed for performing some procedures under sedation alone. Concepts and principles of how to deliver the various drug(s) used to maintain anesthesia are explained in Chapter 6. See examples of anesthesia induction protocols in Table 12.6.

Recovery

At the end of anesthesia, it is wise to ensure completion of all procedures before ending anesthetic administration. Even procures such as bandaging and clipping nails are, in preference, completed during anesthesia. These apparently innocuous procedures can stimulate a patient unnecessarily during recovery and cause a rough recovery (emergence delirium/dysphoria).

Body temperature should be monitored before and during recovery. Hypothermia occurs in over 90% of healthy dogs and cats during general anesthesia and can prolong recovery if no steps are taken to maintain or correct body temperature.

Extubation of the trachea should be performed when there are signs of swallowing (in dogs), indicating that the animal can protect its airway. In cats, laryngospasm is a risk if the swallow reflex has returned at the time of extubation. Generally, cats are extubated when cranial reflexes return, most commonly, a brisk palpebral reflex, ear flick response to touching the hairs on the inner pinna, and increased jaw tone.

Many veterinarians will deflate the cuff of the ET tube and undo ties on the basis of reducing time necessary for extubation in the case of an unexpectedly rapid recovery. The authors prefer not to undo ties when the breathing system is attached, ensuring no drag on the ET tube (leading to inadvertent extubation). Ideally, the animal should be placed in a cage (or recovery area), and once in its recovery position (and the bladder emptied), only then should preparations be made to extubate. The oral cavity should be inspected to make sure it is clear: no pools of saliva, gastric content, tooth polish or blood, etc. (e.g., from oral surgical or dental procedures). A square swab can be used to clear the oral cavity. Deflating the cuff removes protection for the airway. The authors prefer to maintain the cuff inflated until the time of extubation, but

Table 12.5 Examples of drug combinations for sedation (or premedication) in dogs and cats. Doses (mg/kg) are to provide moderate sedation in healthy animals and intended for intramuscular administration. Decreasing or increasing the dose by 50% can result in a lighter or deeper sedation.

Drug combination	Doses		Notes
	Dogs	Cats	
Acepromazine +	0.03	0.03	
opioid (select 1)	Methadone: 0.3	Methadone: 0.2	
	Morphine: 0.3	Morphine: 0.2	
	Buprenorphine: 0.03	Buprenorphine: 0.03	
	Butorphanol: 0.3	Butorphanol: 0.2	Only for nonpainful procedures or animals not in pain
Alpha-2 adrenergic receptor agonist	Medetomidine: 0.01	Medetomidine: 0.03	
(select 1) +	Dexmedetomidine: 0.005	Dexmedetomidine: 0.015	
	Xylazine: 1.0	Xylazine: 1.0	Associated with increased peri-anesthetic mortality in dogs
opioid			Doses of opioids as for Acepromazine + opioid combination
Benzodiazepine (select 1) +	Midazolam: 0.4	Midazolam: 0.2	
	Diazepam: 0.3	Diazepam: 0.2	Recommended to only be given IV after sedation from the opioid is observed
opioid			Doses of opioids as for Acepromazine + opioid combination
Alfaxalone +	1.0	2.0	If volume a concern, then administered SC
Alpha-2 adrenergic receptor agonist +			Doses of alpha-2 adrenergic receptor agonist as in the preceding text
opioid			Doses of opioids as for Acepromazine + opioid combination
Ketamine	5.0	3.0	Recommended in very anxious aggressive animals
Alpha-2 adrenergic receptor agonist +			Doses of alpha-2 adrenergic receptor agonist as in the preceding text
opioid			Doses of opioids as for Acepromazine + opioid combination
Aggressive geriatric animal of unknown cardiovascular status			
Although IM combinations are used, applying a Chill Protocol in planned cases is advised (see Chapter 10)			
Alfaxalone +	1.5	2.0	
[OR Ketamine +]	3.0	3.0	Ketamine can be considered if alfaxalone is not available
Butorphanol +	0.4	0.3	
Midazolam	0.5	0.3	

close vigilance is required. Attention to jaw tone, responses to opening the mouth, and gentle withdrawal of the tongue can indicate that extubation will be soon required. If the ET tube is secured using a tie around the back of the head, this may be pulled forward, over the head, or cut to release rapidly, without requiring untying. Untying knots made in some materials (gauze ribbon or string) can be challenging, especially if the dog or cat has long fur. After

Table 12.6 Examples of anesthesia induction protocols in dogs and cats.

Drug	Level of sedation	Dose		Notes
		Dog	Cat	
IV induction				
Doses are for the initial bolus to be administered IV over 10–30 s. Additional drug should be drawn up into the syringe in case an additional dose needs to be given. Additional doses are usually at 50% of the initial dose.				
Propofol	None	3.0	3.0	
	Light	2.0	2.0	
	Moderate	1.0	1.0	
	Deep	1.0	1.0	Apnea can be frequently observed
Alfaxalone	None	2.0	2.0	
	Light	1.5	1.0	
	Moderate	1.0	0.5	
	Deep	0.5	0.5	Apnea can be frequently observed
Thiopentone	None	7.5	Not recommended	
	Light	5.0	Not recommended	
	Moderate	2.0	Not recommended	
	Deep	1.0	Not recommended	
Ketamine	None	7.5	7.5	Not recommended to be given alone use midazolam or diazepam at 0.4 mg/kg
	Light	6.0	6.0	
	Moderate	5.0	5.0	Might not require midazolam or diazepam
	Deep	2.0	2.0	Might not require midazolam or diazepam
IM induction				
Doses are for drug combination with the intention of inducing general anesthesia. Once the animal is immobilized or under general anesthesia, then an IV cannula should be placed in a peripheral vein.				
Alfaxalone OR	–	2.0	3.0	
Ketamine +	–	7.5	6.0	Apneustic breathing patterns are common
Medetomidine OR		0.015	0.06	
Dexmedetomidine +		0.007	0.03	
opioid (select 1)		Morphine: 0.3	Morphine: 0.2	
		Methadone: 0.3	Methadone: 0.2	
		Buprenorphine: 0.03	Buprenorphine: 0.03	Recommended to give IV once immobilized
		Butorphanol: 0.3	Butorphanol: 0.2	Not recommended for painful procedures or animals

extubation, ensure a patent airway (pharyngeal and laryngeal muscle relaxation can be present which can lead to partial or complete airway occlusion) is present by feeling for airflow from the nares during exhalation or hearing air flow through the larynx. Another method, useful in animals less than 3 kg, is to hold a microscope slide in front of the nares and condensation of air should be seen during exhalation. Observation of inspiratory chest excursions alone is not an indicator that there is airflow during the respiratory cycle.

Antagonism of alpha-2 agonists may be required in shorter duration surgeries. When these drugs are given with ketamine, ensure a minimum of 40 min after ketamine has been administered before antagonism. In longer duration procedures, where some alpha-2 agonist has been eliminated, a half-dose of antagonist may be given.

Ensure a quiet, comfortable, warm place for recovery with suitable observation in this high-risk period.

Peri-anesthetic Plans for Common Scenarios in Dogs and Cats

Spay-neuter Clinics

High-volume spay-neuter clinics often have some special requirements for staff and animals. If animals are stray/feral, they are more likely to be difficult to handle and examine. There is often little follow-up available and the cost of the techniques and drugs can constrain drug options. There may be a lack of equipment in some remote clinics and in some countries. Availability of drugs (and oxygen) will play a factor in some countries (including legalities of transporting drugs and oxygen to remote locations). There may be limited staff support for monitoring and assisting with patient care during the peri-anesthetic period. Therefore, a reliable, standard drug protocol can improve overall safety and decrease peri-anesthetic mortality. The mortality rates for cats (0.05%; 1 in 2000) and dogs (0.009%; 1 in 11111) in high-volume spay-neuter clinics are much lower than those reported from a mix of practice types (see the preceding text). This low mortality rate reflects the combination of multiple factors, including many of the animals being relatively young and healthy and a short duration procedure performed by skilled and experienced people. Regardless of the peri-anesthetic plan, the authors recommend that, at minimum, IV access should be obtained before intra-abdominal surgery is started. The association of shelter veterinarians have compiled guidelines for spay-neuter programs that can be accessed online (https://doi.org/10.2460/javma.249.2.165).

The peri-anesthetic plan for dogs and cats includes a basic, abbreviated clinical examination. In dogs, injecting a drug for premedication, followed by induction and maintenance of anesthesia, can be performed by total intravenous anesthesia using an intermittent bolus technique. Oxygen support is provided when available. Alpha-2 agonists in combination with an opioid are useful as IM sedation of all dogs, especially those that are difficult to handle. In very difficult dogs, ketamine can be included during premedication. Induction and maintenance of anesthesia is usually carried out by intermittent IV doses of propofol, alfaxalone, ketamine, or thiopentone. In some high-volume clinics, inhalational anesthetics are used to maintain anesthesia. Tracheal intubation is recommended due to risk of regurgitation, even if there is not capacity to supply oxygen or inhalational anesthetics. By contrast, general anesthesia in cats is often induced directly, without a premedication phase, using an IM ketamine-, tiletamine- (with zolazepam), or alfaxalone-based drug combination. The primary anesthetic drug is combined with an alpha-2 agonist and an opioid. For high-volume clinics, if the surgery is quick (<10–15 min) there may be no need for additional drugs (injectable or inhalational) to be given for maintenance. Tracheal intubation may be unnecessary in cats that are healthy and undergoing efficient, brief surgery (<30 min). However, suitable equipment for intubation should be available. In dogs and cats, analgesia can be supplemented using a nonsteroidal anti-inflammatory drug (NSAID) and local anesthetic blocks (e.g., splash block in the incision or pre-incisional line block for a spay and testicular block for castrations).

Diabetes Mellitus

Diabetes mellitus is common in dogs and reasonably common in cats. In most cases, patients need to be anesthetized for procedures unrelated to diabetes (e.g., dental procedures, orthopedic surgery, etc.).

As we anesthetize the diabetic animal, we need to consider the disruption to the usual feeding and insulin regimen. Hyperglycemia is common; however, hypoglycemia may easily be overlooked while under anesthesia. Hypotension is more common in diabetic dogs than the normal patient, probably due to osmotic diuresis caused by hyperglycemia subsequently causing hypovolemia. It is increasingly recognized there may be serum potassium disruption too. Commonly, serum potassium is low (approximately 3.0–3.5 mmol/L) and will fluctuate during the day according to insulin levels. However, if the animal is hypovolemic, then a decrease in glomerulus filtration rate can result in an increase serum potassium (even causing hyperkalemia). Low serum potassium levels can result in muscle weakness, especially during recovery, whereas hyperkalemia can result in cardiac arrhythmias and a reduction in cardiac output (see Chapter 17). Measuring this electrolyte during the pre-anesthetic workup is recommended.

Different strategies regarding timing of anesthesia have been suggested. Traditionally, it has been recommended to perform anesthesia first thing in the morning after a longer fasting period (no morning meal). However, some veterinarians advocate providing a morning meal (along with prescribed insulin), followed by a shorter fasting period, and anesthesia in the afternoon. Guidelines from the American Animal Hospital Association suggest a small meal 2–4 h before anesthesia (https://www.aaha.org/globalassets/02-guidelines/2020-anesthesia/aahaanesthesiaguidelines_fastingandtreatmentrecommendations.pdf). Regardless of feeding strategy, it is important to check blood glucose before premedication. There are different suggested peri-anesthetic management strategies, and one option is described in Table 12.7. If the patient has ketoacidosis with diabetes mellitus, then management is more complex; dextrose may need to be supplemented along with short-acting insulin therapy (https://www.aaha.org/aaha-guidelines/diabetes-management/resource-center/tips-and-tricks-for-anesthetizing-diabetic-dogs-and-cats). Patients with complicated diabetes mellitus should be stabilized before elective surgery or, in the event of an emergency, they should be referred to a hospital where there is expertise in managing these patients. However, in every case, a mild hyperglycemia is preferred over hypoglycemia. Importantly, blood glucose must be monitored regularly during anesthesia, at least every 30 min (and more frequently if there is evidence of actual or impending hypoglycemia).

The aim of peri-anesthetic management of diabetic patients is to return the animal to its normal routine as soon as possible. Therefore, a smooth, rapid recovery period and return to feeding and insulin routine is an important aspect of management. With regard to drug selection, for premedication, an opioid will be useful depending on the procedure to be performed. Acepromazine may slightly increase the risk of hypotension in these animals. Alpha-2 agonists reduce insulin release and cause hyperglycemia; this is not generally considered a contraindication to their use provided the level of sedation they provide is useful in a given patient. Induction may be performed as considered appropriate. Maintenance with inhalational anesthetics is probably preferable to injectable drugs to promote a faster recovery.

Hyperadrenocorticism ("Cushing's Disease")

Hyperadrenocorticism is more common in dogs than cats. A surplus of endogenous steroid hormones is produced, either due to a pituitary tumor stimulating release from the adrenal gland or a functional tumor in the adrenal gland itself. The excess of steroid hormones, notably cortisol, is responsible for altered metabolism and redistribution of

Table 12.7 Peri-anesthetic protocol for insulin therapy in dogs or cats with diabetes mellitus.

	Insulin dose			
Blood glucose checks at pre-anesthetic check, during anesthesia and recovery until eating	**Based on pre-anesthetic check if anesthetic is scheduled for the morning in a fasted patient**	**Based on patient administered a full insulin dose in the morning and a small meal given 2–4 h**	**Monitoring frequency during peri-anesthetic period**	**Notes**
<70 mg/dL (3.8 mmol/L)	None	None	15 min	Administer 0.25–0.5 g/kg dextrose bolus[a]
70–90 mg/dL (<3.8–5 mmol/L)	None	None	15–30 min	Consider administer 0.25–0.5 g/kg dextrose bolus[a]
90–144 mg/dL (5–8 mmol/L)	None	None	30 min	Be prepared to treat hypoglycemia if glucose monitoring has a downward trend
144–270 mg/dL (8–15 mmol/L)	Half of the prescribed dose	None	30–60 min	No dextrose therapy required, but if the patient does not eat well post-anesthesia, then continue monitoring an consider short-acting insulin therapy; keep vigilant for the development of diabetic ketoacidosis
>270 mg/dL (>15 mmol/L)	Full prescribed dose	If diabetic ketoacidosis is diagnosed[b] in dogs or cats then consider *short-acting (regular) insulin* therapy administered IM until <270 mg/dL Initial dose 0.2 U/kg and then 1 U/kg every hour	30–60 min	As in the preceding text, but once the blood glucose is <270 mg/dL, then continue with prescribed insulin therapy; animals with diabetic ketoacidosis are critically ill and are often hypovolemic and require isotonic fluid therapy (i.e., 20 mL/kg boluses given hourly until peripheral pulses are felt or arterial blood pressure is within normal range)

[a]When administering a dextrose bolus (i.e., dextrose 50%) first, dilute the solution with normal saline (0.9% NaCl) at a 1:4 ratio and administer over 10–15 min.

[b]Hypovolemia, dehydration, blood pH <7.1, and ketones present on urinalysis.

fat. In dogs, the common clinical manifestation of hyperadrenocorticism is polyphagia, polydipsia, polyuria, heat intolerance, lethargy, abdominal enlargement giving a characteristic "pot-belly" appearance (organomegaly, increased intra-abdominal fat accumulation, and abdominal muscle weakness), panting, obesity, and generalized muscle weakness. Some dogs will present with concurrent diabetes mellitus as a result of insulin antagonism caused by hypercortisolemia. By contrast, in cats, dermatological manifestation is the hallmark characteristic of hyperadrenocorticism, with the development of very thin skin that can incur open wounds from self-grooming. In dogs, alopecia, development of comedones, bruising, calcinosis cutis, and thinning of the skin are common dermatological manifestations. These associated skin conditions and propensity to develop skin infections mean that intravenous cannulation must be done with good aseptic technique, including clipping and cleaning an appropriate area of skin. Pre-anesthetic serum chemistry may reveal increased alkaline phosphatase (ALP) and alanine aminotransferase (ALT), hypercholesterolemia, hyperglycemia, and decrease blood urea nitrogen (BUN). The hemogram is characterized by a reticulocytosis and stress leukogram (mature neutrophilia, lymphopenia, monocytosis, and eosinopenia). Thyroid hormone concentrations and response to thyroid stimulating hormone stimulation are decreased and resemble euthyroid sick syndrome. The commonly measured liver enzyme activity (ALP and ALT) does not indicate overall liver function and its ability to metabolize anesthetic and analgesic drugs (see Chapter 19). Selection of drugs is determined by the patient's cardiovascular and respiratory function rather than hepatic function. Urinalysis is an important pre-anesthetic assessment because urinary tract infections are very common. Hypercortisolemia increases the risk of infection and antimicrobial therapy is warranted for animals undergoing surgery. Dogs are prone to developing a hypercoagulopathy with an increased risk of thrombotic events. There is a general consensus that not all dogs with hyperadrenocorticism require antithrombotic therapy, but if they have additional risk factors for developing a hypercoagulable state, then antithrombotic therapy should be started. The American College of Veterinary Emergency and Critical Care drafted a consensus statement on the Rational Use of Antithrombotics in Veterinary Critical Care (CURATIVE) in small animals (see Further Reading). Therefore, specifically asking about current drug therapy is important in these patients because they may already be receiving antithrombotic therapy, which can result in increased risk of intra-operative hemorrhage.

The clinical manifestations of hyperadrenocorticism have consequences for general anesthesia, which can be managed with particular attention to supporting cardiovascular and respiratory function. Assessing perfusion and intravascular volume status is important because of the potential combined effects of polyuria and withholding water before an anesthetic. In patients with a very pendulous abdomen, providing a 10 mL/kg bolus of isotonic fluids before premedication can help prevent post-induction hypotension, especially if the patient requires mechanical ventilation. Muscle weakness and abdominal enlargement can also result in fatigue soon after induction of anesthesia and mechanical ventilation may be required. Furthermore, in very obese dogs, the functional residual capacity and tidal volumes are smaller than healthy dogs, resulting in more atelectasis. This makes these dogs susceptible to a form of obesity hypoventilation syndrome (Pickwickian syndrome; term adopted from human medicine) in which persistent hypercapnia that worsens after anesthetic induction occurs. These obese patients will almost always require mechanical ventilation. Dogs and cats that have alopecia and muscles that fatigue quickly are unable to generate enough body heat and are prone to developing peri-anesthetic hypothermia, especially during the recovery period where monitoring may be less frequent.

Drug selection for sedation and anesthesia in dogs with mild obesity and normal intravascular volumes are similar to any ASA I or II patient. However, very obese patients, those that do not have good exercise tolerance, would benefit from the use of drugs that have multiple sites of metabolism or those that can be antagonized if the response to the drug is unexpected. Generally, premedication with an opioid, followed by induction with propofol (alone, or with a benzodiazepine), and maintenance using an inhalational anesthetic are common combinations. In very anxious animals, sedation with an alpha-2 agonist or acepromazine (only if normovolemic), along with an opioid, can be considered. The use of locoregional anesthesia should be included, where possible, in all cases. The routine use of NSAIDs in dogs with hyperadrenocorticism is cautioned because of an increased incidence of gastrointestinal ulceration. These drugs should only be used if the dog is stable on medical management, eating well, and hydrated. If needed, other analgesics can be included postoperatively (e.g., opioids and paracetamol).

Hyperthyroidism

Hyperthyroidism is more common in cats than dogs. A hyperthyroid cat will tend to present as thin, excitable, or aggressive and may be difficult to handle. Affected cats usually present with polyphagia and polydipsia. They may also have chronic kidney disease as it is relatively common in older cats. In the early stages of CKD, hyperthyroidism may mask renal disease, which becomes apparent as thyroid function is managed medically. Arterial thromboembolism is more common in cats with hyperthyroidism and concurrent heart disease. Excessive T4 leads to an increased metabolic rate and oxygen consumption. The heart rate is high, and systemic hypertension is identified in some hyperthyroid cats. Contractility of the myocardium is high and over time there is remodeling with hypertrophy of the myocardium. Differentiating hypertrophic changes related to hyperthyroidism and those due to primary cardiac disease may be difficult (see Chapter 17). In either case, stroke volume is reduced and heart rates are often rapid, often exhibiting tachycardia when the cat is at rest (>180 beats per minute). Ventricular filling during rapid heart rates is poor and, together with the left ventricular hypertrophy, a dynamic left ventricular outflow obstruction can further decrease stoke volume. Furthermore, especially in hyperthyroid cats with tachycardia, coronary perfusion is reduced due to the reduction of time in diastole. This may lead to impaired oxygen delivery despite high oxygen use by the myocardium. A key goal of pre-anesthetic stabilization is to reduce the heart rate and ensure normovolemia. Cats require lifelong medication (e.g., methimazole) or surgery (if indicated and available) at least to stabilize (resolution of polyphagia and tachycardia) the cat before thyroidectomy. Some owners will struggle to maintain oral medication at home in these cats, which may affect the control of the disease at the time of presentation for anesthesia.

An event known as a "thyroid storm" is reported in humans, where there is massive release of thyroid hormones. This has been described to occur while palpating a thyroid gland or taking fine needle aspirates and biopsies or during surgical excision. Although questionable whether cats exhibit this phenomenon, at least one suspected case has been reported, suggesting its occurrence is rare (Potter et al. 2020). Sudden additional release of T4 converted to T3 causes tachycardia and hypertension. Manipulation of the thyroid glands may also stimulate hormone release.

Many of these cats will require some sedation before procedures or placing an intravenous cannula. It is preferable to sedate hyperthyroid cats rather than risk tachycardia (and associated complications) as a result of physical restraint. In all cases, minimizing stress, fear, and anxiety are important goals in managing these cats in a hospital environment. Alpha-2 agonists may be beneficial in reducing left ventricular outflow obstruction as a result of increasing afterload. Their effect of decreasing heart rate allows for improved ventricular filling and stoke volume. However, alpha-2 agonists should not be used in hypovolemic cats. When deeper sedation is sought, options include alfaxalone or ketamine in combination with opioids or midazolam. Of these, alfaxalone-butorphanol or ketamine–midazolam, with or without an alpha-2 agonist, are preferred because they can sedate an aggressive, difficult-to-handle cat without causing pronounced cardiovascular and respiratory depression. It is common practice to use an opioid alone or in combination with a benzodiazepine for sedation. However, in cats with hyperthyroidism, the effects of sedation can be unreliable and unpredictable, especially in anxious, fractious cats. Premedication drugs that have vasodilatory effects, such as acepromazine, are best avoided because a decrease in afterload can worsen dynamic left ventricular outflow obstruction. Furthermore, cats that have not been stabilized medically before anesthesia or surgery are at risk of developing peri-operative hypotension because of vasodilation. Hyperthyroid cats are often vasoconstricted and have a contracted intravascular volume; therefore, if vasodilation occurs a relative hypovolemia is unmasked, leading to hypotension. In cats that are not stabilized, providing a 5–10 mL/kg bolus of fluids before premedication can help prevent peri-anesthetic hypotension. If the cat is to undergo thyroidectomy (unilateral or bilateral), serum ionized and total calcium should be monitored for up to three days post-operatively because the parathyroid gland is removed at the same time.

Intravenous induction of anesthesia may be completed with alfaxalone or propofol, and anesthesia maintained with inhalational anesthetics. Inhalational anesthetics (e.g., isoflurane/sevoflurane) cause cardiovascular depression. Providing good pre-operative analgesia, particularly locoregional techniques, results in a dose reduction in inhalational anesthetics that minimizes their cardiovascular depression. Fluid therapy should be administered cautiously with care not to cause fluid overload. An intra-operative isotonic fluid rate of 3 mL/kg/h is recommended (if the patient is normovolemic). For analgesia, opioids (e.g., buprenorphine, morphine, and methadone) can be used as necessary. However, the use of NSAIDs is cautioned, especially if concurrent acute kidney injury is present. Meloxicam and robenacoxib have been administered long term to cats with chronic kidney disease (see Chapter 19). However, if concurrent heart remodeling is diagnosed, then use of NSAIDs is cautioned due to the risk of arterial thromboembolism. Furthermore, as per the CURATIVE consensus statement (see the preceding text), the use of antiplatelet drugs (e.g., clopidogrel and aspirin) is warranted in cats with cardiac remodeling. The use of locoregional analgesia should be used whenever possible to minimize tachycardic responses to surgical stimulation and promote a reduction in anesthetic requirements.

Peri-anesthetic Plan for Common Emergency Procedures

Emergency Cesarean Section

Emergency cesarean section is relatively commonly required for dystocia in bitches and somewhat less common in queens. The peri-anesthetic plan for an elective cesarean section is similar to emergency situations except that dystocia is not occurring and the fetuses are not in distress. The key consideration is selecting the timing of elective cesarean section. The ideal time is when the lungs are developed and able to produce surfactant once the neonate is born. The different techniques for planning the date for an elective cesarian section is outside the scope of this textbook.

Considerations

Regurgitation of gastrointestinal contents is a higher risk than in nonpregnant animals, as gastric emptying is slower in pregnancy, there may not have been time to withdraw food, and intra-abdominal pressure is increased. The bitch may be fatigued, especially if labor is long and unproductive. If this is the case, reduced water intake may lead to dehydration and hypovolemia.

Importantly, there are changes in physiology related to pregnancy, mostly secondary to the effects of progesterone. In normovolemic pregnant animals, cardiac output is increased by up to 40% and there is limited reserve for any further increase. The functional residual capacity and tidal volume of the lungs are reduced due to physical encroachment of abdominal contents onto the diaphragm and increased intra-abdominal pressure, especially in the last weeks of pregnancy. Due to increased oxygen demand, minute ventilation is often higher (reflected by a lower arterial partial pressure of carbon dioxide) than in nonpregnant animals despite these changes, and this is achieved with a higher respiratory rate.

In some species, there are concerns about the gravid uterus pressing on the caudal vena cava when the animal is placed in dorsal recumbency and reducing venous return. Due to the shape and position of the uterine horns in bitches, this is less likely but possible depending on the fetal positions and numbers in the uterus.

The fetuses should always be considered. It is important to maintain placental blood flow and oxygen delivery during anesthesia. Placental transfer of drugs may cause decreased vigor in puppies or kittens on delivery. Therefore, peri-anesthetic drug selection should include drugs that have extrahepatic sites of metabolism or those that have antagonists.

Peri-anesthetic Plan

Parts of the peri-anesthetic plan are presented as a collage in Figure 12.12. Premedication should be carefully considered. Some practitioners avoid premedication; however, this will increase the induction dose(s) required and can also make maintaining a stable plane of anesthesia more difficult as the patient will be more responsive to surgical stimulation. In a very nervous or difficult-to-handle bitch, the alpha-2 agonist [dex]medetomidine ([0.003] - 0.007 mg/kg IV) may be considered in preference to other alpha-2 agonists. Benzodiazepines (diazepam and midazolam) should not be included in the protocol because they are associated with decreased neonatal vigor at birth and increased mortality.

A fluid bolus may be administered before induction of anesthesia (e.g., 5–10 mL/kg over 10–15 min), because most bitches are hypovolemic, especially those that have been demonstrating nesting behavior and have not drunk water in the few hours before surgery. In addition, drugs used for induction and maintenance commonly cause vasodilation and result in relative hypovolemia and hypotension. Pre-oxygenation is useful if tolerated. Clipping and washing the ventral abdomen before induction can be done if the bitch is not anxious and tolerates the response to handling and dorsal recumbency. If the bitch (and often cats) does not tolerate surgical preparation, then further preparation should be stopped to reduce anxiety and stress. Anxious and stressed animals require higher doses of induction drugs and this can be detrimental to the fetuses. Induction of anesthesia should be performed with the aim of securing a protected airway (with a cuffed ET tube) as soon as possible. Maintaining a head-up posture will reduce the chances of regurgitant material reaching the pharynx. An alternative approach is to intubate the trachea with the head positioned downward so that any regurgitant volume is likely to fall out of the oral cavity. Propofol and alfaxalone have both been used for inducing anesthesia, and there is no evidence to suggest a preference of one over the other.

Locoregional anesthesia techniques will provide analgesia and will not cross the placenta to adversely affect the fetuses. However, any procedures should not cause delay, particularly in any situations of fetal distress. Lidocaine has a rapid onset but short duration. An epidural or incisional line block may be used. Vasodilation secondary to epidural local anesthesia may reduce blood pressure. A splash block (incision line and/or ovarian pedicles) or infiltration (around the incision line) at the end of anesthesia is quick to perform and can supplement post-operative analgesia. Once the neonates are removed, a single bolus of a longer acting opioid can be administered (e.g., morphine, methadone, and hydromorphone).

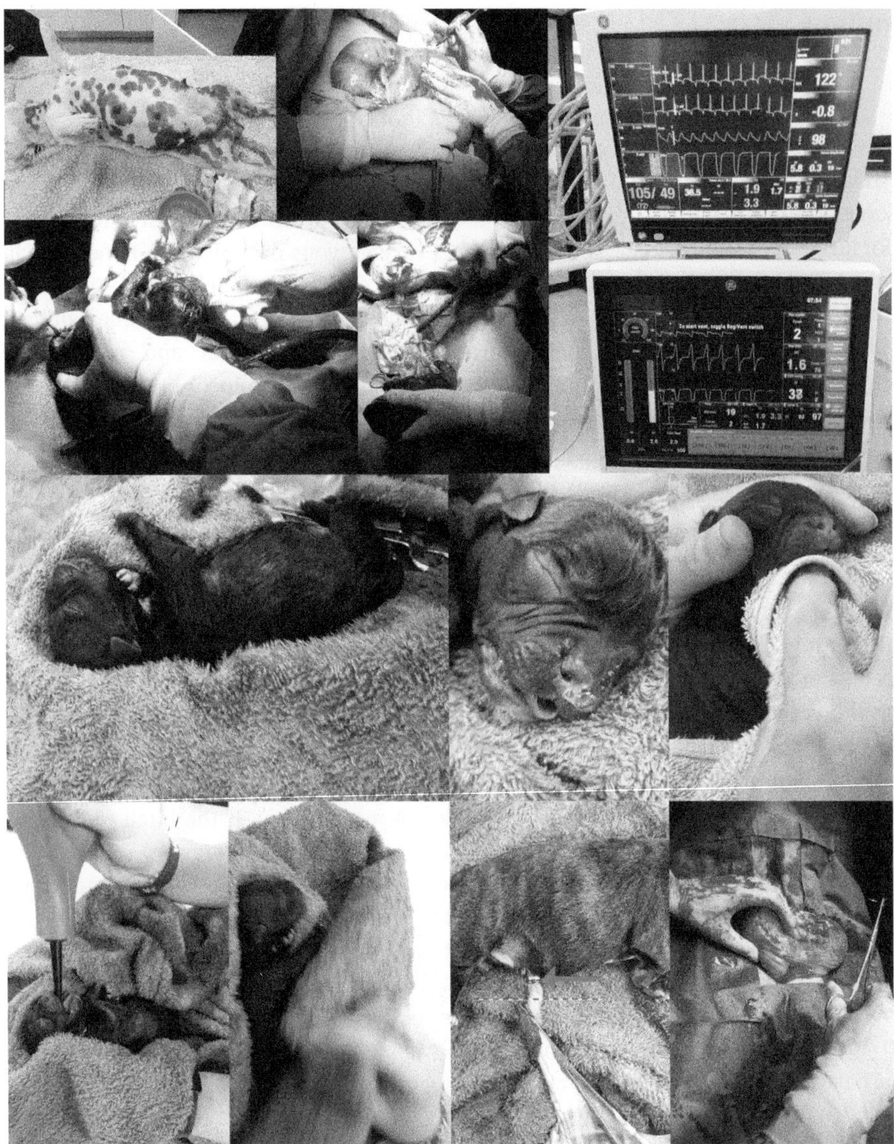

Figure 12.12 Collage of photographs of a bitch undergoing an emergency cesarean section. See text for explanations for preparing the bitch and resuscitating the neonates.

If positioning in dorsal recumbency reduces blood pressure, consider a slight oblique tilt to reduce pressure on the vena cava. A head-up tilt on the table will reduce pressure of the gravid uterus on the diaphragm. In bitches, where the uterus is large, assisting spontaneous ventilation with manual breaths 2–4 times per minute, or starting IPPV, can be useful in promoting gas exchange and delivering inhalational anesthetic to the alveoli.

An assistant (or several, if available, for litters >4 neonates) should be ready to dry neonates and ensure that they start to breathe. It is important to clear the airways of the neonate. This can be done by using a human infant suction bulb nasal aspirator or very gently swabbing the caudal oropharynx. The neonate should never be "swung" to clear the airways because of the risk of causing neural or spinal trauma or accidently dropping (throwing) the neonate on the ground. To stimulate a breath, the neonate can be rubbed along the spine in a caudal to cranial direction against the direction of hair growth. If no breaths are stimulated or crying heard, then endotracheal intubation can be considered (often using an IV cannula without the stylet). Another technique is to use acupuncture stimulation of Governing Vessel 26 (GV26, Jen Chung) that is located in the philtrum of the nose at the border of the nose and the lip. Using acupuncture needles is preferred; however, if none are available then a hypodermic needle can be used. The needle is inserted into the tissue and rotated back and forth around its long axis. Oxygen supplementations is often not required but can be used if the neonate's vigor and breathing does not progressively improve over 2–5 min of resuscitation. If the heart rate is <120 beats per minute, then chest compressions (as fast as possible, over the heart with the resuscitator's thumb and forefinger on opposite sides of the chest) can be started to speed up the heart rate, and oxygen supplementation (by facemask) should be started without delay. External chest compressions also result in movement of gases in and out of the lungs which promotes oxygenation and elimination of inhalational anesthetics, respectively. If [dex]medetomidine was administered to the bitch during premedication, antagonism using atipamezole (0.05 mg/neonate SC) may be required in the neonates.

For post-operative analgesia in the bitch, local anesthetics are useful as there is no transfer in milk to the neonates. Opioids and NSAIDs (specifically meloxicam or carprofen) may pass to the neonates in milk; however, pharmacokinetic studies on these drugs indicate the transferred concentrations are low and unlikely to be significant. A rapid recovery from anesthesia is desirable in order to improve nursing behavior. Before recovery, the ventral abdomen should be rinsed with warm water (avoiding the surgical site) to remove soaps and substances used during the surgical scrub. In general, additional doses of opioids in the recovery period are often not required, but the bitch should be evaluated for pain as individual responses to surgery vary. If painful, an opioid can be administered though care should be taken in dose selection to avoid sedation.

Pyometra

Pyometra is a severe type of endometritis associated with infection. The uterus is inflamed and contains purulent material. More common in the bitch than the queen, pyometra may be open (where there is a discharge from the vulva) or closed. Patient presentation can vary from minimal systemic illness (ASA II) to critically ill (ASA IV or V). Generally, the peri-anesthetic plan of an ASA II patient is similar to that for ovariohysterectomy. In sick patients (>ASA III), pre-anesthetic stabilization is required as described in the following text.

Considerations

The bitch will tend to present with polyuria and polydipsia and may be clinically dehydrated. Concurrent urinary tract infection is common. Renal signs, including azotemia, are often present in dogs but less frequently seen in cats.

The uterus may be fragile, particularly if very distended. This may contribute to difficulty during surgical manipulation but could lead to rupture and a consequent septic abdomen, especially in closed cervix pyometra (Figure 12.13).

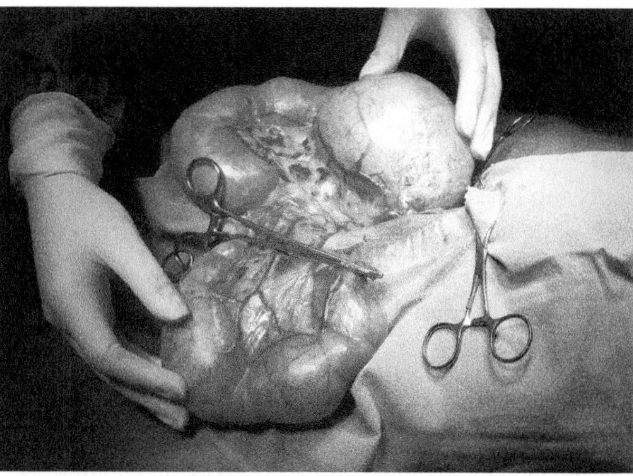

Figure 12.13 The uterus can be very large in animals with a closed cervix pyometra. In this case, the 4.2 kg Pomeranian had a 1.2 kg uterus that was surgically removed by ovariohysterectomy.

Surgical management of a pyometra requires an ovariohysterectomy. Although this is the same surgery as often performed for neutering, it is technically more challenging due to the enlarged, fragile, and inflamed uterus, with an associated increased risk of hemorrhage.

The decision to use NSAIDs should be carefully considered. Dehydration (and hypovolemia) will exacerbate the risk of adverse effects and renal effects are a particular concern. NSAIDs are usually withheld until hypovolemia is corrected and other analgesics (e.g., opioids) used in their place.

Peri-anesthetic Plan

Blood sampling for biochemistry is useful to check for azotemia. Hematology may reveal leukocytosis and possible anemia (nonregenerative). Generous pre-anesthetic fluids (e.g., 10–30 mL/kg bolus over 30–60 min of an isotonic crystalloid) to ensure hydration and correction of uremia (if possible) is advantageous. Opioids used alone for premedication are likely to provide adequate sedation for most animals.

Pre-oxygenation is useful, particularly in individuals with a markedly distended abdomen. Induction of anesthesia may be performed using various induction drugs. Using a co-induction technique (e.g., midazolam + ketamine, midazolam + alfaxalone, or ketamine + propofol) may be useful to decrease doses of individual drugs and associated depressant effects.

During anesthesia, arterial blood pressure should be monitored and supported as necessary to ensure adequate renal perfusion. Local anesthetic drugs may be used (e.g., epidural [not in hypovolemic animals, see the preceding text] and local anesthetic infiltration). If additional analgesia is required, short-acting opioids (e.g., fentanyl) or lidocaine (not in cats) can be administered by IV infusion. Dogs, especially if critically ill, can benefit from IV lidocaine boluses (1–2 mg/kg over 10 min) or a constant rate infusion (1–3 mg/kg/h). The benefit is related to lidocaine's analgesic, anti-inflammatory, and anti-endotoxic properties.

Care should be taken with NSAID use. Older NSAIDs (e.g., ketoprofen and aspirin) were associated with renal dysfunction in animals with pyometra. Although modern drugs (e.g., meloxicam, carprofen, and robenacoxib) are less likely to cause adverse effects, it is important to ensure appropriate hydration, renal perfusion, and correction of uremia before administration. Fluid support should be continued into recovery until the animal is eating and drinking on its own.

Urinary Obstruction

Urethral obstruction is a common problem in male cats but can also occur in male dogs (see Chapter 19). Calculi form in the urine and become lodged in the urethra (common) or ureter (less common). The narrower male urethra (and *os penis* in male dogs) is more likely to become obstructed compared to female cats and dogs (Figure 12.14). Animals may present with a history of stranguria or pollakiuria (ASA II or III), be systemically ill (ASA IV), or moribund (ASA V).

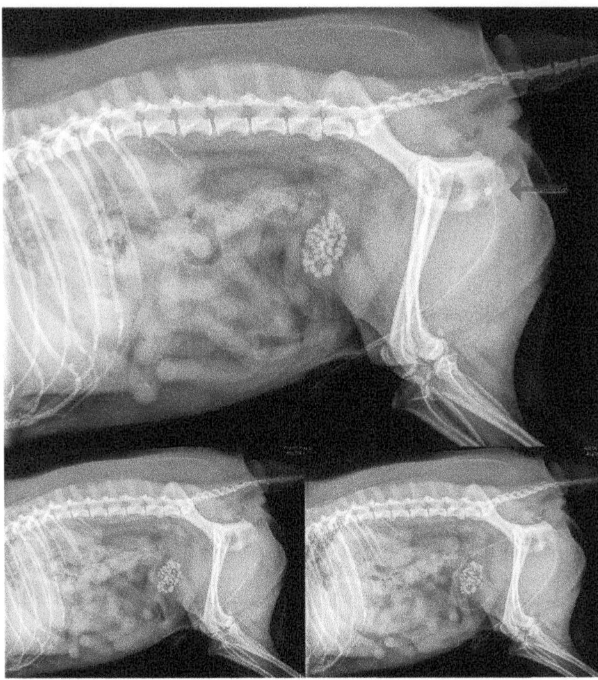

Figure 12.14 Sequential lateral abdominal radiographs of a dog with a calculous blocking the urethra (top) where a urinary catheter could not be advanced into the urinary bladder (which also has calculi). The urethral calculus was hydropulsed back into the urinary bladder (bottom left) before the urinary catheter could be advanced into the bladder (bottom right).

Considerations

Animals with urinary obstruction are often dehydrated and hypovolemic. With post-renal obstruction, there is failure to eliminate urea and creatinine, and they are often elevated on blood biochemistry. The plasma potassium concentration is frequently elevated, which may be worsened by coexisting acidemia. During acidemia, there is an increased concentration of hydrogen ions in the blood and, in an attempt to decrease the hydrogen ion concentration, it is exchanged for intracellular potassium, which can worsen hyperkalemia. Other causes of hyperkalemia are secondary to a decrease in glomerular filtration rate or uroabdomen. Cardiac action potentials may be affected by hyperkalemia, leading to bradycardia and other electrocardiographic changes, such as an absent P wave and a "spiked" or "tented" T wave.

Peri-anesthetic Plan

Parts of the peri-anesthetic plan are presented as a collage in Figure 12.15. Urinary catheterization may be attempted in conscious and obtunded animals, but sedation is usually required. Epidurals using sacrococcygeal and coccygeal approaches are becoming common practice because they contribute to analgesia and relaxation of the urethra, which can facilitate catheterization. The same principles of epidural injection via the lumbosacral approach apply to sacrococcygeal and coccygeal approaches as described in the preceding text (except for a lower risk of hypotension as local anesthetic distribution is more limited). In some cases, where the urinary catheter cannot be passed or if additional procedures are planned, e.g., for retropulsion of calculi and cystotomy, then an anesthetic must be planned.

Before anesthesia, a blood sample should be drawn to check acid–base status, presence of azotemia (or uremia; see Chapter 19), and hyperkalemia. Some stabilization before the procedure is beneficial. Fluids (e.g., initial bolus of 10–20 mL/kg of isotonic crystalloid administered over 30–60 min; the bolus often needs to be repeated 2–3 times) can start to correct hydration (dehydration is corrected over 12–36 h), intravascular volume, and lower potassium, although a plan to void urine should be enacted within 1 h of starting a fluid bolus. If the bladder is very distended, cystocentesis may be required. Most anesthetists are reluctant to anesthetize animals with serum potassium >6–6.5 mmol/L. However, if the heart rate is >150 and >80 in cats and dogs, respectively, then the hyperkalemia may not be associated with an arrhythmia. Ideally, ECG monitoring should be used where available. If heart rates are lower than these values (and the presence of arrhythmias cannot

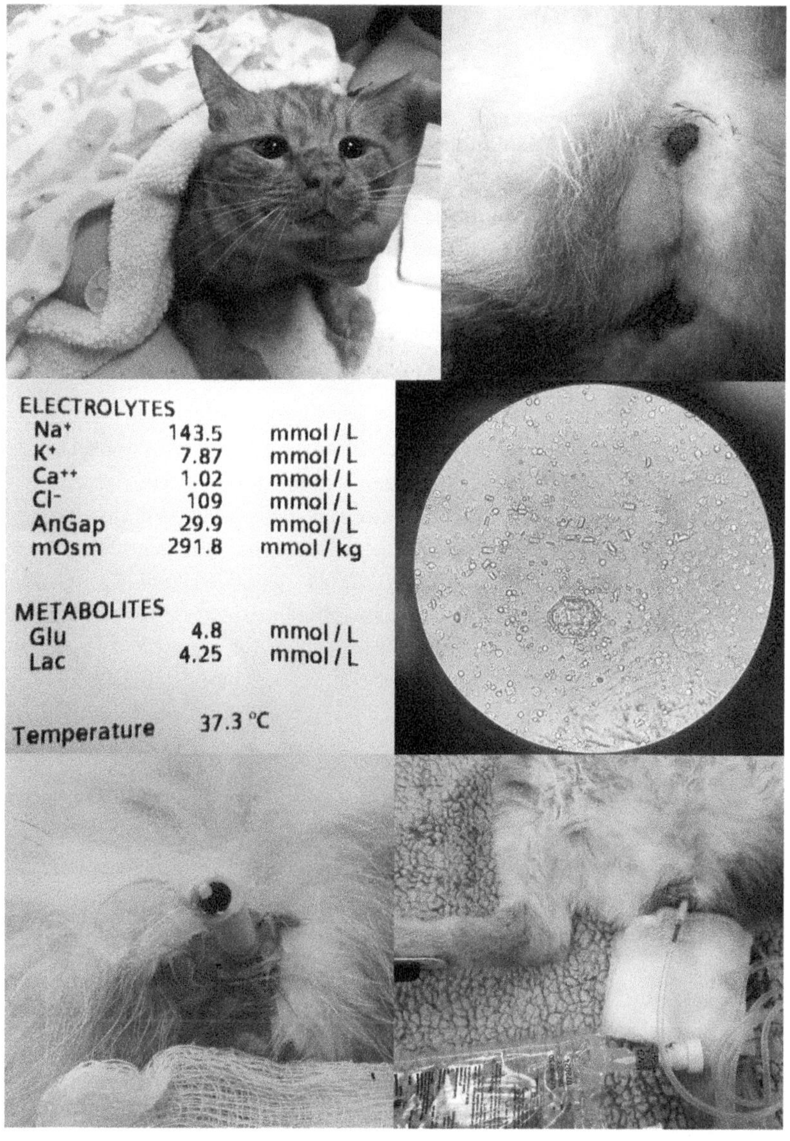

Figure 12.15 A cat that presented with a urethral obstruction causing a "blocked cat" was very depressed and weak. A large (often hard feeling) bladder can easily be palpated and blood tinging of the perineal region is common. Evaluating the electrolytes will often reveal a hyperkalemia and a sediment smear done during the urinalysis might reveal crystalluria (green arrow). A major priority in patient management is to decompress the bladder by placing a urinary catheter and attaching it to a "closed" collection system, such as an IV admin set attached to an empty 200 mL bag.

be ruled out by ECG), then treating hyperkalemia becomes more urgent. The mainstay of treatment is fluids (to dilute) and administration of a glucose bolus (0.5 g/kg dextrose 50%, diluted with normal saline in a 1:4 ratio, given over 10 min) to increase the reuptake of potassium into cells. If this is not effective, then administering short-acting (regular) insulin (0.2 U/kg IM or IV) can be considered. In severe acidemia (blood pH < 7.0) and hyperkalemia unresponsive to standard treatment, sodium bicarbonate (0.5–1 mEq/kg over 60 min) may be administered to increase pH, which will cause a decrease in potassium concentration.

The choice of isotonic fluid for resuscitation has been questioned. Previously, normal saline (0.9% NaCl) was advocated because it does not contain potassium. However, the volume required (often >30 mL/kg) for resuscitation results in a hyperchloremic acidosis. Furthermore, there is no difference in potassium dilution using a balanced electrolyte solution with a buffer (e.g., Hartmanns, Normosol, or Plasma-Lyte) compared to normal saline despite the presence of potassium in these solutions. Therefore, the use of a balanced solution is preferred because they do not contribute to acidemia and, in many cases, increase the plasma bicarbonate concentration, which aids in correcting severe metabolic acidosis. In marked bradycardia related to hyperkalemia, calcium (10% calcium gluconate or 10% calcium chloride; 0.25–1.0 mL/kg IV over 10 min) can be used to stabilize the myocardium, but it is important to be aware that this is a temporary solution that does not correct hyperkalemia.

Ultimately, relief of the obstruction is vital to allow elimination of potassium. Be aware of post-obstruction diuresis, which may increase fluid and electrolyte loss in the recovery period and can last for up to two days.

Analgesia is necessary to relieve discomfort, and repeated attempts at urinary catheterization may also cause pain and inflammation. An opioid may provide adequate sedation in some animals. Intramuscular alfaxalone (e.g., 1–2 mg/kg, with an opioid) may be helpful in cats to obtain IV access. Ketamine and its active primary metabolite, norketamine, are excreted in the urine in cats, and the effect of renal dysfunction on elimination should be borne in mind. Regardless of these concerns, ketamine-based protocols are commonly used as they provide a useful duration that allows for catheterization without needing additional anesthetic drugs. In most cases, keeping the ketamine dose <6 mg/kg can be used without major concerns of a delayed or stormy recovery. Examples of ketamine-based protocols that are commonly used include ketamine–midazolam, ketamine–midazolam–butorphanol, and ketamine–midazolam–buprenorphine. The routine use of alpha-2 agonists is cautioned, especially in cases of hyperkalemia, and should only be reserved for patients (<ASA III) who are normovolemic, normokalemic, and have no preexisting cardiac disease.

Gastric Dilation and Volvulus (GDV)

In this condition, the stomach is distended with a variable degree of torsion. More common in larger-breed and deep-chested dogs, this can present as unproductive vomiting and a rapid development of shock with third space losses of fluid (see Chapter 16). A diagnosis of GDV can be confirmed by a lateral abdominal radiograph to determine if there is dilation, with or without volvulus (Figure 12.16).

Considerations

Many dogs are hypovolemic and may show signs of shock at presentation. Abdominal distension can be marked and results in diaphragm stenting and a reduced tidal volume. In a full volvulus, stomach contents cannot be regurgitated; however, there may be fluid and saliva in the esophagus, which may present an aspiration risk at the time of induction.

Rapid treatment by stabilization (e.g., fluids and administering analgesics) and gastric decompression (often under general anesthesia) is paramount to successful management. There is debate as to whether surgical intervention (i.e., exploratory laparotomy to investigate visceral tissue damage, rupture of short gastric arteries, and gastropexy) should be performed rapidly (within 2–3 h of stabilization) after presentation or delayed until the next day. The treatment protocol is usually established by the hospital and based on previous experience and success rates. However, mortality rates are similar between rapid and delayed surgery, and therefore no clear advantage can be used to promote one treatment protocol over the other. The authors advice that rapid surgical intervention should be opted for in cases where gastric rupture (perforation) is likely or severe hemoabdomen (ultrasound abdominal free fluid score of 3 or 4, i.e., blood found as free fluid in 3–4 quadrants of the abdomen) is diagnosed. This condition is acutely painful. Electrocardiographic changes such as ventricular premature complexes (VPCs) and ventricular tachycardia are not uncommon, during or after anesthesia. The major causes of the VPCs are myocardial hypoperfusion, hypoxemia, and ischemia and can be complicated by release of inflammatory mediators and reperfusion injury. Pain and sympathetic stimulation may increase the likelihood of VPCs, but acidemia and metabolic causes are also relevant.

Peri-anesthetic Plan

If there is rapid in-house testing available, measurements of serum electrolytes, biochemistry, and hematocrit may be beneficial. These pretreatment values can be used to assist in fluid therapy and ongoing management.

At least one large-bore IV cannula will be required, and fluids should be administered rapidly in the initial stabilization phase. Pressurized fluid administration and/or a second IV line may be required to provide adequate rate of fluid administration in large dogs. A total of 30–50 mL/kg over 30–45 min might be required to resuscitate the intravascular compartment. Analgesia (e.g., 0.2–0.4 mg/kg methadone) can be provided at this time. Dogs that are dyspneic have pale mucous membranes, have VPCs or ventricular tachycardia, or signs of cyanosis should be supplemented with oxygen (facemask is less tolerated compared to quickly placing a cannula into the nasopharynx) early on during the resuscitation phase.

After adequate fluid resuscitation (generally indicated by a reduction in heart rate and improved blood pressure), anesthesia may go ahead. However, the fluid bolus administered for resuscitation will only have a transient volume expansion effect and the improved cardiovascular effect will only last for approximately 45–60 min. Therefore, the goal is to decompress the stomach before the transient volume expansion effects wane. Most dogs are unlikely to

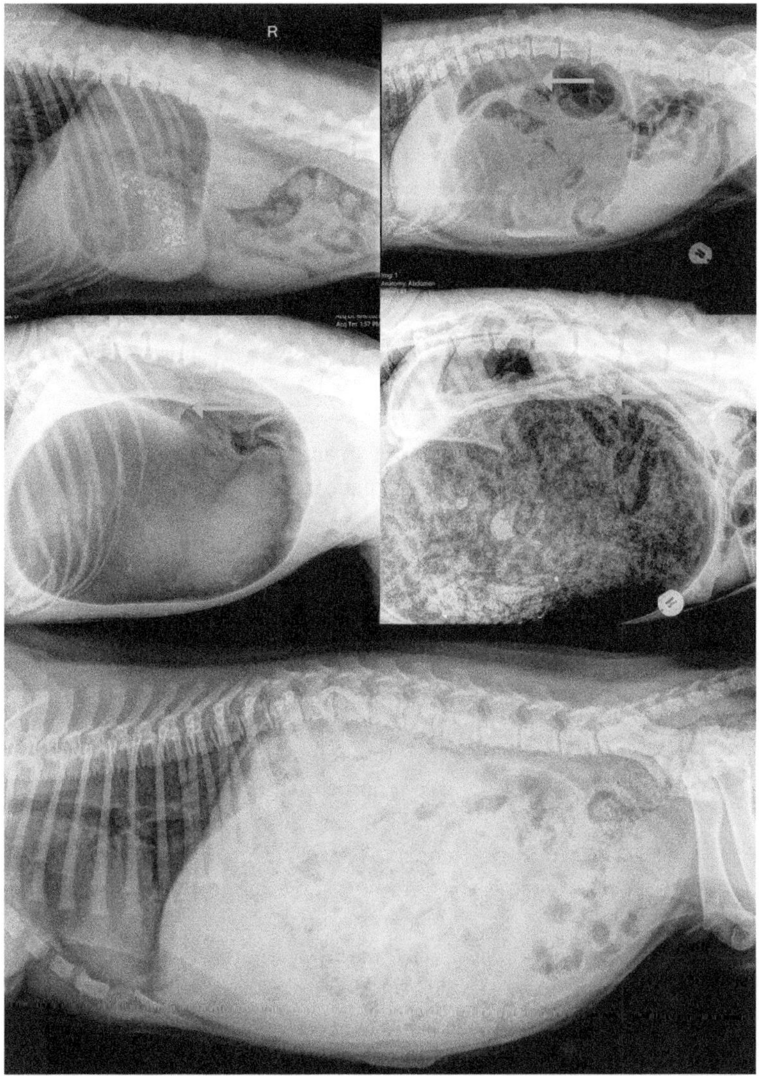

Figure 12.16 Obtaining a lateral abdominal radiograph is helpful in confirming a gastric dilatation and volvulus (GDV) in dogs instead of dilatation alone. The radiographs where the stomach looks like a "boxing glove" are where the pylorus has shifted dorsally (green arrows), which indicates that volvulus has occurred. The first radiograph is dilatation without volvulus and the bottom radiograph is of a puppy that overengorged.

require much if any sedation for premedication, and typically only an opioid, is administered.

A rapid sequence induction should be performed, ensuring intubation of the trachea and cuff inflation before allowing the head to be lowered. An alternative approach that has been described is to intubate the trachea with the head and mouth lower than the shoulders (leaning the head over the edge of the tables used for induction). This head position promotes free flow of saliva and other refluxed fluids out of the oral cavity. The person performing the tracheal intubation must be prepared to clean the oropharynx (e.g., suction, square gauze swabs, etc.) from saliva or gastric fluids, etc., before passing the ET tube into the trachea. If possible, deflate the stomach. Some veterinarians will attempt deflation by stomach tube before induction of anesthesia; however, this may not be possible or tolerated. Moreover, there is a risk of the dog aspirating during conscious decompression because it is fairly common for gastric fluid to exit the esophagus around the stomach tube. If gastric decompression is attempted in a sedated patient, then using a roll of adhesive bandage (50 or 75 mm) with a large-bore spindle as a gag can assist in advancing the stomach tube into the stomach. With the bandage roll in place, positioning the tongue to one side of the jaw allows swallowing, and the gag is advanced until the incisors are at the halfway point, and then the jaws are closed over the gag and taped with easily removable tape. Brachycephalic dogs and those with preexisting respiratory compromise (collapsing trachea) may benefit from being anesthetized for stomach tube placement instead of attempting to pass a stomach tube while sedated. In severely compromised animals with severe gastric dilation, percutaneous puncture, using a large-bore over-the-needle IV cannula, can be performed after aseptic preparation of the puncture site on the left lateral abdomen. Use of ultrasound guidance can minimize the chance of inadvertently piercing other organs (e.g., spleen, liver, and kidney). If ultrasonography is unavailable, then percussing the lateral abdominal wall to find the region that has a tympanic "ping" can be used to identify a puncture site. Once the cannula is inserted, the stylet is removed to prevent organ damage. Applying gentle pressure on the skin around the cannula while the stomach deflates is helpful to prevent dislodgment of the cannula. When placing a stomach tube, the tube should be marked to indicate the insertion depth at which it is expected to enter the stomach. This is measured by marking the distance on the tube from the level of the last rib to the nose. A tip to remedy a tube that is difficult to advance through the lower esophageal sphincter is to blow into the stomach tube while gently retracting and advancing the tube until it slips into the stomach. If the stomach tube will not advance into the stomach, then performing a percutaneous puncture can help deflate the stomach enough to allow advancement of the tube (volvulus will reduce as the stomach deflates).

Monitoring cardiovascular function with ECG and arterial blood pressure are particularly important during anesthesia due to the likelihood of hypotension or arrhythmias. Additional opioid analgesia may be administered or a lidocaine infusion used (e.g., 1 mg/kg bolus followed by 1–3 mg/kg/h). A lidocaine infusion has been associated with less post-operative cardiac arrythmias and improved survival. In addition, lidocaine has analgesic, anti-inflammatory, and anti-endotoxic properties that will benefit the dog during convalescence.

During recovery, monitoring of the ECG and arterial blood pressure should continue. Arrhythmias, particularly VPCs, are commonly observed and may require treatment. Opioids and possibly lidocaine may be used for post-operative analgesia. Most anesthetists will avoid NSAIDs in the immediate peri-operative period due to risk of gastric damage and poor volume status affecting renal perfusion. However, NSAIDs can be given the next day if the patient is normotensive.

Questions and Answers

There are more practice questions and answers available for this chapter on the website. Please visit http://www.wiley.com/go/VeterinaryAnesthesiaZeiler.

Questions

1) A one-year-old Boxer presents to your clinic for a castration. On clinical examination, you find the following:
   - Alert, bouncy, and very excitable
   - Heart rate: 80 beats per minute
   - Respiratory rate: 18 breaths per minute
   - Temperature: 37.7 °C
   - Mucous membranes pink and glistening
   - CRT: 1.5 s

   Which drug(s) would you recommend for pre medication?

   Briefly justify your choice(s) of drugs.
2) List the functions of an endotracheal tube.
3) List complications that can occur with an epidural containing local anesthesia.

Answers

1) Alpha-2 adrenoceptor agonists: dexmedetomidine, medetomidine, etc., provide good sedation. *Mu* agonist (e.g., morphine, methadone, fentanyl, etc.): painful procedure (accept any opioid except butorphanol with justification of analgesia). Some anesthetists choose to avoid acepromazine (Boxer) or benzodiazepine (not for excitable dog). Adding ketamine to the premedication can be helpful in very excitable dogs.
2) Maintains patent airway, protects airways, facilitates administration (and removal) of oxygen and inhalational drugs, and application of IPPV in the case of apnea or hypoventilation.
3) Neural damage/neurotoxicity – spinal trauma, infection (abscess or meningitis), inadvertent spinal injection, inadvertent IV injection (venous sinus puncture), hypotension/bradycardia, Horner's syndrome, respiratory depression, total spinal anesthesia (cranial migration), toxicity (inadvertent subarachnoid injection), urinary retention (opioids), allergic reaction – use preservative-free local anesthetic drugs, pruritus (opioids), and accidental wrong drug administration.

Further Reading

Aona, B.D., Rush, J.E., Rozanski, E.A. et al. (2017). Evaluation of echocardiography and cardiac biomarker concentrations in dogs with gastric dilatation volvulus. *J Vet Emerg Crit Care* 27: 631–637.

Bainbridge, D., Martin, J., Arango, M. et al. (2012). Perioperative and anaesthetic-related mortality in developed and developing countries: a systematic review and meta-analysis. *Lancet* 380: 1075–1081.

Barton-Lamb, A.L., Martin-Flores, M., Scrivani, P.V. et al. (2013). Evaluation of maxillary arterial blood flow in anesthetized cats with the mouth closed and open. *Vet J* 196: 325–331.

Bellini, L. and Seymour, C.J. (2016). Effect of intraoperative constant rate infusion of lidocaine on short-term survival of dogs with septic peritonitis: 75 cases (2007–2011). *J Am Vet Med Assoc* 248: 422–429.

Blunt, M.C., Young, P.J., Patil, A., and Haddock, A. (2001). Gel lubrication of the tracheal tube cuff reduces pulmonary aspiration. *Anesth* 95: 377–381.

Briganti, A., Portela, D.A., Barsotti, G. et al. (2012). Evaluation of the endotracheal tube cuff pressure resulting from four different methods of inflation in dogs. *Vet Anaesth Analg* 39: 488–494.

Brodbelt, D.C., Blissitt, K.J., Hammond, R.A. et al. (2008). The risk of death: the confidential enquiry into perioperative small animal fatalities. *Vet Anaesth Analg* 35: 365–373.

Bruchim, Y., Itay, S., Shira, B.H. et al. (2012). Evaluation of lidocaine treatment on frequency of cardiac arrhythmias, acute kidney injury, and hospitalization time in dogs with gastric dilatation volvulus. *J Vet Emerg Crit Care* 22: 419–427.

Clarke, K.W. and Hall, L.W. (1990). A survey of anaesthesia in small animal practice: AVA/BSAVA report. *J Assoc Vet Anaesthet Great Brit Ire* 17: 4–10.

Colucci, P., Yue, C.S., Ducharme, M., and Benvenga, S. (2013). A review of the pharmacokinetics of levothyroxine for the treatment of hypothyroidism. *Europ Endocrin* 9: 40.

Costa, R.S. and Jones, T. (2023). Anesthetic considerations in dogs and cats with diabetes mellitus. *Vet Clin N Am: Sm Anim Prac* 53: 581–589.

De Cramer, K.G.M., Joubert, K.E., and Nöthling, J.O. (2017). Puppy survival and vigor associated with the use of low dose medetomidine premedication, propofol induction and maintenance of anesthesia using sevoflurane gas-inhalation for cesarean section in the bitch. *Theriogen* 96: 10–15.

Deshpande, D., Hill, K.E., Mealey, K.L. et al. (2016). The effect of the canine ABCB1-1Δ mutation on sedation after intravenous administration of acepromazine. *J Vet Intern Med* 30: 636–641.

Drobatz, K.J. and Cole, S.G. (2008). The influence of crystalloid type on acid–base and electrolyte status of cats with urethral obstruction. *J Vet Emerg Crit Care* 18: 355–361.

Fagerholm, V., Haaparanta, M., and Scheinin, M. (2011). α2-Adrenoceptor regulation of blood glucose homeostasis. *Basic Clin Pharmacol Tox* 108: 365–370.

Fuentes, V.L. and Wilkie, L.J. (2017). Asymptomatic hypertrophic cardiomyopathy: diagnosis and therapy. *Vet Clin: Sm Anim Prac* 47: 1041–1054.

Goggs, R., Blais, M.-C., Brainard, B.M. et al. (2019). American College of Veterinary Emergency and Critical Care (ACVECC) consensus on the rational use of antithrombotics in veterinary critical care (CURATIVE) guidelines: small animal. *J Vet Emerg Crit Care* 29: 12–36.

Harrison, R.L., Clark, L., and Corletto, F. (2012). Comparison of mean heart rate in anaesthetized dachshunds and other breeds of dog undergoing spinal magnetic resonance imaging. *Vet Anaesth Analg* 39: 230–235.

Herbert, G.L. and Murison, P.J. (2013). Eye position of cats anaesthetised with alfaxalone or propofol. *Vet Rec* 172: 365.

Hung, W.C., Ko, J.C., Weil, A.B., and Weng, H.Y. (2020). Evaluation of endotracheal tube cuff pressure and the use of three cuff inflation syringe devices in dogs. *Front Vet Sci* 7: 39.

Itami, T., Aida, H., Asakawa, M. et al. (2017). Association between preoperative characteristics and risk of anaesthesia-related death in dogs in small-animal referral hospitals in Japan. *Vet Anaesth Analg* 44: 461–472.

Kronen, P., Moon-Massat, P., Ludders, J. et al. (2001). Comparison of two insulin protocols for diabetic dogs undergoing cataract surgery. *Vet Anaesth Analg* 28: 146–155.

KuKanich, B., Coetzee, J.F., Gehring, R., and Hubin, M. (2007). Comparative disposition of pharmacologic markers for cytochrome P-450 mediated metabolism, glomerular filtration rate, and extracellular and total body fluid volume of Greyhound and Beagle dogs. *J Vet Pharmacol Therapeut* 30: 314–319.

Lamont, L.A., Bulmer, B.J., Sisson, D.D. et al. (2002). Doppler echocardiographic effects of medetomidine on dynamic left ventricular outflow tract obstruction in cats. *J Am Vet Med Assoc* 221: 1276–1281.

Levy, J.K., Bard, K.M., Tucker, S.J. et al. (2017). Perioperative mortality in cats and dogs undergoing spay or castration at a high-volume clinic. *Vet J* 224: 11–15.

Lhuillery, E., Velay, L., Libermann, S. et al. (2022). Outcomes of dogs undergoing surgery for gastric dilatation volvulus after rapid versus prolonged medical stabilization. *Vet Surg* 51: 843–852.

MacPhail, C.M., Lappin, M.R., Meyer, D.J. et al. (1998). Hepatocellular toxicosis associated with administration of carprofen in 21 dogs. *J Am Vet Med Assoc* 212: 1895–1901.

Martinez, S.E., Andresen, M.C., Zhu, Z., and Papageorgiou, I. (2020). Pharmacogenomics of poor drug metabolism in Greyhounds: cytochrome P450 (CYP) 2B11 genetic variation, breed distribution, and functional characterization. *Sci Rep* 10: 1–19.

Martinez-Taboada, F. and Redondo, J.I. (2017). Comparison of the hanging-drop technique and running-drip method for identifying the epidural space in dogs. *Vet Anaesth Analg* 44: 329–336.

Martin-Flores, M., Moy-Trigilio, K.E., Campoy, L., and Gleed, R.D. (2021). Retrospective study on the use of lumbosacral epidural analgesia during caesarean section surgery in 182 dogs: impact on blood pressure, analgesic use and delays. *Vet Rec* 188: e134.

Matthews, N.S., Mohn, T.J., Yang, M. et al. (2017). Factors associated with anesthetic-related death in dogs and cats in primary care veterinary hospitals. *J Am Vet Med Assoc* 250: 655–665.

Norgate, D.J., Nicholls, D., Geddes, R.F. et al. (2021). Comparison of two protocols for insulin administration and fasting time in diabetic dogs anaesthetised for phacoemulsification: a prospective clinical trial. *Vet Rec* 188: 1–14.

Oliver, J.A., Clark, L., Corletto, F., and Gould, D.J. (2010). A comparison of anesthetic complications between diabetic and nondiabetic dogs undergoing phacoemulsification cataract surgery: a retrospective study. *Vet Ophthalmol* 13: 244–250.

Potter, J.J., Cook, J., and Meakin, L.B. (2020). Suspected thyroid storm in a cat anaesthetised for bilateral thyroidectomy. *Vet Rec Case Rep* 8: e000895.

Ramoo, S., Bradbury, L.A., Anderson, G.A., and Abraham, L.A. (2013). Sedation of hyperthyroid cats with subcutaneous administration of a combination of alfaxalone and butorphanol. *Austr Vet J* 91: 131–136.

Robinson, E.P., Sams, R.A., and Muir, W.W. (1986). Barbiturate anesthesia in greyhound and mixed-breed dogs: comparative cardiopulmonary effects, anesthetic effects, and recovery rates. *Am J Vet Res* 47: 2105–2112.

Sams, R.A., Muir, W.W., Detra, R.L., and Robinson, E.P. (1985). Comparative pharmacokinetics and anesthetic effects of methohexital, pentobarbital, thiamylal, and thiopental in Greyhound dogs and non-Greyhound, mixed-breed dogs. *Am J Vet Res* 46: 1677–1683.

Seneviratne, M., Kaye, B.M., and Ter Haar, G. (2020). Prognostic indicators of short-term outcome in dogs undergoing surgery for brachycephalic obstructive airway syndrome. *Vet Rec* 187: 1–9. https://doi.org/10.1136/vr.105624

Sharp, C.R., Goggs, R., Blais, M.C. et al. (2019). Clinical application of the American College of Veterinary Emergency and Critical Care (ACVECC) Consensus on the Rational Use of Antithrombotics in Veterinary Critical Care (CURATIVE) guidelines to small animal cases. *J Vet Emerg Crit Care* 29: 121–131.

Shoop-Worrall, S.J., O'neill, D.G., Viscasillas, J., and Brodbelt, D.C. (2022). Mortality related to general anaesthesia and sedation in dogs under UK primary veterinary care. *Vet Anaesth Analg* 49: 433–442.

Song, K.K., Goldsmid, S.E., Lee, J., and Simpson, D.J. (2020). Retrospective analysis of 736 cases of canine gastric dilatation volvulus. *Austr Vet J* 98: 232–238.

Tong, J. and Pang, D.S. (2019). Investigating novel anatomical predictors for endotracheal tube selection in dogs. *Canad Vet J* 60: 848.

Van Dijl, I.C., Le Traon, G., van De Meulengraaf, B.D.A.M. et al. (2014). Pharmacokinetics of total thyroxine after repeated oral administration of levothyroxine solution and its clinical efficacy in hypothyroid dogs. *J Vet Intern Med* 28: 1229–1234.

White, D.M., Makara, M., and Martinez-Taboada, F. (2020). Comparison of four inflation techniques on endotracheal tube cuff pressure using a feline airway simulator. *J Fel Med Surg* 22: 641–647.

White, R.S., Sartor, A.J., and Bergman, P.J. (2021). Evaluation of a staged technique of immediate decompressive and delayed surgical treatment for gastric dilatation-volvulus in dogs. *J Am Vet Med Assoc* 258: 72–79.

Zoran, D.L., Riedesel, D.H., and Dyer, D.C. (1993). Pharmacokinetics of propofol in mixed-breed dogs and greyhounds. *Am J Vet Res* 54: 755–760.

13

Approach to Healthy Horse, Donkey, and Mule Anesthesia and Analgesia

John Hubbell, Nora Matthews, and Daniel Pang

The horse has evolved as its relationship to humans and the environment has changed with the development of alternative methods of providing "horsepower" including automobiles, trains, and tractors. Although equidae (horses, donkeys, and mules) are used as beasts of burden and commerce in many parts of the world, veterinary care of the majority of equidae focuses on horses used for pleasure and sport, and in commercial activities (such as breeding and sales). Veterinarians provide services to the horse-owning public on a number of levels including basic preventive and medical care, specialized medical care, and advanced surgical care for a wide range of maladies.

Risk of Anesthetic Mortality in Horses

Veterinary interactions with equidae represent physical risks for the practitioner and the equid. It has been estimated that 50% of large animal veterinarians will suffer a significant physical injury during their career. Before the 1970s, there were a few clinically useful sedative and tranquilizer drugs available for use in equidae. Most procedures included a significant component of physical restraint, a condition that made the interactions perilous for both humans and equidae. The development of suitable sedatives and anesthetic drugs has increased safety for humans and equidae, but present-day reports indicate that the risk of general anesthesia in horses is greater than that of the other common companion animals (dogs and cats) with a mortality rate in the range of 1%. The reason for the increased risk is multifactorial, including the flight-or-fight nature of the species, the weight of an individual, anatomy, the desire of anesthetized horses to stand relatively rapidly upon awakening, and the difficulties associated with managing a recumbent equid, including personnel safety and the potential for the animal to further injure itself.

Personnel Requirements for Safe Anesthesia

Historically, most practitioners have practiced their craft alone with the assistance of the animal owner or trainer. Currently, there is a movement toward employment of veterinary assistants (animal health technologists/nurses/technician assistants) to aid in the performance of both routine and advanced care. It is the opinion of the authors that the use of assistants enhances veterinary care and safety for the veterinarian and the equid through safe restraint for the administration of parenteral medications and other activities. In most practice situations, sedation of equidae is produced via intravenous or intramuscular administration of sedatives. While this often can be accomplished utilizing the animal's owner or other lay personnel, such restraint is often inconsistent and if the assistant is injured, the veterinarian may have liability. When anesthetizing equidae, it is important to monitor depth of anesthesia and cardiopulmonary function and, on occasion, administer additional medications to maintain the anesthetized state. The use of an assistant, while not mandatory, can greatly improve the experience for both the veterinarian and the equid.

Characteristics of Horses, Donkeys, and Mules

Many veterinarians have developed different drug-dosing regimens for different breeds or types of horses based on their experiences and anecdotal reports. For example, the authors believe that draft horse breeds and American Saddlebreds require smaller doses of sedatives to produce useful sedation compared to mustangs, Arabian horses, and Appaloosas. Beyond widespread anecdotal reports, there are few data available to directly support such beliefs.

Fundamental Principles of Veterinary Anesthesia, First Edition. Edited by Gareth E. Zeiler and Daniel S. J. Pang.

Companion Website: www.wiley.com/go/VeterinaryAnesthesiaZeiler

However, studies of breed temperament/demeanor suggest that Thoroughbreds, Arabian horses, Walking horses, cobs, and Welsh ponies are more anxious and excitable than other breeds, such as American Quarterhorses, Paints, Appaloosas, and drafts. The intended use of the animals and the management practices employed by the owners and trainers of the various breeds of horses probably play a larger role in the quality of veterinary interactions with individual animals than the breed of the animal. Miniature horses are small horses that have been bred primarily for companionship but are also used in carriage driving. They are classified by their size. Some genetic lines are associated with a number of genetic defects that should be examined for on physical examination. Ponies are distinct breeds (e.g., Welsh, Shetland, Dartmoor, and Newfoundland) or crosses and are generally classified as small (less than 127 cm at the top of the withers), medium (127–137 cm), or large (137–147 cm).

Donkeys (also called "burros") are of the species *Equus asinus*. Donkeys are registered based on size in the most countries. Miniature donkeys are less than 86 cm at the withers. Standard donkeys range in size from 86 to 137 cm while mammoth donkeys are greater than 137 cm at the withers. Mules are produced from breeding a jackass (male donkey) to a mare (female horse). While both donkeys and mules have long ears, mules will show horse characteristics (i.e., a more refined head, reflecting the breed of horse used) and will have a tail similar to a horse. The donkey will have a tail similar to a cow, with only a switch of hair at the end. Behavioral differences are most evident in donkeys that have had little handling or training. Donkeys do not have the same flight response as the horse; when confronted with something new, they usually become stationary until they become acclimated. Patience is required when trying to get them to perform tasks such as entering a stock. A nose twitch is frequently ineffective in restraining donkeys (in part because it easily slides off the nose). Donkeys may be adequately restrained by snuggly attaching the head rope securely to a stout fixed object. Mules may be more difficult than donkeys (unless well trained), and because of their larger size they are generally more dangerous. It is strongly recommended to have an experienced mule handler available when working around untrained mules. Both mules and donkeys can accurately kick without warning.

Both donkeys and mules are stoic making it difficult to assess pain or illness; they can be much sicker or more painful than casual observation suggests. Donkeys exhibit the same pain behaviors as horses but must be acclimated to their surroundings before they show those behaviors. There is a myth that says that donkeys and mules do not colic. This is not true, but mild bouts of colic are probably never observed because of their impassive nature. The animal may be significantly ill before being presented for treatment or surgery, thus the anesthetic risk may be underestimated.

Treating Acute and Chronic Pain

Pain management in equidae, as in other species, requires at least three components: recognition that the pain exists; a desire to provide relief from the pain; and the ability to provide relief. Behaviors associated with acute pain are a frequent reason for presentation. Equidae that are non-weight bearing on a limb give a good indication of where to start with diagnosis and therapy. Equidae with colic usually present because they are showing signs of abdominal pain whether that be inappetence, looking or kicking at the abdomen, or violently rolling. Further, the lack of response to analgesic administration continues to be a primary indication for the need for an exploratory laparotomy to hopefully correct the problem and relieve the discomfort.

Acute pain usually responds to analgesic administration, at least for a brief period, which can help localize its origin. Chronic pain is often more difficult to localize and treat, particularly when the original inciting cause is not apparent. Animals with chronic pain often develop non-specific coping strategies such as limiting activity, lying down, and altering their gait or posture. Further, the numerous and variable changes within the nervous system associated with chronic pain may make treatment challenging. Treatment of chronic pain may require a combination of drug and other supportive therapies to provide comfort, and trial therapies are often necessary to identify a successful pain management strategy. Some chronically painful conditions, such as laminitis, can have both acute and chronic pain components.

A number of neurons interact with the pain pathways along their route from the periphery to the brain (see Chapter 3). The drugs and techniques used to provide analgesia act on these pathways, interrupting the sensing, transmission, or interpretation of pain. Some drugs act at multiple sites along a pain pathway. Combinations of drugs (e.g., opioids and alpha-2 adrenergic receptor agonists), acting at one or more sites, can produce synergism. When synergism occurs, enhanced analgesia is produced or equivalent analgesia is produced at decreased drug doses. Multimodal analgesia, the use of different classes of analgesic drugs to act at different sites along the pain pathway, is an important approach in providing appropriate analgesia. The treatment of pain is frequently approached using combinations of drugs (multimodal analgesia) in the hope that they will be effective at lower doses and thus produce analgesia with reduced adverse effects, as well as potentially improved pain relief through activity at different sites of the pain pathway. Veterinarians have long used such techniques for standing chemical restraint including the administration of alpha-2 adrenergic receptor agonists with opioids or acepromazine. A rational approach to multimodal therapy is to start with a single drug or drug combination and add other drugs if analgesia is insufficient.

Pain assessment is based on observations of the animal and measurement of physiologic parameters such as heart rate and respiratory rate. When assessing the degree of pain, ask the following questions: Does the animal move freely? Does the animal rest comfortably? Does the animal appear interested in its environment? Does the animal eat and drink normally? If you cannot answer yes to all of these questions, the horse (or donkey or mule) might be painful.

Further determinations of the degree of pain can be made using scoring systems such as the Obel. This system grades lameness from 0 to 4. A score of "0" is a normal horse with no gait abnormality. Horses scoring "1" incessantly shift their weight at rest. They are not "lame" at the walk but they have a short, stilted gait. Grade "2" horses allow their feet to be lifted. They walk in a stilted manner but willingly and are lame at the trot. Grade "3" horses move reluctantly and cannot trot. Grade "3" horses vigorously resent picking up their feet. Grade "4" horses refuse to move unless force is used.

It may be helpful to apply a pain assessment scale to assist in evaluating pain and guiding management (see Further Reading and Chapter 3). Several scales have been developed for acute pain in equidae. Importantly, pain assessment scales are a tool to guide decision-making, in combination with history, physical examination, and the questions listed in the preceding text.

Pain associated with laminitis is one of the more frustrating conditions to treat in equidae. Pain and reluctance to move are frequently the first signs that owners see when their animal develops acute laminitis or other painful conditions. An inability to make the animal comfortable enough to eat and drink normally through the initial insult can lead to euthanasia. Treatment of chronic laminitis includes the systemic use of nonsteroidal anti-inflammatory drugs. These are usually well tolerated but can cause significant adverse effects, primarily related to the gastrointestinal tract and kidney. Providing comfort for the animal is a key part of the successful treatment of laminitis, but complete analgesia like that produced by local anesthetics can lead to overloading and hasten the progression of the disease. A balance must be struck between providing analgesia and limiting the pressure that the animal places on its hooves by constantly standing. Successful long-term management of a laminitic animal requires multiple therapies including those directed at the inciting cause, the management of body weight, the optimization of hoof care, and the provision of analgesia.

Analgesic Drug Classes in Common Use

Nonsteroidal Anti-inflammatory Drugs (NSAIDs)

These drugs provide analgesia and reduce inflammation and fever. NSAIDs are useful in the treatment of mild-to-moderate acute pain and in combination with other drugs to manage more severe pain (see Chapters 3, 7, and 9). They are also used to reduce the pain and inflammation associated with chronic states. The incidence of adverse effects is greatest in foals, in hypovolemic animals, and when the drugs are administered for extended periods. NSAIDs are not controlled; therefore, they do not have to be locked up and extensive record keeping is not required. The goals of NSAID administration should be to provide comfort at the lowest possible dose of drug at a cost that is sustainable by the owner and is well tolerated by the horse. The same NSAIDs can be used in donkeys and mules. Generally, the duration of action is shorter in donkeys than in the horse, so more frequent administration may be warranted dependent on monitoring the animal for signs of pain (Table 13.1). For example, based on pharmacokinetic data, flunixin may need to be given three times a day in miniature donkeys.

There are a number of NSAIDs approved for use in the horse. One of the most widely used, phenylbutazone, is available as tablets, as a paste, and for intravenous injection, and is widely used for both acute and chronic pain. Phenylbutazone, given IV, is frequently the first drug administered in the treatment of acute laminitis and the response to its administration provides some information about the severity of the disease. Doses of phenylbutazone in the range of 4 mg/kg (IV) provide analgesia in chronically lame horses for greater than 12 h. Doubling the dose increases the duration of effect but does not produce further reduction of the lameness. Phenylbutazone (2 mg/kg) is effective dosed orally twice daily. Phenylbutazone may allow some lame horses to live apparently comfortable lives and in some cases permit performance. Chronic administration (longer than one to two weeks) can be associated with significant adverse effects including renal failure, gastrointestinal ulceration (in particular right dorsal colitis), diarrhea, hypoproteinemia, and anemia. For these

Table 13.1 Nonsteroidal anti-inflammatory drugs (NSAIDs) for donkeys, mules, and horses.

		Dosing interval		
Drug	**Dose (mg/kg), route**	**Donkeys**	**Mules**	**Horses**
Phenylbutazone	2.2–4.4, IV, PO	2–3 times daily	Twice daily	Twice daily
Vedaprofen	1.0–2.0, PO	Twice daily	NA[a]	Twice daily
Ketoprofen	2.2, IV	NA[a]	NA[a]	Once daily
Flunixin	1.1, IV, PO	3 times daily	NA[a]	Once daily
Carprofen	0.7, IV, PO	Once daily	NA[a]	Once daily
Firocoxib	1 tablet (57 mg) per 450–600 kg, PO	NA[a]	NA[a]	Once daily
Meloxicam	0.6, IV, PO	2–3 times daily	NA[a]	Once daily

a) No information available.
Note: Please refer to package insert for licensed dosing in country of practice.
IV: intravenous; PO: per *os* (oral).

reasons, once pain appears to be controlled, the dose should be titrated to the lowest dose that appears to be effective. Such effects are not limited to phenylbutazone but are often associated with this NSAID because of its widespread use. Treatment usually involves withdrawal of phenylbutazone and use of another, potentially less toxic NSAID.

Other NSAIDs are available for use in equidae, with licensing varying between countries. Diclofenac is applied topically as a liposome-based cream. It is indicated for control of pain and inflammation associated with osteoarthritis of the tarsal, carpal, and distal joints. Adverse effects are dose dependent and include those described in the preceding text for phenylbutazone. Anecdotal evidence suggests that some NSAIDs are more effective when given in combination, but supporting evidence for this practice is limited. Firocoxib is a newer NSAID with increased selectivity for the inhibition of inducible prostaglandin synthesis and is reported to produce reduced gastrointestinal side effects. Such drugs can be advantageous in young horses or those known to be sensitive to other NSAIDs.

Alpha-2 Adrenergic Receptor Agonists

These drugs produce sedation with muscle relaxation, ataxia, and analgesia. Xylazine, detomidine, and romifidine are approved for use in the horse in most countries. The level of sedation produced by administration of any alpha-2 adrenergic receptor agonist is pronounced and extends beyond the duration of analgesia for all available drugs, limiting their use beyond acute treatment. Intravenous administration produces a rapid onset of action, an increased intensity of effect, but a shorter duration of effect. Intravenous infusions of alpha-2 adrenergic receptor agonists to facilitate standing surgery and to provide analgesia are commonly used. The use of a constant rate infusion reduces the peaks and troughs in plasma drug concentration that result from repeat bolus administration and frequently lowers the total dose of drug administered. Alternatively, intramuscular drug administration is easily accomplished and has a duration of action approximately twice that of an IV bolus.

Opioids

These drugs are used to produce analgesia and augment the effects of sedatives and tranquilizers. When administered alone to pain-free equidae, opioids can cause nervousness and excitability. Signs may include head twitching and pacing. Opioid administration is typically accompanied by a tranquilizer or sedative such as acepromazine or an alpha-2 adrenergic receptor agonist to minimize the risk of these adverse effects. Butorphanol is a synthetic opioid agonist/antagonist that is commonly used in equidae for the treatment of abdominal pain. Butorphanol is less prone to cause excitement than morphine or fentanyl but ataxia can be severe at high doses (0.05–0.1 mg/kg, IV). Periodic head jerks and twitches occur and horses may head press (lean forward). Buprenorphine has a longer duration of action and has been used in a similar manner to butorphanol but experience with its use is limited.

Morphine is the prototypical opioid drug and has the potential to provide profound analgesia through its *mu* receptor agonist activity. As with butorphanol, morphine has the potential to cause excitement which, due to its longer duration of action, may present after sedation has worn off. Naloxone can be used to antagonize morphine and may need to be re-dosed as its duration of action is shorter than that of morphine (Table 13.2). Note that naloxone will also antagonize analgesic effects. Alternatively, sedation (with an alpha-2 adrenergic receptor agonist) may be sufficient to control excitation. In addition, morphine and other opioids produce significant adverse effects with

Table 13.2 Examples of drug antagonists that can be used in an emergency situation or to reverse sedation in an equid.

Drug category	Drug group	Antagonists generic name	Dose (mg/kg)	Route(s)	Comment
Sedative-hypnotic	Benzodiazepine antagonists	Flumazenil	0.01	IV	
Nonopioid analgesic	Alpha-2 adrenergic receptor antagonists	Yohimbine	0.075	IV	May cause excitement, and reversal is incomplete and transient
		Tolazoline	4	IV, IM	May cause hypotension, and reversal is incomplete and transient
		Atipamazole	0.05–0.1	IV, IM	Effects are incomplete and transient
Opioid analgesic	Opioid antagonists	Naloxone	0.015–0.02	IV, IM	Reversal may be transient
		Naltrexone	0.75	IV	

IV: intravenous; IM: intramuscular.

regard to slowing of gastrointestinal motility and increases in vagal tone. Gastrointestinal function must be closely monitored if morphine is administered for extended periods.

Peri-anesthetic use of morphine for treating moderate-to-severe pain has been increasing but remains controversial (see Further Reading). Factors against its use include decreased gastrointestinal function and a lack of a MAC-sparing effect (a standard indicator of analgesic effect in many species). Factors in favor of its use include morphine's established use and efficacy in other mammalian species, and evidence that potential analgesic effects outweigh the risk of developing post-operative colic. The latter is based on the assumption that untreated pain or ineffective analgesia is also associated with decreased gastrointestinal motility and risk of post-operative colic. Fentanyl, another potent opioid with *mu* receptor agonist activity, can be delivered transdermally by the application of a patch. Considerable variation in the rate of absorption occurs, particularly in systemically sick horses, and plasma levels may be below therapeutic levels.

Other Advanced Analgesic Techniques

These techniques frequently require intravenous catheterization and infusions. Lidocaine infusions are used for post-operative pain, particularly in colic patients because of the anti-inflammatory properties and potential to increase gastrointestinal motility (though evidence supporting this latter effect in the large intestine is limited). The administration of lidocaine may have additional benefits in patients with inflammation (e.g., laminitic patients) because of the potential for anti-endotoxin and vascular effects. Lidocaine requires a constant rate infusion to be effective systemically. Ketamine infusions can be incorporated into standing restraint protocols in an attempt to increase analgesia. The dose administered ranges from 0.4 to 0.8 mg/kg/h given at a constant rate. The effectiveness of the technique depends on the type of pain being induced or treated with excellent results seen for patients with burns.

In considering the approach to a painful patient, using laminitis as an example, NSAIDs have frequently been administered as well as acepromazine because of its reputed effects on improving digital blood flow. If comfort is not produced, a lidocaine infusion is a logical addition because of its anti-endotoxic effects. Ketamine and opioids, such as morphine, could also be added if analgesia is insufficient. Gabapentin has been shown to have some utility in chronic pain states though dosing is not well established, and there may be considerable inter-individual variability in responses. A promising new class of drugs for the treatment of pain and inflammation is the soluble epoxide hydrolase inhibitors. These experimental drugs slow the metabolism of soluble epoxides, compounds that are part of the arachidonic acid cascade with analgesic and anti-inflammatory properties.

Intravenous Access

Vascular catheters are frequently placed to provide rapid access for the injection of fluids, obtaining blood samples and administering drugs. The placement of a catheter avoids the restraint and pain associated with multiple needle insertions and helps ensure that substance delivery is intravascular. The jugular veins are most frequently used in horses. They are of a large diameter and have relatively high flow rates which help reduce thrombus formation. Other potential sites for venous access include the cephalic, saphenous, median, and lateral thoracic veins.

Protocols for placement of intravenous catheters should be used to ensure aseptic placement and facilitate securing the catheter in place. The hair over the vein can be clipped and aseptic preparation performed. A small subcutaneous bleb of local anesthetic can be placed over the insertion site to minimize resistance to catheter placement (strongly recommended in donkeys and mules). Three to six inch long, 12–14 gauge over-the-needle catheters should be used for adult horses and 16–20 gauge catheters are suitable for foals. The catheters should be secured with sutures and capped or a short catheter extension can also be used (Figure 13.1). Aseptic technique should be followed when performing injections (clean off any visible dirt and wipe injection port with 70% alcohol before needle insertion). When left in place for longer than six hours, catheters should be flushed with heparinized solutions to help maintain patency.

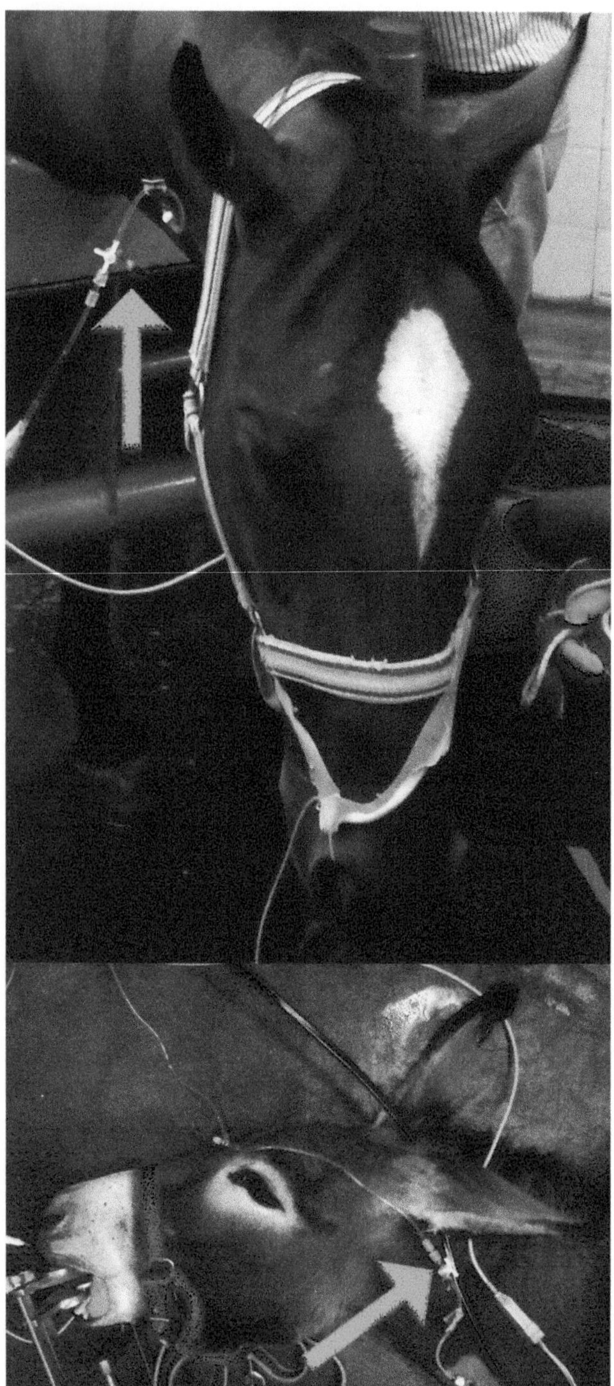

Figure 13.1 An intravenous catheter placed into the jugular of a horse (top) and a donkey (bottom), and both catheters are connected to short catheter extension set fitted with a three-way stopcock (green arrows).

Deciding Between Performing Standing Sedation or General Anesthesia

Many surgical and medical procedures can be accomplished in the standing horse if appropriate combinations of physical and chemical restraint are employed. The ability to perform procedures in the standing position is more important in the horse than in other species because of the greater risk of complications associated with general anesthesia. The goal of most standing restraint is to produce a quiet, calm horse that is immobile and does not react to stimuli or manipulation. Analgesia should be provided if the intended procedure is expected to be painful. The choice of standing sedation or general anesthesia is in part made by the physical qualities and abilities of the individual performing the procedure, thus personal preference and self-assessment play a key role. As an example, a standing castration or tooth extraction in a mature 500 kg horse would be feasible for most veterinarians but would be a challenge if the patient was a 50 kg miniature horse. By contrast, procedures such as abdominal exploratory surgery are usually performed via a ventral midline incision, thus dorsal recumbency and general anesthesia are required (Figure 13.2).

The temperament of the animal is another consideration. The veterinarian should determine the level of restraint that the animal is accustomed to before attempting a standing procedure. Questions to ask include: Will the horse stand in place when held by a halter and lead rope? Is the animal accustomed to being tied to a wall? Will the horse stand in cross ties? Does the horse throw itself (become recumbent) if it becomes excited? Does the horse strike or kick when restrained? Equidae that are used to standing in place or in confined spaces for extended periods are better candidates for standing procedures. Another consideration is the available physical facilities including nonslip flooring and appropriate stocks. In the authors' experience, standing procedures in foals and small horses

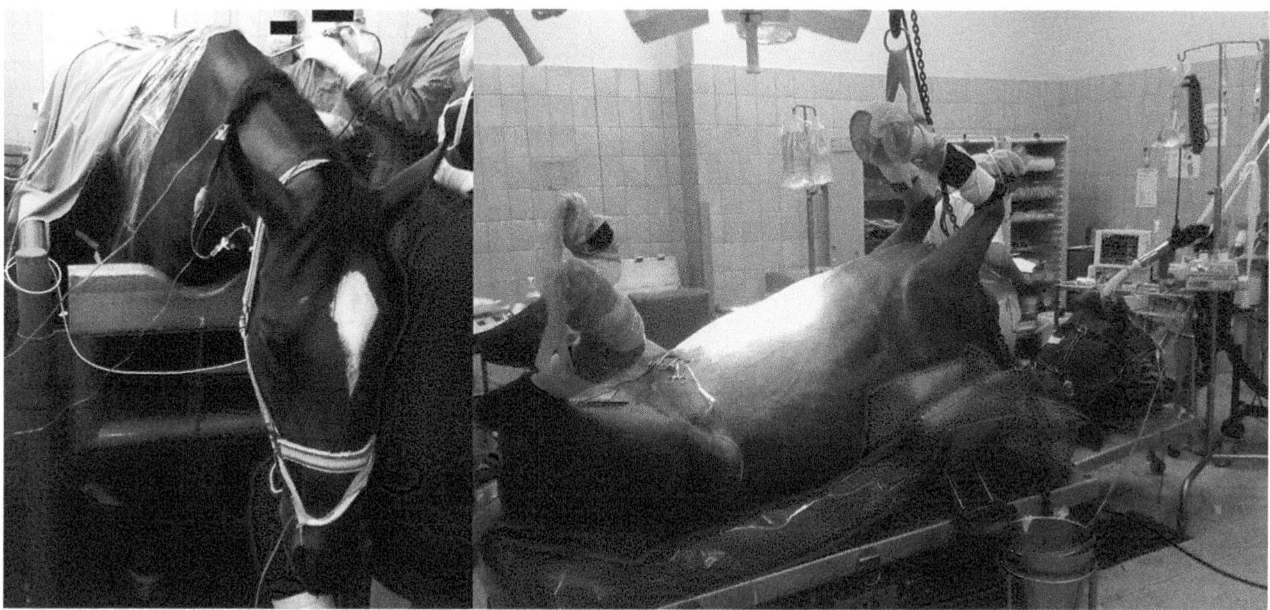

Figure 13.2 Surgery can be performed during standing sedation (left) or general anesthesia (right). See text for details on how to decide which technique to use.

are more difficult. Foals tend to lie down when sedated, thus it is advisable to account for this possibility. It is recognized that anesthesia of draft horses and other large (greater than 600 kg) horses is more perilous than for smaller horses, in part because it is harder to assist recovery.

Concurrent Diseases

The presence of concurrent diseases in equidae may increase the risk of anesthesia, so pre-anesthetic assessment should be carried out. This pre-anesthetic exam is focused on the cardiopulmonary system in young, apparently healthy equidae (including mucous membrane color, palpation of peripheral pulses, and auscultation of the heart and lungs). It may be necessary to ask questions about herd health or genetic predisposition (e.g., hyperkalemic periodic paralysis in horses and renal insufficiency) depending on age and breed of the patient. Obvious concurrent problems such as severe arthritis, chronic obstructive lung disease, and poor body condition (or obesity) may need to be further investigated before anesthesia. Older equidae frequently have heart murmurs, which should be noted, while younger animals may be in atrial fibrillation when presented for "routine" procedures (see Chapter 17 and Figure 13.3). Either condition could increase the risk of anesthesia and should therefore be further evaluated, particularly in animals with a history of exercise intolerance.

Anticipated Duration

It is important for the practitioner to objectively and accurately predict how long a procedure will take so that the appropriate anesthetic techniques can be used. For example, padding and positioning that would be acceptable for a short procedure can lead to catastrophic consequences for a long procedure (i.e., neuropathy and myopathy). Additionally, repeated injections of anesthetic drugs may become cumulative when repeated numerous times, producing prolonged and rough recoveries.

Concept of Return to Function

It may be necessary to consider how long it will take the patient to return to normal after sedation or general anesthesia. In most instances, food should be withheld until the animal is fully awake after any administration of a sedative. All sedative, analgesic, and anesthetic drugs will slow the gastrointestinal tract of the horse; return to normal eating, drinking, and defecation may be variable but need to be carefully monitored in the post-operative period. Post-operative colic can occur; early recognition and intervention is critical to successful treatment. For procedures performed outside a clinic, veterinarians should be aware of any country-specific legal requirements surrounding when an animal can be left under the care of its owners.

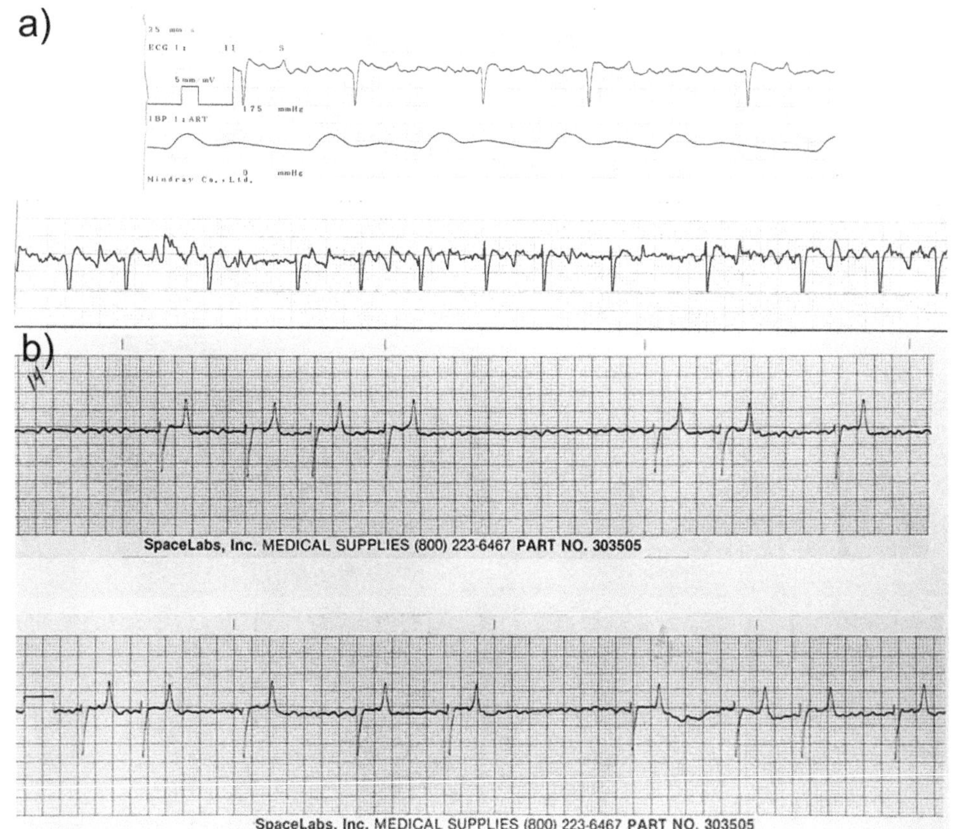

Figure 13.3 Electrocardiogram (ECG) tracings from a multiparameter physiological monitor used during general anesthesia in horses with atrial fibrillation (a), and the ECG tracing and invasive blood pressure (IBP) tracing show that each QRS–T complex is associated with a pulse wave. Another example of atrial fibrillation (b). These arrhythmias should be ruled out in horses older than 10 years of age during the pre-anesthetic examination. (Source: John Hubbell, Chapter Contributor).

Common Drug Protocols and Techniques for Performing Standing Sedation

Drug protocols are summarized in Table 13.3. No single drug produces "ideal" standing chemical restraint for every patient. The majority of veterinarians use drugs in combination, with the goal of optimizing the onset, quality, and duration of the alteration in mentation while minimizing potentially deleterious adverse effects. It is important to allow sufficient time for drugs to take effect and minimize disturbance or interactions during this period to maximize sedation quality.

Phenothiazine Tranquilizers

The most commonly used drug is acepromazine and they are used to produce calming. They do not produce analgesia, but they do enhance the analgesic activity of other drugs such as alpha-2 adrenergic receptor agonists and opioids. Phenothiazines can be given orally, intramuscularly, and intravenously. Alpha-1 adrenergic receptor blockade caused by these drugs can lead to arterial hypotension. This is of particular concern in excitable horses (activation of the sympathetic nervous system causes vasoconstriction) and in horses that have hemorrhaged or are dehydrated. Phenothiazines do not significantly affect respiration, but respiratory rate frequently decreases. Following administration, it is common for the penis to be exteriorized outside the sheath, returning to its normal position within 2–4 h. In stallions, phenothiazine administration rarely causes priapism (prolonged erection) or persistent penile paralysis (paraphimosis). For this reason, some anesthetists prefer to avoid using acepromazine in stallions, particularly those used for breeding.

Acepromazine is commonly supplied as a 1 or 2.5% solution (10 or 25 mg/mL) for injection. Following IV and IM administration, onset of action occurs within 15–30 min but peak effects may not be seen for up to 45 min, a factor that may limit its use as a sole drug in clinical practice. Duration of sedation depends on the dose but may last for

Table 13.3 Drugs for standing chemical restraint in horses.

Drug	Dose and route	Onset of effect and duration	Comments
Acepromazine	0.02–0.05 mg/kg, IM, IV	20–40 min IV, IM Duration: 4–6 h.	Use cautiously in stressed or hypotensive horses Potential for penile prolapse/paraphimosis and priapism in males
Xylazine	0.2–1.0 mg/kg, IV 1.0–2.2 mg/kg, IM	3–5 min, IV 10–20 min, IM Duration: 20–30 min, IV	Ataxia produced and head-down posture Start with low dose and repeat as needed
Detomidine	0.01–0.02 mg/kg, IV 0.02–0.04 mg/kg, IM 0.06 mg/kg, PO Infusion (IV) 0.01 mg/kg bolus followed by 0.5 mcg/kg/min for 15 min, then 0.3 mcg/kg/min for 15, and then 0.1 mcg/kg/min	3–5 min, IV 10–20 min, IM 30–45 min, PO Duration: 45–60 min, IV Decrease infused dose when procedures are prolonged	Ataxia produced and head-down posture Start with low dose and repeat as needed Dosing at constant rates prolong effects
Romifidine	0.04–0.120 mg/kg IV	2–5 min, IV Duration: 2–3 h, IV	Less head-down posture Reduced ataxia and reduced analgesia
Butorphanol	0.02–0.04 mg/kg, IV Infusion: 0.01–0.015 mg/kg/min	3–5 min Duration: 1–2 h, IV	Usually used in combination with a sedative or tranquilizer Some twitching Improves well-being after colic surgery
Buprenorphine	0.006 mg/kg, IV	10–20 min Duration:	Longer acting opioid Use in conjunction with xylazine or detomidine
Morphine	0.05–0.1 mg/kg, IV	3–5 min Duration: 2–6 h, IV	Sedate with xylazine or detomidine prior to administering morphine Potential for excitement Reversible with naloxone

IV: intravenous; IM: intramuscular; PO: per os (oral); min: minutes.

6–10 h. Acepromazine cannot be relied upon to make an aggressive horse a malleable patient. Increasing the dose does not usually produce a greater effect but may increase the duration of effect. The best index of the degree of sedation with acepromazine is the presence of protrusion of the penis in male horses. In addition, the eyelids will droop and the third eyelid will protrude. Hypovolemic horses administered acepromazine may become acutely hypotensive, faint, and become recumbent. Treatment of hypotension should include large volumes of intravenous fluids (5–10 L for an adult).

Alpha-2 Adrenergic Receptor Agonists

These drugs produce sedation with muscle relaxation, ataxia, and analgesia, when given transmucosally, intravenously, or intramuscularly. The alpha-2 adrenergic receptor agonists produce a number of cardiorespiratory and other adverse effects. Arterial blood pressure is initially increased due to drug-induced increases in peripheral vascular resistance (vasoconstriction). Hypertension may be sustained (20–60 min), particularly when the longer acting alpha-2 adrenergic receptor agonists, detomidine and romifidine, are used. In response to vasoconstriction, the heart rate decreases and sinus arrhythmia and first- and second-degree atrioventricular blockade are commonly observed. Decreases in heart rate and increases in peripheral vascular resistance produce significant decreases in cardiac output, often to levels 50% of pre-drug values. Respiratory rate is usually decreased, but tidal volume increases in compensation. Relaxation of the muscles of the upper airway occurs and can predispose the horse to stridor. This may be exacerbated by mucous membrane congestion if the head is lowered secondary to sedation. Providing head support can be useful in maintaining a patent airway during prolonged (>1 h) standing procedures (Figure 13.4). The administration of an alpha-2 adrenergic receptor agonist decreases salivation, gastric secretions, and gastrointestinal motility and increases urine volume. Swallowing is depressed, and thus passage of nasogastric tubes may be more difficult. Other incidental effects of alpha-2 adrenergic receptor agonist administration include increases in intrauterine pressure, hyperglycemia, and hypoinsulinemia.

The level of sedation produced by administration of an alpha-2 adrenergic receptor agonist is more pronounced than that produced by phenothiazine administration. Depending on the dose and drug administered, horses assume a "head-down" or "saw horse" stance and frequently shift their weight from side to side (Figure 13.5). Care should be taken when performing procedures when alpha-2 adrenergic receptor agonists have been given alone. Equidae can appear profoundly sedated (extreme head-down posture) but respond unexpectedly to stimuli (e.g., touch), including kicking. The addition of an opioid (commonly butorphanol) improves sedation quality. Unprovoked aggression has been reported after the administration of xylazine or detomidine. Combining alpha-2 adrenergic receptor agonists with other drugs (i.e., acepromazine and/or butorphanol) often permits the use of reduced doses, lessening the head-down posture, and causing the horse to stand more squarely on all four feet.

Detomidine is approximately 100 times more potent than xylazine and has a duration of action approximately

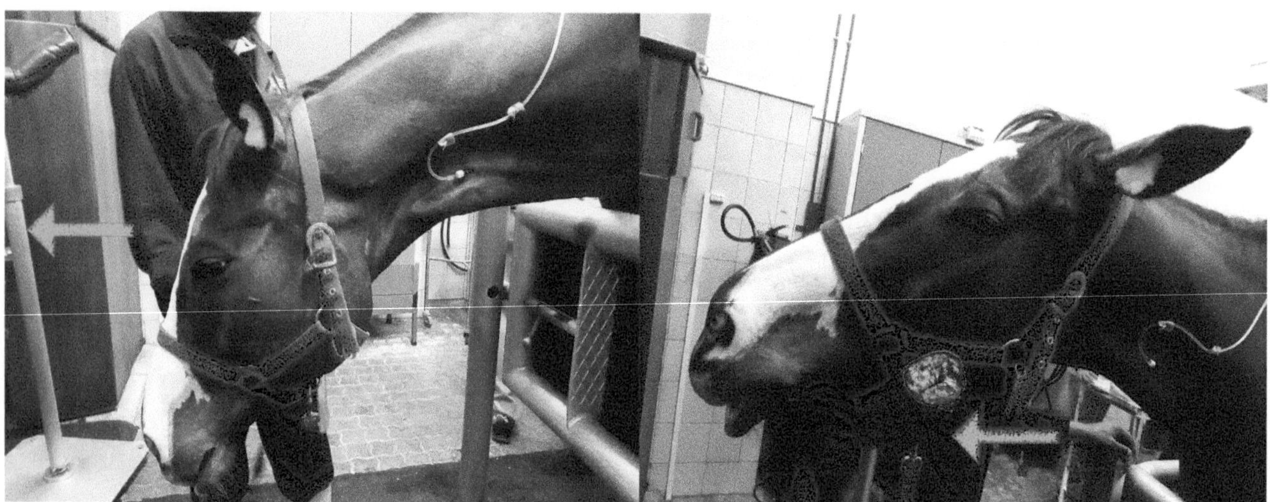

Figure 13.4 A deeply sedated horse (left) with the head carriage lower than the heart and at risk of forming nasal edema that can cause a partial airway obstruction in these obligate nasal breathing animals. To remedy or prevent nasal edema, the head should be rested on a head stand (green arrows).

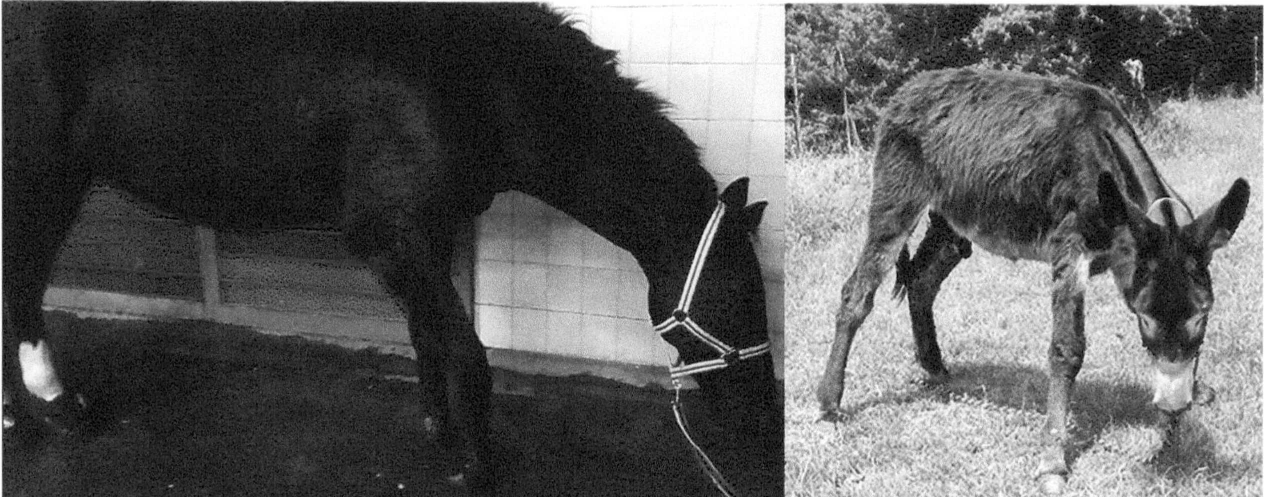

Figure 13.5 Deeply sedated horse (left) and donkey (right). Deeply sedated equids have a wide base stance, head is lowered, and they shift weight from limb to limb.

twice as long. Detomidine is used alone and in combination with opioids (butorphanol and morphine) to produce standing chemical restraint for a wide variety of procedures. Romifidine causes dose-related sedation when administered intravenously or intramuscularly with a rapid onset of action and a duration of action similar to detomidine. Sedation with romifidine is associated with less lowering of the head and less ataxia than with other alpha-2 adrenergic receptor agonists. This can make it an attractive choice for standing dental procedures.

Intramuscular drug administration is easily accomplished but the onset of drug action is slower than after intravenous administration (less than 5 min for IV compared to 10–15 min for IM). The intensity of the cardiorespiratory adverse effects after intramuscular injection is reduced, presumably due to the lower plasma concentration of unbound drug. Intravenous administration produces a quicker onset of action, an increased intensity of effect, but a shorter duration of effect. Currently, oral transmucosal administration of alpha-2 adrenergic receptor agonists is saved for occasions when the horse is not amenable to injections because of inconsistent effects. In some countries, paste formulations containing alpha-2 adrenergic receptor agonists are licensed for oral transmucosal use in horses. Oral transmucosal administration of detomidine (0.06 mg/kg body weight) has been shown to produce profound sedation 45 min after administration. The analgesia produced by opioids alone or in combination with alpha-2 adrenergic receptor agonists is insufficient to blunt the pain of procedures involving incisions so local or regional anesthetic blocks should be incorporated.

Alpha-2 Adrenergic Receptor Agonists in Combination with Other Drugs

Buprenorphine can be used in a similar manner to butorphanol. Other opioids, including morphine, have been used to produce standing chemical restraint. The combination of an alpha-2 adrenergic receptor agonist and morphine can produce a profoundly sedated animal. Alpha-2 adrenergic receptor agonist administration should precede morphine to prevent opioid-induced excitement. Horses remain sensitive to touch so local anesthesia should be incorporated with this technique for potentially painful procedures.

The combination of acepromazine with an alpha-2 adrenergic receptor agonist allows for a reduction in the dose of both drugs, reducing cardiopulmonary side effects and ataxia. Typically, 0.02–0.03 mg/kg of acepromazine is combined with 0.2–0.5 mg/kg of xylazine. The drugs can be combined in the same syringe and are usually given IV. The placement of an intravenous catheter should be considered if the duration of a procedure is expected to last longer than 30 min. This is because it is likely that supplementation of the initial dose of sedative will be required, which is facilitated by the presence of a catheter.

Estimating the Required Level of Restraint and Analgesia

These need to be based on the size and temperament of the patient and the procedure to be performed. A particular challenge is sedation or anesthesia of feral equidae, which can be extremely difficult to sedate or anesthetize. In these animals, one must consider whether it is possible to contain them in a pasture, pen or chute, and the size of available area. Large or uncontained areas will require dart administration which is a skill that requires training to develop proficiency. In smaller areas, IM administration of drugs by manual injection may be possible. Second, drug doses usually have to be significantly higher unless animals are depressed or ill, and body weights are only estimates. It is likely that sedation with alpha-2 adrenergic receptor agonists would require 2–3 times the usual dose and ketamine doses would be increased by 2–3 times. To limit injectate volumes, it may be necessary to source higher concentrations of drugs from a compounding pharmacy. Veterinarians should be aware of relevant legal restrictions to sourcing compounded drugs.

Donkeys and Mules

Sedation with tranquilizers, sedatives, and analgesics discussed in the preceding text are also used for sedation and analgesia in donkeys in mules. Donkeys usually respond to horse doses, but mules require increased doses (about 50% more) of alpha-2 adrenergic receptor agonists. Drug doses required will also depend on the degree of handling and training the donkey or mule has received. Feral donkeys must be handled using the same techniques used for feral horses.

Intravenous General Anesthesia

Drugs used in equidae during the peri-anesthetic period are summarized in Table 13.4. Intravenous administration of ketamine is the most widely used technique for induction and maintenance of short-term (<60 min) anesthesia in the horse. The original technique used xylazine given IV 5 min before ketamine. Recumbency occurs within 30–60 s of ketamine administration and anesthesia lasts approximately 15–20 min with recovery to standing occurring 10–20 min later. The quality of recovery is excellent, with most horses standing on their first attempt. Hemodynamic variables, including cardiac output and

Table 13.4 Drugs for premedication, induction, and maintenance in donkeys, mules, and horses.

Drug	Dose: donkeys (mg/kg IV)	Dose: mules (mg/kg IV)	Dose: horses (mg/kg IV)
Pre-anesthetics			
Xylazine	0.6–1.0	1.0–1.6	0.5–1.0
Detomidine	0.005–0.02	0.01–0.03	0.005–0.02
Romifidine	0.1	0.15	0.1
Butorphanol	0.02–0.04	0.02–0.04	0.02–0.04
Morphine	0.05–0.2[a]	0.05–0.2	0.05–0.2
Acepromazine	0.05	0.05–0.1	0.05
Induction			
Ketamine	2.2[b]	2.2[b]	2.2
Thiopental	5.0	5.0	5.0
Tiletamine–zolazapam	1.1	1.1	1.1
Guaifenesin	50 with ketamine or thiopental	50 with ketamine or thiopental	50 with ketamine or thiopental
Diazepam[c]	0.03	0.03	0.05–0.1
Midazolam[c]	0.06	0.06	0.05–0.1
Propofol	2.2	NA[d]	2.2
Maintenance			
Propofol	0.2–0.3 mg/kg/min	NA	0.2–0.3 mg/kg/min
G-K-X[e]	1.1 mL/kg/h	1–2 mL/kg/h	1–2 mL/kg/h
Guaifenesin with thiopental[f]	"To effect" with careful monitoring of respiration		"To effect"

[a] Recent evidence suggests that higher doses of morphine (0.5 mg/kg) may be more effective in donkeys without adverse effects (Maney et al. 2022).
[b] More rapidly metabolized than in the horse; must re-dose at shorter intervals.
[c] Suitable for sedation in foals.
[d] No information available.
[e] 50 mg/mL; 1–2 mg/mL; and 0.5 mg/mL.
[f] 50 mg/mL; 3mg/mL.

ventilation, are maintained while arterial oxygenation is decreased. Analgesia and muscle relaxation are generally good. Modifications of the original technique include the use of other alpha-2 adrenergic receptor agonists (detomidine, romifidine, and medetomidine) and the addition of butorphanol to improve the quality of sedation and analgesia.

The addition of a muscle relaxant such as guaifenesin or a benzodiazepine (diazepam and midazolam) to the xylazine–ketamine combination improves muscle relaxation with minimal additional cardiovascular depression. Guaifenesin (50 mg/kg, IV) is a centrally acting skeletal muscle relaxant that is administered intravenously after sedation just before the bolus of ketamine. A large volume (250–500 mL; approximately 1 mL/kg of a 5% solution) is required and there may be a period of ataxia at induction. Guaifenesin is administered fairly quickly (over 3–5 min), with a pressure bag or a ventilated fluid administration set (flutter valve); see Figure 13.6. If using a pressure bag, care should be taken to not give more than is needed. Guaifenesin produces some sedation, but it is primarily used to augment muscle relaxation. Diazepam is a sedative and centrally acting skeletal muscle relaxant, and improves the quality of surgery. Diazepam is given at a dose of 0.025–0.1 mg/kg intravenously immediately before or in combination with the standard dose of ketamine (2.2 mg/kg, IV). The addition of diazepam increases the duration of anesthesia to 20–25 min. Midazolam is a water-soluble benzodiazepine similar to diazepam but more potent. Midazolam is dosed at the lower end of the diazepam dose range (0.05 mg/kg, IV).

The proprietary combination of tiletamine and zolazepam administered after alpha-2 adrenergic receptor agonists produces qualitatively similar anesthesia to xylazine–diazepam–ketamine and is of longer duration, but the quality of recovery is reduced. Propofol, a commonly used drug in other species, is not widely used in

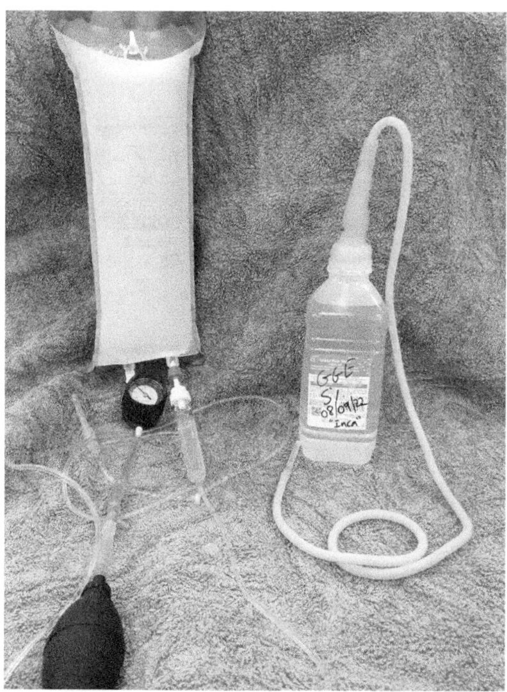

Figure 13.6 A pressure bag (left) or a flutter valve (right) assembly can be used to rapidly infuse GGE to clinical effect during the induction phase of general anesthesia in an equid.

horses. Initial reports suggested that propofol, after xylazine, was a satisfactory technique, but subsequent investigations raised concerns with excitement on induction, significant respiratory depression, and hypoxemia. More recently, the combination of propofol (dosed at approximately 0.5 mg/kg IV, used in place of a benzodiazepine) and ketamine after xylazine sedation has been investigated and may have some application, particularly in hospital settings where ventilation can easily be assisted.

Extending Anesthesia Beyond 20 min

While short procedures can be accomplished with a single IV injection of xylazine and ketamine administered via needle stick (i.e., "off the needle"), if anesthesia needs to be extended because of unforeseen circumstances, such as encountering a hernia while castrating a stallion, an additional dose of xylazine–ketamine can be administered. The drugs are given at the rate of 30–50% of the initial dose (e.g., xylazine 0.5 mg/kg and ketamine 1.1 mg/kg), combined in the same syringe. The administration of a second dose of the combination extends the anesthetic period by approximately 10 min. The administration of additional doses beyond a single redosing is discouraged because the quality of the anesthetic state and recovery from anesthesia worsen. Seizure-like activity has been observed if the combination is repeatedly re-dosed.

Guaifenesin combinations are one of the most popular methods of producing intravenous anesthesia for up to 60 min. Following induction of general anesthesia with the xylazine–diazepam–ketamine technique described in the preceding text, anesthesia is extended using a guaifenesin-based drug combination. Guaifenesin (5%) solution is combined with xylazine and ketamine to produce a solution known as "Triple Drip." Triple Drip is formulated by taking 1 L of 5% guaifenesin solution and adding 1000–2000 mg of ketamine and 500 mg of xylazine. The combination is administered to effect up to a rate of 2 mL/kg/h. The combination produces excellent muscle relaxation and analgesia. The degree of muscle relaxation and lack of movement are the best indicators of the depth of anesthesia. Tearing, blinking, and palpebral reflexes remain active throughout the anesthetic period. The quality of recovery is generally good if the anesthetic duration is kept under 60 min. Triple Drip should not be used for anesthetics greater than one hour in duration unless oxygen supplementation and respiratory support are provided. It is strongly recommended to administer Triple Drip through an IV catheter as guaifenesin is irritating if given into perivascular tissue.

Midazolam can be used to replace guaifenesin in Triple Drip. The usual quantities of xylazine (500 mg) and ketamine (1000–2000 mg) are added to 1 L of isotonic fluids. Midazolam (25–50 mg) is used in place of guaifenesin. The resultant solution is dosed at the same rate as conventional Triple Drip (up to 2 mL/kg/h, IV). The effects are similar to conventional Triple Drip and the cost may be less expensive depending on the source of guaifenesin.

Care Pathway to Prepare for Induction of General Anesthesia

Horses being prepared for general anesthesia should have an intravenous catheter placed in order to reduce stimulation of the animal at the time of induction. The mouth should be rinsed with water to facilitate endotracheal (ET) intubation and reduce the chance of aspirating foreign material. Often, analgesics, such as an NSAID, and tetanus toxoid are administered before induction. Antimicrobials, if desired, should be administered before induction of anesthesia because they can cause hypotension and adverse systemic reactions (that might not be obvious if administered during anesthesia).

Principles of Tracheal Intubation

Endotracheal intubation maintains the airway and allows insufflation of oxygen and inhalant anesthetics. Orotracheal intubation is facilitated by use of a mouth gag (Figure 13.7). A mouth speculum may be used or a mouth gag may be made from plumbing piping (40–60 mm diameter) wrapped in tape to minimize slipping. The gag is placed between the horse's incisors after induction of anesthesia. Orotracheal intubation is usually accomplished by extending the horse's head and neck at the level of the shoulders. An endotracheal tube of the appropriate size (26–30 mm internal diameter for adult horse, with smaller tubes for smaller horses) is introduced over the horse's tongue through the oral cavity and oropharynx and into the trachea. Introducing the ET tube into the larynx can be facilitated by rotating the tube as it is advanced, timing insertion with inspiration (when arytenoid cartilages are abducted). Proper positioning is confirmed by feeling for air flow when the horse breathes and a lack of resistance as the tube passes down the trachea. If intubation is difficult (as in the instance of a horse with a paralyzed arytenoid or if muscle relaxation is profound), a clean stomach tube or endoscope may be passed through the endotracheal tube and into the trachea acting to guide the ET tube into place. Intubation should always be as gentle as possible to avoid damage to the pharynx, larynx, and trachea.

Nasotracheal Intubation

For certain surgical procedures where the presence of the ET tube in the oral cavity makes surgery more difficult (e.g., dental procedures), a smaller tube may be passed into the trachea via the nasal passages. A smaller tube

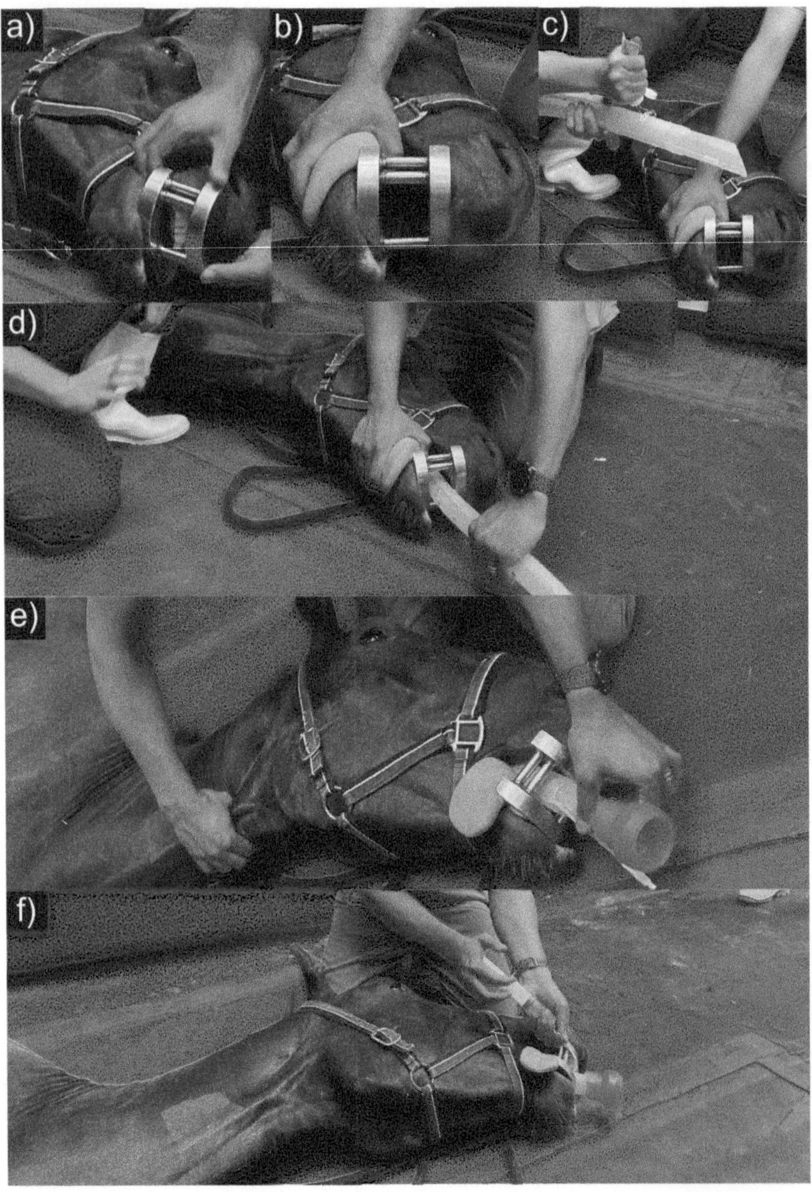

Figure 13.7 Orotracheal intubation of the trachea is performed in a horse in lateral recumbency with its head and neck fully extended. First, a mouth gag is placed (a), and the tongue retracted to one side (b) before a lubricated (water-based lubricant used to improve the seal of the endotracheal tube within the trachea once the cuff is inflated) endotracheal tube is advanced into the oral cavity (c). The tube is advanced to the caudal oropharynx where it enters the trachea via the *rima glottidis* (d), and the tube can be gently rotated back and forth through 180° as it is advanced. Advancement can be timed with inspiration to improve the success of entering the trachea. Once positioned in the trachea, the endotracheal tube can be palpated within the trachea while gently advancing and retracting the tube (e), or by pushing on the thorax, while a second person confirms air exiting the endotracheal tube (with their hand). Once in place, the cuff can be inflated with air (f).

(20–24 mm internal diameter) is required, and it is helpful to soak the tube in warm water and lubricate it generously before intubation. The tube is passed up the nose, via the ventral meatus, carefully (to avoid contact with the nasal turbinates which produce a nosebleed) and into the trachea (Figure 13.8).

Tracheostomy

Horses with collapse of the upper airway may require a temporary tracheostomy for safe anesthesia. Horses are obligate nasal breathers so surgical procedures such as ethmoid hematoma removal or sinusotomy that may require packing of the nasal cavity to effect hemostasis should have a tracheostomy performed before removal of the orotracheal tube. Preferably, the tracheostomy should be performed before the surgical procedure.

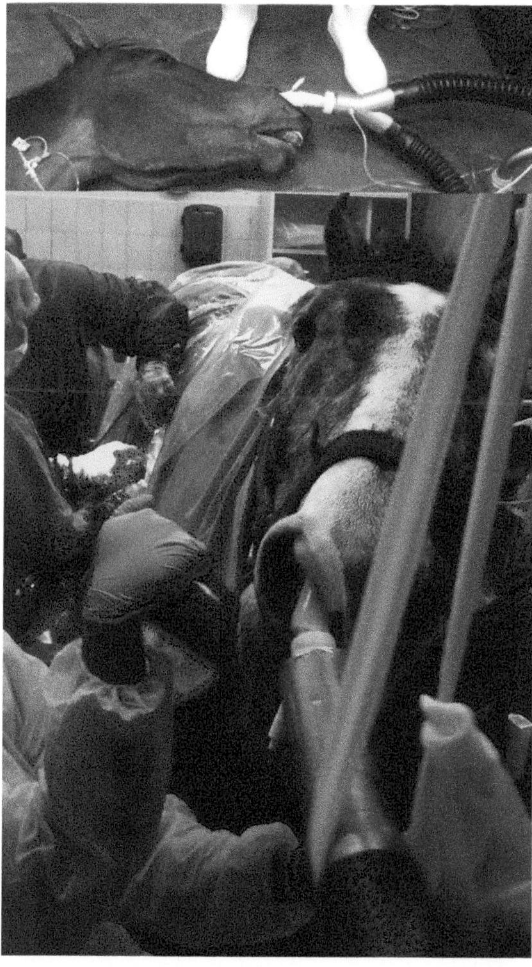

Figure 13.8 Nasotracheal intubation by passing a smaller diameter endotracheal tube via the ventral meatus, through the *rima glottidis* into the trachea in a horse undergoing a dental procedure (top) or a standing thoracotomy (bottom).

Facility and Equipment Requirements for General Anesthesia

Monitoring and Recordkeeping

Any sedated or anesthetized horse should be monitored and records kept of what drugs were administered (name, dose, route, and time) and the vital signs of the horse. Keeping records may be legally required but are also good practice. An anesthetic record does not have to be extensive, but should clearly identify the patient, drugs administered, duration of sedation or anesthesia, problems encountered and their treatment, and how the patient was monitored. Guidelines for monitoring horses during anesthesia can be found on the American College of Veterinary Anesthesia and Analgesia website, and anesthetic records are available to download from the Association of Veterinary Anaesthetists website (see Further Reading). While monitoring injectable anesthesia in the field may consist of watching respiratory rate and palpating a peripheral pulse, additional monitoring should be used for inhalant anesthesia. Numerous monitors have been used and can be used (see Chapter 4); however, some means of monitoring cardiovascular function, such as blood pressure, is recommended. Arterial blood pressure should be measured directly using an arterial catheter connected to aneroid manometer or transducer. As horses commonly hypoventilate under inhalational anesthesia, capnography is commonly used to guide ventilation. Additional monitors (e.g., anesthetic gas analyzer and blood gas machine) are recommended for prolonged or invasive surgeries; the reader is directed to the monitoring guidelines mentioned in the preceding text.

Field Considerations

If anesthesia is to be performed in the field, the practitioner needs to evaluate what help is available for induction and recovery as well as the best site for laying the horse down (Figure 13.9). Ideally, the horse will be anesthetized on a padded or soft surface, but a heavy, loose surface (such as shavings) may not be optimal if present as a deep layer. Nonslippery footing is also important. A flat, grassy area, free of debris/equipment, is optimal. A solid fence may be useful to push the horse against for induction, while a tree or post may be useful for restraining the horse's head during induction. It should be possible to have all equipment close by but not in the immediate induction area. Depending on weather conditions, cover or shade may be important depending on how long the horse will be anesthetized.

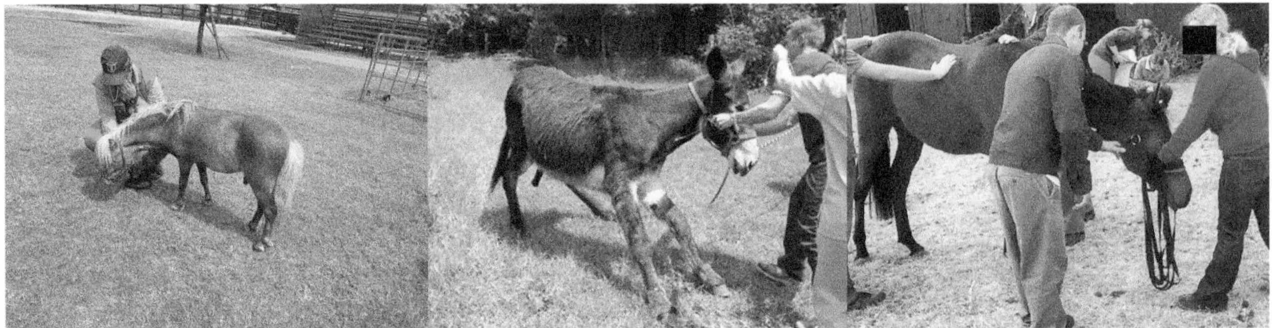

Figure 13.9 Considerations for field anesthesia of an equid include a large, soft, level area free of obstacles and buildings. These procedures are best performed in a grassy region of the property. For large equidae, it is helpful to have experienced assistants supporting the lumbar and pelvic region of the horse during the induction of general anesthesia; however, if only untrained people are available, they should stay clear of the horse during induction of anesthesia.

Checklist for Key Considerations in Preparing for a Field Anesthesia Procedure

1) Physical examination and history performed?
2) Does local environment provide a safe area for anesthetic induction and recovery?
3) Have temperament and predicted procedure duration been considered when selecting drug protocol?
4) Is all necessary anesthetic and surgical equipment available and functioning (e.g., surgical instruments and monitoring equipment)?
5) Is emergency/support equipment available (e.g., drug antagonists, endotracheal tube, and oxygen supply)?

Considerations for In-hospital Procedures

Most in-hospital anesthetics and procedures are performed in specially designed spaces (Figure 13.10). The safety of the attending personnel and the patient should be a primary consideration in the design. Facilities handling feral equidae should include a chute system so the animals can be moved with minimal human contact.

The most perilous parts of anesthesia are induction and recovery. The area where anesthesia is induced needs to be large enough to provide an "escape route" for personnel and provide access to a hoist and surgical table with appropriate padding for procedures lasting longer than 30 min. The induction stall may serve as the surgical preparation area so it must also be large enough to fit the anesthesia machine and monitoring equipment unless the horse will be moved to a different area for surgical preparation.

Hoists

Different types of hoists can be used to lift the recumbent horse from the induction stall floor onto the surgical table or cart used to move the horse. A tracking hoist can be used to carry the horse from induction to surgery and then to recovery, or a stationary hoist may be used in induction and recovery. Usually, the hoist will have a 2–3-ton capacity to facilitate safe lifting of larger horses and wear and tear of repeated use. Some type of safety mechanism for power outages and stuck chains is also essential.

Surgery

Surgical suites for equine surgery generally require a room large enough for the horse on the table, anesthesia machine with monitoring equipment, surgical equipment, and equipment tables. Good ventilation is important, as is the ability to disinfect the room. Disinfecting a room usually requires large-bore floor drains for draining the large volumes of water and disinfectant used for cleaning. Nonslip flooring and good lighting are also important.

Required Equipment

Most surgeries on horses are facilitated using inhalant anesthetics. Guidelines for inhalant anesthesia of equidae formulated by the American College of Veterinary Anesthesia and Analgesia state that when inhalant anesthesia is used, there should be equipment available to assist or control ventilation, and directly monitor arterial blood pressure. Considerations on the purchase of anesthetic machines with ventilators and monitoring equipment is beyond the scope of this chapter, and the reader is directed to the Further Reading section. Several types of surgical tables are commercially available, which feature different configurations for dorsal versus lateral positioning (i.e., head and leg board versus braces for holding the patient in dorsal recumbency). Newer tables also facilitate lifting the horse to different heights and tilting.

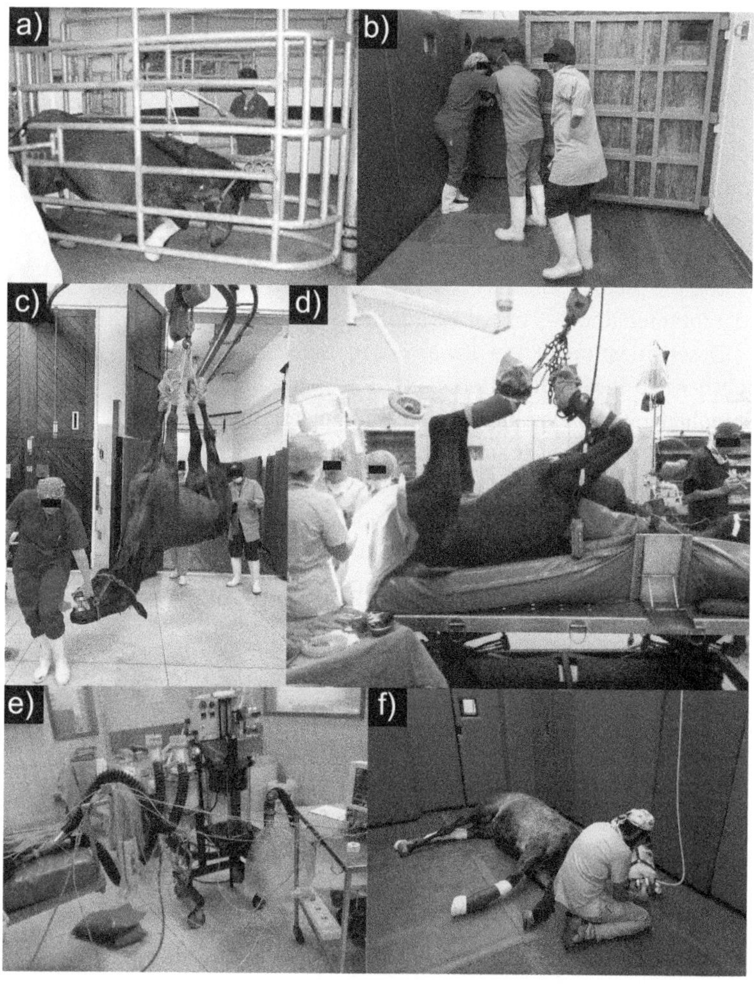

Figure 13.10 The in-hospital facilities may include a chute-type system, especially if feral horses are frequently presented (a), and the induction room (or box) should be large enough to allow for free movement and escape of personnel when required, and for moving anesthetic equipment into the area if it is used as a surgical preparation area ((b), swing door system in use). The facility should have some form of overhead hoist system to move the equid to the surgical room (c). This hoist system can be used to suspend limbs when the horse is in dorsal recumbency (d). The surgical table should be adequately padded to prevent myopathies and neuropathies. The surgical room should be large enough to accommodate the anesthetic equipment, patient, and personnel (e). The recovery box should allow for a number of techniques to be used safely (hand recovery, rope-assisted recovery, and unassisted recovery) and should have a means to provide oxygen supplementation during recovery (f). The person in (f) is in a dangerous position (in the path of the horse should it move, and he is kneeling, which will impede moving quickly). This person should be positioned at the dorsal side of the horse's head and neck so that if the horse raises its head and attempts to stand he would not be knocked over.

Local Anesthesia

Local anesthetics provide a method to desensitize pain receptors and/or block the transmission of pain impulses both peripherally and centrally. Local anesthetics are widely used in combination with sedatives and analgesics to facilitate standing procedures and are increasingly utilized during general anesthesia to reduce inhaled anesthetic requirements. The use of local anesthetics is encouraged as part of pain management protocols. Regional techniques are also useful, but it should be noted that techniques that cause weakness or loss of proprioception to the degree that the animal's ability to stand is compromised should be employed with caution.

Lidocaine (0.5, 1, and 2%) and mepivacaine (1, 1.5, and 2%) are amide-linked local anesthetics, produce minimal irritation of tissues, and have durations of action of approximately two hours. Bupivacaine (0.2, 0.5, 0.75, and 1%) and ropivacaine (0.2, 0.75, and 1%) are newer local anesthetics with anesthetic durations of 4–6 h and are approximately four times more potent than lidocaine. All of these drugs can be used for local infiltration, line block, conduction (nerve) block, intra-articular block, and epidural and spinal anesthesia and analgesia. Alpha-2 adrenergic receptor agonists and opioids are also given by the epidural route to provide analgesia without the risk of motor blockade associated with larger volumes of local anesthetic deposited in the epidural space. Total doses of lidocaine should be kept below 10 mg/kg, and aspiration should be performed before injecting any local anesthetic to minimize the risk of intravascular injection.

Local Anesthesia of the Head

Akinesia of the upper eyelid is produced by blockade of the auriculopalpebral nerve, producing motor blockade of the upper eyelid enabling surgery. Importantly, the eyelid is immobilized but not desensitized. The supraorbital nerve must also be blocked to desensitize the upper eyelid. The auriculopalpebral nerve is palpated in a slight depression on the temporal aspect of the zygomatic arch. Five to eight milliliters of 2% lidocaine is administered subcutaneously. Remember to protect the eye until motor function returns.

Desensitization of the upper eyelid is accomplished via blockade of the supraorbital nerve, a branch of the frontal nerve. The nerve is blocked at the level of the supraorbital foramen that is palpated midway between the upper and lower borders of the supraorbital process, about 5–6 cm above the medial canthus of the eye. A needle is placed into the foramen and 3–5 mL of 2% lidocaine is injected.

Desensitization of the lower eyelid is usually accomplished via local infiltration. Sensation to the lower lid is supplied by the zygomatic nerve (except for the medial canthus), a terminal branch of the maxillary branch of the trigeminal nerve. The nerve enters the eyelid just rostral to the lateral canthus. It is difficult to block on the floor of the orbital socket, so local infiltration is usually employed.

Desensitization of the upper lip, nose, and the upper dental arcade is accomplished by blockade of the infraorbital nerve. The infraorbital is a branch of the maxillary division of the trigeminal nerve. The nerve exits the infraorbital foramen under the *levator nasolabialis superioris* muscle. Within the canal, the nerve supplies the maxillary teeth, their alveoli, and the gums. The infraorbital foramen can be found approximately 4 cm above and just in front of the rostral end of the facial crest. If blockade of the teeth is desired, use a 5 cm (2 inch), 20 gauge needle and advance the needle into the canal after desensitizing the skin over the opening. Occlude the opening of the canal with a finger as you inject (under pressure) 4–6 mL of local anesthetic. The local anesthetic is distributed caudally and can produce anesthesia of all of the upper molars and the maxilla itself. If only desensitization of rostral superficial structures is required, the nerve can be blocked as it exits the infraorbital foramen. The maxillary nerve can also be blocked within the orbit prior to its entry into the bony canal.

Desensitization of the lower lip and the lower dental arcade is accomplished by blockade of the mandibular nerve. The mental nerve is a continuation of the alveolar branch of the mandibular division of the trigeminal nerve. The mental foramen is located just ventral to the middle of the interdental space on the lateral aspect of the mandible. The foramen is covered by the *depressor labiinferioris* muscle that can be deflected in order to palpate the bony lip of the opening. To block the lower cheek teeth, insert a 20 gauge, 5 cm (2 inch) needle into the canal and inject 4–7 mL of local anesthetic under pressure (occlude the opening). If only the rostral, superficial structures required desensitization, simply desensitize the nerve as it exits the foramen. Then, mandibular nerve can also be blocked on the medial side of the mandible proximal to its entrance into the bony canal.

Local Anesthesia for Other Anatomical Regions

The inclusion of a local anesthetic block in the anesthetic technique for castration improves surgical conditions by decreasing the risk of movement. If general anesthesia is employed, the local anesthetic technique of choice can be applied immediately after induction of anesthesia so that the block can take effect during the surgical scrub. Injection into the spermatic cord is easily accomplished. Ten milliliters of lidocaine (2%) in each cord is sufficient. It is necessary to wait a short time after injection (30–60 s) for the local anesthetic to take effect. The addition of the local anesthetic reduces the likelihood of a reaction when the emasculator is applied and may reduce post-operative pain. A number of procedures (neurectomy and curettage of the third phalanx) can be facilitated by applying commonly used sensory blocks in anesthetized horses. The benefits of intra-articular administration of local anesthetics or opioids are unclear but generally considered low risk.

Epidural Anesthesia and Analgesia

Caudal epidural anesthesia is useful for surgery of the rectum, anus, perineum, tail, vulva, vagina, penis, and inguinal region. It can also be used for pain relief, reduce straining, and to allow obstetrical manipulations. Single injection techniques are most commonly employed. Clip the area over the injection site and prepare it aseptically. Subcutaneous administration of a small quantity of rapid acting local anesthetic (usually lidocaine 2%) should be used to facilitate placement of the spinal needle. The site for injection is located by moving the tail up and down and palpating the junction between the first and second coccygeal vertebrae on the dorsal surface. An 18 gauge, 7.5 cm (3 inch) spinal needle is inserted perpendicular to the skin at the middle of the intercoccygeal space. The needle is advanced until there is an abrupt loss of resistance to further advancement. Correct placement is confirmed by injecting a small quantity of air or injectate with little to no resistance. When using injectate, a bubble of air is commonly introduced into the syringe. This provides visual feedback that there is minimal resistance to injection, as the air bubble maintains its shape (i.e., it is not compressed during injection). The air bubble is not injected into the patient. Lidocaine (6–10 mL of 2%) is commonly used, producing 90 min of anesthesia with an initial onset of action within 5 min. The duration of the blockade can be dramatically extended (2–4 times longer) by using xylazine (0.17 mg/kg diluted to 6 mL with 0.9% NaCl/450 kg) or combining lidocaine (2%, 5 mL) with xylazine (10%, 1 mL) and administering the combination at a rate of 6 mL/450 kg.

Nonmedical Considerations in the Sedation and Anesthesia of Horses

Most performance horses are subject to restricted drug usage, with some jurisdictions maintaining "drug free" policies. It is important to communicate to the owner/trainer how long any anesthetic/analgesic drugs are expected to be present in horse's system. This information may not be published, but most governing bodies provide withdrawal guidelines in order to prevent residual drug levels being present at the time of competition. Modern drug testing techniques can identify drugs in picogram concentrations; horses should not return to race or show until they test negative. Additionally, some drugs may reside in fatty or muscle tissue for prolonged periods. The labels for most drugs approved for use in horses carry the warning "Not to be used in animals intended for food."

Questions and Answers

There are more practice questions and answers available for this chapter on the website. Please visit http://www.wiley.com/go/VeterinaryAnesthesiaZeiler.

Questions

1) Anesthetic mortality in horses is in the range of
   a) 5%
   b) 1%
   c) 0.1%
   d) 0.01%
2) Response to drug-dosing regimens in equines:
   a) does not vary from breed to breed
   b) does not vary from individual to individual
   c) does not vary from horses to mules
   d) varies widely from breed to breed and individual to individual
3) Regarding pain assessment in equines, which of the following is false?
   a) horses are stoic and their high pain tolerance rarely requires pain relief
   b) heart and respiratory rate are helpful parameters for assessment
   c) owner's observations may be helpful, especially in donkeys and mules
   d) reluctance to move may indicate pain
4) Standing surgery might be preferred over recumbent general anesthesia in
   a) a young foal
   b) a draft horse weighing 1000 kg
   c) an unhandled horse
   d) for an abdominal exploratory

Answers

1) b
2) d
3) a
4) b

Further Reading

Andersen, M.S., Clark, L., Dyson, S.J., and Newton, J.R. (2006). Risk factors for colic in horses after general anaesthesia for MRI or nonabdominal surgery: absence of evidence of effect from perianaesthetic morphine. *Equine Vet J* 38: 368–374.

Bussières, G., Jacques, C., Lainay, O. et al. (2008). Development of a composite orthopaedic pain scale in horses. *Res Vet Sci* 85: 294–306.

Dalla Costa, E., Minero, M., Lebelt, D. et al. (2014). Development of the Horse Grimace Scale (HGS) as a pain assessment tool in horses undergoing routine castration. *PLoS ONE* 9: e92281.

De Oliveira, M.G.C., de Paula, V.V., Mouta, A.N. et al. (2021). Validation of the Donkey Pain Scale (DOPS) for assessing postoperative pain in donkeys. *Front Vet Sci* 8: 671330.

Figueiredo, J.P., Muir, W.W., and Sams, R. (2012). Cardiorespiratory, gastroinetestinal, and analgesic effects of morphine sulfate in conscious healthy horses. *Am J Vet Res* 73: 799–808.

Gleerup, K.B. and Lindegaard, C. (2016). Recognition and quantification of pain in horses: a tutorial review. *Equine Vet Educ* 28: 47–57.

Johnston, G.M., Eastment, J.K., Wood, J., and Taylor, P.M. (2002). The confidential enquiry into perioperative equine fatalities (CEPEF): mortality results of Phases 1 and 2. *Vet Anaesth Analg* 29: 159–170.

Maney, J.K., Dzikiti, B.T., Escobar, A. et al. (2022). Morphine in donkeys: antinociceptive effect and preliminary pharmacokinetics. *Eq Vet J* online. https://doi.org/10.1111/evj.13912.

Mircica, E., Clutton, R.E., Kyles, K.W., and Blissitt, K.J. (2003). Problems associated with perioperative morphine in horses: a retrospective case analysis. *Vet Anaesth Analg* 30: 147–155.

Regan, F.H., Hockenhull, J., Pritchard, J.C. et al. (2014). Behavioural repertoire of working donkeys and consistency of behaviour over time, as a preliminary step towards identifying pain-related behaviours. *PLoS ONE* 9: e101877.

Senior, J.M., Pinchbeck, G.L., Allister, R. et al. (2006). Post anaesthetic colic in horses: a preventable complication? *Equine Vet J* 38: 479–484.

Senior, J.M., Pinchbeck, G.L., Dugdale, A.H.A., and Clegg, P.D. (2004). Retrospective study of the risk of colic in horses after orthopaedic surgery. *Vet Rec* 155: 321–325.

Skrzypczak, H., Reed, R., Barlett, M. et al. (2020). A retrospective evaluation of the effect of perianesthetic hydromorphone administration on the incidence of postanesthetic signs of colic in horses. *Vet Anaesth Analg* 47: 757–762.

Taylor, P.M., Hoare, H.R., de Vries, M. et al. (2016). A multicentre, prospective, randomised, blinded clinical trial to compare some perioperative effects of buprenorphine or butorphanol premedicaion before equine elective general anaesthetia and surgery. *Equine Vet J* 48: 442–450.

van Dierendonck, M.C., Burden, F.A., Rickards, K., and van Loon, J.P.A.M. (2020). Monitoring acute pain in donkeys with the Equine Utrecht University Scale for Donnkeys Composite Pain Assessment (EQUUS-DNBKEY-COMPASS) and the Equine Utrecht University Scale for Donkey Facial Assessment of Pain (EQUUS-DONKEY-FAP) Animals 10. https://doi.org/10.3390/ani10020354.

van Dierendonck, M.C. and van Loon, J.P. (2016). Monitoring acute equine visceral pain with the Equine Utrecht University Scale for Composite Pain Assessment (EQUUS-COMPASS) and the Equine Utrecht University Scale for Facial Assessment of Pain (EQUUS-FAP): a validation study. *Vet J* 216: 175–177.

Van Loon, J.P. and van Dierendonck, M.C. (2015). Monitoring acute equine visceral pain with the Equine Utrecht University Scale for Composite Pain Assessment (EQUUS-COMPASS) and the Equine Utrecht University Scale for Facial Assessment of Pain (EQUUS-FAP): a scale-construction study. *Vet J* 206: 356–364.

Van Loon, J.P. and van Dierendonck, M.C. (2019). Pain assessment in horses after orthopaedic surgery and with orthopaedic trauma. *Vet J* 246: 85–91.

Anesthetic monitoring guidelines and monitoring forms: https://ava.eu.com/resources/checklists https://acvaa.org/veterinarians/guidelines.

14

Anesthesia and Analgesia of Healthy Exotic Companion Mammals, Ruminants, and Pigs

Hugo van Oostrom, Samantha Swisher, and Gareth Zeiler

Exotic Companion Mammals

Risk of Peri-anesthetic Mortality

Exotic companion mammals (exotics), such as rabbits, ferrets, guinea pigs, chinchillas, hamsters, and rats, are widely perceived to have much higher rates of peri-anesthetic mortality than dogs and cats, though research to support this supposition and identify underlying causes is limited (Figure 14.1). In 2008, Brodbelt et al. reported that peri-anesthetic death rates in rabbits were significantly higher than in dogs and cats (0.73% of rabbits believed to be healthy and 7.37% of sick rabbits), but the numbers of other exotic species included in the study were insufficient to draw firm conclusions. The causes of peri-anesthetic death in exotics are likely multifactorial; however, in many cases, they can be attributed to technical challenges, failure to identify underlying illness, or a combination of both. The major challenges of exotic companion mammal anesthesia are summarized in Concept Box 14.1.

Technical challenges in exotic anesthesia result mostly from their small size, which complicates intubation, intravenous (IV) catheter placement, monitoring, and maintenance of normothermia. Some species also have unique anatomy or physiology that present challenges during anesthesia, such as the palatial ostium in the guinea pig, which complicates intubation. These challenges are compounded by the fact that most anesthetists have less experience performing anesthesia in exotics than traditional companion animals.

Failure to identify underlying illness or appreciate the severity of known illness in exotics is also an important contributing factor to the higher peri-anesthetic mortality observed in these species. This has historically been attributed to the natural inclination of prey species to "hide" signs of illness, but it is perhaps more accurate to say that the signs of illness in these species are often subtle and can be difficult to detect, especially for a less experienced veterinarian or technician. Other plausible reasons for not identifying illness include the challenges of performing diagnostics (physical examination, blood sampling, radiographs, etc.) in conscious animals, and in some cases, lack of familiarity with normal species behaviors. Because signs of illness can be subtle, especially to the untrained eye, it is critical to collect a thorough history and be alert to subtle behavioral abnormalities at home or during the exam. General signs of illness that apply to most exotic species include hyporexia (decreased appetite), hiding behavior, abnormal response to handling, lack of appropriate alertness in a new setting (e.g., the veterinary clinic), hunched posture, poor grooming, piloerection (especially in rodents), and orbital tightening. Hypothermia is very common in sick exotics and has been associated with a poor prognosis in rabbits and guinea pigs; thus, measuring rectal temperature before administering anesthetic drugs can be helpful if it can be performed without causing too much stress to the animal. Except in the most extreme emergencies (such as uncontrolled hemorrhage), almost all sick exotic patients will benefit from taking extra time to ensure that they are warm and well hydrated before proceeding with anesthesia.

While low-stress handling is important for the welfare of all patients, it is especially critical for sick exotics. It is very common for animals that seem only mildly ill at home to decompensate on presentation to the veterinary clinic from the combination of stress of transportation and handling by unfamiliar people. Exotics should be housed in a quiet area of the hospital with good footing and low lighting, and

Fundamental Principles of Veterinary Anesthesia, First Edition. Edited by Gareth E. Zeiler and Daniel S. J. Pang.

Companion Website: www.wiley.com/go/VeterinaryAnesthesiaZeiler

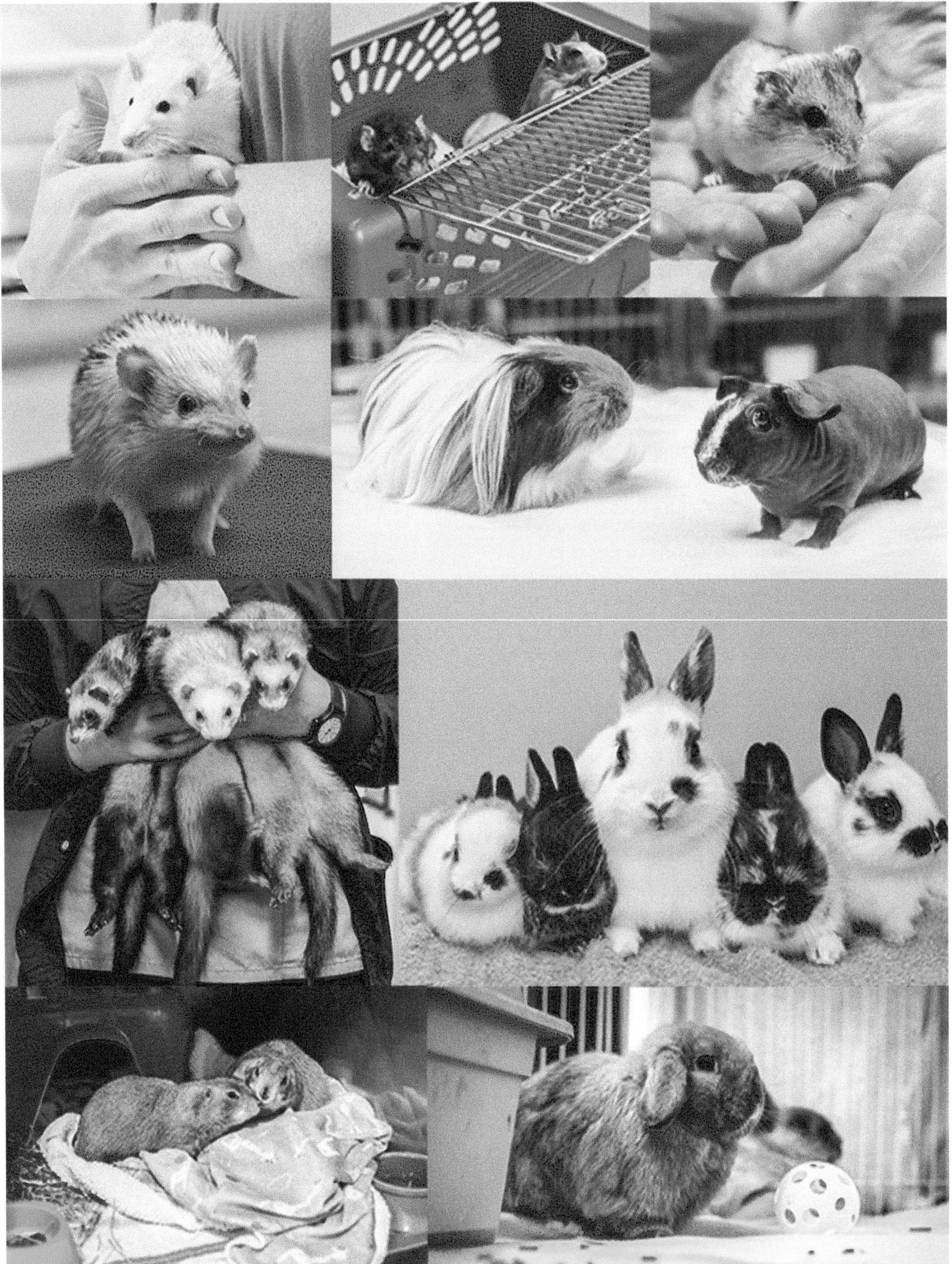

Figure 14.1 Collage of exotic companion mammals that can present to a veterinary clinic for treatment. From left to right, top row: a white rat, two rats in a blue enclosure, and a hamster; second row: a hedgehog, and a hairy and a naked guineapig; third row: three ferrets, a family of rabbits; fourth row: two prairie dogs and two rabbits. (*Source:* Courtesy of Ms. Katie Lennox-Philibeck.)

Concept Box 14.1

The three major challenges of exotic companion mammal anesthesia.

Hypothermia

- Challenges:
  - High surface-area to volume ratio allows rapid heat loss.
  - Some common heat support devices obscure anesthetist's view of the patient.
- Tips and tricks:
  - Provide heat support in the cage while premedication is taking effect and pre-warm surgery table and recovery area. If diagnostic imaging is required, bring heat support with you.
  - Use warmed IV/SC fluids and scrub solutions, and dry patients thoroughly after procedure.
  - Insulate areas prone to heat loss (e.g., rabbit ears and rat tails).

Apnea

- Challenges:
  - Many exotic species are not routinely intubated and are difficult to intubate quickly in an emergency.
  - When patients are intubated, the small size of the tubes makes the tube prone to obstruction, kinking, and displacement.
  - Surgical draping makes visual monitoring of small patients difficult.
- Tips and tricks:
  - Use a capnograph for intubated patients to monitor tube placement and patency.
  - If using a mask for anesthetic maintenance, ensure that the mask fits properly and the reservoir bag is appropriately sized to facilitate mask ventilation if needed. Note that some capnographs detect breaths when used with a tight-fitting mask.
  - Use clear drapes to allow the anesthetist to visually monitor breathing. Clear drapes also reduce the risk of the surgeon inadvertently compressing the thorax with their hand or instruments (by maintaining awareness) and help trap heat.

Hypotension

- Challenges:
  - Indirect blood pressure monitoring techniques are unreliable in some species and not feasible at all in others.
  - Catheter placement is more challenging and many not be routinely performed in some species.
  - There is limited data about the efficacy and appropriate dosing for pressors in exotics. Available information suggests that they are often ineffective at the doses recommended for dogs and cats, and higher doses may be required, titrating to effect.
- Tips and tricks:
  - Become familiar with other changes that may accompany hypotension, including bradycardia, low respiratory rate, hypothermia, and/or slow anesthetic recovery.
  - If not placing a catheter in advance, be sure that someone other than the surgeon is comfortable placing an IO catheter in case of emergency. Regular practice in cadavers can be helpful to gain and maintain proficiency.
  - Steps to address hypotension are similar to those recommended for other species and include reducing anesthetic gas/reversing injectable drugs (if possible) and/or giving fluid boluses.

prey species should be out of visual or olfactory contact with predator species. Ideally, exotics would be housed separately from dogs and cats; if this is not possible, many clinics choose to house exotics in their feline ward, which is generally quieter. All supplies should be prepared in advance to reduce handling time. While many clinicians are reluctant to sedate sick exotics for fear of adverse outcomes, it is important to understand that in many cases the negative effects of the stress that results from not sedating the animal may outweigh the risk of achieving mild–moderate sedation, with analgesia.

Vascular Access Sites

Adjunct Therapy to Facilitate Vascular Access

Premedication is required to facilitate catheter placement in all but the most debilitated exotics. For IV catheters, it may be helpful to apply local anesthetic cream (e.g., EMLA™ cream) topically to the catheter site at least 30–45 min before placement. Rates of percutaneous systemic absorption of these products have not been determined for most species, so caution should be used when applying to very small patients and to those that are prone to grooming themselves to avoid toxicity. Placement of a small bandage over the site may help to prevent ingestion.

If applying local anesthetics topically is not possible, then the anesthetist could consider injecting a small volume of rapid-onset injectable local anesthetic drug (i.e., lidocaine or mepivacaine) around the site. This method provides faster onset of analgesia compared to topical application, but can impair visualization of the vessel, and some animals may react (suspected stinging sensation) during or shortly after injection. Thus, this practice should be reserved for situations when catheter placement is expected to be difficult and the benefit of injecting the local anesthetic outweighs the initial discomfort of transcutaneous catheter puncture. Local anesthesia should always be provided before intraosseous catheter placement.

Intravenous Catheterization

Appropriate catheter sizes for exotics range from 30-gauge diameter in very small rodents (mice and hamsters) to 18 gauge in large rabbits. Catheterization of the cephalic vein is usually possible in rabbits (26–20 gauge, depending on the size of the rabbit), ferrets (26–24 gauge), and guinea pigs

(26–24 gauge), and may be possible in other species with practice. In rabbits, additional veins that can readily be catheterized include the lateral saphenous vein (26–18 gauge) and the marginal ear veins (not the central artery; 26–22 gauge). The lateral saphenous vein is often the easiest vein to catheterize in rabbits but is difficult to maintain in an awake animal. Thus, this vein is best reserved for situations when the catheter is expected to be removed shortly after anesthesia. Some anesthetists avoid placing catheters in the ear because of the risk of thrombosis and subsequent ear necrosis; however, in laboratory animal research, ear catheters are commonly used and a very few complications are reported. In rabbits and ferrets, intact males and individuals with adrenal tumors may have very thick skin, so puncturing the skin first with a hypodermic needle (one size larger than the catheter) is often helpful to minimize potential for damage to the tip of the catheter during placement.

Intraosseous Catheterization

Intraosseous (IO) catheterization using a hypodermic needle or IO needle provides an alternative to intravenous catheterization, especially in very small or debilitated patients. The pharmacokinetics of IO injection of drugs are similar to IV injection. Appropriate needle sizes range from 25 to 18 gauge, depending on the size of the patient (e.g., 20–18 gauge for a large-breed rabbit and 25–22 gauge for a ferret). It is recommended to use the largest needle size possible, as smaller needles are prone to bend, break, or block. Recommended placement sites include the proximal tibia, the proximal humerus, or the proximal femur. Placement in the proximal tibia is usually the most straightforward because the landmarks are easily palpable in most exotics. However, rats have a more curved tibia than other exotics, making placement of a needle in the tibia more difficult compared to the humerus or femur. If the needle becomes obstructed with bone during placement, the bone core can be dislodged with the stylet from an IV over-the-needle catheter. If a stylet is not available, it is often possible to remove the clogged needle and place a new needle through the same entry site. Correct placement should always be confirmed with orthogonal radiographs. Many electronic fluid pumps struggle with the increased resistance produced by small diameter needles used for IO access, so manual intermittent fluid administration using a syringe may be required.

General Anesthesia

Patient Preparation

Withholding of Food (Fasting) and Water

When developing pre-anesthetic fasting protocols, it is important to consider patient size, anatomy, physiology, and underlying medical conditions. Many small herbivores (e.g., rabbits, guinea pigs) are not anatomically capable of vomiting except when gastric pressure is very high. These species may benefit from a short (1–4 h) fast to reduce the amount of food in the oral cavity, but prolonged fasting is not necessary. Guinea pigs tend to hold food material in their mouths for long periods of time, and the oral cavity should always be cleared of food material using cotton tipped applicators and/or oral rinses. Fasting is recommended for young, healthy ferrets, but can be relatively short (four hours is usually sufficient) because of their rapid gastrointestinal transit time. Fasting older ferrets (>3–4 years old) is controversial because of the high prevalence of insulinoma in this population. Blood glucose monitoring should be strongly considered before, during, and after anesthesia for older ferrets, and an IV catheter should be in place to allow prompt intervention if needed. Water is generally not withheld in any exotic species, but access is prevented once premedication is administered.

Preparing Small Drug Volumes

In most standard syringes, the hub of the syringe introduces inaccuracy in drug measurement when multiple drugs are drawn up in to one syringe. This inaccuracy is a problem both when drugs are being drawn up (the first drug to be drawn up is present in a larger volume because it fills both the hub and the barrel of the syringe) and when drugs are administered (a small volume of the mixture remains in the hub after injection). These inaccuracies are likely inconsequential in larger patients but may represent a safety concern for small exotics patients. There is no perfect solution to this problem, but options to mitigate it include the following:

1) Using more dilute solutions, when possible, especially if the drug is to be administered IV or SC. When administering drugs IM, the discomfort produced by a larger injection must be considered.
2) Drawing up the least potent drug (e.g., a benzodiazepine) first and mixing thoroughly before administration. Listing injectable drugs from least to most potent in drug orders can help to remind staff to do this.
3) Using “hubless” syringes, which have a modified plunger to minimize dead space in the hub.

See Chapter 6 for an in-depth discussion and worked examples of how to dilute a drug.

Prokinetics

Many clinicians routinely administer prokinetic drugs (e.g., metoclopramide, cisapride, ranitidine) before and after anesthesia in small herbivores to preempt the development of ileus in the post-operative period. There is little evidence to support this practice so decisions of whether to use prokinetics and which drug to use are a matter of veterinarian preference.

Antimicrobial Therapy

Pre-operative antimicrobial prophylaxis should be considered for clean-contaminated surgery (e.g., gastrointestinal surgery) and those involving placement of implants. First-generation cephalosporins (e.g., cefazolin) are commonly used for this purpose in other species, but many veterinarians are reluctant to use them in small herbivores due to concerns over the risk of gastrointestinal dysbiosis. Available evidence suggests that beta-lactams (i.e., penicillins and cephalosporins) are well tolerated in exotics when given parenterally, but the substitution of a fluoroquinolone (e.g., ciprofloxacin) can also be considered, especially if continued oral administration is expected to be necessary after surgery.

Drugs Used During the Peri-anesthetic Period

Commonly used drugs during the peri-anesthetic period are presented in Table 14.1. When using formularies (see Further Reading) to select doses for anesthetic drugs (particularly ketamine and [dex]medetomidine), it is important to consider the source of dosing information; many higher doses are from laboratory animal literature where it is more common to use injectable drug protocols to induce general anesthesia, and these higher doses are rarely used in companion exotics.

Drugs Used During the Pre-anesthetic Period

Historically, concerns about the "fragility" of exotic patients caused many anesthetists to avoid injectable anesthetic drugs, preferring to use only inhalational anesthesia so that patients could be recovered more quickly. Just as this practice is no longer recommended in dogs and cats, it is becoming clear that this approach is inappropriate for

Table 14.1 Drugs and doses (mg/kg, unless otherwise stated) that are commonly used during the peri-anesthetic period management of exotic companion mammals.

Drug	Ferrets	Rabbits	Guinea pig/chinchilla	Rats, mice, and hamsters
Premedication, sedation, or IM induction of anesthesia				
Benzodiazepines				
Midazolam	0.25–0.5	0.25–1	0.5–1	0.5–1
Opioids				
Hydromorphone	0.05–0.2	0.1–0.3	0.3–2	0.1–0.3
Methadone	0.1–0.3	0.1–0.3	0.3–0.5	0.3–0.5
Morphine	0.5–2.0	1.2–5	2–4	2–4
Buprenorphine	0.01–0.03	0.01–0.05	0.05–0.2	0.05–0.2
Butorphanol	0.05–0.5	0.5–2	0.5–2	1–2
Other				
Alfaxalone	1–2	1–4	1–4	1–4
Dexmedetomidine	0.005–0.01	0.005–0.01	0.01–0.01	0.01–0.02
Ketamine	5–15	5–15	5–15	10–20
Intravenous (or intraosseous) induction				
Alfaxalone	1–4	0.5–3	0.5–2	1–2
Ketamine + midazolam	5 (K) + 0.2 (M)	5 (K) + 0.5 (M)	5 (K) + 0.5 (M)	10 (K) + 0.5 (M)
Propofol	3–6	2–6	3–5	3–5 (IV/IO access not easy to establish)
Isotonic crystalloid fluids and constant rate infusions				
Maintenance fluid rate	60–70 mL/kg/day	100–150 mL/kg/day	GP: 100 mL/kg/day Chin: 60 mL/kg/day	Rats: 22–33 mL/adult/day Mice: 5–8 mL/adult/day Hamster: 50–150 mL/adult/day

(*Continued*)

Table 14.1 (Continued)

Drug	Ferrets	Rabbits	Guinea pig/chinchilla	Rats, mice, and hamsters
Anesthetic fluid rate	10 mL/kg/h			
Resuscitation bolus volume	10–20 mL/kg			
Fentanyl CRI	2–5 mcg/kg loading 5–10 mcg/kg/h	5–10 mcg/kg loading 10–40 mcg/kg/h	5–10 mcg/kg loading 10–30 mcg/kg/h	5–10 mcg/kg loading 30–60 mcg/kg/h
Lidocaine CRI	1–2 mg/kg/h	2 mg/kg loading + 3–6 mg/kg/h	-	-
Local anesthesia (maximum recommended doses)				
Lidocaine	2.0			
Bupivacaine	1.0			
Post-operative analgesia				
Opioids				
Methadone	0.2–0.3 (q 2–3 h)	0.1–0.3	0.3–0.5	0.3–0.5
Hydromorphone	0.05–0.2 (q 6–8 h)	0.05–0.3 (q 6–8 h)	0.3–2 (GP: q 6–8 h; Chin: q 2–4 h)	0.1–0.3 (q 2–4 h)
Buprenorphine	0.01–0.03 (q 8–12 h)	0.01–0.05 (q 6–12 h)	0.05–0.2 (q 6 h)	0.05–0.2 (q 6–8 h)
Meloxicam	0.1–0.2 (q 24 h)	1 (q 24 h)	0.5 –1 (q 24 h)	1–2 (q 24 h)
Tramadol	*Not recommended*			
Gabapentin	3–10 (PO q 8–12 h)	5–15 (q 8–12 h)	*Conflicting efficacy data*	
Other drugs that can be used during the peri-anesthetic period				
Drug	**Indication**	**Dose**	**Route**	**Notes**
Atropine	Bradycardia and hypotension	0.04–0.1	IV (preferred in emergencies) IM	May be less effective in rabbits because some individuals possess serum atropinases but still appropriate to try if glycopyrrolate unavailable
Glycopyrrolate	Bradycardia and hypotension	0.01–0.02	IV (preferred in emergencies) and IM	Preferred for rabbits if available
Epinephrine	Cardiac arrest	0.01–0.1	IV	Higher doses only if there is a prolonged arrest (>10 min)
Doxapram	Respiratory stimulation	1–10	IV	Generally not recommended for use; use only when manual ventilation is not possible
Atipamezole	Reversal of α_2 agonists	0.01–0.03	IM	Commonly used if there is a prolonged recovery
Flumazenil	Reversal of benzodiazepines	0.01–0.05	IV (emergencies) IM/SC (prolonged recovery)	Commonly used if there is a prolonged recovery; re-sedation possible

Note: The doses provided in this table are based on published literature and the author's (S.S.) experience, but the appropriate dose for an individual patient is affected by many factors, including the patient's species, age, other drugs administered, and underlying medical conditions.

The authors acknowledge and thank Dr. Juliette Raulic (University of Montreal) for guidance in completing information presented in this table.

exotics as well. Appropriate use of sedation reduces patient stress, supports hemodynamic stability by reducing the minimum alveolar concentration for inhalant anesthetics, and, depending on the drugs selected, may also provide analgesia. Drugs that are injected should be administered quickly and efficiently using low-stress handling techniques (e.g., wrapping the patient in a towel), and the patient should be returned to a quiet, dark cage until the drugs have taken effect. Hypothermia may develop quickly in small patients, so pre-emptive active heat support (i.e., electric heating blanket, heating lamp, etc.) during this period is beneficial.

The only circumstance in which the use of inhalational anesthetics without premedication is still widespread is for routine wellness exams and grooming for unsocialized hedgehogs. Sedation using injectable drugs could also be used for this purpose, but many clinicians prefer inhalational anesthetic for these routine appointments to reduce client wait time and shorten the recovery period. There is a widespread misconception that injectable anesthetic drugs cannot be used in hedgehogs because the leg muscles are not readily accessible and drugs are not well absorbed from the mantle area. In the author's (S.S.) experience, however, injecting drugs into the epaxial muscles (identified through palpation with a cotton tipped applicator or similar instrument) is just as effective as it is in other species (Figure 14.2).

Minimally invasive procedures such as venipuncture, radiography, and bandage changes can be performed under sedation using injectable drugs. More invasive procedures

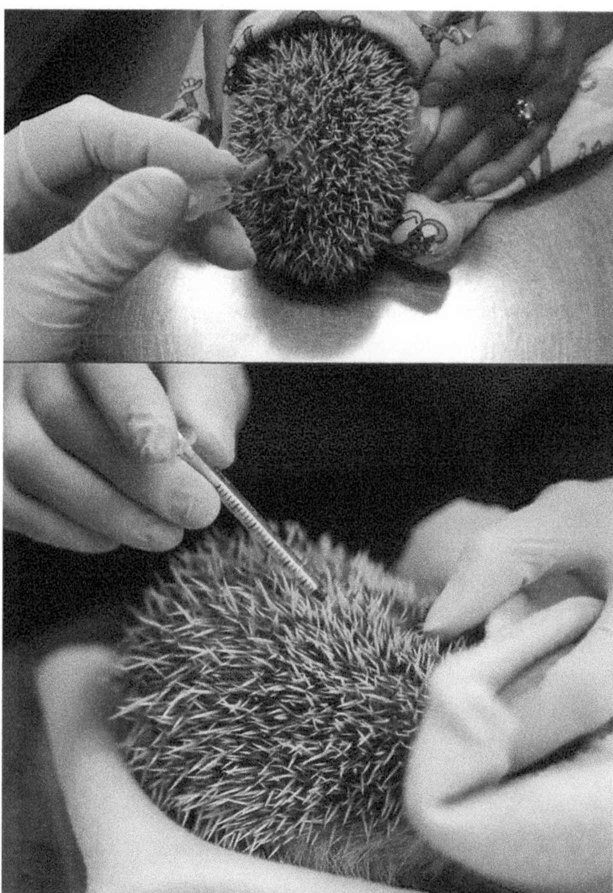

Figure 14.2 Performing an intramuscular injection into the epaxial musculature of a hedgehog. The muscle can be identified by palpating with a cotton tipped applicator (or similar). (*Source:* Courtesy of Ms. Katie Lennox-Philibeck.)

(wound care, digit or tail amputation, IO catheter placement, skin biopsy, or minor mass removal) may also be possible with sedation and good analgesia (an opioid and a local anesthetic block) but without inhalational anesthesia.

Premedication of ASA I and II Patients ASA I and II patients typically receive a benzodiazepine and an opioid for premedication, but in many cases will require additional drugs for sedation to facilitate low-stress induction of anesthesia. For induction, ketamine and (dex)medetomidine were commonly used, but in recent years, the use of intramuscular (IM) alfaxalone has become increasingly popular. While some published doses extend as high as 4 mg/kg IM for alfaxalone alone, 1–2 mg/kg is usually sufficient when used in combination with a benzodiazepine and an opioid. Because the onset of action for alfaxalone is relatively rapid, some clinicians prefer to administer the benzodiazepine and opioid first, followed by alfaxalone about 10 min later. In the author's (S.S.) experience, the onset of action of alfaxalone is often rapid and very abrupt in guinea pigs and chinchillas, so these patients should be monitored especially closely. Inclusion of alfaxalone increases the likelihood that general anesthesia is induced (rather than sedation), increasing the risk of hypoxemia. Therefore, it is good practice to provide supplemental oxygen as soon as the patient is suitably sedated and monitor oxygenation with pulse oximetry.

Premedication of ASA III to V Patients For systemically sick or critically ill patients, it is most common to use midazolam and an opioid for premedication. Generally, these medications are given IM to facilitate catheter placement, but if a catheter is already present, they can also be given IV (or IO). Midazolam is used more commonly than other benzodiazepines in exotics because its aqueous formulation allows it to be administered IM, but other benzodiazepines could be considered if IV/IO access is available. Exotics tend to require higher doses of midazolam than dogs and cats (0.5–1 mg/kg IM for all but the sickest patients), and the paradoxical excitatory response sometimes observed in healthy dogs and cats is rarely seen in exotics. If patients experience a prolonged recovery after anesthesia, reversal of the benzodiazepine with flumazenil (0.01–0.05 mg/kg IV, IM, or SC) is often helpful. The duration of effect of flumazenil is typically shorter than that of midazolam, so patients should be monitored for re-sedation, especially if flumazenil is given soon after midazolam dosing.

Opioids are the mainstay of analgesia in exotics undergoing surgical procedures. Some veterinarians attempt to avoid opioids in herbivores due to concerns about inducing gastrointestinal stasis. However, poorly controlled pain is also a common cause of decreased gastrointestinal motility in these species, and the benefits of opioid administration generally outweigh the risks. The choice of opioid is dependent on availability and veterinarian preference. Common choices include hydromorphone, methadone, or fentanyl for very painful procedures/conditions and buprenorphine for less painful procedures/conditions. Morphine use in exotics has fallen out of favor compared to the other opioids because of a perception that it causes more adverse effects, such as anorexia and gastrointestinal stasis, though there is little experimental evidence to support this. In the author's (S.S.) experience, morphine does seem to be associated with higher rates of vomiting in ferrets. Butorphanol usually provides better sedation than full- or partial-*mu* agonists; however, there is limited data about its analgesic efficacy in most exotic species, so this opioid should be reserved for less painful procedures. Exotics often require much higher doses of opioids than dogs and cats, with the exception of ferrets, who are very sensitive to opioids (especially butorphanol) and may have prolonged recoveries when high doses are given. Identifying the appropriate opioid doses for different exotic species is an active area of research, and it would be prudent for those who work with exotics to check the literature periodically for the latest recommendations or to contact a specialist when dealing with infrequently encountered species.

Drugs Used During the Anesthetic Period

Historically, most exotics were induced using inhalational anesthetics delivered by facemask or using an induction chamber, often without adequate (or any) premedication. This method does not allow for close monitoring of the patient's condition (since patients are either enclosed in an induction chamber or tightly restrained in a towel) and tends also to result in struggling and breath-holding in many species. Use of an induction chamber also increases occupational exposure to anesthetic gases. If a facemask is to be used for induction, the veterinarian should aim to ensure that the patient is heavily sedated to reduce stress, and increasing the inhalational anesthetic concentration gradually can sometimes help to reduce breath-holding. If an IV catheter is present, the use of an injectable protocol to induce general anesthesia is preferred. Alfaxalone, propofol, etomidate, and ketamine/midazolam have all been used in exotics. Alfaxalone and propofol should be administered slowly (one quarter of calculated total dose as a bolus, delivered over 15 s, followed by further doses as required) and with careful respiratory monitoring as they can cause hypoventilation and apnea. Alternatively, as described in the preceding text, anesthesia can be induced by adding an anesthetic drug (ketamine or alfaxalone) to the drug combination used for IM premedication.

Drugs Used During the Recovery Period

Meloxicam is the most commonly used nonsteroidal anti-inflammatory drug (NSAID) analgesic in exotics. For omnivorous/insectivorous/carnivorous exotics (ferrets, sugar gliders, hedgehogs, etc.), very little evidence is available to support a specific dose, but most clinicians use 0.1–0.2 mg/kg. For rabbits and rodents, however, there is increasing evidence that much higher doses are required, ranging from 0.5 to 1 mg/kg. Undiagnosed renal disease is relatively common in older rabbits (>6 years) and rats (>12 months), and this must be considered when deciding whether to prescribe meloxicam (or other NSAIDs) for these patients. In many cases, meloxicam is well tolerated for chronic pain management in a stable geriatric patient. Administration of NSAIDs during the pre-anesthetic or anesthetic period is generally not recommended when arterial blood pressure monitoring is not possible. However, NSAIDs often can still be given during recovery, when the blood pressure is expected to return to normal in most patients. If NSAIDs are administered for longer than five days, then monitoring renal function and administering the lowest effective dose are recommended.

While some veterinarians use tramadol in exotic mammals, there is limited evidence to support this practice, and clear evidence in dogs and cats indicates that there is considerable inter-species variation in efficacy (see Chapter 3). Studies in rabbits and chinchillas found that tramadol did not produce analgesia when used at the 1–4 mg kg dose typically used in dogs and cats, and in chinchillas it caused neurologic signs, including tremors and muscle fasciculation, at higher doses. The author (S.S.) has also observed neurologic signs (tremors and profound sedation) in ferrets given doses of less than 4 mg/kg PO q 12 h. There is limited evidence to support the efficacy of gabapentin for analgesia in exotics, but it is generally well tolerated.

Oral transmucosal buprenorphine has been studied in rabbits, guinea pigs, and rats and was either ineffective or required unreasonably high volume and dosing frequency. The effect of sustained-release formulations of buprenorphine has been mixed, possibly in part because multiple formulations are available with different pharmacokinetic profiles and bioavailability. Reported complications include sedation, hyporexia, and decreased fecal production. In the author's (S.S.) experience, rats and guinea pigs often exhibit significant sedation, to an extent that complicates patient status assessment and limits normal activities. Rabbits tend to tolerate the medication better, but sedation and decreased appetite are observed in some individuals.

The use of acupuncture in exotics is increasing and may be helpful as an adjunctive therapy if a licensed practitioner familiar with exotics is available. However, supporting literature is highly variable in quality (lack of appropriate controls), so acupuncture should not be the mainstay of any analgesic plan.

Practical Advice on Patient Recovery

There is increasing recognition across species of the importance of careful monitoring and supportive care during the recovery period to reduce peri-anesthetic complications and mortality. The considerations for exotics during this period are similar to those for other species and include supporting a return to normal physiological states, such as maintaining appropriate body temperature and blood pressure, as well as careful assessment of the patient's analgesic needs. Temperature monitoring is especially critical for exotics because their small size (large surface-area-to-volume ratio) predisposes them to rapid changes in body temperature, including both hypothermia and iatrogenic hyperthermia if heat support is provided to a sedated patient without adequate monitoring. As discussed in the preceding text, blood pressure monitoring is challenging in smaller exotics, so it is not uncommon to give a trial fluid bolus to patients that are not recovering (i.e., moving into sternal recumbency and responsive) within approximately 15 min.

Because of their small airways, even mild laryngeal swelling from intubation trauma can be life-threatening. If a patient was intubated and there is any reason to suspect airway trauma (blood on the tube, audible breathing, increased respiratory effort, and visualization of swelling/hemorrhage with an endoscope), they should be recovered slowly in a quiet, oxygen-enriched incubator, and extubation should be delayed for as long as possible. Steroids are generally avoided in exotics, when possible, but the author (S.S.) has given a single low dose of dexamethasone (0.03 mg/kg IV) to rabbits with laryngeal trauma without observing any negative effects.

For most exotic species, it is critical that the patient begin eating as soon as possible. Food should be offered as soon as it is deemed safe to do so, and syringe feeding is recommended if the patient does not begin eating on their own within a few hours. Cages should be designed to make patients feel secure, while allowing for visual monitoring. If possible, it is often beneficial to monitor patients by camera as many exotics will hide signs of pain and be reluctant to eat when unfamiliar people are present. Pair-bonding is common in many exotic mammal species (with the exception of hamsters and hedgehogs), so it is important to ask the owner if the patient has a companion kept in the same enclosure. Pair-bonded animals should be returned to their bonded partners as soon as it is safe to do so.

Self-mutilation of surgical incision sites is uncommon in most exotic species with the exception of sugar gliders, prairie dogs, and occasionally, rats. Preventive techniques such as Elizabethan collars and body wraps are stressful for most exotics, so these are typically only used if a patient demonstrates that they are needed. Bitter substances used for lick prevention in dogs and cats may not be as effective in many exotics because herbivores tend to have a higher tolerance for bitter tastes. In the author's (S.S.) experience, the most common times for self-mutilation to occur are (1) as the patient is recovering from sedation or anesthesia, (2) the first night in the hospital after the procedure, and (3) the first day after the patient returns to their usual environment. Heightened monitoring is recommended during these times.

Principles of Airway Management

Tracheal Intubation

As for other species, tracheal intubation of exotics offers numerous benefits, including protecting the airway, facilitating manual or mechanical ventilation, and allowing more effective intervention in case of emergency. However, intubation can be significantly more challenging in some exotic mammal species, leading to increased risk of trauma and longer anesthetic times associated with multiple failed attempts. For smaller species that require short, small diameter endotracheal tubes (e.g., rat, hedgehog, hamster, and small guinea pigs), the risk of tube displacement or occlusion (e.g., mucoid or saliva plug, twisting, or kinking tube) is significant. For these reasons, it is important that the anesthetist carefully consider each case to determine whether the benefits of tracheal intubation outweigh the risks of complications and have clear, predetermined criteria for switching to other methods if problems arise in the placement or maintenance of the endotracheal tube, or an unacceptably long time has passed during intubation attempts (Figure 14.3). Factors to consider when deciding whether to attempt tracheal intubation include the species, the duration (>30 min) and type of procedure (i.e., complex dental procedures and invasive procedures where a body cavity is entered), preexisting medical conditions, and the experience level of the anesthetic team. Intubation of ferrets and rabbits should be considered the standard of care for all but very short duration or minimally invasive procedures. Other exotic mammal species are intubated on a case-by-case basis with consideration of the factors listed in the preceding text.

As in other species, the application of lidocaine (common veterinary formulations are 2%; i.e., 20 mg/mL) onto the glottis can help facilitate tracheal intubation in exotics. Because of the small size of many exotics, it is advisable to avoid

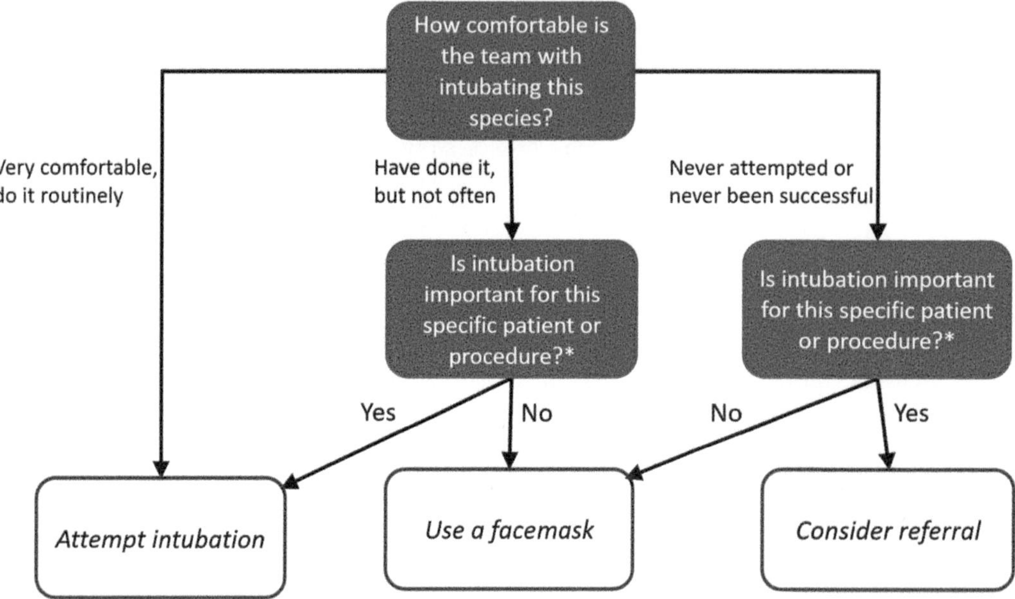

Figure 14.3 Flow diagram to assist decision-making for performing endotracheal intubation in exotic companion mammals undergoing general anesthesia. Footnote: *Examples of situations where intubation might be important include long/complex dental surgeries, procedures where fluid is introduced into the oral cavity (e.g., dental prophylaxis) or anesthesia in patients with obstructed nasal cavities. If intubation is the goal, a predetermined limit should be set (e.g., based on time or number of attempts) to minimize the risk of fixating on this goal, before moving on to an alternative plan (e.g., facemask, abort procedure, get help, change technique, etc.).

devices that deliver lidocaine in metered sprays (often 10 mg per delivery/actuation) in favor of manual administration from a syringe (attach a 24-gauge IV catheter to the end to facilitate reaching the oropharynx and to decrease the size of the drops delivered), which allows delivery of smaller doses. For very small patients, even one drop of lidocaine may represent an overdose; in these cases, the lidocaine can be diluted to a 1% (10 mg/mL) concentration.

Ferrets

Orotracheal intubation of ferrets is performed similarly to dogs and cats (see Chapter 12). Standard uncuffed endotracheal tubes ranging from 2.0–3.0 mm are appropriate, depending on the size of the ferret. For larger ferrets, cuffed endotracheal tubes can also be used. Because of the small size of the ferret mouth, choosing a small laryngoscope blade (size 0 Miller or Macintosh blade) and having an assistant use a 25 mm gauze strip (or string; string can cause damage to the gingiva causing pain and hemorrhage, especially if there is periodontal disease) to hold the mouth open can assist in visualization of the caudal oropharynx and *rima glottidis*.

Rabbits

Intubation of rabbits is challenging because their narrow oropharyngeal cavity, relatively large tongue, and prominent incisors can cause difficulty visualizing the glottis. Many different techniques have been described, but the most common are blind intubation and endoscope-assisted intubation. Endotracheal tubes range from 2.0 mm (appropriate for rabbits under 2 kg) to 3.5–4.0 mm (appropriate for larger breeds, e.g., Flemish Giant and New Zealand White).

For blind intubation, the neck is extended with the nose directed toward the ceiling (Figure 14.4). The tube is advanced until it is close to the level of the *rima glottidis* (identified by hearing loud breath sounds when the anesthetist's ear is held at the endotracheal tube connector), and then gently advanced, while slowly rotating the tube until it enters into the trachea. If the tube does not enter the larynx (either because the larynx is closed or the tube enters the esophagus), the tube is retracted and another attempt made. Experienced practitioners can often locate the glottis by feel, but there are a variety of techniques that help to locate the glottal opening, including the following:

1) Listening for breath sounds at the proximal end of the endotracheal tube as it is advanced, either by simply placing an ear at the end of the tube or by magnifying the sound using stethoscope earpieces attached via an elbow connector or a Beck Airway Airflow Monitor (BAAM) device.
2) Using a capnograph to guide placement.

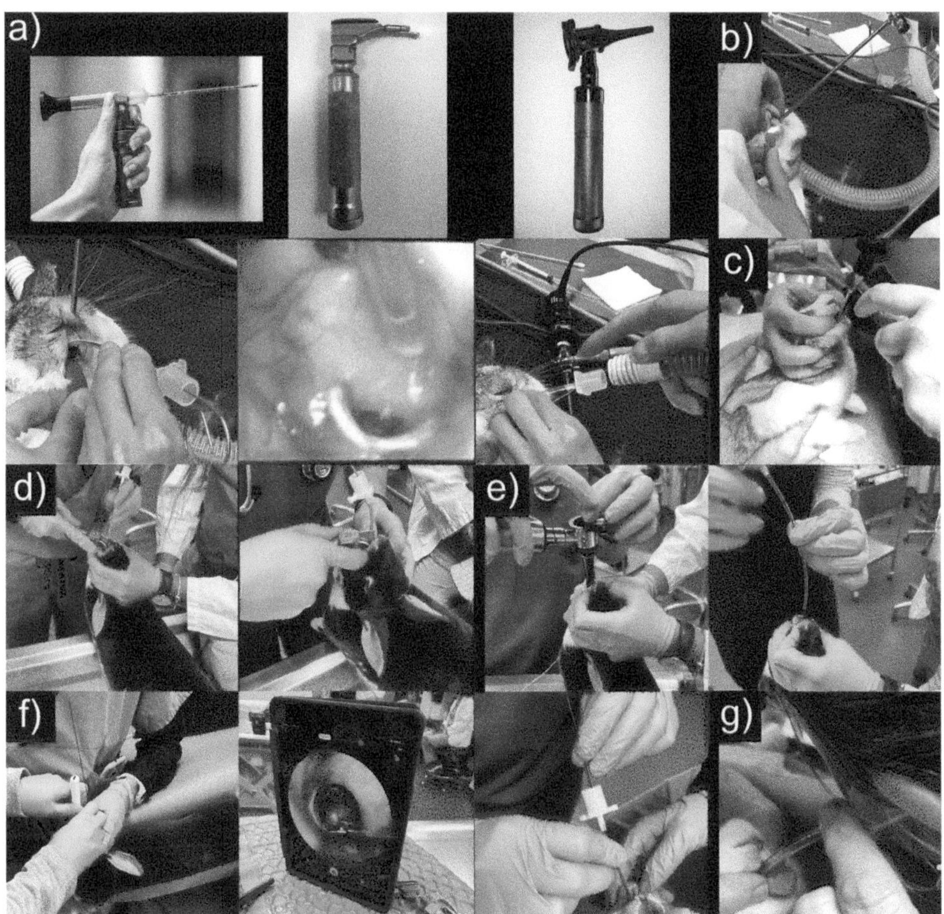

Figure 14.4 Equipment used to facilitate intubating the trachea of rabbits includes (from left to right) (a) a handheld battery-operated rigid endoscope, a small size (size 0) Miller blade laryngoscope, or an otoscope. Two techniques for using a rigid endoscope are the side-by-side technique (b), where the endoscope is placed into the oropharynx and then shifted laterally to observe the endotracheal (ET) tube being advanced down the center of the oral cavity and into the trachea, and the "railroad" or "over-the-scope" technique (c), where the endotracheal tube is positioned over the endoscope and both endoscope and ET tube advanced together until just past the *rima glottidis*. Then, the ET tube is advanced off the endoscope and into the trachea. A laryngoscope (d) can be used in larger rabbits, in the same way as in other species, to visualize the larynx. Here, an intubating stylet is placed within the endotracheal tube to help support and guide the ET tube into the airway. An otoscope (e) can be used to visualize the *rima glottidis* and an endotracheal tube introducer (boogie and intubating stylet) can be advanced through the otoscope and into the trachea. Then, the otoscope is removed, with the introducer maintained in place, and the endotracheal tube is "railroaded" into the trachea over the introducer. Other advanced equipment includes a flexible bronchoscope (f) attached to a portable video screen (or cell phone) and a similar procedure as described for (e) is followed. Blind intubation (g) is also possible, where endotracheal tube positioning and placement are guided by listening for breath sounds. If the endotracheal tube is advanced into the esophagus, no breath sounds will be heard. If advanced into the trachea, breaths sounds will be audible. (*Source:* Rigid scope: Courtesy of Ms. Katie Lennox-Philibeck; photos (c) and (g): Courtesy of Dr. Dorianne Elliot, Bird, and Exotic Animal Hospital; photos (b), (d), (e) and (f): Courtesy of Dr. Javier Benito; Université de Montréal.)

Endoscope-assisted intubation can be performed either by threading the endoscope through the endotracheal tube (the "railroad" or "over-the-scope" technique) or by using a side-by-side technique. In the author's (S.S.) experience, the over-the-scope technique seems to be more intuitive for most users. While a diagnostic endoscope can be used for this purpose, there are smaller, semi-flexible, handheld endoscope developed specifically for this purpose, which have the advantage of being more convenient and also reduce the risk of damage to a more expensive diagnostic endoscope (Figure 14.4). With the appropriate scope, the over-the-scope technique can be used with tubes as small as 2.0 mm. The tube should be cut to length that allows the tip of the endoscope to align with the tip of the tube for optimal visibility. Patient positioning is similar to that used for blind intubation. Extension of the neck usually frees the tip of the epiglottis from the soft palate (it is normally positioned with the tip dorsal to the soft palate). If it does not, the end of the endoscope can be used to gently displace the soft palate dorsally, allowing visualization of the *rima glottidis*. Ideally, before attempting endoscopic-assisted intubation, IV access should be established and anesthetic drugs be readily available to deepen the anesthetic if the rabbit reacts (head avoidance, chewing, etc.) during the intubation procedure. Rabbits that are inadequately anesthetized during intubation attempts may launch forward unexpectedly, which presents a risk for airway trauma. Practicing with a cadaver first can be very helpful and is recommended for those learning how to perform orotracheal intubation using this technique.

If the tube is advanced gently, the risk of damage to the *rima glottidis* using either method of intubation should be minimal. However, attempts to intubate should be aborted if (1) prolonged efforts are unsuccessful, (2) the patient moves in a way that causes the tube to impact the epiglottis with great force, (3) respiration becomes labored, or (4) blood is observed on the endotracheal tube (Figure 14.5). Correct placement often results in a cough; this can help confirm correct placement (some anesthetists avoid topical lidocaine during blind intubation for this reason), but can also displace the tube, so the anesthetist should be prepared to hold the tube in place until it is secured and quickly attach the patient to the anesthetic breathing circuit. Regardless of the method of intubation used, proper placement is preferably confirmed with a capnograph after the tube is tied in place.

An alternative to orotracheal intubation is nasotracheal intubation, where the endotracheal tube is passed through the ventral meatus of the nasal cavity, through the nasopharynx and into the trachea. This method is especially helpful for dental procedures where an orotracheal tube could interfere with the assessment of the dental arcade occlusion or access to the caudal oral cavity (see Further Reading).

Rodents

Intubation of guinea pigs and chinchillas is complicated by the need to pass the endotracheal tube through the palatial ostium to access the glottis, which is quite small. Larger guinea pigs and chinchillas can be intubated with a 2.0 mm endotracheal tube, but smaller animals may require specialized tubes. Intubation is generally easier with endoscopic guidance, and placing the patient on a dental rack may help to facilitate visualization (Figure 14.6). Guinea pigs tend to hold large amounts of food in their oral cavity, and this should be removed before intubation is attempted. Guinea pigs tend to produce abundant and relatively thick oral and respiratory secretions, so the tube should be monitored closely for signs of obstruction, such as increased expiratory effort or declining SpO_2.

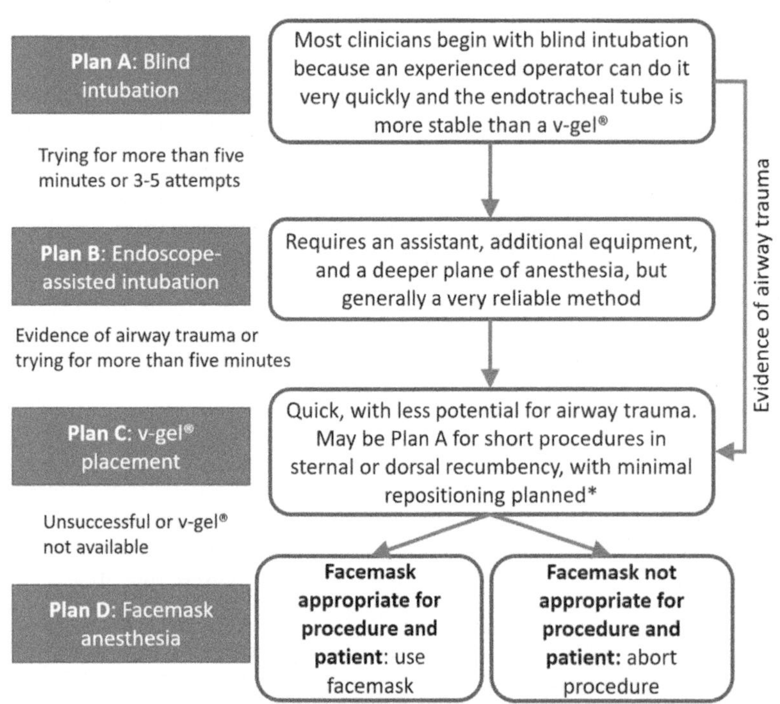

Figure 14.5 A decision flowchart for intubating the trachea of a rabbit.

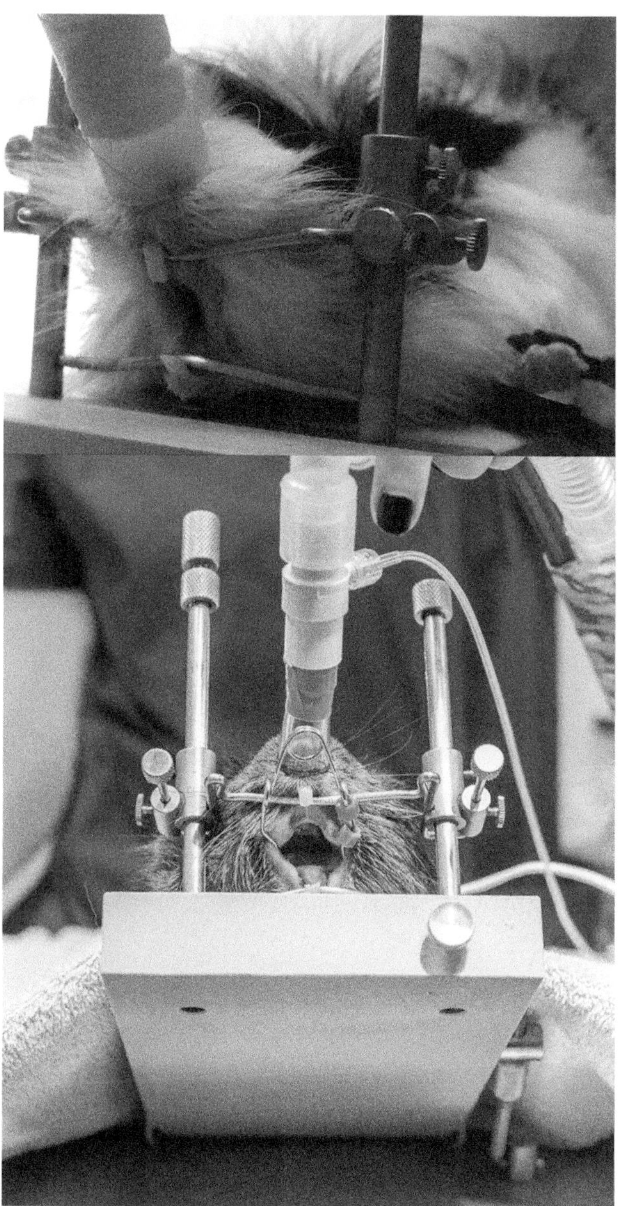

Figure 14.6 A dental rack can be used to position the patient to facilitate endotracheal intubation. These photos are of exotic companion mammals placed in a dental rack but have a nose cone (very small facemask) to deliver oxygen and inhalational anesthetics. (*Source:* Courtesy of Ms. Katie Lennox-Philibeck.)

Intubation of smaller rodents, such as rats and hamsters, is possible and is performed routinely in some laboratory settings, but it is a technique that requires special equipment and practice (Figure 14.7). Because of the small diameter of the tubes used (often 20–18-gauge IV catheters attached to a 15 mm connector), they clog and kink easily and can be difficult to maintain. Most short-stay IV catheters are constructed from relatively stiff material, so they may be more likely to cause airway trauma, especially if the tube is not secure and with changes in patient positioning. Hamsters often store food in their cheek pouches, and they should be emptied before tracheal intubation or mask anesthesia.

Supraglottic Airway Devices

Supraglottic airway devices are available for rabbits in a variety of sizes (Figure 14.8). Advantages include ease of placement (placement can be achieved within 30 s by novice anesthetists) and reduced potential for airway trauma. Disadvantages include the risk of the device being dislodged if the patient is moved (especially when the patient is placed in dorsal recumbency) and the need for capnography to monitor placement. To place the device, the patient's tongue is extended, and the device is advanced along the hard palate with the airway channel facing lingually until resistance is encountered, indicating that the channel should be seated over the *rima glottidis*. It is strongly recommended to use capnography during placement and throughout the procedure to ensure that the device remains properly positioned. The capnograph trace will become distorted or disappear if the device moves out of position. Relying on increased respiratory noise is an insensitive means of identifying partial/complete airway obstruction associated with supraglottic airway device placement.

Facemasks

Delivery of inhalational anesthesia by facemask is common in many exotic species because of the challenges associated with tracheal intubation (Figure 14.9).

Since the patient's airway will not be protected, it is important to ensure that the oral cavity is free from debris/food material (e.g., guinea pigs and hamsters). Canine and feline facemasks can be appropriate for larger exotics, but it is important to choose the smallest facemasks available to improve fit and minimize mechanical dead space. A facemask can be fashioned out of a plastic bottle with its base cut off and an examination glove stretched over the cut end to provide a seal, if no suitable facemask is available. However, for practices that routinely see smaller patients, specialized facemasks should be purchased. The facemask selected should form a tight seal with the patient's face in order to minimize exposure of the surgical team to anesthetic gas and to allow effective manual ventilation in the event of apnea. A properly fitted facemask may also allow for capnography readings in some cases. Many practitioners find it helpful to secure the facemask in place by threading a loop of gauze, dental floss or suture through the facemask, and looping it around the patient's incisors before securing the facemask to the anesthetic tubing (Figure 14.10). Note that rabbits and hystricomorph (i.e., guinea pigs and chinchillas) rodents are obligate nasal

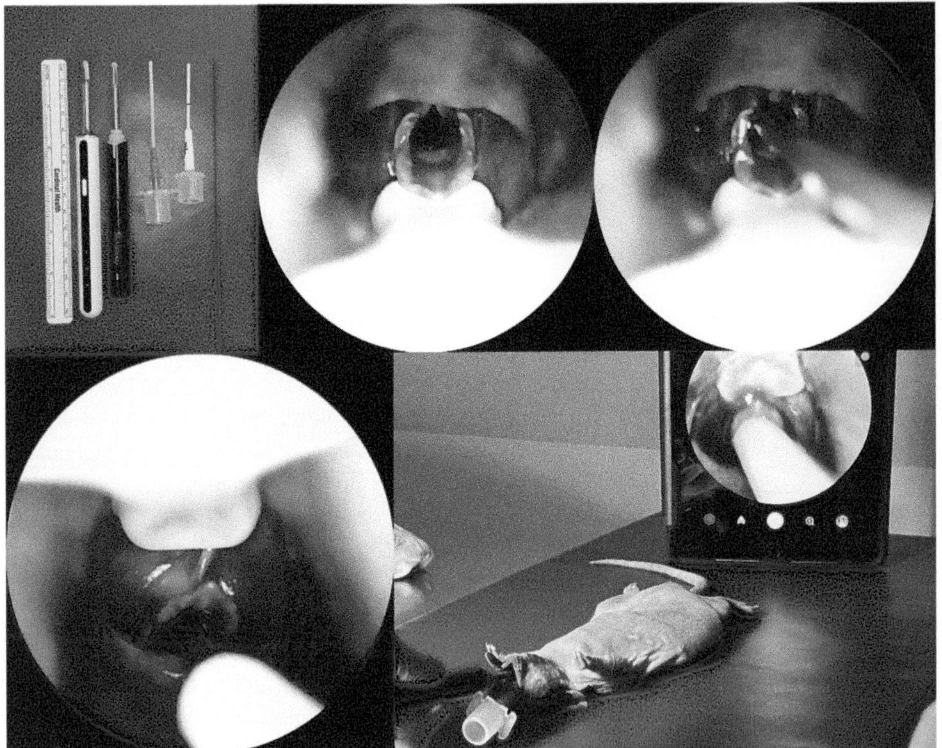

Figure 14.7 Tracheal intubation of a rat using a handheld camera otoscope and intubating stylet. From left to right, the equipment that can be used, a video image of the *rima glottidis*, the intubating stylet being advanced into the trachea, the over-the-needle intravenous catheter being used as an endotracheal tube is advanced over the intubating stylet into the trachea, and a photograph of a rat with the intravenous catheter endotracheal tube in place (inset is view provided by handheld otoscope). (*Source:* Courtesy of Dr. Javier Benito; Université de Montréal.)

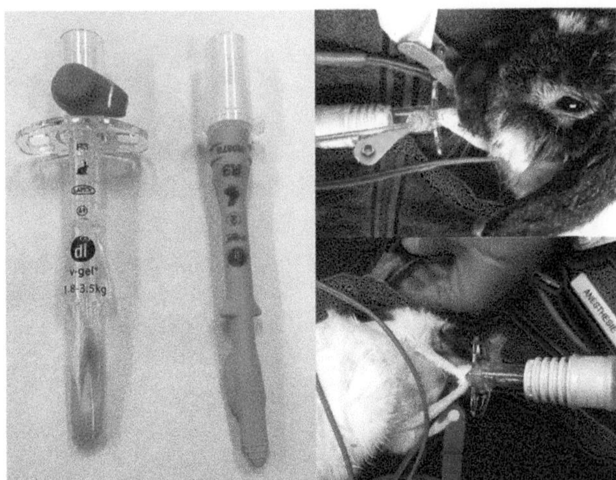

Figure 14.8 Left: Two different versions of a size 3 supraglottic airway device designed for rabbits (original version on the left and current version on the right). A rabbit with the supraglottic airway device secured in place and attached to the breathing circuit of an anesthetic machine (photographs on the top right and bottom). (*Source:* Photographs on the right: Courtesy of Dr. Javier Benito; Université de Montréal.)

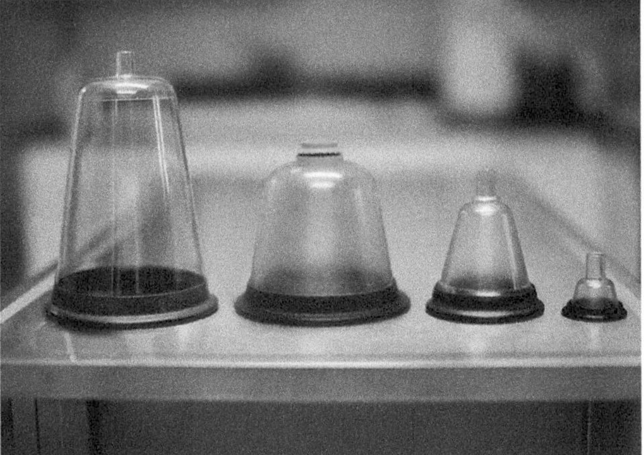

Figure 14.9 Different sizes of transparent facemasks that can be used on exotic companion mammals to either supplement oxygen or to deliver an inhalational gas mixture to maintain general anesthesia. (*Source:* Courtesy of Ms. Katie Lennox-Philibeck.)

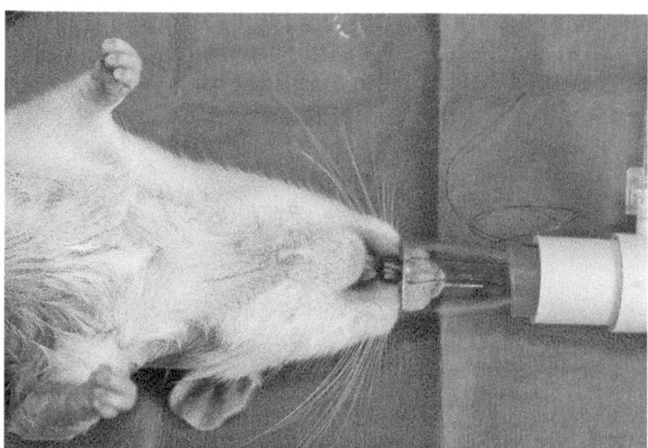

Figure 14.10 Photograph illustrating how a suture (or an elastic band) can be used to secure a facemask (or nose cone) to a patient. Suture is looped behind upper incisors and the ends passed through the facemask so the facemask connection holds the suture in position. (*Source:* Courtesy of Ms. Katie Lennox-Philibeck.)

breathers, allowing anesthetic gas to be delivered through a small facemask placed only over the nose during short oral procedures.

Management of Apnea

Respiratory rate and quality should be closely monitored as respiratory changes are often an early indicator of an anesthetic complication. If apnea occurs, the patient should be ventilated while the cause is identified and treated. If the patient is intubated, apnea can be managed as in other species with manual assisted ventilation. If the patient is not intubated, facemask ventilation can be attempted by pressing the facemask firmly against the patient's face and providing a forceful burst of air (or oxygen-rich gas mixture) from the reservoir bag. The effectiveness of this technique is highly dependent on the fit of the facemask. For hamsters, it is important to prevent the air from being misdirected into the cheek pouches by applying external pressure at the angle of the jaw during ventilation. In rabbits, if the cause of apnea is cardiac arrest, there is evidence that outcomes are similar with assisted ventilation through an endotracheal tube or a facemask. For this reason, it is generally not recommended to delay facemask ventilation by attempting intubation in an apneic rabbit. If ventilation is being performed as part of cardiopulmonary resuscitation (CPR), it is important to remember that facemask ventilation will be ineffective if administered while the patient is actively receiving chest compressions because compression of the thorax can cause the air (or oxygen-rich gas mixture) to be diverted into the esophagus rather than filling the lungs. This is doubly harmful because not only is the ventilation ineffective, but the resulting gastric distension may decrease venous return. For these reasons, chest compressions should be briefly interrupted every 30 compressions to provide two breaths via facemask ventilation.

Doxapram is sometimes used to stimulate ventilation in an apneic patient. However, there is controversy about its use because it increases global oxygen consumption. This author (S.S.) typically does not use doxapram during CPR or in apneic patients that are intubated because they can be effectively ventilated. However, its use may be appropriate in some cases for facemask-ventilated patients who develop apnea under anesthesia from unknown causes or as a result of accidental anesthetic drug overdose.

Anesthetic Monitoring Techniques

The principles of anesthetic monitoring for exotics are similar to those for other species though modifications in technique may be required in some cases to accommodate small patient size. An electrocardiogram (ECG) and pulse oximeter can be used in the same manner as in other species. Note that many veterinary pulse oximeters can only detect pulse rates up to 300–350 beats per minute. This is adequate for larger exotics, but for smaller patient like small rodents or sugar gliders, it is advisable to purchase a machine capable of measuring higher heart rates. If the equipment fails in smaller species, a Doppler ultrasound probe (see Chapter 4) can be placed directly over the heart for cardiac monitoring (Figure 14.11).

Temperature monitoring is also performed similarly to dogs and cats, though exotics may require more aggressive thermal support because of their large surface area relative to their body size and consequent predisposition to hypothermia. Some exotics (sugar gliders, hedgehogs, and many rodents) have normal body temperatures that are significantly lower (35.8–37.5 °C; 96.4–99.5 °F) than anesthetists

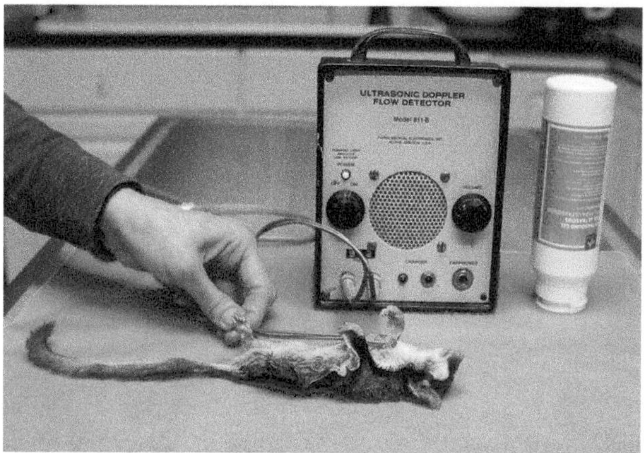

Figure 14.11 Photograph of a Doppler probe placed on the thorax to auscultate the heart of a sugar glider. This device can be used in any exotic companion mammal to listen to the heartbeat. (*Source:* Courtesy of Ms. Katie Lennox-Philibeck.)

may expect based on their experience with dogs and cats. It is therefore important to be familiar with species-specific reference intervals. Temperature monitoring should extend into recovery; hypothermia is major contributor to prolonged recovery in exotics.

Respiratory and blood pressure monitoring often present significant challenges. Most anesthetists use sidestream capnography with pediatric adaptors in exotics because of the decreased mechanical dead space. Sidestream capnographs with lower gas sampling flow rates (<50 mL/min) should be used, when possible, instead of typical sampling flow rates (150–200 mL/min) to prevent sampling the airway gases meant for breathing, especially if the patient is not receiving supplemental oxygen. Mainstream capnographs may be used, but are not preferred, as their increased weight can cause unintended extubation, partial or complete occlusion by bending the ET tube, or airway trauma through traction on the ET tube. For patients receiving facemask ventilation, it is sometimes possible to obtain a reasonably good capnograph tracing with a tight-fitting facemask, but the end-tidal CO_2 values underestimate the true value. With experience, a subjective visual assessment of respiratory quality can be made; for this reason, clear plastic surgical drapes should be used in small patients to improve visualization of thoracic movement.

Options for monitoring blood pressure vary by species. For rabbits, direct blood pressure monitoring via the central auricular artery is a relatively straightforward procedure and should be considered in sick patients. In ferrets, the coccygeal artery can be used for catheter placement. Indirect blood pressure monitoring using a Doppler technique or oscillometric monitor is an option for exotics with limbs large enough for available cuffs, such as rabbits and ferrets. Using the pelvic limb for oscillometric readings in exotics should be avoided because readings are inaccurate compared to invasive measurements. In rabbits, the thoracic limb should be used. In ferrets, either the thoracic limb or the tail can be used. When using Doppler measurements, the value obtained most closely represents the systolic arterial blood pressure. The accuracy of indirect blood pressure monitoring varies by species, by blood pressure status, and by monitor. For this reason, most sources recommend monitoring for trends rather that exact values; however, values less than 60 mmHg are usually a cause for concern (suggestive of hypotension). Note that the fur on the bottom of a rabbit's feet should never be clipped to facilitate Doppler probe placement as this fur is slow to regrow and removing it can result in pododermatitis. Instead, shaving the hair on the dorsal aspect of the metatarsal region to place the probe over the dorsal pedal artery could be considered. Use of indirect blood pressure monitoring in smaller species is limited by the lack of appropriately sized pressure cuffs. Nonetheless, placing a Doppler probe is a valuable indirect monitor of cardiac function and pulsatile blood flow.

Routine Local Anesthetic Block Techniques

As in dogs and cats, local anesthesia increases anesthetic safety by reducing the dose of injectable and inhalational anesthetic required. In some cases, it may even allow a procedure that would otherwise require general anesthesia to be performed under sedation. Total lidocaine and bupivacaine doses of 2 mg/kg and 1 mg/kg, respectively, are generally safe for all exotic mammal species. Because of the small size of many exotics, dilution with saline is often required to obtain a volume practical for injection.

Common techniques for performing local anesthesia include ring blocks for digit or tail amputation, local infiltration for cutaneous mass removal or wound care, and "splash blocks" around the incision site during wound closure. The application of lidocaine gel can also be helpful to facilitate at-home wound care. For anesthetists interested in more advanced techniques, landmarks have been described for epidural anesthesia in many species, sciatic and femoral nerve blocks in rabbits and guinea pigs, and dental blocks in rabbits (see Further Reading).

Examples of Peri-anesthetic Protocols

Examples of peri-anesthetic protocols for rabbits, ferrets, guinea pig, chinchilla, and rats are presented in Table 14.2.

General Aspects of Ruminant and Pig Anesthesia

Before addressing the "what" and "how" of anesthesia in ruminants and pigs, an important aspect to consider is that members of these species are usually classified as food-producing animals. Consequently, specific legislation applies to these animals with respect to the drugs that are allowed to be used and withdrawal times after administering drugs before milk, meat, and potentially other products of these animals are allowed to enter the food chain.

In general, only drugs that are licensed for a specific species and specific indication should be used. Under specific conditions, however, extra-label (off-label) use of drugs is permitted. For the United States of America, this is written in the Animal Medicinal Drug Use Clarification Act (AMDUCA), which is an amendment of the Federal Food, Drug, and Cosmetic Act (FD&C Act). In Europe, the regulations are laid out in EU directive 37/2010 and the "Cascade." As legislation and regulations differ in different

Table 14.2 Peri-anesthetic protocols that can be used in exotic companion mammals presenting for selected procedures.

Species and procedure	Notes
Rabbits	
Castration *(ASA I, short procedure)*	
Pre-anesthetic considerations:	Fast 1–4 h, water available. If patient is a mature male (>8–12 months), be prepared for thick skin, which may damage small needles or IV catheters. Pre-anesthetic blood work recommended but not required.
Premedication:	Hydromorphone (0.3 mg/kg) OR Buprenorphine (0.05 mg/kg) OR Methadone (0.2 mg/kg) PLUS Midazolam (1 mg/kg) PLUS Ketamine (10 mg/kg) PLUS Dexmedetomidine (0.01) mg/kg All given as a single injection IM
Anesthetic induction and maintenance:	Option 1: Facemask induction and maintenance Option 2: Facemask induction + supraglottic airway device Option 3: Induction with alfaxalone (1–2 mg/kg) or propofol (1–2 mg/kg) slowly (over 60 s) IV to effect Anesthetic maintenance: isoflurane (1–2% vaporizer setting) OR sevoflurane (2–3% vaporizer setting)
Vascular access:	Strongly recommended for Option 3, optional for Options 1 and 2 in the preceding text
Monitoring and fluids:	Temperature support and monitoring throughout (from sedation until sternal and normothermic). ± SC isotonic crystalloid fluids (30 mL/kg).
Analgesic plan:	• Testicular + incisional block with – Lidocaine (2 mg/kg) • Meloxicam (1 mg/kg SC at extubation, continue 1 mg/kg PO once daily for 2–3 days) • Cold compress incision site during recovery
Recovery:	Offer food as soon as patient is able to maintain sternal recumbency
Ovariohysterectomy *(ASA I, moderate length procedure)*	
Pre-anesthetic considerations:	Fast 1–4 h, water available If patient is a mature female (3+ years old), consider performing thoracic radiographs before surgery to screen for metastatic neoplasia. Pre-anesthetic blood work recommended but not required.
Premedication:	Hydromorphone (0.3 mg/kg) OR Buprenorphine (0.05 mg/kg) OR Methadone (0.2 mg/kg) PLUS Midazolam (1 mg/kg) PLUS Ketamine (10 mg/kg) PLUS Dexmedetomidine (0.01 mg/kg) All given as a single injection IM
Anesthetic induction and maintenance:	Induction: alfaxalone or propofol (both 1–2 mg/kg slowly IV to effect) Maintenance: isoflurane (1–2% vaporizer setting) OR sevoflurane (2–3% vaporizer setting) via endotracheal tube or supraglottic device

(Continued)

Table 14.2 (Continued)

Species and procedure	Notes
Vascular access:	Recommended Lateral saphenous catheter and removed immediately after surgery
Monitoring and fluids:	Temperature support and monitoring throughout (from sedation until sternal and normothermic). ± SC isotonic crystalloid fluids (30 mL/kg).
Analgesic plan:	• Incisional block with – Lidocaine (2 mg/kg) OR – Bupivacaine (1 mg/kg) • Meloxicam (1 mg/kg SC at extubation, continue 1 mg/kg PO once daily for 3–5 days) • Cold compress incision site during recovery
Recovery:	Offer food as soon as patient is able to maintain sternal recumbency
Dental occlusal adjustment *(ASA II–III, short procedure)*	
Pre-anesthetic considerations:	Patients are usually anorexic, so fasting not required. For severely debilitated patients, consider supportive care (analgesia and syringe feeding) first until patient is stable and hydrated. For patients on chronic meloxicam, do not administer in 24 h prior to anesthesia. Pre-anesthetic blood work strongly recommended, especially for more debilitated patients.
Premedication:	Hydromorphone (0.3 mg/kg) OR Buprenorphine (0.05 mg/kg) OR Methadone (0.2 mg/kg) OR Butorphanol (0.5 mg/kg) (minor trims only) PLUS Midazolam (0.5 mg/kg) Given IM as a single injection THEN 5–10 min later Alfaxalone (2 mg/kg) IM
Anesthetic induction and maintenance:	Induction: facemask induction OR Alfaxalone or propofol (1–2 mg/kg slowly IV to effect) Maintenance: isoflurane (1–2% vaporizer setting) OR sevoflurane (2–3% vaporizer setting) delivered through a small facemask held over patient's nose only
Vascular access:	Recommended for debilitated patients
Monitoring and fluids:	Temperature support and monitoring throughout (from sedation until sternal and normothermic). ± SC isotonic crystalloid fluids (30 mL/kg) OR IV fluids (10 mL/kg/h), depending on patient condition.
Analgesic plan:	• Buprenorphine (0.05 mg/kg q 6–12 h) • Meloxicam (1 mg/kg SC in recovery, continue 1 mg/kg PO q 24 h as needed)
Recovery:	Offer food as soon as patient is able to maintain sternal recumbency. Expect that many patients will require syringe feeding for several days.
Ferrets	
Exploratory laparotomy *(ASA III-IV, longer procedure)*	
Pre-anesthetic considerations:	Pre-anesthetic blood work is strongly recommended. If blood glucose is low or borderline, do not fast and consider checking blood glucose with a glucometer periodically throughout anesthesia and recovery.

Table 14.2 (Continued)

Species and procedure	Notes
Premedication:	Hydromorphone (0.2 mg/kg) OR Methadone (0.2 mg/kg) OR Buprenorphine (0.02 mg/kg) PLUS Midazolam (0.3 mg/kg) Given IM as a single injection If sedation inadequate for IV catheter placement after 5–10 min, THEN alfaxalone (1 mg/kg) IM Note: For gastrointestinal surgery or other clean-contaminated surgery THEN cefazolin (22 mg/kg slow IV, ideally 30–60 min before first incision and every 90 min thereafter)
Anesthetic induction and maintenance:	Alfaxalone or propofol (1–3 mg/kg slowly IV to effect) Intubate and maintain isoflurane (1–2% vaporizer setting) OR sevoflurane (2–3% vaporizer setting)
Vascular access:	Vascular access strongly recommended IV catheter possible in most cases For severely debilitated patients, may need IO access
Monitoring and fluids:	Temperature support and monitoring throughout (from sedation until sternal and normothermic). IV fluids at 10 mL/kg/h (+1.25 to 2.5% dextrose supplementation, if needed).
Analgesic plan:	• Incisional block with – Lidocaine (2 mg/kg) OR – Bupivacaine (1 mg/kg) • Buprenorphine (0.01–0.02 SC/IV q 6–8 h) • ± Meloxicam (0.1–0.2 mg/kg SC at extubation, continue PO once daily for 3–5 days; avoid in dehydrated or debilitated patients or those with suspected gastrointestinal ulcers)
Recovery:	Post-operative hyperthermia and blood glucose derangements are relatively common, so consider monitoring these parameters longer than you would in other species. Ferrets tend to recover more slowly than other species. This is not necessarily cause for concern, as long as the patient rouses when stimulated. Syringe feeding is recommended for older patients that do not immediately start eating on their own. Anti-emetics at typical canine/feline doses may also be beneficial if patient shows signs of nausea (lip licking and hypersalivation). Ferret skin bruises easily, so consider applying cold compresses to the incision site if patient is not hypothermic.
Guinea pig and chinchilla	
Small mass removal/castration *(ASA I-II, short procedure)*	
Pre-anesthetic considerations:	Healthy guinea pigs often have large amounts of food in their oral cavity. Fast for 1–4 h and manually remove debris from oral cavity with cotton swabs and/or irrigation. Blood collection in awake animals can be challenging but consider collecting blood after sedation.
Premedication:	Hydromorphone (0.5–1 mg/kg) OR Methadone (0.3 mg/kg) OR Buprenorphine (0.05–0.1 mg/kg) PLUS Midazolam (0.5–1 mg/kg) PLUS Ketamine (10 mg/kg; GP only) Given IM as a single injection OR Alfaxalone (1–2 mg/kg; GP or Chin) given IM 5–10 min later The effects of alfaxalone tends to present suddenly and are very pronounced, so monitor closely after administering is advised

(Continued)

Table 14.2 (Continued)

Species and procedure	Notes
Anesthetic induction and maintenance:	Induction: facemask induction Maintenance: isoflurane (1–2% vaporizer setting) OR sevoflurane (2–3% vaporizer setting) via facemask Swab oral cavity periodically to remove excess fluid (especially for guinea pigs)
Vascular access:	Optional. Gaining access can be challenging, so often omitted for short procedures.
Monitoring and fluids:	Temperature support and monitoring throughout (from sedation until sternal and normothermic). SC isotonic crystalloid fluids (30 mL/kg).
Analgesic plan:	• Meloxicam (1 mg/kg SC in recovery, continue 0.5 mg/kg PO q 24 h as needed)
Recovery:	Offer food as soon as patient is able to maintain sternal recumbency
Dental occlusal adjustment (ASA II–III, short procedure)	
Pre-anesthetic considerations:	Patients are usually anorexic, so fasting not required. For severely debilitated patients, consider supportive care (analgesia and syringe feeding) first until patient is stable and hydrated. For patients on chronic meloxicam, do not administer in 24 h before anesthesia. Blood collection in awake animals can be challenging but consider collecting blood after sedation.
Premedication:	Hydromorphone (0.5–1 mg/kg) OR Buprenorphine (0.05–0.1 mg/kg) OR Methadone (0.3 mg/kg) OR Butorphanol (0.5–1 mg/kg) (only for very minor trims) PLUS Midazolam (0.5–1 mg/kg) Given IM as a single injection THEN 5–10 min later Alfaxalone (1–2 mg/kg) IM The effects of alfaxalone tends to present suddenly and are very pronounced, so monitoring closely after administering is advised
Anesthetic induction and maintenance:	Induction: facemask induction Maintenance: isoflurane (1–2% vaporizer setting) OR sevoflurane (2–3% vaporizer setting) delivered through a small mask held over patient's nose only
Vascular access:	IV/IO catheter placement optional for short procedures but recommended for longer procedures in debilitated patients
Monitoring and fluids:	Temperature support and monitoring throughout (from sedation until sternal and normothermic). SC isotonic crystalloid fluids (30 mL/kg) OR IV fluids (10 mL/kg/h), depending on patient condition.
Analgesic plan:	• Meloxicam (0.5 mg/kg SQ in recovery, continue 0.5 mg/kg PO q 24 h as needed) • ± Opioids, depending on severity of disease
Recovery:	Offer food as soon as patient is able to maintain sternal recumbency. Expect that many patients will require syringe feeding for a few days or even weeks (especially chinchillas).
Rat	
Mass removal *(ASA II–III, short to moderate length procedure)*	
Pre-anesthetic considerations:	Fast 1–2 h, water available until sedation. Many rats with mammary masses are older, and this population has a high prevalence of chronic subclinical respiratory disease that could affect anesthesia or flare up during recovery. Consider starting antimicrobials (enrofloxacin, doxycycline, or azithromycin) a few days before the procedure for patients with a known history of respiratory disease. If the mass is large and you are not placing a catheter, consider proactively administering subcutaneous fluids to help offset any fluid loss from intra- or post-operative bleeding. A blood chemistry panel (collected from the sedated patient) can be beneficial but must be carefully considered, in light of the potential for additional blood loss during surgery.

Table 14.2 (Continued)

Species and procedure	Notes
Premedication:	Hydromorphone (0.3 mg/kg) OR Methadone (0.3 mg/kg) OR Buprenorphine (0.05 mg/kg) PLUS Midazolam (0.5–1 mg/kg) Given IM as a single injection THEN 5–10 min later Alfaxalone (2 mg/kg) IM
Anesthetic induction and maintenance:	Isoflurane (1–2% vaporizer setting) OR sevoflurane (2–3% vaporizer setting) via facemask
Vascular access:	IO catheter placement should be considered for large masses, when significant hemorrhage is possible but can be challenging in this species because of the shape of the tibia
Monitoring and fluids:	Temperature support and monitoring throughout (from sedation until sternal and normothermic). Take care not to get the patient any wetter than necessary when scrubbing large masses and dry thoroughly before returning to cage. SC or IV fluids as detailed in the preceding text.
Analgesic plan:	• Incisional block with – Lidocaine (2 mg/kg) OR – Bupivacaine (1 mg/kg) • Meloxicam (0.1–0.2 mg/kg SC at extubation, continue PO once daily for 3–5 days) • ± Opioids depending on severity of disease
Recovery:	Offer food as soon as patient is able to maintain sternal recumbency (fruit baby food is often well received). Monitor closely for hemorrhage and self-mutilation of the incision site.

parts of the world, anesthetists must be familiar with local requirements regarding drug use in food-producing species (Table 14.3).

Restrictions in drug use in food-producing species are sometimes regarded as frustrating. However, with the drugs and techniques that are allowed to be used, all aspects of the peri-anesthetic period can still be served.

This chapter addresses the important considerations for anesthesia in ruminants and pigs, the drugs that are *likely* to be allowed to be used, and relevant species-specific techniques.

Common Procedures Performed During Standing Sedation or General Anesthesia

Sheep and Goats

Common procedures in general practice for which sedation or general anesthesia may be needed are husbandry procedures, such as disbudding, castrations, and tail docking, or emergency procedures, such as wound management and Cesarean sections.

Cattle

Due to their size, and limited facilities for general anesthesia in the field (or at most production or mixed-animal practices), many procedures are performed under standing sedation and locoregional analgesia in adult cattle. These include dehorning, ocular surgeries, castrations, assisted delivery of calves or Cesarean sections, digit amputations or other painful procedures on the digits, management of teat and udder trauma, abomasum replacement, or explorative laparotomies. In younger calves, general anesthesia may be used to facilitate umbilical hernia repairs (simple hernias can be repaired with appropriate sedation, analgesia, and restraint). Depending on the specifics of each procedure and available resources, a recumbent and restrained animal or an animal under general anesthesia can be desirable.

Pigs

Most husbandry procedures in commercially farmed pigs are, unfortunately, still performed with rudimentary or no analgesia/anesthesia. However, surgical procedures requiring sedation or general anesthesia are increasingly common in pet pigs. Examples include claw trimming, dental procedures, ovariohysterectomy, and orchidectomy.

Standing Sedation

The mainstay of a successful standing procedure is good locoregional anesthetic technique, so that adequate

Table 14.3 Legislation of drug use in food-producing animals.

Country or region	Legislation document	URL
USA	Animal Medicinal Drug Use Clarification Act of 1994 (AMDUCA)	https://www.fda.gov/animal-veterinary/guidance-regulations/animal-medicinal-drug-use-clarification-act-1994-amduca
EU	Commission Regulation (EU) No. 37/2010 of 22 December 2009 on pharmacologically active substances and their classification regarding maximum residue limits in foodstuffs of animal origin	http://data.europa.eu/eli/reg/2010/37(1)/oj and https://ec.europa.eu/food/animals/animal-health/vet-meds-med-feed_en
UK	The Animals and Animal Products (Examination for Residues and Maximum Residue Limits) Regulations 1997 as amended (the "Residue Regulations") and the Veterinary Medicines Regulations 201	https://www.gov.uk/guidance/managing-livestock-veterinary-medicines
Canada	The Veterinary Drugs Directorate (VDD) applies the Food and Drug Regulations under the authority of the Food and Drugs Act	https://www.canada.ca/en/health-canada/services/drugs-health-products/veterinary-drugs.html
Australia	The legislative and regulatory environment of veterinarians can be complex and depend on their location and type of work	https://www.ava.com.au/library-journals-and-resources/ava-other-resources/legislation-for-veterinary-professionals and https://www.ava.com.au/library-journals-and-resources/ava-other-resources/prescribing-guidelines
South Africa	Medicines and Related Substances Act (previously Drugs Control Act) 101 of 1965 and Fertilizers, Farm Feeds, Seeds and Remedies Act 36 of 1947	https://www.gov.za/documents/drugs-control-act-7-jul-1965-0000 and https://www.gov.za/documents/fertilizers-farm-feeds-seeds-and-remedies-act-28-may-2015-1101

analgesia is provided at all times. In a cooperative animal, a locoregional anesthetic technique on its own may suffice although additional sedation may be beneficial in providing anxiolysis and facilitating restraint. It is important to remember that, although locoregional anesthetic techniques render a surgical area completely desensitized (see Chapter 3), sensation will return as the anesthetic effects of the block wear off. Therefore, it is advantageous to administer systemic analgesia before the effects of any locoregional technique dissipate.

When it is preferred to perform a procedure on a recumbent animal but without general anesthesia, casting the animal with a rope, preferably after administering a sedative or anxiolytic drug, can be a very useful technique.

The use of standing procedures can have several advantages compared to general anesthesia, which are described in the following text.

Concept of Return to Function

During a standing procedure, physiology is considerably less disrupted compared to general anesthesia. This helps ensure adequate circulation and ventilation, and a faster return to normal function after the procedure. In addition, in ruminants, extended periods of recumbency can lead to myopathy, neuropathy, and bloat. Furthermore, although recovery from general anesthesia in ruminants is usually calm, there is always a risk of animals injuring themselves when returning to a standing position.

Access to Equipment and Facilities

When performing general anesthesia, specific equipment, such as a well-padded table or platform, hoist, oxygen source, and an inhalational anesthetic delivery device may be needed. Equipment for extended general anesthesia (>45 min) can be expensive and difficult to transport, making it less suitable for use under field conditions. Shorter duration procedures (<45 min) on recumbent animals, either involving a general anesthetic or adequate sedation and mild restraint, are possible even in field settings.

Estimating the Pain Experience of the Procedure

When an animal is sedated or anesthetized for an invasive procedure, attention should be given to adequate analgesia. Alpha-2 adrenergic receptor agonists, ketamine, nonsteroidal anti-inflammatory drugs (NSAIDs), and local anesthetics can all be used to provide pain relief and are often administered in combination (see Chapter 3). In estimating what pain relief is needed, the analogy "what is painful in humans is also painful in animals" should be used. This sentiment is important to follow because, for a long time, it has erroneously been thought (and taught) that ruminants and pigs do not require analgesia. It is now evident that there is a lack of familiarity with evaluating and observing signs associated with pain in these species. Pain identification in these species is an important, active area of research. Experience with, and outcomes of, previous procedures can help further refine analgesic protocols. An analgesic plan (choice of drug(s), route, dosing interval, and duration) should be drafted for each case.

Drug Protocols and Techniques for Standing Sedation in Production Animals

Species-specific information on sedatives commonly used for livestock species will be provided here (see Tables 14.4 and 14.5). Drug pharmacology is explained in Chapters 6–10.

Table 14.4 Recommended doses of drugs used for standing sedation in small ruminants, cattle, and pigs.

Drugs for standing sedation (mg/kg; IV preferred to IM, except in pigs where IM is most practical initially) Check local legislation to ascertain drugs are allowed to be used in your target species

	Xylazine	Detomidine	"Ketamine stun"	Butorphanol	Azaperone	Diazepam[a]/midazolam
Small ruminants	0.05–0.2	0.005–0.010		0.1–0.2		0.05–0.2
Cattle	0.05–0.1	0.005–0.010	0.05–0.1	0.1–0.2[b]		0.05–0.1
Pigs	2	0.005–0.010		0.1–0.2	0.4–2	0.1–0.3 (0.2 intranasal midazolam)

[a]Diazepam should not be administered by the intramuscular route.
[b]If a ketamine stun is planned for, then the butorphanol dose should be reduced to 0.1 mg/kg.

Table 14.5 Examples of drug combinations for various procedures performed under standing sedation in production small ruminants, cattle, and pigs.

Procedure	Suggested drug combinations	Route(s) of administration
Foot/tooth trim in a production pig	Recumbent sedation: Xylazine + ketamine OR Detomidine + ketamine	Drugs can be mixed in one syringe and given as a deep IM injection
Udder laceration repair in cow	Standing sedation: Butorphanol + xylazine OR Butorphanol + detomidine AND Local infiltration of udder wound area with lidocaine AND Ketamine stun can be added in noncooperative animals	Drugs can be mixed in one syringe and be given either as an IV or IM injection. Doses for the IM route are usually higher compared to IV route. Low-dose ketamine can be given IV in small increments to effect. Be prepared for the cow to move into sternal recumbency.
Calf disbudding	Recumbent sedation: Xylazine alone AND Cornual nerve block with lidocaine	Xylazine can be administered IV using the jugular vein.
Radiograph for bladder stones in a goat	Recumbent sedation: Butorphanol + xylazine OR Butorphanol + detomidine AND Low-dose ketamine can be added in noncooperative animals	Drugs can be mixed in one syringe and administered IV using the jugular vein. Low-dose ketamine can be given IV in small increments to effect.

Alpha-2 Adrenergic Receptor Agonists

Xylazine and detomidine are the most commonly used drugs of this class. Care is advised when administering these drugs, especially xylazine, to ruminants in the last trimester of gestation as they may induce uterine contractions, which could lead to abortion or premature delivery of the fetus (see Further Reading).

Compared to other species, ruminants are more sensitive to the sedative effects of xylazine (require a tenth of the dose), whereas the sedative effects are similar to other species for other licensed drugs within this drug class (see Further Reading). This means that a typical dose of xylazine to achieve sedation is in the region of 0.05–0.1 mg/kg given IV or IM.

In sheep, these drugs can induce acute pulmonary inflammation that can lead to clinically significant hypoxemia (see Further Reading). However, the risk of this adverse effect is difficult to predict and may vary between breeds and individuals.

When planning a standing procedure, these drugs should be titrated to achieve the desired effect (using incremental dosing, preferably IV, and allowing time for peak effect before deciding on additional doses; see Chapter 6). A small increase in dose can result in recumbency and it is good practice to plan for this unintended outcome.

When needed, the effects of alpha-2 adrenergic receptor agonists can be antagonized with the drug atipamezole. Atipamezole (5× the dose of the agonist given administered IM) will antagonize both the analgesic and sedative effects of any alpha-2 adrenergic receptor agonist drug.

Ketamine

Ketamine is regularly used to induce deep sedation or general anesthesia. In very low doses, it can be used to augment a standing or recumbent sedation. The addition of a low-dose ketamine will increase the level of analgesia and allows for reduction of the dose of other sedatives (e.g., xylazine and butorphanol) used. When adding a low dose of ketamine to the sedation protocol, noncooperative animals can suddenly become amenable. When performing a standing sedation, ketamine must be given slowly and in low doses to mitigate the risk of the animal becoming recumbent. Colloquially, the addition of ketamine to a standing sedation protocol is known as "ketamine stun" (see Further Reading). Ketamine stun was initially described for use in cattle but it can be used in small ruminants and possibly pigs.

Benzodiazepines and Opioids

Short-acting benzodiazepines (e.g., midazolam) and opioids (e.g., butorphanol) are valuable additions to sedation protocols, and these drug classes are not licensed for use in food-producing animals in many countries. Butorphanol is sometimes used, within the limits of legislative guidelines (such as the cascade framework) as it is licensed for use in horses (for food production) in some parts of the world. Benzodiazepines provide a useful level of sedation in ruminants with a greatly reduced risk of recumbency compared to alpha-2 adrenergic receptor agonists.

Azaperone

Azaperone is specifically licensed as an anxiolytic for pigs and has minor sedative effects. To maximize the quality of effect, pigs should be left undisturbed for approximately 20 min after administration. For good-quality sedation, it is best combined with an alpha-2 adrenergic receptor agonist, benzodiazepine, or ketamine.

General Anesthesia

When the species or the procedure does not allow for standing sedation, then general anesthesia will be required. General anesthesia can be induced by a single injection of a combination of drugs or by stepwise approach, where initial sedation (premedication) of the animal is followed by administration of an anesthetic drug to induce general anesthesia.

Drug Combinations for Short Procedures (<30 min)

General anesthesia for short procedures in ruminants and pigs can be achieved by a single IM or IV injection of a combination of ketamine with either xylazine or detomidine (Table 14.6).

In pigs, azaperone can be added for a more reliable effect because they are not very sensitive to the sedative effects of the alpha-2 adrenergic receptor agonists. For additional sedation and mild analgesia, butorphanol can be added. Other opioids, such as morphine and buprenorphine, have been administered to pigs with moderate-to-severe pain, but they are not licensed in most parts of the world for production animals. If opioids are given to a pig that is not experiencing pain, there is a chance that excitement can occur, especially during recovery. Therefore, recovery should take place in a quiet and warm environment. General anesthesia protocols for pigs undergoing gonadectomy are presented in Table 14.7.

Drug Combinations for Longer Procedures (>30 min)

For longer procedures, or short procedures that take longer than anticipated, general anesthesia can be maintained by redosing ketamine (IV) every 15–20 min. Unlike many other species, ruminants do not experience muscle rigidity, prolonged recoveries, moderate-to-severe ataxia, or seizure-like activity when ketamine is used to maintain

Table 14.6 Recommended drug doses (mg/kg) to achieve general anesthesia in small ruminants, cattle, and pigs and suggested drugs doses for constant rate infusion (CRI; mg/kg/h). Note that lower doses can be used when adding butorphanol and or azaperone. Intravenous route of administration in ruminants and intramuscular doses for pigs until intravenous access is obtained.

Species	Xylazine + ketamine	Detomidine + ketamine	Ketamine re-dose	Xylazine + ketamine CRI	Detomidine + ketamine CRI
Small ruminants	0.05–0.2 + 3–5	0.005–0.01 + 3–5	0.5–1	0.25 + 2.5	0.01 + 2.5
Cattle	0.05–0.2 + 3–5	0.005–0.01 + 3–5	0.5–1	0.25 + 2.5	0.01 + 2.5
Pigs	1–2 + 5–7	0.001–0.002 + 5–7	0.5–1	2.5 + 2.0	0.01 + 2.0

Table 14.7 General anesthetic protocols for gonadectomy in pigs kept as companion animals.

Procedure	Considerations	Suggested protocol
Ovariohysterectomy	Hypoventilation, hypothermia, hypotension, hemorrhage, and pain Brachycephalic pig breeds such as the Vietnamese pot-bellied and Kunekune pigs can have upper airway obstruction when sedated or anesthetized	General anesthesia using Ketamine 10 mg/kg PLUS Xylazine 2 mg/kg OR Midazolam 0.5 mg/kg PLUS Butorphanol 0.25 mg/kg All given as a single IM injection Or Ketamine 10 mg/kg PLUS Detomidine 0.02 mg/kg PLUS Butorphanol 0.25 mg/kg All given as a single IM injection Followed by additional bolus of ketamine IV (1 mg/kg) Or Isoflurane in oxygen to extend the duration of the anesthetic
Orchidectomy	Hypoventilation, hypothermia, hypotension, hemorrhage, and pain Brachycephalic pig breeds such as the Vietnamese pot-bellied and Kunekune pigs can have upper airway obstruction when sedated or anesthetized	Sedation using: Ketamine 5 mg/kg PLUS Xylazine 2 mg/kg OR Midazolam 0.5 mg/kg PLUS Butorphanol 0.25 mg/kg All given as a single IM injection Or Ketamine 5 mg/kg PLUS Detomidine 0.02 mg/kg PLUS Butorphanol 0.25 mg/kg All given as a single IM injection Followed by additional bolus of ketamine IV (1 mg/kg) Or Isoflurane in oxygen to extend the duration of the anesthetic IN COMBINATION WITH Lidocaine intratesticular at a maximum total dose of 4 mg/kg

Note: These drugs cannot be used in some countries because even pigs kept as companion animals are still considered food-producing animals.

anesthesia. To ensure a fast time of onset, ketamine is best administered IV (see "Intermittent hand bolus technique" in Chapter 6). Alternatively, general anesthesia can be maintained by inhalational anesthesia using drugs like isoflurane, when an anesthetic machine is available (see Chapters 5 and 8). However, as with other species being given inhalation anesthetics, the chances for hypotension and hypoventilation are always concerns. Therefore, if an inhalational technique is used, these patients must be appropriately monitored.

Constant Rate Infusion of Drugs

Instead of repeatedly dosing ketamine to maintain anesthesia, it can also be administered as an intravenous infusion. With this approach, ketamine is often combined with either xylazine or detomidine. The constant rate infusion is usually started immediately after induction of general anesthesia and after 1.5–2 h of infusion, the rate should be decreased by 25% per hour to prevent prolonged recoveries. For drug calculation examples, see the "Intravenous infusion technique" in Chapter 6.

Intravenous Access Sites and Procedures

Although sedation and general anesthesia can be obtained by administering drugs via the IM route, having IV access is always preferred. When a vein is catheterized, clipping of hair and aseptic preparation of the skin overlying the vein is recommended to reduce the risk of infection. Achieving IV catheterization can be facilitated by IM sedation.

Small Ruminants

Venous access is relatively easy to obtain in small ruminants. The cephalic vein is easily catheterized even in nonsedated animals. Another easily accessible vein is the jugular vein. The jugular vein lends itself for both IV catheter placement and so-called "off-the-needle" injections. The former is preferable as it ensures proper IV administration of drugs, reduces the risk of thrombophlebitis when administering irritant substances (by reducing likelihood of inadvertent perivascular administration), allows IV fluid therapy, and maintains venous access for the duration of a procedure.

Cattle

If an animal is cooperative, IV access is relatively easy to obtain via the auricular vein. Off-the-needle injections are possible, but for longer procedures and administration of fluids it is prudent to place an IV catheter. Alternative sites of venous catheterization are the jugular and cephalic veins (as for small ruminants). The cranial epigastric vein ("milk vein") and medial coccygeal vein ("tail vein") are less suitable due to the risk of thrombophlebitis, which can cause significant damage to the mammary gland or tail.

Pigs

Due to their temperament and anatomy, venous access is not readily accessible in unsedated pigs. Placement of an IV catheter is often only possible after sedation in healthy pigs. Due to their usually large subcutaneous fat deposits, attempted IM injections can easily end up in the adipose tissue. In the pelvic limb (biceps femoris, semimembranosus, or semitendinosus muscles) and just behind the ear (brachiocephalic muscle), muscle tissue is more easily accessed. (Note: In production animals, the pelvic limbs should be avoided so as not to affect the meat quality.) Intramuscular injections are therefore preferably performed in the neck, just behind the ears. Care must be taken to use a sufficiently long needle (18-gauge 1.5 inch or longer needle for a pig up to 70 kg). Pigs are most easily injected when using low-volume flexible extension tubing between the needle and the syringe (Figure 14.12). Gentle insertion of the needle is often better tolerated than rapid insertion ("darting"). Finally, distracting the animal with food (e.g., an apple or hard sweet like candy) or by scratching its back with a plastic garden rake (raking/forking) is often a successful strategy to facilitate IM injection. Once the animal is adequately sedated, venous access is possible via an auricular vein in most breeds. In breeds with smaller ears (e.g., Vietnamese pot-bellied pigs), cephalic, lateral saphenous, and dorsal metatarsal veins can be assessed. Ultrasound guidance can be valuable to locate veins (cephalic and jugular) and guide catheter placement.

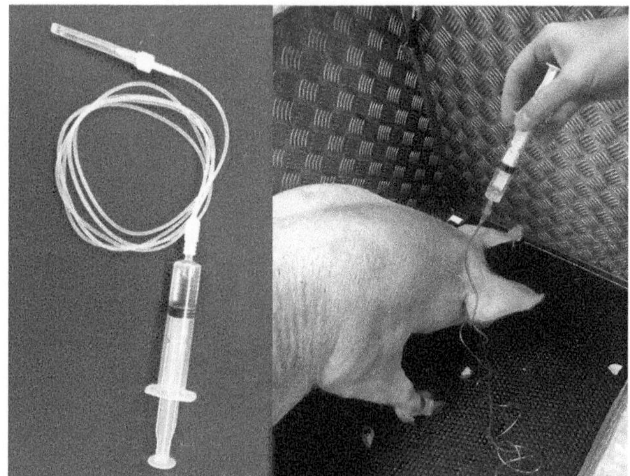

Figure 14.12 Needle and syringe configuration using a low-volume extension set (left) to aide in intramuscular injection of pigs (right). (*Source:* Photograph on right: Courtesy of Drs. Julia Deutsch and Paul MacFarlane; Langford Vets, University of Bristol.)

Principles of Endotracheal Intubation

Orotracheal intubation is recommended for animals undergoing general anesthesia. It facilitates oxygen supplementation, provides a means of administering inhalational anesthetics when used to maintain general anesthesia (without the workplace pollution associated with facemasks), and, especially in ruminants, it reduces the risk of aspiration of saliva and regurgitated ruminal contents.

When performing field anesthesia in or around an animal enclosure, ensure that the animal does not inhale fine particulate matter such as straw, or other bedding material, through the endotracheal tube, once intubated and in lateral recumbency. Often, placing the animal's head and proximal end of the endotracheal tube on a towel will minimize the risk of inhaling foreign material.

If intubation is not performed in anesthetized ruminants, care must be taken to prevent regurgitation and aspiration. When the animal is in lateral recumbency, this is best performed by placing some padding under the neck of the animal directly behind the angle of the jaw. This way, the neck of the animal will be tilted up, impeding flow of regurgitated material into the oropharynx, while the mouth of the animal points downward, allowing saliva and any regurgitated material to drain away from the larynx (Figure 14.13).

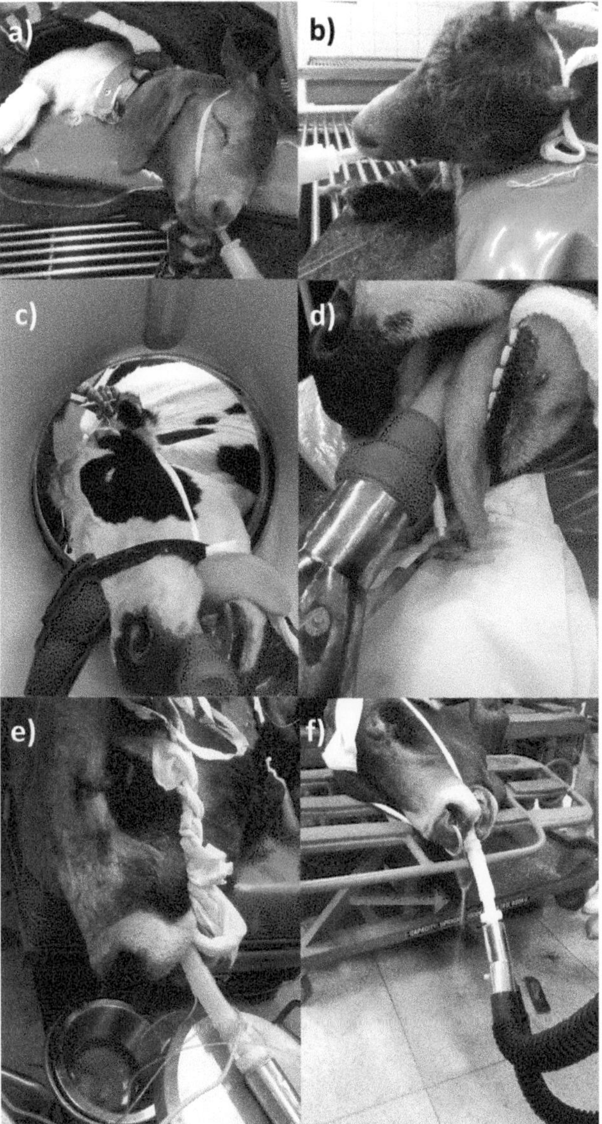

Figure 14.13 Head positioning in an anesthetized (a, b) goat kid, (c) cow undergoing a computed tomography scan of the head, (d) a close-up view of saliva draining from the cow, and (e) a bull undergoing an operation. The reason for swift intubation is to prevent aspiration of ruminal content (f): in this case, water was not withheld before anesthesia by mistake and the error was not discovered until after anesthetic induction and a large volume of fluid was regurgitated (blue arrow). The same head position should be used in sedated, nonintubated ruminants.

Small Ruminants

The process of orotracheal intubation in small ruminants is relatively straightforward but requires assistance and a good-quality illuminated laryngoscope with a long, straight blade (Miller blade). The blade should have a minimum length equivalent to the distance from the incisors to the angle of the mandible. If necessary, blade length can be extended by welding an extension to the tip of a regular Miller blade. Due to the high risk of regurgitation (and subsequent aspiration) during intubation, the animal is ideally kept in a sternal position or sitting upright ("dog sit" position). The risk of regurgitation is higher if intubation is attempted when depth of anesthesia is light. With the animal sitting upright between the legs of the assistant, the assistant can stretch the neck upward and open the mouth of the animal with two pieces of cotton tape (or light rope). One around the mandible and one around the maxilla. Due to the lack of upper incisors in small ruminants, which help keep the tape in place, care must be taken to avoid it slipping off. The oropharynx of small ruminants is rather narrow but sufficient visualization of the caudal pharynx and larynx can usually be achieved by pulling on the cotton tape. The tongue can be extended and fixed under the lower cotton tape though care should be taken not to damage it on the sharp lower incisors. With the laryngoscope pressing down firmly on the base of the tongue, the epiglottis and *rima glottidis* can be visualized provided the laryngoscope blade is sufficiently long and the light source is functioning. Direct contact of the laryngoscope blade with the epiglottis and *rima glottidis* is best avoided as these structures are easily traumatized. It is advised to work swiftly during the intubation process as the copious saliva production quickly leads to pooling of saliva in the laryngeal area, precluding adequate vision of the larynx and enhancing the risk of subsequent aspiration of saliva. Once the *rima glottidis* is visible, the trachea should be gently intubated as the laryngeal mucosa is easily abraded. With the endotracheal tube in place, its cuff should be inflated to secure the airway. If an anesthetic machine is available, adequacy of cuff inflation can be confirmed by providing a few positive pressure breaths (see Chapter 5). The endotracheal tube can be tied in place using one of the cotton bands used for opening the mouth. During attempted intubation, if the endotracheal tube obscures the view of the *rima glottidis* to an extent that prevents intubation, a stylet can be inserted into the trachea first, over which the endotracheal tube is subsequently "railroaded" into the trachea (Figure 14.14).

Cattle

Orotracheal intubation in calves can be performed using the same approach as described for small ruminants. In large ruminants, this is not feasible because the length of the oral cavity is too long. The mouth of a large ruminant

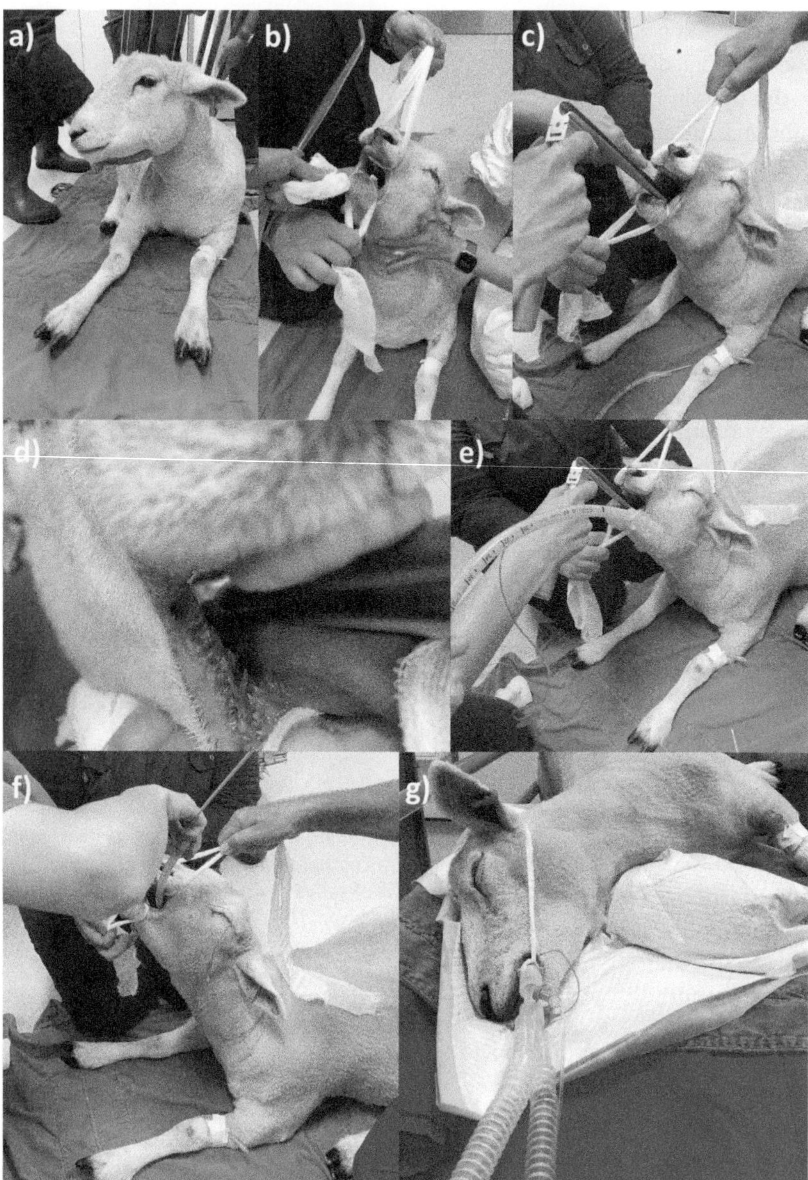

Figure 14.14 Photographs showing the order of events for intubating a sheep (a). General anesthesia was induced by intravenous injection, followed by opening the mouth using gauze bandage (b). A laryngoscope with a Miller blade is being introduced, and suctioning of saliva from the oropharynx is being performed (c). The Miller blade is gentle advanced toward the oropharynx with the tip of the blade positioned at the base of the tongue immediately rostral to the epiglottis (d). An intubating stylet is advanced through the endotracheal tube (e). Then, the tip of the stylet is advanced into the trachea via the *rima glottidis* and the endotracheal tube is "railroaded" off the stylet, which is subsequently withdrawn (f). The endotracheal tube is connected to the breathing circuit of an anesthetic machine, and the cuff of the endotracheal tube is inflated and the head positioned to promote saliva flow out of the oral cavity (g). (*Source:* Courtesy of Drs. Julia Deutsch and Paul MacFarlane; Langford Vets, University of Bristol.)

should be opened with an appropriate adjustable mouth gag (use of a gag is recommended to protect the operator's fingers from the molar teeth). Intubation can be performed blind; however, there is a risk of intubating the esophagus and stimulating the esophagus increases the risk of regurgitation. An alternative, straightforward approach is manual guidance of the endotracheal tube into the larynx. One hand (with any jewelry and watch removed), enveloping the distal end of the tube, is advanced through the mouth toward the larynx. The index finger of this hand can be placed in the laryngeal inlet and, subsequently, the endotracheal tube can be advanced, using the finger to direct the tube into the trachea. As the edges of the molars can be very sharp, care should be taken not to cut oneself or the cuff of the endotracheal tube when advancing through the oral cavity. Alternatively, one hand can be advanced into the oral cavity until the larynx is palpated, at which point the endotracheal tube can be introduced into the oral cavity and guided forward to the hand placed alongside the larynx. This technique may be easier if there is a tight fit when trying to introduce the endotracheal tube and forearm simultaneously into the oral cavity.

A further method is to insert a stomach tube into the trachea first using digital palpation to guide placement. This stomach tube is then used as a guide, over which the endotracheal tube is subsequently "railroaded" over the stomach tube into the trachea. It is important to adequately lubricate the outside of the stomach tube to ensure smooth passage of the endotracheal tube.

Finally, endoscopic guidance can be used to facilitate endotracheal intubation. A flexible endoscope can be threaded through the endotracheal tube, after which both the scope and the endotracheal tube can be advanced together through the oral cavity. Using the scope image, the scope can be maneuvered into the trachea of the animal, after which the endotracheal tube can be slid into the trachea using an "over-the-scope" method. With the current availability of long and relatively cheap flexible scopes that can connect to a smartphone, this technique has become a viable option (Figure 14.15).

Pigs

Endotracheal intubation in pigs is often described as difficult, which relates to the specific anatomy of the larynx. It has a curve in it ("U" or "V" shaped), which makes it more difficult for the endotracheal tube to pass through. With the right technique and practice, however, pigs are easily intubated. Intubation is possible under direct laryngoscopy provided a sufficiently long laryngoscope blade and quality light source are used. The trachea of pigs is small relative to their total body weight (7.5 mm internal diameter endotracheal tube for 25–30 kg pig; 9.0 mm internal diameter for >80 kg pig).

Pigs can be positioned in dorsal or sternal recumbency for endotracheal intubation as determined by user preference. Sternal positioning is described here, but the concept is the same for dorsal positioning. With the pig in a sternal position, an assistant can open the mouth by using two cotton tapes, one behind the incisors of the maxilla and one behind the incisors of the mandible. The tongue can be protracted and placed under the lower cotton band to fixate it; however, care should be taken not to damage it on the lower incisors. With the head sufficiently lifted (same position as for intubating the trachea of a dog), it should be possible to visualize the epiglottis with the aid of a laryngoscope. The tip of the epiglottis is often dorsal to the soft palate and can be freed using the tip of the laryngoscope blade or a stiff stylet. Once freed, the laryngoscope blade (Miller [straight] blades are generally preferred) can be gently placed on top of the epiglottis to gently press it downward (ventrally), revealing the *rima glottidis*. Care should be taken to do this gently as the mucosa of the laryngeal structures is easily abraded. Once the *rima glottidis* is visible, the endotracheal tube, threaded over an intubation stylet, can be gently introduced. By letting the distal end of the stylet extend beyond the tip of the endotracheal tube, the stylet can be introduced into the larynx first. With the stylet held in place, the endotracheal tube can be advanced gently so that it slides over the stylet. When resistance to advancing the tube is encountered, the tube should be rotated 180° and advanced further. It can be very helpful to use a plastic-coated wire stylet. This type can be pre-shaped into a gentle curve, approximating the shape of a banana or ice-hockey stick. This shape aids in directing the endotracheal tube upward after the 180° rotation is performed. Pre-shaping also has the advantage of usually not requiring the tip of the stylet to extend beyond the endotracheal tube, reducing the risk of damage to the trachea. If the technique is unsuccessful, using a smaller endotracheal tube size is often the solution (Figure 14.16).

Practical Tips for Peri-anesthetic Management

Small Ruminants and Cattle

Practices with regard to fasting ruminants vary widely, generally ranging from no fasting at all to fasting times of up to 24 h (see Chapter 2), largely guided by the size and age of the animal. Fasting reduces the total volume of the rumen which can be beneficial for the respiratory and circulatory physiology of the animal as there will be less pressure on the diaphragm and lungs, and the large blood vessels, when the animal is recumbent. Fasting the animal also reduces the risk of gas distension. Fasting is unlikely to reduce the risk of regurgitation as fasting leads to a more liquid ruminal content, which might even increase the risk of regurgitation.

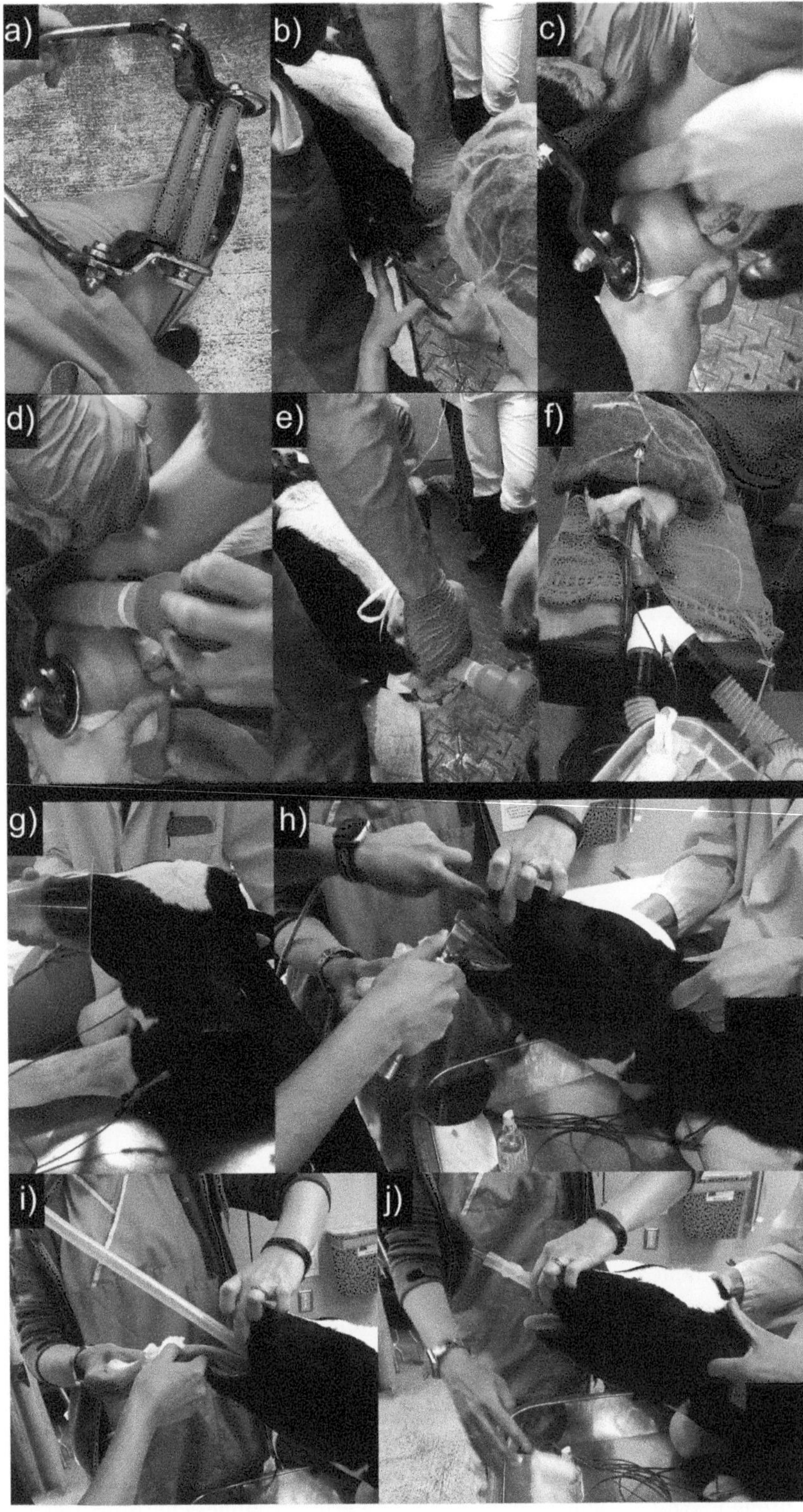

Figure 14.15 Photographs showing the order of events for tracheal intubation of an adult cow. A mouth gag (a) is used to open the jaws and protect the person performing intubation (b) before a person reaches into the mouth to palpate the *rima glottidis*. An endotracheal tube is advanced into the oropharynx with the free hand (c), and it is guided through the arytenoid cartilages and into the trachea (d). The endotracheal tube is secured (e) and connected to the breathing circuit of the anesthetic machine (f). Tracheal intubation in a calf can be carried out by direct visualization, using a laryngoscope with a long Miller blade. In calves, pre-oxygenation can be performed (g), before general anesthesia is induced. Following induction, the mouth is opened and the blade of the laryngoscope placed on the base of the tongue immediately cranial to the epiglottis. An endotracheal tube exchanger (a long intubating stylet) is advanced through the *rima glottidis* (h), and then the laryngoscope is removed and the endotracheal tube advanced into the trachea over the endotracheal tube exchanger (i) and secured in position (j) after removing the endotracheal tube exchanger. (*Source:* Photographs (a) to (f): Courtesy of Dr. Javier Benito; Université de Montréal.)

In very young animals that are not eating solids yet, fasting is generally unnecessary, and may lead to hypoglycemia. Monitoring blood glucose and potential intravenous supplementation are recommended in ruminants <1-month old.

Due to decreased frequency (or absence) of eructation under general anesthesia and continued fermentation in the rumen, ruminants are prone to develop distension or bloat during general anesthesia. Placement of an orogastric tube at the start of the anesthetic can help in channeling liquid and gas out of the rumen, preventing distension. In case of significant bloat, not prevented by placing an orogastric tube, transcutaneous puncture of the rumen with a trocar or wide bore intravenous

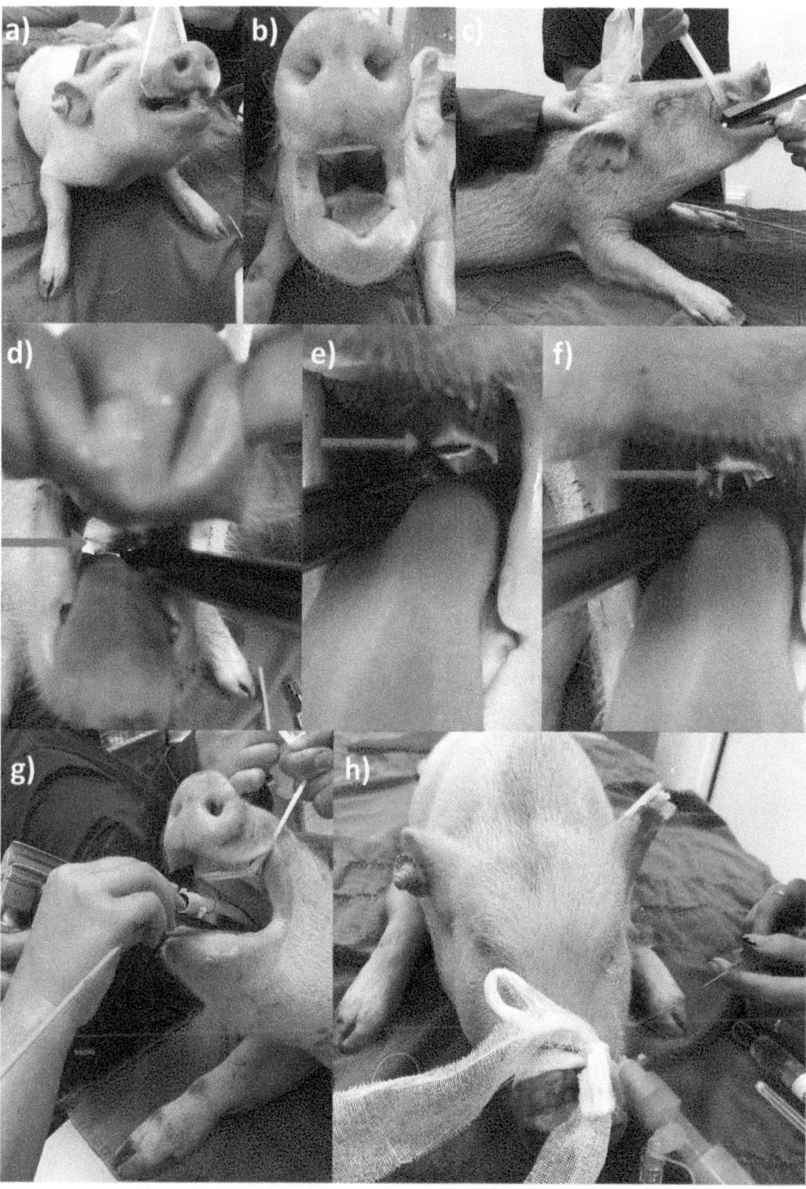

Figure 14.16 Photographs showing the order of events for tracheal intubation of an anesthetized pig. The head is supported and the mouth opened using gauze bandage looped around the maxilla (a, b). Then, the operator grasps the tongue, using square swabs if required, and a laryngoscope with a Miller blade is inserted into the oral cavity and advanced to the oropharynx (c). The Miller blade is advanced until the epiglottis cartilage can be seen, often caudal to the soft palate, indicated by the blue arrow (d). The tip of the Miller blade is tilted ventrally to disengage the tip of the epiglottis from the soft palate (e), to reveal the arytenoid cartilages (f), indicated by the blue arrows. An endotracheal tube is advanced into the oral cavity and through the *rima glottidis* into the trachea with (as shown here) or without the aid of an intubating stylet (g). The endotracheal tube is connected to a breathing system of an anesthetic machine and the endotracheal tube cuff is inflated (h). (*Source:* Courtesy of Drs. Julia Deutsch and Paul MacFarlane; Langford Vets, University of Bristol.)

catheter is usually an effective solution. The trocar or catheter can be left in place for the remainder of the procedure, if necessary. At the end of the procedure, the trocar or catheter can be removed without consequence. Provided distension does not cause impairment of ventilation (secondary to increased intra-abdominal pressure) or circulation (secondary to reduced venous return), it may be left untreated.

Whenever performing a procedure on a large ruminant, workplace safety (personnel and animal) is an important consideration. Before undertaking a procedure, the area should be cleared of any potential hazards and escape routes identified.

Historically, pain has not been readily recognized and was therefore often undertreated in ruminants. There is growing literature on pain assessment in ruminants that is guiding the use of analgesia in these species. However, as of yet, the number of licensed analgesic drugs is limited (see Further Reading). Within these constraints, every effort should be made to provide ruminants with proper analgesia. Whenever pain is identified or suspected, analgesia should be provided, usually in the form of administering an NSAID and applying locoregional anesthesia.

Pigs

Practices regarding fasting pigs vary widely, ranging from no fasting at all to fasting times of up to 12 h (see Chapter 2). Pigs are easily stressed and every effort should be taken to keep the animal calm. Pigs are highly trainable and, with adequate planning and time, positive reinforcement training can be used to facilitate tolerance of intramuscular injection.

As they mostly lack hair, pigs easily develop hypothermia during anesthesia. Heat loss can be mitigated by covering the animal with a blanket or bubble wrap, placing it on an electrical heating mat or forced warm air blanket, and using hot water bottles. Use a thin layer of padding between electrical heating mats or hot water bottles and the skin of the animal to avoid skin burns. Pigs usually recover calmly; however, enough padding or bedding should be provided as their skin is easily damaged if they experience excitement during recovery. Loud noises, bright lights, and excessive handling during the recovery period can precipitate stress and excitement during recovery.

Like ruminants, pain in pigs is probably underappreciated and undertreated. Pig-specific pain scales have been developed (see Further Reading) and can be used to guide analgesia management. Due to the limitations of available licensed analgesic drugs, the use of locoregional analgesia is strongly recommended during the peri-operative period. Blocks can be repeated immediately before recovery to extend their duration into the recovery period (paying attention to not exceed toxic doses of the local anesthetic).

Routine Local Anesthetic Block Techniques

Standing procedures with the potential to cause pain must not be performed without an adequate locoregional anesthetic technique. During general anesthesia, the same locoregional anesthetic techniques can be valuable adjuncts to analgesia for the animal. Lidocaine (2%; 20 mg/mL) is the most commonly used, and licensed, local anesthetic drug used in production animal anesthesia. In each case, the maximum recommended dose to avoid toxicity should be calculated in order to ensure that the recommended volumes of injection in Table 14.8 do not exceed this limit. To avoid toxicity, the following maximum doses are recommended: sheep and goats: 5 mg/kg; cattle: 6 mg/kg; pigs: 4 mg/kg.

Table 14.8 Selected local anesthetic blocks performed in ruminants and pigs.

Site	Technique	Indication	Location	Drug(s)
Head	Auriculo palpebral nerve block	Eye exam and eyelid surgery	• Deposit local anesthetic at dorsal edge of caudal aspect of zygomatic arch just cranial to base of ear • Nerve itself palpable where it runs over zygomatic arch	Lidocaine, approx. 5 mL
	Supraorbital nerve block	Eyelid and frontal face surgery	• Supraorbital foramen found by placing thumb and middle finger on medial and lateral canthus of eye. Index finger will "automatically" be placed on supraorbital foramen. • Deposit local anesthetic over foramen while applying gentle pressure onto foramen.	Lidocaine, approx. 5 mL
	Petersen eye block	Surgery of the eye	• Block skin overlying the junction of the supraorbital process and the zygomatic arch. • Insert 14-gauge 4 cm long needle in horizontal plane caudal to supraorbital process and dorsal to zygomatic arch. • Insert 18-gauge 9 cm long needle through previously placed needle. Advance in horizontal but slightly dorsal direction until encountering coronoid process of the mandibula. • Walk needle off rostral aspect of coronoid process and advance further in slightly ventral direction until hitting bony plate of the foramen orbitorotundum. • Withdraw needle a few millimeters before injecting.	Lidocaine, 15–20 mL
	Four-point block	Surgery of the eye	• Bend a 18-gauge 9 cm needle into a halve circle • Insert needle between globe and orbital rim at the 12, 3, 6, and 9 o'clock • "Thug" on eye is noted when needle is in ocular cone where injection should be made	Lidocaine, approx. 5–10 mL per site
	Retrobulbar block	Enucleation	• Variant of four-point block, where needle is inserted at only one point of the eye • Injection made into the ocular cone	Lidocaine up to 20 mL
	Cornual nerve block	Dehorning	• Zygomaticotemporal nerve at the temporal ventral border of the upper third of the temporal ridge • Infra-trochlear nerve roughly halfway on an imaginary line between the medial canthus of the eye and the medial side of the base of the horn • Additional ring-block around the base of the horn may be needed	Lidocaine up to 10 mL per site Calculate max total dose of 4 mg/kg in small ruminants

Table 14.8 (Continued)

Site	Technique	Indication	Location	Drug(s)
Hind quarters/ Flank/ Abdomen	Epidural	All surgery caudal from the umbilicus	• In cattle at sacrococcygeal intervertebral space (S5–Co1) or first intercoccygeal intervertebral space (Co1–Co2) found by moving tail upward and downward and feeling for indentation/pivoting point at proximal end of tail. • In small ruminants and pigs at L/S junction (L6/7–S1), found by palpating cranial edges of iliac wings with thumb and middle finger. Place index finger halfway thumb and middle finger. Index finger will be over L/S junction. • Confirm correct needle placement with "hanging drop" or "loss of resistance" method.	Lidocaine up to 4 mg/kg Ketamine 1 mg/kg Xylazine 0.1 mg/kg Combinations of drugs can be used
	Paravertebral	Surgery of the flank	• Proximal block: Insert needle in dorso-ventral direction just cranial to transverse process of T13, L1, and L2, just lateral from the spine • Use long needle to also block ventral branches • Distal block Insert needle in latero-medial direction dorsal and ventral from tips of transverse processes L1, L2, and L4	Lidocaine up to 4 mg/kg
	Inverted L-block	Surgery of the flank	• Infiltrate a vertical line cranial to the surgical area and an intersecting horizontal line dorsal to the surgical area, making an inverted L	Lidocaine up to 4 mg/kg
	Local infiltration	All (minor) surgeries	• Infiltrate local tissues	Lidocaine up to 4 mg/kg
	IVRA	Surgery of the foot or distal limb	• Place IV catheter in distal part of limb that needs to be anesthetized • Apply Esmarch's bandage from distal to proximal minimally 10 cm proximal to area that needs to be anesthetized • At the proximal end, make Esmarch's bandage into tourniquet • With tourniquet in place, remove Esmarch's bandage from distal to proximal, leaving tourniquet and previously placed IV catheter in place • Verify absence of peripheral pulse in exposed distal limb • Inject local anesthetic through the previously placed IV catheter • Leave tourniquet for a maximum time of 90 min • When releasing tourniquet, analgesia wears off quickly	Lidocaine up to 4 mg/kg

Questions and Answers

There are more practice questions and answers available for this chapter on the website. Please visit http://www.wiley.com/go/VeterinaryAnesthesiaZeiler.

Questions

Exotic Mammal Questions

1) Which of the following administration routes is a comparable alternative to intravenous injection in exotic species?
   a) Intraosseous
   b) Subcutaneous
   c) Oral gavage
   d) Intramuscular
2) For an ovariohysterectomy surgery in a female rabbit, place the following methods of providing oxygen and inhalational anesthetic agent in order, from most to least preferred: facemask, supraglottic airway device (e.g., laryngeal mask airway), and endotracheal intubation.
3) Which is the following methods is the gold standard method for confirming endotracheal (ET) tube placement in the trachea in a rabbit or ferret?
   a) Listening for breath sounds at the end of the ET tube.
   b) Looking for condensation on a cold surface held to the end of the ET tube.
   c) Looking for movement in plucked hair/fur held to the end of the ET tube.
   d) Use of a sidestream or mainstream capnograph.

Ruminants and Pig Questions

1) Regurgitation is common in ruminants under anesthesia. Describe three methods to reduce the risk of anesthetized ruminants aspirating regurgitated contents.
2) What condition can sheep and goats develop after administering xylazine?
3) What is the longest period of fasting in an adult pig before anesthesia?

Answers

Exotic Mammal Questions

1) a
2) Endotracheal intubation > supraglottic airway device > facemask
3) d

Ruminants and Pig Questions

1) Appropriate starving times (food and water) Intubate and inflate the cuff/do not deflate cuff until swallowing Head positioning during surgery (head occiput higher than mouth)
2) Pulmonary edema and pulmonary hypertension
3) Up to 12 h

Further Reading

Exotic Mammals Section

Aguiar, J., Mogridge, G., and Hall, J. (2013). Femoral fracture repair and sciatic and femoral nerve blocks in a guinea pig. *J Sm Anim Prac* 55: 635–639.

Buckley, G.J., DeCubellis, J., Sharp, C.R., and Rozanski, E.A. (2011). Cardiopulmonary resuscitation in hospitalized rabbits: 15 cases. *J Exot Pet Med* 20: 46–50.

Carpenter, J. and Marion, C. (2017). *Exotic Animal Formulary*, 5e, 1–776. Saunders, USA.

D'Ovidio, D., Rota, S., Noviello, E. et al (2014). Nerve stimulator–guided sciatic-femoral block in pet rabbits (*Oryctolagus cuniculus*) undergoing hind limb surgery: a case series. *J Exot Pet Med* 23: 91–95.

Di Girolamo, N., Toth, G., and Selleri, P. (2016). Prognostic value of rectal temperature at hospital admission in client-owned rabbits. *J Am Vet Med Assoc* 248: 288–297.

Freijs, E. (2016) Comparison of plasma levels and analgesic effect between oral transmucosal and subcutaneous administration of buprenorphine in rabbits. Swedish University of Agriculture Sciences, Veterinary Medicine Programme, 1–24.

Hawkins, M.G. and Pascoe, P.J. (2021). Chapter 37 Anesthesia, analgesia and sedation of small mammals. In: *Ferrets, Rabbits, and Rodents, Clinical Medicine and Surgery*, 4e (ed. K.E. Quesenberry, C.J. Orcutt, C. Mans, and J.W. Carpenter), 536–558. Elsevier Inc..

Levy, I.H., Di Girolamo, N., and Keller, K.A. (2021). Rectal temperature is a prognostic indicator in client-owned guinea pigs. *J Small Anim Pract* 62: 861–865.

Lichtenberger, M. and Ko, J. (2007). Anesthesia and analgesia for small mammals and birds. *Vet Clin N Am Exot Anim Prac* 10: 293–315.

Rousseau-Blass, F., Cribb, A.E., Beaudry, F., and Pang, D.S. (2021). A pharmacokinetic-pharmacodynamic study of intravenous midazolam and flumazenil in adult New Zealand white-californian rabbits (*Oryctolagus cuniculus*). *J Am Assoc Lab Anim Sci* 60: 319–328.

Rufiange, M., Leung, V.S.Y., Simpson, K., and Pang, D.S.J. (2021). Pre-warming following premedication limits hypothermia before and during anesthesia in Sprague-Dawley rats (*Rattus norvegicus*). *Can J Vet Res* 85: 106–111.

Sadar, M.J., Knych, H.K., Drazenovich, T.L., and Paul-Murphy, J.R. (2018). Pharmacokinetics of buprenorphine after intravenous and oral transmucosal administration in guinea pigs (Cavia porcellus). *Am J Vet Res* 79: 260–266.

Schuster, C.J. and Pang, D.S.J. (2018). Forced-air pre-warming prevents peri-anaesthetic hypothermia and shortens recovery in adult rats. *Lab Anim* 52: 142–151.

Thompson, A.C., Kristal, M.B., Sallaj, A. et al (2004). Analgesic efficacy of orally administered buprenorphine in rats: methodologic considerations. *Comp Med* 54: 293–300.

Zhang, E.Q., Knight, C.G., and Pang, D.S. (2017). Heating pad performance and efficacy of 2 durations of warming after isoflurane anesthesia of Sprague-Dawley rats *(Rattus norvegicus). J Am Assoc Lab Anim Sci* 56: 786–791.

Ruminants and Pig Section

Abouelfetouh, M.M., Salah, E., Ding, M., and Ding, Y. (2021). Application of α 2-adrenergic agonists combined with anesthetics and their implication in pulmonary intravascular macrophages-insulted pulmonary edema and hypoxemia in ruminants. *J Vet Pharmacol Ther* 44: 478–502.

Abrahamsen, E.J. (2008). Chemical Restraint in Ruminants. *Vet Clin Food Animal* 24: 227–243.

Celly, C.S., McDonell, W.N., Young, S.S., and Black, W.D. (1997). The comparative hypoxaemic effect of four alpha 2 adrenoceptor agonists (xylazine, romifidine, detomidine and medetomidine) in sheep. *J Vet Pharmacol Ther* 20: 464–471.

Coetzee, J.F., Gehring, R., Tarus-Sang, J., and Anderson, D.E. (2010). Effect of sub-anesthetic xylazine and ketamine ('ketamine stun') administered to calves immediately prior to castration. *Vet Anaesth Analg* 37: 566–578.

Di Giminiani, P., Brierley, V.L., Scollo, A. et al (2016). The assessment of facial expressions in piglets undergoing tail docking and castration: toward the development of the piglet grimace scale. *Front Vet Sci* 14: 100.

Leblanc, M.M., Hubbell, J.A., and Smith, H.C. (1984). The effects of xylazine hydrochloride on intrauterine pressure in the cow. *Theriogen* 21: 681–690.

Robles, I., Arruda, A.G., Nixon, E. et al (2021). Producer and veterinarian perspectives towards pain management practices in the US cattle industry. *Animals* 11: 209.

Törneke, K., Bergström, U., and Neil, A. (2003). Interactions of xylazine and detomidine with alpha2-adrenoceptors in brain tissue from cattle, pigs and rats. *J Vet Pharmacol Ther* 26: 205–211.

Viscardi, A.V., Hunniford, M., Lawlis, P. et al (2017). Development of a piglet grimace scale to evaluate piglet pain using facial expressions following castration and tail docking: a pilot study. *Front Vet Sci* 4: 51.

15

Approach to Neonatal, Pediatric, and Geriatric Patients

Sabine Kästner and Gareth Zeiler

With the changing human–animal bond and animals being considered lifelong family members, more procedures are requested in very young and very old animals. In these patients, immaturity and dysmaturity or aging processes influence the ability of the patient to compensate for the effects of drugs used during the peri-anesthetic period and the anesthetic risk is increased in these age groups. Studies have shown that foals less than 1 month of age and horses above 15 years of age have an increased risk for anesthetic death. In cats and dogs, an increased anesthetic risk is associated with an age >12 years.

Neonates and Pediatric Patients

Difference in Physiology Compared to the Healthy Adult

The physiology of neonates differs from adults and results in differences in the pain experience and differences in drug pharmacokinetics and pharmacodynamics that contribute to altered responses to anesthesia. The degree of maturation at birth greatly varies between precocial (born in a relatively developed state, e.g., foals and calves) and altricial (born in a relatively undeveloped state, e.g., puppies and kittens) species, but also between breeds and individual animals. As a simple guide, in kittens and puppies, the first 6 weeks of life are considered the neonatal phase followed by the pediatric period from 6 to 12 weeks. Foals and calves are precocial animals with a true neonatal phase of 1–2 weeks and can be considered physiologically mature by 4–6 weeks of age. Kittens and puppies rarely undergo surgery during their first days or weeks of life, whereas in foals and calves, umbilical, urachal, and vesical surgeries (for example) are performed in the neonatal period. Many drugs used in veterinary anesthesia are not licensed for neonatal or pediatric animals (<6 months) and are used extra-label (off-label) or according to legislation within the country of practice. Furthermore, legislation and drug licensing for food animals can vary between countries (see Chapters 6, 7, and 11).

Neonatal physiology and physiologic differences related to body composition and organ function result in altered pharmacokinetics and clinical pharmacology of anesthetics. These differences can contribute to increased anesthetic risk if not appreciated by the anesthetist. The consequences relating to different organ system function are summarized in Table 15.1.

Body Composition

The body composition of neonates and young animals is different from adults with a relative high water and low fat content (Figure 15.1). For example, in neonatal foals, total body water content takes up 75% of body mass (BM) compared to 67% in adult horses. This results in a ratio of extracellular to intracellular fluid twice as high as in adults (43% of BM in foals versus 22% of BM in adults). Total body fat comprises 2–3% in foals compared to 5% in adult horses. In puppies, fat content is very low (2–3%) in newborns and increases rapidly during the first month of life.

These differences in body composition can influence the distribution of hydrophilic and lipophilic drugs and their associated effects:

- Low body fat results in a smaller adipose tissue compartment for drug distribution of lipophilic drugs (like most sedatives and anesthetics) resulting in increased plasma concentrations and consequently lower dose requirements. In neonates, drugs being given intravenously (IV), the lowest recommended dose of drug should be administered and then titrated to effect after waiting a sufficient amount of time to reach an onset of action (usually up to one minute for drugs used for induction). For drugs administered intramuscularly (IM), they

Fundamental Principles of Veterinary Anesthesia, First Edition. Edited by Gareth E. Zeiler and Daniel S. J. Pang.

Companion Website: www.wiley.com/go/VeterinaryAnesthesiaZeiler

Table 15.1 Consequences of different organ system function in neonates and pediatrics compared to adults.

Organ system	Consequences	Practical advice
Hepatic system	Immature hepatic function means: • Increased availability of active, unbound drug • Limited drug elimination capacities in neonates, especially those that require phase II biotransformation (see text for detail)	Neonate patients: • Administer drugs at the lowest recommended dose in neonates • Try to administer drugs that are preferentially metabolized by phase I biotransformation in the liver. Pediatric patients: • Liver function reaches maturity, which often implies they require drug administration at the higher recommended dose • Drug duration of effect is often shorter than expected. Thus, drawing up 50–100% more of an induction drug based on initial calculations is prudent
Renal system	Immature renal function means: • Poor ability to concentrate urine • Poor ability to excrete a water load • Susceptibility to dehydration and overhydration • Poor acid–base regulation • Poor potassium excretion in young puppies • Prolonged effects of drugs, which depend on renal excretion • Glucosuria and proteinuria is common in neonatal puppies	• Careful calculation and use of fluids (ins-and-outs of fluid requirements) • Use a Buretrol, an infusion pump or a syringe driver to avoid overinfusion and guarantee infusion of calculated volumes • Careful calculation and monitoring with use of IV potassium supplementation • Avoid renally cleared drugs with narrow margin of safety (i.e., NSAIDs)
Cardiovascular system	Immature cardiovascular system means: • Poor ability to respond to sudden and/or large changes in blood volume or pressure (i.e., poor hemodynamic stability and minimal cardiovascular reserve) • Prone to hypotension • Poor response to inotropes and vasopressors • Intrapulmonary or intracardiac shunting of blood is possible	• In neonates, a mean arterial blood pressure between 40 and 50 mmHg can be considered acceptable • In pediatrics, a mean arterial blood pressure above 50 mmHg (50–70 mmHg) should be expected • Treatment of hypotension should be aimed to treat the underlying cause (fluid depletion, bradycardia, low myocardial contractility, and vasodilation) • Maintaining physiologic body temperature, euglycemia, and oxygenation is crucial for avoiding bradycardia and vasodilation • In neonates, fluid boluses should not exceed 20 mL/kg with careful re-evaluation to avoid volume overload • The response to inotropes (e.g., dobutamine) and vasopressors (e.g., norepinephrine and phenylephrine) is age dependent and can be unpredictable and poor. Therefore, carefully titrate drug to effect while monitoring for adverse effects (e.g., tachycardia with dobutamine) • Neonates are more prone to shunts (intrapulmonary, extra-cardiac, and intra-cardiac) compared to pediatrics. Thus, heart rates and vessel tone should be maintained within normal ranges for the species and breed to mitigate formation of a right-to-left shunt
Respiratory system	Immature respiratory system means: • Prone to hypoxemia • Prone to atelectasis • Prone to respiratory fatigue • High alveolar minute ventilation with low functional residual capacity speeds up anesthesia induction with inhalational anesthetics	• Pre-oxygenation is recommended, if tolerated • Careful monitoring of anesthetic depth during mask induction is necessary • Be prepared to assist ventilation • Animals may profit from immediate mechanical ventilation to avoid atelectasis formation and increased work of breathing • Be careful to not overinflate the lungs (pliable rib cage)

Table 15.1 (Continued)

Organ system	Consequences	Practical advice
Thermoregulatory system	Hypothermia develops easily because: • Immature thermoregulatory system • High body-surface to body-mass ratio • Limited glycogen stores • Limited muscle mass to produce heat by shivering • Low amount of insulating subcutaneous fat • Limited ability to vasoconstrict to prevent heat dissipation	• Monitoring of the body temperature (rectal temperature, esophageal temperature, and nasal temperature in the intubated patient) is prudent to avoid hyper- or hypothermia • Begin warming as early as possible, i.e., use blankets or pre-warming strategies, start active warming as early as possible. However, in small-body-mass patients, be cautious of overheating • Use warm infusion as well as flushing fluids • Use of lowest safe fresh gas flow for inhalational anesthesia is recommended
Hematopoietic system	• In neonates even minor hemorrhage can reduce the oxygen-carrying capacity because they have a lower hematocrit (related to hemoglobin concentration) compared to pediatrics and greatly affect oxygen delivery	• Patients should ideally have a hematocrit above 20% before anesthesia because most sedatives and anesthetic drugs cause a decrease in hematocrit • If the hematocrit is less than 20% patients will be prone to developing hypoxemia despite providing pre-oxygenation and 100% oxygen support when anesthetized

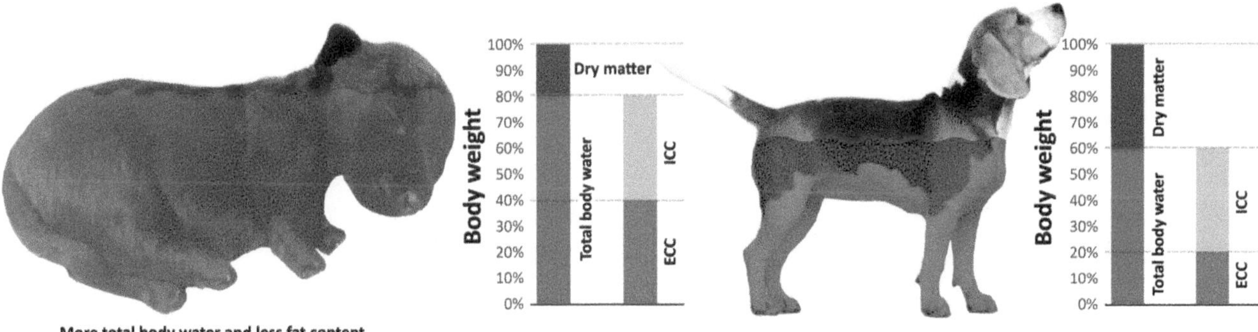

Figure 15.1 The body composition of neonates (left) compared to adult animals (right) includes a higher water content and less fat content.

should also be dosed at the lowest recommended dose of the dosing range. Pediatric patients do not have the same limitations, and once physiologically mature, normal adult dose ranges can be used.

- The absolute and relatively larger extracellular fluid volume results in a greater apparent volume of distribution for water-soluble drugs that are highly ionized in plasma or relatively polar (e.g., nonsteroidal anti-inflammatory drugs [NSAIDs], aminoglycoside antimicrobials). As a consequence, despite a lack of neonatal pharmacokinetic and pharmacodynamic information, it is recommended to use the lowest dose on published drug dose ranges in neonates. Pediatric patients can often be given drugs according to the published adult dose range.

A higher proportion of extracellular water also translates to higher daily water requirements, so not only rapid dehydration but also rapid fluid overload can easily occur in neonates. In addition, the low muscle mass in puppies and kittens restricts the volume for IM administration of drugs. Although not specifically investigated, and no consensus has been reached, a recommendation of a maximum volume of 0.25 mL/kg per injection site is advocated. Larger volumes can be distributed over more than one injection site if necessary.

Neurologic Function, Brain, and Blood–Brain Barrier

The neurologic system of precocious species is well developed as they require the immediate ability to ambulate and function independently. The degree of nerve myelination is higher compared with altricial species of the same age. In contrast, puppies and kittens are born deaf and blind and initially spend 90% of the day sleeping, with minimal ambulation. In the neonatal stage, there is a lower general and local anesthetic requirement to produce general and local anesthesia, respectively. Drug requirements increase with aging, reaching adults level (and sometimes even higher requirements) earlier in precocious species than in altricial species.

In general, neonatal and pediatric animals go through an intensive phase of brain development with reorganization of neural networks by synaptogenesis and apoptosis. During this phase, increased apoptosis and loss of neurons have been seen in laboratory animal studies in response to the majority of inhalational and injectable anesthetics. This is known as "anesthetic neurotoxicity." The greatest vulnerability seems to be associated with the phase of the most intense synapatogenesis or the "brain growth spurt," with temporal variation between different species. The clinical relevance for human and veterinary anesthesia of this observation is not clear at present as some of the observed changes could be related to hypoxemia and hypercapnia and not the drugs per se.

Behavioral and physiologic/pathophysiologic responses to pain or (nerve) injury differ between neonatal, pediatric, and adult animals. For a long time, this difference has led to the erroneous idea that neonates feel less pain and require less analgesia as compared to an adult. Research has shown that untreated or long-standing pain in neonates and pediatric animals can lead to persistent changes in the pain pathways and phenotype expressions, which can alter their behavior, including long-term effects.

The highly selective, semipermeable blood–brain barrier composed of the capillary wall, astrocytes, pericytes, and transport proteins undergoes development in neonatal animals and has higher permeability. This means that a larger percentage of a drug dose can reach the brain and the required dose for centrally acting drugs (e.g., anesthetics and sedatives) is reduced.

The neuromuscular junction in juvenile animals is smaller than in adults, but this is compensated by a larger number of neuromuscular junctions with a similar distribution explaining a greater resistance to neuromuscular blocking agents.

Liver Function

The liver of neonates has poor gluconeogenic abilities and limited glycogen stores at birth. In combination with a high metabolic rate, neonates are therefore very susceptible to hypoglycemia.

Biliary function is not fully developed at birth, leading to a mild physiologic cholestasis; however, bile flow reaches normal adult rates in puppies by 4–6 weeks of age.

Hepatic cytochrome P450 content and enzymatic activity are reduced at birth, but hepatic function matures rapidly within 1–2 weeks in foals and calves. In puppies and kittens, it takes longer to reach adult levels (between about 3–4 and 12 weeks of life). At birth, hepatic metabolism by oxidation is the most effective pathway of phase I, whereas hydrolysis and reduction and phase II activity (conjugation, e.g., glucuronidation) are reduced. This can lead to prolongation of drug effects in cases where drug elimination depends on hepatic biotransformation, such as the benzodiazepines, opioids, propofol, and NSAIDs for example (see Chapter 6).

In puppies and kittens, a variable degree of hypoalbuminemia can be present in the neonatal period. Adult albumin levels are attained by about 16 weeks. Low albumin results in a greater proportion of unbound, free (active) drug in highly protein-bound substances. Unbound active drug can increasingly pass into the brain and may lead to an increased response to drugs like barbiturates, ketamine, etomidate, benzodiazepines, and NSAIDs. Healthy foals are rarely hypoalbuminemic and total protein is close to adult levels after the first day of life, though this may differ in sick foals and protein levels should be confirmed in this population.

After weaning, cytochrome P450 activity can rise above adult levels, which may lead to increased hepatic clearance of some drugs in pediatric patients. During this growth period, more frequent dosing of some drugs, especially the induction drugs (propofol and alfaxalone), may be necessary; however, this has not been investigated thoroughly.

Kidney Function

Kidney function matures more rapidly in precocious animals than in altricial species. In foals and calves, glomerular filtration rate (GFR) is at adult levels by 2–4 days, whereas renal tubular function (secretion, reabsorption) requires about 4–6 weeks to be fully functional.

Nephrogenesis in puppies (and probably kittens) is not complete until the third week of life; the outer cortical nephrons are the last ones to become fully functional. Therefore, GFR develops over the first 2–3 weeks of life accompanied by slower tubular secretion for the first 4–8 weeks of life. The high total body water content and increasing function of the kidneys over time make recommending appropriate fluid rates (by bolus or infusions) challenging in neonates. The risks of underhydration and overhydration are real concerns, and fluid status should always be monitored. In neonatal animals, assessment of underhydration (dehydration or hypovolemia) is difficult to assess because of their differences in physiological function and body composition. Dehydration is usually based on clinical suspicion where there is vomiting and diarrhea (increased fluid losses) or poor nursing (poor milk quality, low milk volumes, and failure to suckle) causing a decreased intake. Weighing the neonate on a regular basis (2–3 times a day) on an appropriate scale will help determine neonatal weight against acceptable breed standards and age. Rapid changes in weight could indicate rapid changes in total body water. Expected signs of dehydration in pediatric animals are similar to adult animals (tacky mucous membranes, skin tenting, sunken ocular globes, etc.), but these signs are not reliable in neonates. Assessment of hypovolemia in neonates is focused on mucous membrane color (pale pink to white), capillary refill time (delayed), pulse quality (difficult to feel femoral or dorsal pedal pulses), and jugular vein distensibility (hard to raise or feel). Overhydration (hypervolemia and volume overload) is also difficult to evaluate in neonates, but serous nasal discharges, chemosis, tachypnea (or other altered breathing patterns), restlessness, coughing (with or without auscultating pulmonary crackles), ascites, and polyurea are strong indicators of overhydration.

Cardiovascular Function

The parasympathetic system is fully functional shortly after birth, while sympathetic function is incomplete. This predisposes the neonate to pronounced vagal responses and poor vasomotor control with an inadequate hypotension-induced baroreceptor response, which needs to undergo resetting from fetal conditions after birth. Arterial blood pressures and vascular tone increase and heart rate decreases from birth to infancy and adulthood. As an example, in awake puppies, MAP increased from 49 ± 15 mmHg at one month to about 60 mmHg at three months and 94 ± 2 mmHg at nine months, reaching a plateau at about seven months. In awake pony foals, MAP increased from 50 ± 8 mmHg on day 1 to 61 ± 15 mmHg, 74 ± 11 mmHg, and 75 ± 16 mmHg at one week, four weeks, and 3 months, respectively.

Sympathetic adrenergic stimulation (endogenous or exogenous agonists) results in a limited increase in heart rate and contractility, which means potentially poor responses to vasopressors, positive inotropes, and anticholinergics, with a generally unpredictable response depending on the age and stage of development.

The neonatal heart contains a higher proportion of fibrous tissue relative to contractile tissue compared to an adult heart and has limited compliance, making the heart less able to respond to volume loading with an increased cardiac output. In the neonate myocyte, the T-tubules and sarcoplasmic reticulum, responsible for calcium ion storage and release, are not fully developed and myocyte contraction is highly dependent on plasma ionized calcium. Because of the limited ability to increase stroke volume and contractility, cardiac output is largely dependent on heart rate. Therefore, bradycardia is poorly tolerated and results in hypotension, with a poor ability to compensate (immature sympathetic system not able to increase the heart rate or force of ventricular contraction).

The resting cardiac output is high in neonates and is very close to maximal cardiac output, leaving only a minimal cardiac reserve. An adult heart can increase output by 300%, whereas the neonatal heart can only increase output by 30%. Neonatal oxygen requirements (reflecting an increased metabolic rate) are also much greater than in the adult, which requires the neonatal heart to function at near maximal capacity all the time.

In very young puppies (<4 days of age), hypoxia leads to bradycardia instead of a compensatory tachycardia. In addition, puppies below two weeks of age do not respond to atropine with an increase in heart rate. For young puppies, and likely other altricial neonates with bradycardia, treatment with oxygen and warming, rather than atropine, is recommended.

Before complete anatomic closure (3–4 weeks after birth) of the *foramen ovale* (FO) and *ductus arteriosus* (DA), functional closure occurs. In foals, puppies, and kittens, an associated heart murmur can still be heard for 3–4 and 1–2 days after birth, respectively. This reflects the time to achieve functional closure. In rare cases, neonates can revert to a fetal pattern of circulation when they are under physiological stress causing an increase in sympathetic tone and changes in systemic or pulmonary resistance. This can lead to an extra-cardiac transpulmonary (or intracardiac, via the FO) shunting of blood via the patent DA in either direction (Figure 15.2).

Left-to-right shunting leads to recirculation of oxygenated blood from the arterial system into the lungs, whereas right-to-left shunting leads to circumvention of the lungs of deoxygenated blood. In the short term, the former is often unnoticed, whereas the latter leads to systemic hypoxemia and cyanosis. Therefore, in neonates, the physiological pressure gradients (high-pressure arterial system and low-pressure venous system) need to be maintained to prevent shunt reversal, which means maintaining arterial vascular tone and avoiding fluid overload (because it increases venous pressure).

Lactate is the primary fuel source for the immature myocardium, in contrast to the adult myocardium, which utilizes fatty acids for energy. Thus, if the lactate concentration

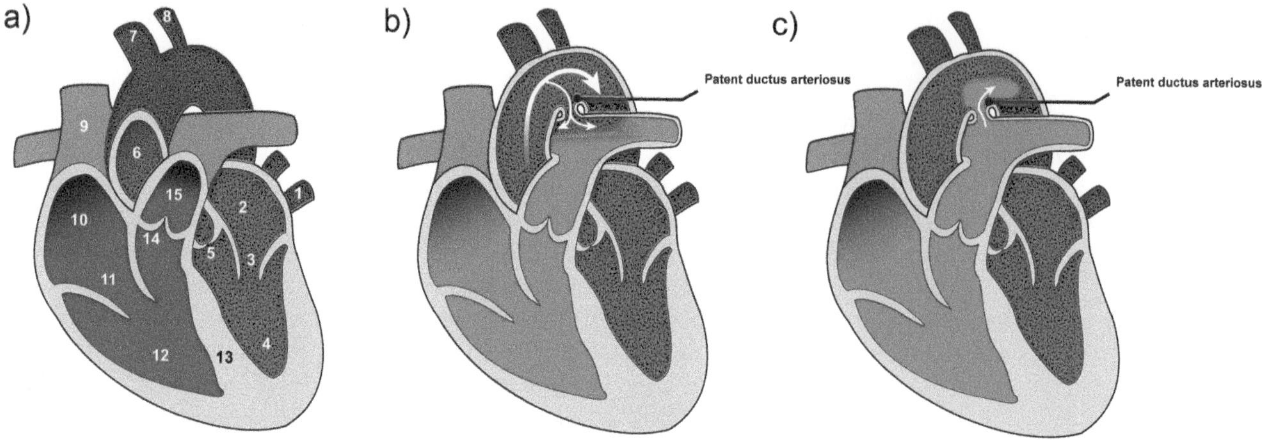

Figure 15.2 Normal cardiac anatomy (a): 1, pulmonary vein; 2, left atrium; 3, mitral valve; 4, left ventricle; 5, aortic valve; 6, aorta; 7, brachiocephalic trunk; 8, left subclavian artery; 9, cranial vena cava; 10, right atrium; 11, tricuspid valve; 12, right ventricle; 13, interventricular septum; 14, pulmonic valve; 15, main pulmonary artery. The left side of the heart carries oxygenated blood (red). The right side of the heart carries deoxygenated blood (blue). Compared to a normal heart but with the extra-cardiac *ductus arteriosus* that is still patent. The oxygenated blood exits the heart via the aorta at a higher pressure compared to the pulmonary artery and thus some of this blood re-enters the pulmonary circulation. While the aortic pressure is higher than the pulmonary pressure, it causes a left-to-right shunting of blood (b) However, when the pulmonary pressure is higher than aortic pressure (i.e., pulmonary hypertension) then deoxygenated blood bypasses the lungs and enters the systemic circulation and causes a right-to-left shunting of blood (c). This shunt leads to hypoxemia and cyanosis.

is high in neonates, then it may be normal. However, if the lactate concentration is greater than 5 mmol/L, then further investigation should be performed to determine if there is an increased production or a decrease in hepatic metabolism.

Respiratory Function

In puppies and kittens, the tongue is large relative to the oral cavity and can obstruct the oropharynx and air passage through the upper airways when the muscles relax with sedation or anesthesia.

Neonates have a high resting metabolic rate, which means high oxygen consumption requiring high minute ventilation. The chest wall of young animals is very compliant leading to less negative pleural pressure and a tendency toward lung collapse. The lungs are less air filled with a lower functional residual capacity (FRC) compared to an adult lung, making neonatal lungs prone to collapse and atelectasis. This limits the tidal volume that can be obtained and makes minute ventilation more dependent on respiratory rate. A high respiratory rate and the compliant rib cage can result in an increased work of breathing, making neonates prone to respiratory fatigue (see Chapter 18).

In very young puppies (<4 days of age), the response to hypoxia can be biphasic with a transient increase in respiratory rate followed by decreased respiratory rate or apnea. This seems to be related to a fetal "shut down" response to hypoxia with reduced muscle activity, bradycardia, and bradypnea.

Thermoregulation

Neonates have a high metabolic rate and use brown fat metabolism to produce heat. However, they develop hypothermia very quickly and more so under sedation and anesthesia (which decrease metabolism) because of their large surface-area-to-body-mass ratio, which promotes heat loss. Hypothermia leads to increased CNS depression (manifested as increased anesthetic depth) and prolonged recovery times (delayed clearance of drugs by metabolism).

Hemopoietic System (Red Blood Cells and Oxygen-carrying Capacity)

In puppies and kittens, hematocrit decreases by more than 30%, from approximately 35% to 25% in the first four weeks of life. By contrast, in foals, hematocrit decreases by approximately 20%, from 45% to 35% within the first week of life and then remains quite stable between 36% and 38% for the first six months. This drop in red blood cells (and thus hemoglobin) is related to reduced production of erythropoietin secondary to increased blood oxygenation via the lungs, reduced lifespan of fetal red blood cells, and rapid expansion of plasma volume, resulting in hemodilution. The hemoglobin of newborn foals and adult horses has been shown to be structurally identical. The main difference between fetal and adult hemoglobin in some species, such as horses, dogs, and rabbits, is the content of 2,3 diphosphoglycerate (2,3-DPG). An immediate rise in red blood cell 2,3-DPG occurs leading to normal (maternal) levels within five days allowing the foal to keep up with the mother because of better oxygen offloading in the metabolizing tissues compared to the fetal stage. The hemoglobin of cats, small ruminants, and cows does not interact significantly with 2,3-DPG and rely on other mechanisms to adapt oxygen affinity to extrauterine life.

Immune System

The immune system, consisting of humoral and cellular immunity, is not fully functional after birth. Within the first 24–48 h, the number of leucocytes increases followed by a decrease in the first months and a consecutive gradual increase. The number of leukocytes and the percentage of granulocytes and lymphocytes making up the leukocyte count vary among species and change from birth to adulthood with large individual variation.

In mammals, total protein concentrations are low at birth, increase dramatically after absorption of colostrum, and then decrease over 1–5 weeks as colostrum is metabolized.

Humoral immunity and the transfer of maternal immunoglobulins to the fetus vary with the type of placentation. Immunoglobulin A (IgA) antibodies do not cross the placenta, while immunoglobulin G (IgG) and immunoglobulin M (IgM) antibodies can be transferred in species with hemochorial placentation (primates, rabbits, rats, and mice) but is limited with endotheliochorial placentation, like in carnivores. Therefore, neonatal puppies are nearly agammaglobulinemic, with IgG serum levels of 0.3 g/L at birth, while adult dogs have 8–25 g/L. In puppies, 5–10% and in kittens approximately 25% of maternally derived IgG, and possibly IgM, may be transferred transplacentally. The epitheliochorial type of placentation in horses, pigs, and ruminants further restricts the transfer of maternal IgG antibodies to the fetus. Intake of colostrum, containing large concentrations of maternal antibodies, and intestinal permeability for immunoglobulins (pinocytosis) within the first hours of life are crucial for survival in cats and dogs and more so in horses, cattle, goats, sheep, and pigs.

Maximal uptake of IgG occurs at around 8 h after birth, and maximal IgG concentrations in plasma are reached between 12 and 18 h (Table 15.2). Keep in mind that during the time of increased intestinal permeability for immunoglobulins an increased uptake of drugs can occur (i.e., NSAIDs from mother, but a single dose has no clinically relevant consequence for the newborns).

Failure of passive transfer (FPT) of IgG leads to high susceptibility to infections (pneumonia, septic arthritis, omphalitis, etc.) and can result in severe debilitation. In all neonates with general weakness, an infection or septicemia, FPT has to be considered. Affected foals or calves might have to undergo various procedures requiring general anesthesia (joint lavage and omphalectomy). By the time FPT is usually diagnosed, it is too late to benefit from colostrum administration. Therefore, timely treatment by oral or ideally intravenous plasma transfusion is required. In foals, high-quality normal plasma with at least 15 g/L IgG (fresh and fresh frozen) or hyperimmune plasma should be used. Plasma also provides colloid support in neonates with FPT-related septicemia. Frequent retesting of IgG concentrations and administration to effect is required to treat FPT effectively/sufficiently. In foals with total FPT, it can be expected that 2 L of normal plasma needs to be transfused. In kittens or puppies, plasma can be delivered by the SC, intraperitoneal (IP), or intraosseous (IO) routes if IV access is difficult. A worked example on how to calculate the volume of plasma for intravenous transfusion in animals with FPT can be found in Concept Box 15.1.

Table 15.2 Normal levels of IgG (g/L) and cutoff values for failure of passive transfer (FPT) in common domestic neonates.

Species	Total FPT	Partial FPT	Minimum protective plasma concentration	Ideal 12–18 h after birth
Puppies	–	<2.3 at 2 days	–	>2.3 at day 2
Kittens	<0.2 Pre-suckling	–	–	(1) 26.5 ± 10.5 at day 1 or (2) 8.2 ± 0.4
Foals	<2	2–4	4–6	8–12
Calves	<10	10–17.9	18–24.9	>25
Sheep	<15	–	–	30–40

"–" indicates no value found to report.

Concept Box 15.1

Example calculation for required volume of normal plasma for intravenous transfusion in neonates with failure of passive transfer (FPT).

A 50 kg foal with total FPT will be used as an example:

The first step is to calculate the volume of plasma in a normovolemic foal:

$$\begin{aligned}\text{Volume of plasma} &= \text{body weight }(\text{kg})\times 60\text{ mL/kg}\\ &= 50\text{ kg}\times 60\text{ mL/kg}\\ &= 3000\text{ mL or 3 L of plasma}\end{aligned}$$

However, any plasma that is administered intravenously will have its components, specifically IgG in this example, redistribute to the extravascular space (i.e., interstitial and intracellular space) over a 24 h period. The distribution is approximately a 1:1 ratio between the extravascular and intravascular spaces. Therefore, doubling the calculated plasma volume is recommended to ensure enough IgG is given.

$$\begin{aligned}\text{Calculating redistributed plasma volume in the patient} &= 2\times\text{calculated plasma volume}\\ &= 2\times 3\text{ L}\\ &= 6\text{ L}\end{aligned}$$

The required amount of IgG should be calculated. The desired IgG concentration to reach is 6 g/L.

$$\begin{aligned}\text{Required IgG to be transfused} &= \begin{pmatrix}\text{redistibuted plasma}\\ \text{volume}\end{pmatrix}\times\begin{pmatrix}\text{desired IgG}\\ \text{cocntration}\end{pmatrix}\\ &= 6\text{ L}\times 6\text{ g/L}\\ &= 36\text{ g of IgG}\end{aligned}$$

Horse plasma must have at least 15 g/L of IgG, and this value is used to calculate the volume of plasma required for transfusion.

$$\begin{aligned}\text{Volume of plasma to be transfused} &= \begin{pmatrix}\text{Requried IgG to}\\ \text{be transfused}\end{pmatrix}\Big/\begin{pmatrix}\text{donar plasma}\\ \text{IgG g/L}\end{pmatrix}\\ &= 36\text{ g}/15\text{ g/L}\\ &= 2.4\text{ L of donor plasma needs to be transfused}\end{aligned}$$

Gastrointestinal Tract

The lower esophageal sphincter is not fully functional for the first weeks after birth and contributes to increased incidence of regurgitation in neonatal puppies and kittens. Postnatal development of the gastrointestinal tract and milk feeding can affect enteral absorption of oral drugs. Factors such as gastric pH, gastrointestinal motility, mucosal absorbing area, microbial population, and milk feeding significantly influence the degree of ionization and the absorption of orally given drugs. In the early neonatal phase (0–24 h), colostrum can pass across the intestine by pinocytosis; in this phase, orally given drugs can also be taken up more easily.

Considerations for Neonatal and Pediatric Anesthesia

Pre-operative Assessment and Preparation

As in adults, a thorough pre-operative assessment with a focus on the cardiopulmonary system should be performed. In neonatal puppies and kittens, this can be challenging and a comparison to the development of littermates can be helpful.

When blood tests become necessary in puppies and kittens, only small sample volumes can be taken (<1.0 mL) to avoid an excessive reduction in blood volume. Pre-anesthetic blood glucose testing can be useful for monitoring of potential hypoglycemia. Glucose, ideally, should not be given without testing as iatrogenic hyperglycemia can induce detrimental effects by deranging metabolism, promoting osmotic diuresis, and, after brain injury, promote secondary damage to neurons. Pre-operative stress can lead to normal or even elevated glucose levels, whereas hypoglycemia develops with anesthetic duration.

An accurate bodyweight with an appropriate weigh scale (human infant scale or kitchen scale) needs to be taken to allow accurate dosing of anesthetic drugs. Careful dosing might require dilution of commercial drug formulations and using appropriate syringe sizes to avoid inadvertent overdosing. Dilution mathematics can be found in Concept Box 15.2.

Nursing neonates should not be fasted, to avoid hypoglycemia, but a milk-filled stomach immediately before anesthetic induction should also be avoided as neonatal puppies and kittens are prone to regurgitation. A short waiting period of 30–45 min after feeding is recommended. This allows for gastric emptying.

Depending on the size of the animal, vascular access can be challenging in neonates. Pediatric kittens and puppies can be very active or difficult to handle, which makes

Concepts Box 15.2

How to dilute a drug to prepare for small-volume injection of drugs.

The goal of diluting a drug for injection is to give an injectable volume that can be accurately measured and delivered. A general guideline is that volumes less than 0.05 mL are not easy to confidently administer intramuscularly. With IV injections, especially for drugs that are titrated to a desired effect (e.g., drugs used during IV induction of anesthesia), a minimum volume of 0.5 mL is desirable, but volumes greater that 0.1 mL are acceptable (when using an appropriately sized syringe).

Example mathematics:
You need to inject a 0.1 kg puppy with combination of alfaxalone (2 mg/kg) and buprenorphine (0.02 mg/kg) IM to induce general anesthesia.

Commercially formulated drug concentrations:
Alfaxalone 10 mg/mL
Buprenorphine 0.3 mg/mL

Therefore, volumes of injection:

$$\begin{aligned}\text{Alfaxalone} &= (\text{BW} \times \text{dose}) / \text{formulation strength}\\ &= (0.1 \times 2.0) / 10\\ &= 0.02\ \text{mL}\\ \text{Buprenorphine} &= (\text{BW} \times \text{dose}) / \text{formulation strength}\\ &= (0.1 \times 0.02) / 0.3\\ &= 0.007\ \text{mL}\end{aligned}$$

These injection volumes cannot be accurately injected into the puppy or even accurately prepared (see Chapter 6).

The only way to increase the volume of injection is to dilute the drugs. A common method is to perform a 10× dilution. A few diluents are available. Sterile water for injection is likely the best to use because there are no ions that could interfere with the drug formulation. A second, common option, is to use normal saline (0.9% NaCl). Also, 5% dextrose in water might be available in the practice and should be used in preference to normal saline because there are no ions that could interfere with drug formulation. Ideally, calcium-containing fluids (e.g., lactated Ringer's solution) should not be used as a diluent as it is a common cause of drug precipitation.

Performing a 10× dilution. It is important to select a starting drug volume that can be accurately measured.

$$\begin{aligned}\text{Alfaxalone} &= \begin{pmatrix}\text{0.1 mL of}\\ \text{alfaxalone}\end{pmatrix} + \begin{pmatrix}\text{0.9 mL sterile}\\ \text{water for injection}\end{pmatrix}\\ &= 1.0\ \text{mg/mL}\\ \text{Buprenorphine} &= \begin{pmatrix}\text{0.1 mL}\\ \text{buprenorphine}\end{pmatrix} + \begin{pmatrix}\text{0.9 mL sterile}\\ \text{water for injection}\end{pmatrix}\\ &= 0.03\ \text{mg/mL}\end{aligned}$$

The new formulation strengths of the drugs can now be drawn into 1 mL syringes fitted with a small gauge needle (24–26 gauge). The new volumes are

$$\begin{aligned}\text{Alfaxalone} &= (\text{BW} \times \text{dose}) / \text{formulation strength}\\ &= (0.1 \times 2.0) / 1.0 = 0.2\ \text{mL}\\ \text{Buprenorphine} &= (\text{BW} \times \text{dose}) / \text{formulation strength}\\ &= (0.1 \times 0.02) / 0.3 = 0.07\ \text{mL}\end{aligned}$$

obtaining vascular access challenging without sedative premedication or desensitizing the skin using a eutectic mixture of local anesthetics (EMLA cream). Pediatric foals can also, at times, be difficult to handle to obtain vascular access and might require sedation.

Premedication/Sedation

Depending on general condition, character, and age of the patient, it must be decided if a sedative premedication is necessary and, if so, what doses are appropriate. Neonates or obtunded pediatric animals usually do not require sedation to achieve IV access. Dose selection needs careful consideration. In pediatric patients, the combination of mature organ function (drug clearance is efficient and rapid) and possible lack of habituation to humans or handling may result in a requirement for increased drug doses (similar to, or greater than, adult doses). Suggested doses for sedation and premedication in neonatal and pediatric animals are found in Tables 15.3 and 15.4, respectively.

Phenothiazines and butyrophenones (e.g., acepromazine and azaperone, respectively) interfere with thermoregulation, cause vasodilation, have a long duration of action, their effects cannot be antagonized, and they should therefore be avoided in neonates. In healthy, older pediatrics, they can be useful at low doses, for anxiolysis in conjunction with opioids.

Alpha-2 adrenergic receptor agonists produce profound sedation, but this comes at the cost of marked bradycardia, and thereby significant reduction in cardiac output, especially in neonates and pediatric puppies and kittens under 12 weeks old. They should be avoided in neonates and cardiovascularly unstable pediatric animals. In healthy, active

Table 15.3 Suggested doses for sedation and premedication in neonatal and pediatric small animals (puppies and kittens).

Drug	Dose (mg/kg)	Route	Comment
Diazepam	0.05–0.2	IV	Combined with opioid
Midazolam	0.05–0.2	IV/IM	Combined with opioid
Methadone	0.2–0.3	IM/SC	
	0.1–0.2	IV	
Levomethadone	0.1–0.15	IM/SC	
	0.05–0.1	IV	
Pethidine (meperidine)	0.05–0.1	IM	
Morphine	0.1–0.3	IM/SC	Dilute for IV use (histamine release)
	0.1–0.2	IV	
Hydromorphone	0.05–0.1	IV/IM/SC	
Buprenorphine	0.005–0.02	IV/IM/OTM	
Butorphanol	0.2–0.3	IM	
	0.1–0.2	IV	
Acepromazine	0.01–0.2	IM/SC	Avoid in neonates
	0.005–0.01	IV	
Dexmedetomidine	0.0005	IV	Avoid in neonates
	0.001–0.003	IM/SC	
Medetomidine	0.001	IV	Avoid in neonates
	0.002–0.005	IM/SC	

IV: intravenous; IM: intramuscular; SC: subcutaneous; OTM: oral transmucosal.
Legislation and drug licensing for food animals can vary between countries (see Chapters 6, 7, and 11).

Table 15.4 Suggested doses for sedation and premedication in neonatal and pediatric large animals.

Species	Drug	Dose (mg/kg)	Route	Comment
Foals, calves, kids, and lambs	Diazepam[a]	0.05–0.1	IV	Mostly combined with butorphanol
Foals, calves, kids, and lambs	Midazolam[a]	0.05–0.1	IV/IM	Mostly combined with butorphanol
Calves and kids	Brotizolam[a]	0.01	IV/IM	Uncommon drug, but when available it is mostly combined with butorphanol
Foals and calves	Methadone	0.05–0.1	IV/IM	
Foals, calves, and piglets	Levomethadone	0.025–0.05	IV	
		0.1–0.2	IM	
Foals	Morphine	0.1	IV/IM	Dilute for IV use (histamine release)
Foals	Buprenorphine	0.003–0.007	IV/IM/OTM	
Foals, calves, lambs, and kids	Butorphanol	0.01–0.05	IV	The younger the animal the more reliable the sedation achieved
		0.05–0.1	IM	
Piglets		0.1–0.2	IM	
Foals	Acepromazine	0.01–0.02	IM/SC	Avoid in neonates
		0.005–0.01	IV	
Piglets	Azaperone	1–2	IM	
		0.5	IV	
Foals	Dexmedetomidine	0.0015–0.002	IV/IM	Avoid in neonates
Foals	Medetomidine	0.003–0.005	IV/IM	Avoid in neonates

Table 15.4 (Continued)

Species	Drug	Dose (mg/kg)	Route	Comment
Foals	Romifidine	0.03–0.1	IV	Avoid in neonates
Foals,	Xylazine	0.3–1	IV/IM	Avoid in neonates
calves,		0.01–0.1	IM	Alpha-2 adrenergic receptor agonists should be given IM in calves, kids, and lambs to reduce the bradycardic effect
lambs,		0.01–0.1	IM	
and kids		0.005–0.01	IM	
Foals	Detomidine	0.005–0.01 IV	IV	Avoid in neonates
and calves		0.01–0.2	IM	Alpha-2 adrenergic receptor agonists should be given IM in calves, kids, and lambs

IV: intravenous; IM: intramuscular; SC: subcutaneous; OTM: oral transmucosal.
[a]Goats and calves respond well to benzodiazepines alone, and moderate to deep sedation can be achieved. Analgesia must still be provided for invasive or potentially painful procedures.
Legislation and drug licensing for food animals can vary between countries (see Chapters 6, 7, and 11).

young animals, they can be helpful to reduce stress, improve handling, and reduce anesthetic dose requirements. To speed recovery, their effects can be antagonized with atipamezole.

Benzodiazepines, in combination with an opioid, are generally a good option in neonatal and pediatric animals, especially in sick animals. By contrast with adults, they induce effective sedation in younger animals, have minimal cardiopulmonary effects, and their effects can be antagonized with flumazenil should excessive sedation or slow recovery occur. Combination with an opioid improves reliability and quality of sedation and provides analgesia.

Foals

Because foals rapidly mature after birth, the following guide can be used to select a sedation protocol:

<1 week: diazepam or midazolam (0.1 mg/kg) and butorphanol (0.05 mg/kg) IV. Unlike in adult horses, butorphanol alone causes sedation in neonatal foals.

1–6 weeks: reduced dose (25–50% reduction) of alpha-2 adrenergic receptor agonist depending on demeanor and health status ± butorphanol.

> 6–8 weeks: treat like an adult horse; alpha-2 adrenergic receptor agonist to effect ± butorphanol.

If possible, the foal should be premedicated and anesthetized in the presence of the mare to avoid unnecessary stress (to mare and foal). Also, for personnel safety, the mare should be sedated before being separated from the foal and sedation may need to be repeated throughout the separation period. A common approach for the mare is to use acepromazine (0.02 mg/kg, IV) combined with detomidine (5–10 mcg/kg, IV), to provide a longer duration of sedation (see Chapter 13).

Small Animals

Depending on health status and temperament/demeanor, a premedication guide for kittens and puppies could be the following:

<8 weeks: benzodiazepine and opioid combination.

8–12 weeks: benzodiazepine and opioid combination or low doses of other sedatives.

>12 weeks: dosing as for an adult.

Analgesia

Neonates and pediatric animals perceive pain, but might display a different behavioral response compared with adults; therefore, careful observation is necessary to assess efficacy of analgesics.

Opioids

As described in the preceding text, the blood–brain barrier is more permeable in neonates, so opioids exert their desired effects, but also adverse effects, at lower doses compared to adult animals. Pediatric animals often require adult doses because the blood–brain barrier is less permeable compared to in neonates. A pragmatic approach is to start at the lower end of the dose range and increase it as required, or to begin with a reduced recommended adult dose of 30%. The additional time that may be necessary to achieve sedation should be taken into account when planning a procedure.

Opioids can be excreted into the milk, but oral bioavailability is low. In humans, morphine has been recommended if an opioid becomes necessary to use in a nursing mother because of its low lipophilicity compared other opioids. Recent studies show that breastfed babies were exposed to less than 1% of the calculated buprenorphine dose of the mother (per kg bodyweight).

Nonsteroidal Anti-inflammatory Drugs

Nonsteroidal anti-inflammatory drugs should not be given in animals less than six weeks of age because of the limited renal and hepatic elimination with the risk of cumulation to toxic doses. Also, inhibition of the cyclo-oxygenase-2 enzyme interferes with renal development and electrolyte regulation as well as the complex regulation of *ductus arteriosus* closure. Many NSAIDs are not licensed for animals less than six months of age. If an NSAID is deemed necessary (i.e., in severe tissue trauma or situations where the animal might benefit from the additional anti-inflammatory effect), a careful risk–benefit assessment is recommended. An NSAID mainly metabolized by phase I enzymes of liver biotransformation (oxidation), such as meloxicam, might be a good choice as this pathway is functional early in hepatic development.

Nearly all drugs transfer into milk to some extent, which is influenced by protein binding, lipid solubility, lipid content of the milk, and ionization as well as active transporters. Drugs excreted into milk are taken up by the nursing animal, the extent depending on oral bioavailability of the drug. In the very early neonatal phase (0–24 h) when colostrum is taken up by pinocytosis, orally given drugs might have an increased bioavailability. The weight-adjusted relative dose a neonate is exposed to via milk feeding varies among drugs. Most NSAIDs are highly protein bound and transfer into milk is low. The risk of harming neonates by treating the mother with an NSAID is extremely low and should not lead to their avoidance, for example after cesarean section. Cimicoxib given to whelping bitches on day 0 and day 28 as a single dose of 2 mg/kg was transferred into the milk with a milk:plasma ratio of 1.7–1.9, but the transfer into the suckling puppies was very low and no abnormalities occurred. Similarly, the concentration of carprofen in milk was one-tenth of a 2 mg/kg dose in whelping bitches (without mastitis). Thus, carprofen has a low excretion into milk and can be safely used in lactating bitches (see Further Reading).

Locoregional Anesthesia

A good choice for neonatal and pediatric peri-operative analgesia is applying a locoregional anesthesia technique (see species-specific chapters). Incomplete myelination of nerve fibers might lead to a more rapid onset of effect. Because of reduced metabolism of amino–amide local anesthetics in the liver (lidocaine, bupivacaine, ropivacaine, and mepivacaine), with an increased risk of reaching toxic doses, careful calculation of the total dose on a weight basis is necessary. Dilution of commercial products to avoid overdose might be useful. However, care should be taken to remain within an effective concentration range of the local anesthetic. Diluting the local anesthetic too much might make the block ineffective when the concentration difference is too low to promote diffusion of the drug into nerve fibers. The lowest recommended drug concentration is 5 mg/mL (0.5%) for lidocaine and 2.5 mg/mL (0.25%) for the other amino–amide local anesthetics.

When using an epidural anesthesia technique, the possibility of the spinal cord extending beyond the puncture site (typically, L7-S1) needs to be considered. Depending on the puncture site chosen, there is a risk of injury to the spinal cord or possible drug injection into the subarachnoid (intrathecal) space or both. In foals and calves, the sacrococcygeal space or intercoccygeal access can be used without concern of injecting into the subarachnoid space because the spinal cord ends (cauda equina) cranial to these locations (Figure 15.3). However, in puppies and especially kittens, the cauda equina is often within the sacrum, and if performing an epidural at the lumbosacral region, there is a risk of puncturing the dura mater and injection into the subarachnoid space (i.e., spinal anesthesia instead of epidural anesthesia).

Induction and Maintenance of General Anesthesia

Induction of general anesthesia with inhalational anesthetic drugs (e.g., isoflurane) is an appealing option in neonates. This is because of (1) their minimal metabolism, (2) ability to make rapid changes to anesthetic concentration

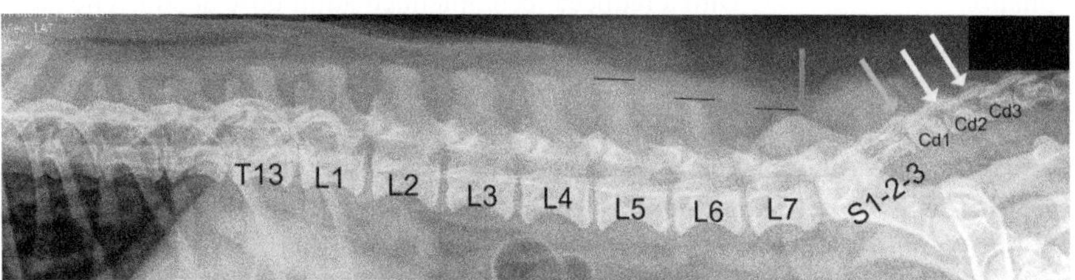

Figure 15.3 A right lateral radiograph of a dog spine demonstrating the puncture sites for performing an epidural, which include lumbosacral (blue arrow), sacrococcygeal (green arrow), and intercoccygeal (yellow arrows) spaces. There are species differences in number of the different types of vertebrae.

and subsequent anesthetic depth, and (3) quick recovery. Importantly, however, depending on the health status and body mass of the neonate (for example foals and calves), induction of anesthesia via mask or nasotracheal intubation poses considerable stress to the animal until loss of consciousness is achieved. Furthermore, in foals, induction of anesthesia using inhalation anesthetics is associated with an increase in mortality. Therefore, a careful selection of the anesthetic induction method is necessary. Neonatal animals have a lower minimum alveolar concentration (MAC) requirement for inhalational anesthetics; MAC increases with age until adulthood and then declines when geriatric ages are reached.

Overall, lower doses of anesthetics are required in neonates, though this changes rapidly with increasing age, underscoring the importance of monitoring anesthetic depth and dosing drugs to effect. Even if the metabolism and elimination of injectable anesthetics may be reduced in neonates, a single induction dose does not necessarily prolong recovery significantly as the duration of effect from a single bolus dose depends on distribution into extravascular tissues. Therefore, in animals with vascular (or intraosseous) access, induction of anesthesia with ketamine (plus a benzodiazepine), propofol, or alfaxalone is an appropriate choice. For very small patients, the drugs can be diluted with saline or 5% dextrose. Care must be taken not to disrupt the emulsion of propofol and more than a 5× dilution of induction drugs is not recommended. Another advantage of diluting propofol is that the total dose administered is lower when slowly titrated to the desired clinical effect. Maintenance of anesthesia is ideally achieved with inhalational anesthetics, as repeated injection or TIVA in neonates results in prolonged recovery times because of delayed metabolism and elimination. In pediatric animals, selected TIVA protocols can be used if normothermia (supportive of hepatic perfusion and drug distribution and elimination) and ventilatory management (to offset respiratory depression associated with some TIVA combinations; see Chapters 6 and 7) are available. Suggested doses and drug protocols for induction and maintenance of anesthesia in neonatal and pediatric small and large animals are found in Tables 15.5 and 15.6, respectively.

Table 15.5 Suggested doses for anesthesia induction and short-term TIVA and PIVA in small animals (puppies and kittens).

Drug(s)	Dose (mg/kg)	Route	Comment
Benzodiazepine, ketamine, and opioid[a]	Mix ketamine (10%) and diazepam or midazolam (0.5%) at 1:1 (v:v), give 0.05–0.1 mL/kg of this mixture in increments to effect	IV	IV mixed syringe, slowly to effect, opioid prolongs and deepens anesthesia, re-dose as required
Midazolam, ketamine, and opioid[a]	0.1–0.2 5	IM	Opioid prolongs and deepens anesthesia
Medetomidine, ketamine, and opioid[a]	0.002–0.005 2–4	IM	Older pediatrics, juvenile animals, deeper plane of anesthesia, and opioid prolongs and deepens anesthesia
Ketamine	1–3	IV	After premedication
Ketamine for PIVA	0.6–1 mg/kg/h	CRI	Additional analgesia
Alfaxalone	2–4 1–3 2–4	IV without premed IV with premed IM (off-label in some countries)	Given slowly to effect premedication, reduces the dose Re-dose as required, give oxygen, and keep ETT ready
Propofol	2–6 1–4	IV without premed IV with premed	Given slowly to effect Premedication and dilution[c] reduce the dose, re-dose as required, always give oxygen, and intubation recommended
Isoflurane	2–3%[b] vol in oxygen, to effect	Induction Maintenance	Induction and/or maintenance of anesthesia Without or with premedication and additional analgesia required for painful procedures
Sevoflurane	3–4%[b] vol in oxygen, to effect	Induction Maintenance	Sevoflurane has a more rapid induction and is less pungent than isoflurane
Naloxone	0.004–0.04 0.01–0.1	IV IM	To antagonize opioid effects and shorten recovery but consider effect on reversing analgesia (plan for additional analgesia)

(Continued)

Table 15.5 (Continued)

Drug(s)	Dose (mg/kg)	Route	Comment
Flumazenil	0.01–0.03	IV to effect	To antagonize benzodiazepine effects to shorten recovery and reduce respiratory depression
Atipamezole		Very slowly IV/IM	In general, 5× administered dose of medetomidine or 2.5× dexmedetomidine dose but depends on timing of initial injection To shorten recovery and reduce bradycardia Should only be used in emergency situation (imminent cardiac arrest) Avoid use intra-operatively

[a] Any opioid can be selected and added to the proposed drug combination; please refer to Table 15.3 for drug and dose information.
[b] Recommended vaporizer setting to use when a rebreathing circuit is used on the inhalation anesthetic delivery device (see Chapter 8).
[c] See Concept Box 15.2 for details about drug dilution.
IV: intravenous; IM: intramuscular; CRI: constant rate infusion.
Legislation and drug licensing for food animals can vary between countries (see Chapters 6, 7, and 11).

Table 15.6 Suggested doses for anesthesia induction and short-term TIVA and PIVA in large animal neonates and pediatric animals.

Species	Drug	Dose (mg/kg)	Route	Comment
Foals, calves, lambs, and kids	Benzodiazepine, ketamine, and butorphanol	0.05–0.1 1–2 0.05	IV mixed in same syringe Increments to effect	Light anesthesia for nonpainful procedure. Opioid prolongs and deepens anesthesia. Re-dose ketamine–benzodiazepine as required.
	Benzodiazepine, ketamine, and butorphanol	0.05–0.1 2–4 0.05	IV mixed in same syringe Increments to effect	Anesthesia. Opioid prolongs and deepens anesthesia. Re-dose ketamine–benzodiazepine as required or maintain with inhalant.
Foals, calves, lambs, kids, and piglets	Midazolam, ketamine, and opioid	0.1–0.2 5	IM	Opioid prolongs and deepens anesthesia.
Foals	Xylazine, ketamine, and opioid	0.2–0.4 2–3	IV	Older pediatrics, juvenile animals, deeper plane of anesthesia, and opioid prolongs and deepens anesthesia.
Calves/lambs	Xylazine Ketamine	0.01–0.02 3–4	IM	
Kids	Xylazine Ketamine	0.005 3–4	IM	
Piglets	Azaperone Ketamine	2 10–15	IM	
Foals, calves, lambs, and kids	Ketamine Ketamine for PIVA In combination with inhalant	2–4 0.5–2 mg/kg/h	IV CRI	After premedication. Additional analgesia.
Foals	Alfaxalone	2–3 1–3	IV without premed IV with premed	Given slowly to effect. Premedication reduces the dose.
	TIVA in older foals	6 mg/kg/h	CRI, with premedication	Re-dose as required, give oxygen, be prepared to intubate.
Foals, (calves, lambs, kids, and piglets)	Propofol TIVA	2–3 1–3 18–24 mg/kg/h	IV without IV with premed CRI	Given slowly to effect. Premedication and dilution reduce the dose, re-dose as required, always give oxygen, and intubate. Be prepared to assist ventilation. Requires additional analgesia, not suitable for field anesthesia.

Table 15.6 (Continued)

Species	Drug	Dose (mg/kg)	Route	Comment
Foals, calves, lambs, kids, and piglets	Isoflurane	Vaporizer setting 3–5 vol% in oxygen To effect	Induction Maintenance	Induction and/or maintenance of anesthesia. Without or with premedication. Additional analgesia required for painful procedures. Adapt initial dose to health status.
	Sevoflurane more rapid induction, less stinging than isoflurane	Vaporizer setting 6–8 vol% in oxygen To effect	Induction Maintenance	
Foals, calves, lambs, kids, and piglets	Naloxone	0.01–0.04	IV/IM	There can be species differences; therefore, IV titration to the desired effect (shorten recovery) is recommended.
Foals, calves, lambs, kids, and piglets	Flumazenil	0.01–0.025	IV to effect/IM	In general, 1 mg of flumazenil can reverse effects of 10 mg of diazepam or midazolam.
Foals, calves, lambs, and kids	Atipamezole Tolazoline Yohimbine	0.06–0.1 4.0 0.1	IV very slowly to effect, IM	Depends on given dose, timing, and species. Availability and legal aspects vary between countries.

TIVA: total intravenous anesthesia; IV: intravenous; IM: intramuscular; CRI: constant rate infusion.
Legislation and drug licensing for food animals can vary between countries (see Chapters 6, 7, and 11).

Small Animals (Puppies and Kittens)

In puppies, kittens, and other small mammals, if vascular access is difficult, induction of anesthesia can be achieved via a close-fitting facemask and a nonrebreathing system (see Chapter 5) with sevoflurane or isoflurane carried in oxygen (or an oxygen–air mixture). Sevoflurane achieves anesthetic concentrations faster, and is less pungent, than isoflurane, and therefore preferred for facemask induction of anesthesia in humans and this is perhaps the same in animals (see Chapter 8). As inhalation anesthetic concentrations can change very rapidly in neonates, vaporizer settings of 3–4% sevoflurane or 2–3% isoflurane are usually sufficient in combination with close monitoring for loss of consciousness.

If endotracheal intubation is not possible, anesthesia can be maintained via a close-fitting facemask or a supraglottic airway device (e.g., laryngeal mask).

Endotracheal intubation in very small animals can be achieved with commercial cuffless endotracheal tubes, intravenous catheters (potentially traumatic because the tip of the catheter is rigid and sharp), or cut-to-size nasogastric feeding tubes/urinary catheters (Figure 15.4). The tongue is relatively large in nursing puppies and kittens and can obscure/obstruct the larynx during intubation. With the use of smaller tubes for orotracheal intubation, anesthetists should be particularly aware of the risk of obstruction by airway secretions, and should check ventilation and oxygenation regularly (direct observation for changes in respiratory effort, capnography, and pulse oximetry). The reservoir bag of a breathing system should hold a volume of approximately 5–6 times the tidal volume. The smallest commercial standard reservoir bag contains 500 mL. Alternatively, small latex or rubber party balloons can be used (Figure 15.5).

Once anesthesia is induced, and the maintenance of anesthesia has begun, it is always recommended to obtain IV access, especially for patients undergoing a procedure lasting longer than 30 min. An alternative to IV access is intraosseous access.

The selection of the breathing system is important to minimize the resistance to breathing and equipment dead space.

- Use nonrebreathing systems (Mapleson E, F, or D, and Bain).
- Use pediatric low dead space adapters for capnography, gas sampling, and connection to endotracheal tube. If these are not available, consider inserting a needle connected to the sampling line and inserted into the endotracheal tube.
- Use correct length of endotracheal tube (pre-measure between nose and thoracic inlet) and avoid long tubes that add to mechanical dead space (tube can be cut to size).
- Use appropriately sized reservoir bags (5–6× tidal volume). In very small patients, party balloons can be considered.
- Mechanically or manually assist ventilation to avoid high work of breathing.
- Provide a high fraction of oxygen of at least 60% (to meet oxygen requirements). This is achieved by using an oxygen–medical air mixture; some anesthetic machines allow for oxygen concentrations to be adjusted (see Chapter 5).

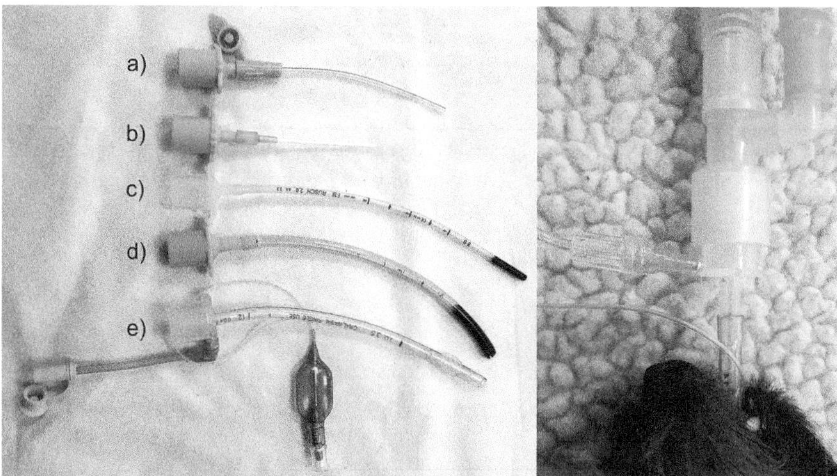

Figure 15.4 Different methods of securing a patent airway in neonates which include (a) a cut-to-size nasogastric feeding tube fitted to a 4.5 mm connecter; (b) and intravenous over-the-needle cannula fitted to a 4.0 mm connecter; (c) 2 mm and (d) 3.5 mm noncuffed endotracheal tubes fitted to standard connecters; and (e) a 3.5 mm cuffed endotracheal tube fitted to a low-volume connecter that allows for gas sampling (e.g., sidestream capnography). The connecters can be attached to patient breathing circuits via a T-piece or Y-piece (Wye-piece).

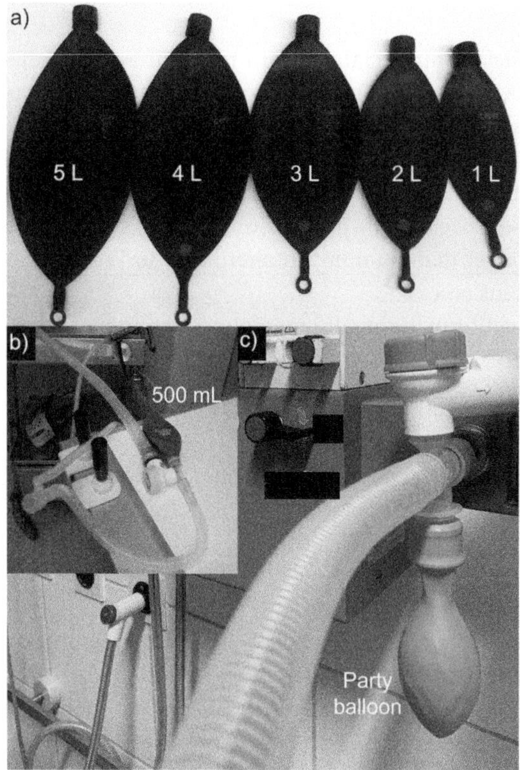

Figure 15.5 Examples of different sizes of rebreathing bags used in a breathing circuit (a). The nonrebreathing circuits are often fitted with a 500 mL bag (b), and if this volume is too large for the patient, then a part balloon could be used (c).

Large Animals (Foals and Calves)

In large animal neonates, obtaining venous access is less challenging than in smaller mammals and can usually be obtained with or without sedation so that general anesthesia can be induced by intravenous injection.

Regardless of drug choice, it is advisable to administer induction drugs slowly to prevent overdosing and to allow oxygen supplementation during the induction process. In contrast to adult horses, intravenous induction of anesthesia can be safely titrated to effect in foals.

Inhalation induction with a facemask or nasotracheal tube is possible but can cause considerable distress and struggling and should therefore be restricted to premedicated animals or patients that are very compromised and moribund (Figure 15.6). In foals, long cuffed endotracheal tubes up to a size 18 mm (inner diameter) are available to fit a standard 15 mm small animal circle circuit breathing system connector.

Maintenance of anesthesia of more than 30 min is preferably performed with an inhalational anesthetic (isoflurane and sevoflurane) to allow rapid recovery (in contrast to risk of drug accumulation with repeated dosing of injectable agents), especially in neonates. For procedures requiring up to 60 min of anesthesia, an injectable technique can be used in pediatric animals, with longer anesthesia times resulting in longer recovery times. In pediatric animals, TIVA protocols containing ketamine, alfaxalone, or propofol could be used (adhering to the food animal drug regulations of the country of practice).

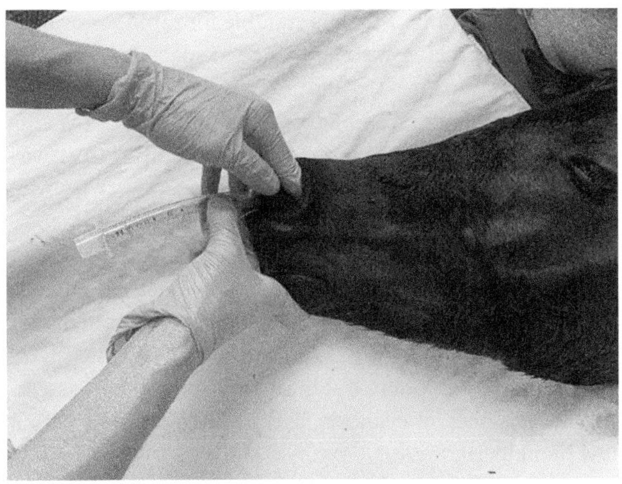

Figure 15.6 Nasotracheal intubation in a foal can be performed by gently guiding the tube down the ventral meatus, into the nasopharynx, and, with the neck in extension, into the trachea. Placement into the trachea can be confirmed by palpation of the cervical neck to confirm feeling only one tube-like structure (i.e., the trachea), or feeling inspired and expired gases freely passing through the endotracheal tube, or even, in some foals, a cough when entering the trachea. Esophageal intubation is identified by palpating two tube-like structures in the cervical neck.

Fluid Support

As venous access in small neonates can be challenging, especially in dehydrated animals, the intraosseous route into a medullary cavity (femur, iliac crest, humerus) using a spinal needle, intraosseous catheters, or large-bore hypodermic needle (16–20 gauge depending on patient size) is an alternative means to supply fluids into the circulation.

As neonates are very sensitive to both dehydration (see body composition and renal function) and overhydration, careful calculation and administration of fluid is necessary. Ideally, a syringe pump/driver is used for accurate volume administration. If available, gravity administration sets that deliveries of 60 drops/mL or a prefilled burette are simple (and cheap) alternatives.

Hypoglycemia is a concern in neonates, especially if preanesthetic fasting times and anesthesia time is long. Therefore, fluids containing 2.5–5% dextrose are recommended. Blood glucose should be monitored during anesthesia to guide use of such fluids.

Fluids should be titrated according to the needs of the patient, keeping in mind that fluid boluses will have minimal influence on cardiac output and hypotension because of the limited compliance of the myocardium in neonates. Starting rates of 3–5 mL/kg/h increasing to 10 mL/kg/h, as needed, seem suitable for neonates of all species. Importantly, the volume of fluids used to "flush" in drugs that are given IV should be factored into fluid calculations: the hub of the catheter and attached injection port can easily contain >0.2 mL of volume. This volume increases if IV fluid administration sets that have a y-port for injection are used; these may require 2–4 mL of "flush" to ensure that the injectate volume is delivered to the bloodstream. Repeated flushing of lines following drug delivery can result in overhydration and should be taken into consideration when selecting a fluid rate during anesthesia. If a syringe driver is not available but fluids must be administered in very small patients, under 3 kg, it is recommended to provide fluid support through timed hand-injection boluses of 2 mL/kg per 20 min, for example.

Monitoring

Monitoring in neonates, especially in those that are very small, is often hampered by limited physical access to the animal beneath surgical drapes, including placement (and checking) of monitoring sensors. Additionally, common measurement ranges of standard monitoring devices may not be sufficient for high respiratory and heart rates. Therefore, a sensible choice of available equipment and useful variables to monitor (see the following text) should be made. In larger neonates (foals, calves), there are usually no such limitations and standard monitoring devices can be used (see Chapter 4).

Heart Rate

Heart rate is an important variable to monitor in neonates as it is a major determinant of cardiac output and oxygen delivery, and bradycardia should be avoided (Table 15.7).

Heart rate can be determined by auscultation, electrocardiogram (ECG), pulse oximetry, or placing a Doppler probe over an artery or directly over the heart. Audible signals

Table 15.7 Lower acceptable limit for heart rates (in beats per minute) in anesthetized neonates and pediatrics.

Species	Neonate	Pediatric
Puppy		
• Large	150	70
• Medium	170	90
• Small breed	180	100
Kitten	180	100
Foal	70	40
Calf	80	50
Lamb/kid	90	60

These values are a general guideline, keep in mind that heart rate is also influenced by the general status of the animal, arterial blood pressures, and the drugs used for sedation or anesthesia.

(esophageal stethoscope, pulse oximetry, or Doppler probe) can give information on heart rate, rhythm, and blood flow. Care should be taken if ECG electrodes are used, and ensure that their attachment does not injure the skin of neonates. Suitable alternatives are atraumatic clamps and adhesive electrodes (attached to footpads). Transmission pulse oximetry probes can be placed on nonpigmented areas of the skin, i.e., the toe web or tail base if the probe is too large for the tongue or the tongue cannot be protracted. Placing a damp (wetted) gauze between the tongue and the sensor can improve the quality of the reading by ensuring that emitted light is directed toward the sensor. Reflectance pulse oximetry probes can be placed in the rectum, the hard palate, or the esophagus.

Systemic Arterial Blood Pressure

In larger species, blood pressure can be measured invasively via arterial catheterization; however, anesthesia time should not be prolonged for the sole purpose of achieving arterial access. In very small neonates, available blood pressures cuffs may be too large to be usable. Overall, noninvasive blood pressure (NIBP) devices (oscillometric, Doppler) are considered reliable but do not display valid measurements. This means the displayed values do not accurately represent true arterial pressure, but the devices indicate changes in pressure, so that trends can be followed and used to guide management. Arterial blood pressure in neonates is lower compared to adults due to lower vascular resistance and an immature sympathetic innervation. Transferred from recommendations for human medicine and values from awake animals, a mean arterial blood pressure of 40–50 and 55–60 mmHg is considered acceptable in neonates and pediatrics, respectively.

Ventilation and Respiratory Rate

Respiratory rate can be determined by counting thoracic excursions (directly or via reservoir bag) or via capnography. Attaching monitoring devices to the endotracheal tube increases the amount of dead space. Information about tidal volume and its relationship to dead space can be found in Chapters 5 and 18. Depending on the size of the animal, low dead space adaptors (for endotracheal tubes <5 mm internal diameter) for sidestream capnographs can be useful. Ideally, microstream technology with low sampling rates (50 mL/min, compared to >120 mL/min in standard machines) should be used. Higher sampling rates can withdraw a significant amount of gas from the breathing circuit and this should be taken into consideration when setting the flowmeter, especially in small patients. The sampling line of sidestream capnographs can also be either attached to a facemask or placed in the nares to obtain a respiratory rate. Mainstream capnographs have a rapid response time, which is suitable for rapid respiratory rates, but can increase apparatus dead space (especially if adult adaptors are used). Additionally, they add weight and bulk, leading to a risk of inadvertent extubation or twisting of the endotracheal tube in the trachea (resulting in airway obstruction and possible tracheal damage).

Oxygenation

Oxygenation can be monitored by evaluating mucous membrane color, or using pulse oximetry, or, in larger species, by arterial blood gas measurements. Mucous membrane color is a popular, but insensitive method for assessing the presence of cyanosis, especially in animals with a low hematocrit.

Body Temperature

Neonates are prone to hypothermia; therefore, continuous monitoring of body temperature is especially important in this age group. Temperature can be taken from the rectum, esophagus, or nasopharynx (if the animal is intubated and there is no air flow through the nose).

Actions to avoid hypothermia in neonates are as follows:

- Minimal fasting of no longer than 30–45 min before anesthesia.
- Avoid excessive clipping of hair/fur and disinfectant use (fluids for preparing surgical sites can be warmed).
- Provide warm environment during sedation and preparation for procedure:
  - Passive insulation with blankets (active warming preferred whenever possible).
  - Infrared heat lamps.
  - Place on warm surface, using heating pads and warm water pads (caution is advised when using these uncontrolled warming techniques because they often give poor performance [under- or overheating patients] and may increase the risk of burning; regular, preferably continuous, monitoring of body–heat pad surface interface temperature [to be maintained <42 °C] could avoid burns).
- Airway heating and humidification, and using the lowest safe fresh gas flow rates during inhalational anesthesia.
- Use warm fluids for flushing body cavities.
- Use of adhesive plastic surgical drapes: surgical incision can be made through plastic while adhesion maintains a seal, trapping warm air around the patient.
- Active warming during surgery.
  - Warm water bottles, wheat bags, heat packs, etc. (see comment in the preceding text on safe use and risk of causing burns).
  - Thermostatic-controlled electric or water heating blankets.
  - Forced-air warming devices with inflatable blankets.

Direct contact of warm/hot surfaces with skin should be avoided (insulate the warming surface with drapes or towels) to prevent or minimize burns. Hot air warming devices have been shown to be the most effective method of maintaining peri-anesthetic body temperate. Other methods are not as effective. A device with built-in accurate thermostatic control is strongly recommended over all other forms of heating. Care should be taken not to overheat small animals as temperature uptake in the small body can be very quick.

Recovery

In neonates, rapid recovery and early return to nursing is important. Recovery should be monitored until return of airway protective reflexes. Warming and, if necessary, dextrose supplementation should be continued until fully recovered (generally considered when the animal is able to move and nurse).

An analgesic plan should be in place and the patient monitored regularly for signs of pain (Chapter 3).

If recovery is delayed by prolonged drug effects, such as may occur with benzodiazepines, alpha-2 adrenergic receptor agonists, and opioids use, these can be antagonized by flumazenil, atipamezole (or yohimbine), and naloxone, respectively.

If the neonate is still with the mother, the patient should be returned as early as possible. During long anesthetic procedures (i.e., fracture repair), milking the mother may be necessary.

Geriatric Patients

At the other end of the lifespan lies the geriatric period. In veterinary medicine, no clear age limits have been given for the term "geriatric" but, in general, *geriatric patients* are defined as those that have reached 75–80% of their expected lifespan. This definition respects the species- and breed-specific differences in lifespan. For example, a Great Dane is "old" long before a Dachshund or Jack Russell Terrier. There are numerous parallels to humans with regard to age-related changes. Adverse drug reactions are reported to be 2–3 times higher in elderly humans compared to younger adults. Even if some of this risk can be attributed to patient confusion and errors in dosing, pharmacokinetic and pharmacodynamic factors play a major role. The pharmacodynamics of a drug can be influenced by age-related changes in the expression and function of drug target sites (receptors, ion channels, etc.), but changes in body composition, organ function, and compensatory physiologic responses are often more relevant. In addition, with increasing age, animals are more likely to have multiple coexisting diseases. The implications of this are twofold. First, the disease processes may directly alter drug pharmacokinetics, and second, polypharmacy may produce drug interactions that alter both pharmacokinetics and pharmacodynamic response of the drugs used during anesthesia.

Difference in Physiology Compared to the Healthy Adult

The consequences of altered organ function are summarized in Table 15.8.

Body Composition

With age, an increase in fat and a decrease in muscle mass and body water occurs (Figure 15.7). These changes alter the tissue distribution of active ingredients and their elimination time. Depending on the lipophilicity of the drug the associated effect can vary:

- For nonpolar, lipophilic drugs, like most injectable anesthetics, distribution into fat can lead to lower plasma concentrations, possibly followed by prolonged recovery times as redistribution occurs from fat into the vascular space after repeated dosing or long drug infusion times.
- For polar, water-soluble drugs with poor fat distribution, like aminoglycoside antimicrobials, dosing should be based on metabolic body weight. Metabolic weight = body weight (kg) to the power of 0.75 ($BWkg^{0.75}$). Alternatively, an empirical dose reduction by 15–20% can be used.
- A decreased muscle mass may lead to increased plasma concentrations of drugs that normally distribute to skeletal muscle or are metabolized in the muscle (e.g., increased sensitivity to remifentanil in old animals, which is significantly metabolized by muscle esterases).

Neuronal Function, Brain, and Blood–Brain Barrier

With increasing age, loss of neurons and synapses lead to reduced sensory functions, behavioral changes, and altered responsiveness to sedatives and analgesics.

- Changes in CNS neurotransmitters and related receptors (e.g., gamma-aminobutyric acid A [GABA-A] and dopamine), diminished cardiovascular responses, and decreased drug elimination probably contribute to the observation that elderly animals require much lower doses of most anesthetics. Furthermore, these factors can also explain why some geriatric patients experience prolonged dysphoria or phases of cognitive dysfunction during and after recovery.

Table 15.8 Consequences of different organ system function changes in geriatrics.

Organ system	Consequences	Practical advice
Hepatic system	Aged hepatic system means: • Reduced liver size • Reduced liver blood flow • Reduced albumin production • Reduced protein binding of drugs • Prolonged elimination of drugs • Reduced gluconeogenesis	• Reduced protein binding can lead to increased availability and effects of many sedatives and anesthetics; therefore, careful titration of drugs to effect is recommended • Reduced liver size and activity contributes to loss of core body temperature; therefore, effective temperature management is desirable to prevent overly long recovery • Consider dose reduction of analgesics (25–50%)
Renal system	• Aged kidney means:Nephron loss • Reduced GFR and renal tubular secretion • Reduced creatinine clearance diminishes reduced ability to concentrate urine and to excrete acids • Changes in acid–base balance alter plasma protein binding and drug activity	• If the renin–angiotensin system is already activated (e.g., as a consequence of dehydration, heart failure or chronic kidney failure), the risk of nephrotoxic effects of NSAIDs is significantly increased • Careful risk–benefit assessment for NSAID prescription • Avoid pre-anesthetic NSAIDs if blood pressure monitoring is not available
Cardiovascular system	• Increased incidence of cardiac disease (see Chapter 17) • Even without overt disease, cardiac reserve decreases with age	• Careful calculation of fluid requirements • Avoid inadvertent fluid excess by using an infusion pump or appropriately sized fluid bags and manual drop administration set • If necessary, pre-anesthetic stabilization and treatment with cardiac medication • Avoid high doses of angiotensin-converting enzyme (ACE) inhibitors immediately before anesthesia to avoid hypotension • Careful monitoring for arrhythmias, signs of hypoxemia, and hypotension
Respiratory system	• Aged lung means:Weaker respiratory muscles • Reduction in vital capacity • Decreased compliance • Higher incidence of pulmonary hypertension • Lower resting arterial oxygen partial pressure • More susceptible to aspiration	• Preoxygenate, if tolerated • Low thoracic compliance requires higher inspiratory pressures to obtain sufficient tidal volume • Consider intermittent positive pressure ventilation to support gas exchange and maintenance of inhalational anesthetics • Rapid intubation and avoid premedication protocols that promote vomiting (like SC opioids/alpha-2 adrenergic receptor agonists) *Ventilator settings*: Small animals: Positive end expiratory pressure: 4–6 cmH_2O Peak inspiratory airway pressure: 8–10 cmH_2O but <20 cmH_2O Large animals: Positive end expiratory pressure: 10–15 cmH_2O Peak inspiratory airway pressure: 12–20 cmH_2O but <40 cmH_2O
Nervous system	• Aged peripheral and central nervous systems means:Lower drug doses needed • Prolonged recovery • Prone to dysphoria in recovery • Prolonged behavioral changes after anesthesia • Cognitive dysfunction • Prone to neuropathic pain • Prone to sensory deficits	• Titrate drugs to effect • Benzodiazepines can have overly long effects because of reduced elimination, consider flumazenil to reduce benzodiazepine-induced dysphoria • Careful positioning during anesthesia to avoid overextension of arthritic joints and fibrotic muscles
Gastrointestinal system	• Prone to reflux and esophagitis • Gastrointestinal tract more sensitive to NSAIDs	• Avoid overly long fasting (reduces tone of esophageal sphincter) • Careful risk–benefit consideration for NSAID use

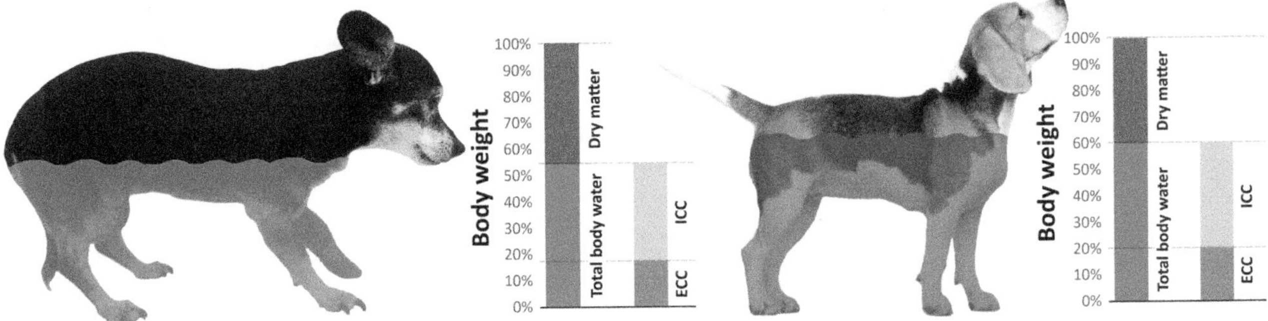

Figure 15.7 The body composition of geriatrics (left) compared to adult animals (right) includes a lower water content and muscle mass and a higher fat content.

For the recognition and classification of pain, changes in behavior and posture are taken into account. Particular attention should be paid to age-related features in this context.

- For example, in dogs it can be very difficult to discern signs of maladaptive (chronic) pain from the cognitive dysfunction syndrome/geriatric disconnection syndrome. Often a combination of osteoarthritis pain and cognitive dysfunction is present in old dogs. If in doubt, an analgesic treatment plan for osteoarthritis can be diagnostic.
- Age-dependent behavioral patterns of animals should be considered. For example, in geriatric patients, hypoactivity can be age-related or disease-related (e.g., due to heart failure).

Liver Function

The production of cytochrome P450 and expression of its enzymes (CYP enzymes; see Chapter 6) and other drug-metabolizing enzymes are fairly well conserved; however, decreased liver size and reduced blood flow to the liver can lead to decreased clearance of some drugs in geriatric patients.

- "Flow-limited" drugs are very efficiently metabolized once they reach the liver but depend on high liver blood flow for efficient clearance. Such drugs include meperidine (pethidine), fentanyl, and (dex)medetomidine, for which lower doses should be used in older patients in conjunction with sedation or general anesthesia. For example, (dex)medetomidine is more rapidly eliminated in young adult ponies than in old ponies. Long-term treatment with propranolol or amitriptyline might also require lower doses or less frequent dosing. Propofol is also a "flow-limited" drug, and its clearance is diminished in geriatric dogs (> 8–9 years old), with higher plasma drug concentrations that can result in more frequent events of apnea in older dogs.
- Reduced hepatic (and renal; see the following text) clearance can affect the elimination of opioids and NSAIDs. In humans, the dose for opioids requires reduction in elderly patients, due to delayed elimination, by 25–50%.

The concentration of plasma proteins can change with an overall increase in total protein because the total body water, ergo plasma volume, is less compared to adult dogs. However, there is a simultaneous reduction in albumin synthesis. Changes in plasma protein binding can have a significant impact on the distribution of NSAIDs as the majority of these are highly plasma protein bound (>95%).

- At high protein binding rates, a small reduction in binding makes a considerable difference (increase) in the unbound, free concentration of active drug. In healthy adults, the increased free active drug concentration is counteracted by an increase in liver clearance; however, in geriatric animals, liver clearance is diminished, hence the dose reduction recommendation (30–50% dose reduction).

Other concerns that require consideration are that gluconeogenesis and production of clotting factors can also be reduced in geriatric patients.

Renal Function

Age-related renal insufficiency is the most important factor affecting drug elimination. Nephron loss leads to diminished GFR and renal tubular secretion of drugs. Creatinine clearance diminishes steadily with age, reflecting reduced renal function. The prevalence of renal insufficiency in older dogs and cats has not been established but appears to be higher in cats. Because of the large functional renal reserve (approximately 75% of nephrons need to be nonfunctional before standard urea and creatinine are increased; see Chapter 19), even patients without overt azotemia are likely to have decreased GFR associated with aging.

- This may lead to decreased elimination and increased toxicity of renally cleared drugs, such as aminoglycoside and fluoroquinolone antimicrobials. Aminoglycosides should be avoided whenever possible in geriatric patients. If they must be used, they should always be accompanied by fluid administration and daily urine sediment evaluation for granular casts.
- In cats, repeated or high ketamine doses can lead to prolonged (and sometimes incoordinated and "stormy" recoveries).

Tubular changes lead to a decreased ability to concentrate urine and to excrete acids.

- Old animals are less tolerant of fluid deficits.
- Changes in acid–base balance alter plasma protein binding and drug activity.

Nephron loss and the consequent changes in pharmacokinetics and pharmacodynamics exacerbate the effects of anesthesia and surgery in geriatric patients, making them more sensitive to further renal damage due to hypotension and hypoperfusion.

- With NSAIDs, preexisting reductions in kidney function must also be taken into account with regard to renal side effects. The reduction in renal blood flow and increased retention of sodium, potassium, and water caused by decreased prostaglandin production (e.g., using NSAIDs) should be given particular attention in geriatric patients. If the renin–angiotensin–aldosterone system (RAAS) is already activated, e.g., as a consequence of dehydration, heart failure, or chronic kidney failure, the risk of nephrotoxic effects of NSAIDs is significantly increased.

Cardiovascular Function

Old animals have an increased incidence of cardiac disease (see Chapter 17). Even without overt disease, cardiac reserve decreases with age, indicated by a reduced maximum heart rate. The sensitivity to endogenous circulating catecholamines is diminished and myocardial fibrosis or myxomatous valvular disease may decrease the ability to increase cardiac output.

- Old dogs, in particular, have an increased incidence of valvular lesions with regurgitation of blood flow. This leads to a reduced stroke volume. Myocardial work and myocardial oxygen consumption are increased to maintain cardiac output. In combination with less effective forward flow, end-diastolic volume increases and can lead to volume overload, requiring therapeutic intervention.
- Decreased baroreceptor responsiveness, decreased circulating blood volume, and decreased vagal tone result in an elevated resting heart rate and an impaired response to preload changes and blood pressure changes.
- Old animals appear to be more sensitive to exogenous catecholamines (i.e., steroidal drugs such as prednisolone) and to anesthetic-induced arrhythmias.
- Impairment of cardiovascular function can result in an altered distribution and elimination of drugs.

Respiratory Function

With increasing age, fibrotic changes of the lung occur, and the respiratory muscles are weakened, contributing to a reduction in vital capacity, decreased compliance, and small airway closure. Also, calcification of terminal bronchioles can result in narrowing of the terminal airways. Related to cardiac disease, old dogs have a higher incidence of pulmonary hypertension with consequent ventilation–perfusion mismatch, reduced diffusing capacity (edema), and venous admixture, leading to increased risk of hypoxemia and hypoxic pulmonary vasoconstriction (all mammals have this response, but there is species variation in its magnitude with the greatest response found in cattle and pigs > horses > dogs and sheep).

- Protective laryngeal and pharyngeal reflexes may be impaired and render old animals more susceptible to aspiration.

Thermoregulation

Reduced metabolic rate, thyroid function, liver size, and muscle mass all combine to make geriatric animals prone to anesthesia-induced hypothermia.

- Hypothermia results in prolonged recovery from anesthesia. Other adverse sequelae of hypothermia have been documented in humans (increases in discomfort, post-operative oxygen requirement, hospital stay, surgical site infection, and arrhythmias) but have not been clearly established in animal species.

Gastrointestinal Function

Lower esophageal sphincter tone can be reduced, making geriatric animals prone to reflux and esophagitis. Geriatric animals are more likely to have chronic intestinal problems and malabsorption of iron and vitamin B12, both of which contribute to anemia. Changes in the gastrointestinal tract with atrophy of the gastric mucosa and of intestinal macro- and microvilli cause an increased sensitivity to gastrointestinal adverse effects of NSAIDs. If these effects of NSAIDs are observed (vomiting, melena, and diarrhea), then the drug should be stopped and misoprostol or a proton pump inhibitor (e.g., omeprazole or pantoprazole) should be given as soon as possible. An adverse response to one NSAID does not preclude use of another. A different NSAID may be selected and started after the adverse effects have resolved (see Chapter 9). Selecting an appropriate NSAID, based on the individual patient response, is important because these patients are often maintained on long-term NSAID treatment. Once a compatible NSAID is identified, titrating the dose downward to the lowest effective dose is recommended.

Polypharmacy Therapy

Long-term drug therapy is commonly implemented in geriatric patients due to existing disease (e.g., diabetes mellitus, heart disease, chronic kidney injury, maladaptive pain, etc.). In this context, the veterinarian may face a complex situation of polypharmacy that requires careful consideration of potential pharmacokinetic and pharmacodynamic interactions. Drug interactions can alter the desired and adverse effects of the combined drugs. These effects may be additive, antagonistic, or synergistic in nature. Common drug combinations and the potential consequences are summarized in Table 15.9.

Considerations for Geriatric Patient Anesthesia

In geriatric patients, anesthetic management considerations include both age-related changes and underlying or coexisting disease(s).

Pre-operative Assessment and Preparation

A thorough pre-operative assessment is crucial, including a good history regarding exercise tolerance, polyuria/polydipsia, known diseases and current medications, and physical examination. In approximately 30% of older dogs (>7 years), previously undiagnosed diseases were revealed by blood work and resulted in a delay of the planned procedure in 10% of the animals. Therefore, because of the increased likelihood of undiagnosed disease and reduced functional reserve in old animals, assessment of packed cell volume, complete blood count, total protein, urea creatinine, glucose concentration, and liver enzymes is warranted and recommended. Further diagnostic tests (e.g.,

Table 15.9 Common drug combinations used in geriatric patients.

Drugs	Indication	Interaction	Consequences
NSAIDs and angiotensin-converting enzyme (ACE) inhibitors	• Osteoarthritis and other maladaptive pain • Chronic heart failure (CHF) mainly valvular disease in dogs • Chronic kidney disease (CKD) and hypertension reduction of proteinuria	By inhibiting the formation of angiotensin II, ACE inhibitors prevent vasoconstriction of the efferent arteriole. Prostaglandins cause vasodilation of the afferent arteriole, but NSAIDs block the formation of prostaglandins which prevents afferent arteriole vasodilation.	The combination of ACE inhibitors and NSAIDs significantly lower transglomerular hydrostatic pressure, and hence glomerular filtration rate. In combination with hypovolemia or anesthesia, the risk of inducing AKI or CKD is increased.
NSAID ACE inhibitor furosemide	• Osteoarthritis and chronic pain • CHF • Plus/minus CKD	NSAIDs interfere with both pharmacokinetics and pharmacodynamics of furosemide. NSAIDs compete for proximal tubular secretion, shift the dose–response curve and impair natriuresis and increased renal blood flow induced by furosemide.	When NSAIDs are taken with a diuretic, the effect of the diuretic is reduced and heart failure may be exacerbated. Both the control of hypertension by ACE inhibitors and diuretics and their unloading effects in heart failure are antagonized by NSAIDs. If CKD is present, check hydration status before starting therapy and monitor plasma creatinine and packed cell volume during therapy.
NSAID Pimobendan NSAIDs and all other drugs with high protein binding	• Osteoarthritis and chronic pain • CHF	Competition for plasma protein binding.	Possibly increased availability and toxicity. Consider reduction of dose of NSAID.
Insulin protocol Alpha-2 adrenergic receptor agonists	• Diabetes mellitus • Sedation and anesthesia	Glucose homeostasis is profoundly disrupted in the peri-anesthetic period resulting in glycemic variability. Alpha-2 adrenergic receptor agonists inhibit insulin release.	Alpha-2 adrenergic receptor agonists can exacerbate undiagnosed diabetes. However, low doses of dexmedetomidine can stabilize glucose levels in diabetics by reducing stress and cortisol (humans)

diagnostic imaging, ECG) should be performed as indicated by the pre-operative assessment.

Fasting times should not be excessively long (>12 h; see Chapter 2) despite the possibility of reduced gastrointestinal motility and a slower gastric emptying time in old animals. Specific feeding and medication protocols need to be followed in diabetic animals (see Chapter 12) to avoid excessive hypo- or hyperglycemia. Animals receiving heart medications should receive their standard treatment to avoid rebound effects with withdrawal (see Chapter 17 for further recommendations).

Most other long-term medications should also not be withdrawn before anesthesia, but careful assessment of the individual case should be performed. Osteoarthritis patients on long-term NSAIDS can receive their daily dose as long as a good hydration and blood pressure monitoring (and management) is available. Additional doses of NSAIDs should not be given as part of peri-operative analgesia in these cases.

When handling old animals, impairment of their senses (deafness, blindness, etc.) should be considered as this may influence their reactions to being approached. Positioning for intravenous catheter placement or surgical positioning should take pain, restricted joint motion, and stiffness due to osteoarthritis into account (e.g., placing a catheter in a standing position [using the saphenous vein] in dogs). Excessive joint or vertebral column extension during surgery can contribute to post-operative pain and delayed recuperation.

Premedication/Sedation

The choice of sedative premedication (Tables 15.10 and 15.11) needs to be based on health status and character of the animal. Light sedation can reduce stress and contribute to smooth induction of anesthesia. However, in very old or very compromised animals, reduced doses are necessary or sedation may be avoided altogether.

Benzodiazepines alone or in combination with an opioid have a more reliable sedative effect in old animals compared to younger adults. Because of their minimal cardiovascular effects, they are well suited for geriatric small animal patients; however, they can exert more pronounced respiratory depression as in neonatal animals. In addition, especially in dogs, these drugs can contribute to prolonged post-operative or post-sedative cognitive dysfunction and dysphoria, which can outlast the duration of the antagonist, flumazenil.

Alpha-2 adrenergic receptor agonists, in large animals, are usually administered by intravenous injection and titrated upward to the desired clinical effect. Lower doses are usually sufficient to achieve the desired effect, taking

Table 15.10 Suggested doses for sedation and premedication in geriatric small animals.

Drug	Dose (mg/kg)	Route	Comment
Diazepam	0.05–0.2	IV	Combination with opioid
Midazolam	0.05–0.2	IV/IM	Combination with opioid
Pethidine (meperidine)	0.1	IM	
Methadone	0.2–0.3	IM/SC	
	0.1–0.2	IV	
Levomethadone	0.1–0.15	IM/SC	
	0.05–0.1	IV	
Morphine	0.1–0.3	IM/SC	Dilute for IV use (histamine release)
	0.1–0.2	IV	
Hydromorphone	0.05–0.1	IV/IM/SC	
Buprenorphine	0.005–0.02	IV/IM/OTM	
Butorphanol	0.2–0.3	IM	
	0.1–0.2	IV	
Acepromazine	0.01–0.1	IM/SC	
	0.005–0.01	IV	
Dexmedetomidine	0.0005	IV	
	0.001–0.003	IM/SC	
Medetomidine	0.001	IV	
	0.002–0.005	IM/SC	

IV: intravenous; IM: intramuscular; SC: subcutaneous; OTM: oral transmucosal.
Legislation and drug licensing for food animals can vary between countries (see Chapters 6, 7, and 11).

Table 15.11 Suggested doses for sedation and premedication in geriatric large animals.

Species	Drug	Dose (mg/kg)	Route	Comment
Cattle Small ruminants	Diazepam[a]	0.05–0.1	IV	Mostly combined with butorphanol
Cattle Small ruminants	Midazolam[a]	0.05–0.1	IV/IM	Mostly combined with butorphanol
Cattle and small ruminants	Brotizolam[a]	0.01	IV/IM	Uncommon drug but, when used, it is mostly combined with butorphanol
Horse and cattle	Methadone	0.05–0.1	IV/IM	
Horse, cattle, and pigs	Levomethadone	0.025–0.05 0.1–0.2	IV IM	
Horse	Morphine	0.1–0.3	IV/IM	Dilute for IV use and administer over 5–10 min (histamine release)
Horse	Buprenorphine	0.003–0.007	IV/IM/OTM	
Horse, cattle, and small ruminants Pigs	Butorphanol	0.01–0.05 0.05–0.1 0.1–0.2	IV IM/IV IM	
Horse	Acepromazine	0.01–0.02 0.005–0.01	IM/SC IV	
Pigs	Azaperone	1–2 0.5	IM IV	
Horse	Dexmedetomidine	0.0035–0.010	IV	
Horse	Medetomidine	0.005–0.007	IV/IM	
Horse	Romifidine	0.03–0.08	IV	
Horse Cattle Sheep Goats	Xylazine	0.3–1 0.01–0.1 0.01–0.1 0.005–0.01	IV/IM IM IM IM	
Horse and cattle	Detomidine	0.005–0.02 0.01–0.03 0.04	IV IM OTM (horse)	Maximal effect after OTM 40 min

IV: intravenous; IM: intramuscular; SC: subcutaneous; OTM: oral transmucosa.
[a] Goats and calves respond well to benzodiazepines alone, and moderate to deep sedation can be achieved. Analgesia must still be provided for invasive or potentially painful procedures.
Legislation and drug licensing for food animals can vary between countries (see Chapters 6, 7, and 11).

into account variability in demeanor. In small animals without overt cardiac disease, low or very low doses (e.g., <2 mcg/kg dexmedetomidine) ± reduced dose of a benzodiazepine often provide sufficient sedation.

Phenothiazines (e.g., acepromazine) depend on hepatic metabolism, which may be reduced in geriatric patients; therefore, reduced doses are recommended to avoid overly long sedation and compromise of thermoregulation. In animals receiving ACE inhibitors, acepromazine should be avoided to reduce the risk of hypotension.

Analgesia

Good analgesia is important in geriatric animals because maladaptive pain (e.g., pain from osteoarthritis or neoplasia) can influence recovery quality. Locoregional techniques are preferred as they are well tolerated and will reduce anesthetic requirements. In geriatric patients, bone formation or calcification of intervertebral ligaments can complicate access to the epidural or subarachnoid space, which makes epidural and spinal blocks more challenging to perform. In addition, performing regional local anesthetic blocks of the limb undergoing surgery will preserve motor function of the other limbs, unlike neuraxial blockade.

The elimination half-life of NSAIDS or opioids is prolonged in geriatric animals, and care should be taken with repeated administration to avoid accumulation or reaching toxic doses. With opioids, careful pain scoring and redosing as needed can be used. With NSAIDs, a single peri-operative dose is well tolerated when hydration and blood pressure are maintained during anesthesia. With repeated doses, a reduction to 70–80% of the initial dose in combination with pain scoring and monitoring renal function is a practical approach.

Induction and Maintenance of Anesthesia

The principles of careful monitoring and giving sedatives and anesthetics to effect are particularly important in geriatric animals as the response to anesthetic drugs can be variable and difficult to predict. In large animals, sedatives can usually be given to effect, whereas for practical and safety reasons the induction of anesthesia continues to be based upon delivery of a single predefined bolus. Titration of induction drugs to effect in large animals is only possible in very compromised, recumbent animals, and care should be taken to not compromise personnel safety.

Small geriatric patients can benefit from pre-oxygenation if it does not cause distress. Pre-oxygenation will increase pulmonary oxygen reserve and protects against hypoxemia during induction and tracheal intubation (especially brachycephalic breeds).

Maintenance of anesthesia is best performed with an inhalational anesthetic (isoflurane and sevoflurane). These drugs are administered and titrated to effect (see Chapter 8). Maintenance of anesthesia with injectable drugs is more difficult to achieve due to unpredictable metabolism and potential for accumulation, which can lead to unintended deep anesthesia, and long and incoordinated recovery.

Fluid Support

In geriatrics, fluid support during anesthesia with a balanced isotonic crystalloid solution is necessary to avoid hypovolemia and maintain GFR and renal function. Unmasking hypovolemia is common in geriatric animals following induction of general anesthesia, especially if water has been withheld (or animal has not been drinking) for longer than eight hours before anesthesia. Depending on the pre-anesthetic volume status and response to drugs, infusion rates between 2 and 10 mL/kg/h are recommended.

Monitoring

In geriatric patients, no sensor size or sampling rate restrictions are present, and available standard monitoring can be used. However, adult animals less than 3 kg could still be a challenge to monitor, and the guidelines for neonatal/pediatric patients described in the preceding text can be followed. Because of the unpredictable responses to drugs and restricted organ functional reserves, it is important to keep cardiopulmonary variables and body temperature close to, or within, normal physiologic ranges for the species.

Recovery

The recovery phase also requires close monitoring and fluid support until complete recovery (return of protective airway and cardiovascular reflexes, and ability to stand [as appropriate]). In small animals, 50–60% of peri-operative fatalities occur in the immediate post-operative period (within four hours of anesthesia). Reduced monitoring and observation, compared to the intra-operative period, are likely contributing factors. A warm, dry, and quiet environment, and a pain-free patient are crucial to promote smooth recovery. Hypothermia leads to prolonged recovery and can induce shivering (increasing oxygen requirements).

Depending on the anesthetic protocol used, overly long recoveries (>1 h) can be shortened by administering antagonists (naloxone, atipamezole/yohimbine or flumazenil) in low incremental doses until the animal shows signs of recovery (opening eyes without nystagmus, lifting head, swallowing, and trying to move into a sternal position). Repeated dosing of antagonists may be necessary.

Questions and Answer

There are more practice questions and answers available for this chapter on the website. Please visit http://www.wiley.com/go/VeterinaryAnesthesiaZeiler.

Questions

1) In neonatal animals, lower doses of sedatives and anesthetics are required to obtain surgical anesthesia. What are the reasons for these lower anesthetic requirements?
   a) Altered distribution of lipophilic drugs, incomplete blood–brain barrier, and reduced liver metabolism.
   b) Altered distribution of hydrophilic drugs, incomplete blood–brain barrier, and reduced liver metabolism.
   c) Altered distribution of hydrophilic drugs, incomplete blood–brain barrier, and reduced renal excretion.
   d) Altered distribution of lipophilic drugs, incomplete blood–brain barrier, and increased pro drug metabolism.

2) In neonates, alpha-2 adrenergic receptor agonists such as xylazine or dexmedetomidine should be avoided or used very cautiously because:
   a) Neonates develop malignant hyperthermia with alpha-2 adrenergic receptor agonist.
   b) Neonates do not respond to alpha-2 adrenergic receptor agonists.
   c) Neonates mainly depend on heart rate to maintain cardiac output.
   d) Neonates excessively vomit in response to alpha-2 adrenergic receptor agonists.
3) In geriatric patients, sedation or premedication with a benzodiazepine, such as diazepam or midazolam, is effective and well tolerated because of minimal cardiovascular effects. What are possible adverse effects that mainly occur in geriatric patients?
   a) Vomiting and regurgitation and exacerbation of cognitive dysfunction.
   b) More pronounced respiratory depression and exacerbation of cognitive dysfunction.
   c) More pronounced respiratory depression and loss of appetite.
   d) Hyperglycemia and loss of appetite.

Answers

1) a
2) c
3) b

Further Reading

Alef, M., von Praun, F., and Oechtering, G. (2008). Is routine pre-anaesthetic haematological and biochemical screening justified in dogs? *Vet Anaesth Analg* 35: 132–140.

Bettschart-Wolfensberger, R., Freeman, S.L., Bowen, I.M. et al. (2005). Cardiopulmonary effects and pharmacokinetics of i.v. dexmedetomidine in ponies. *Equine Vet J* 37: 60–64.

Bidwell, L.A. (2013). Anesthesia for dystocia and anesthesia of the equine neonate. *Vet Clin North Am Equine Pract* 29: 215–222.

Boller, E. and Boller, M. (2015). Assessment of fluid balance and the approach to fluid therapy in the perioperative patient. *Vet Clin North Am Small Anim Pract* 45: 895–915.

Boothe, D.M. (2012). Factors affecting drug disposition. In: *Small Animal Clinical Pharmacology and Therapeutics*, 2e (ed. D.M. Boothe), 34–70. München: Elsevier.

Brodbelt, D. (2009). Perioperative mortality in small animal anaesthesia. *Vet J* 182: 152–161.

Brodbelt, D.C., Blissitt, K.J., Hammond, R.A. et al. (2008). The risk of death: the confidential enquiry into perioperative small animal fatalities. *Vet Anaesth Analg* 35: 365–373.

Brodbelt, D.C., Pfeiffer, D.U., Young, L.E., and Wood, J.L. (2007). Risk factors for anaesthetic-related death in cats: results from the confidential enquiry into perioperative small animal fatalities (CEPSAF). *Br J Anaesth* 99: 617–623.

Bunn, H.F. (1971). Differences in the interaction of 2,3-diphosphoglycerate with certain mammalian hemoglobins. *Sci* 4: 1049–1050.

Davis, A.L., Carcillo, J.A., Aneja, R.K. et al. (2017). American College of Critical Care Medicine clinical practice parameters for hemodynamic support of pediatric and neonatal septic shock. *Crit Care Med* 45: 1061–1093.

Fantoni, D. and Shih, A.C. (2017). Perioperative fluid therapy. *Vet Clin North Am Small Anim Pract* 47: 423–434.

Ferrari, D., Lundgren, S., Holmberg, J. et al. (2022). Concentration of carprofen in the milk of lactating bitches after cesarean section and during inflammatory conditions. *J Theriogen* 181: 59–68.

Fielding, C.L., Magdesian, K.G., and Edman, J.E. (2011). Determination of body water compartments in neonatal foals by use of indicator dilution techniques and multifrequency bioelectrical impedance analysis. *Am J Vet Res* 72: 1390–1396.

Godden, S.M., Lombard, J.E., and Woolums, A.R. (2019). Colostrum management for dairy calves. *Vet Clin North Am Food Anim Pract* 35: 535–556.

Groot AC, G.-D., Strengers, J.L., Mentink, M. et al. (1985). Histologic studies on normal and persistent ductus arteriosus in the dog. *J Am Coll Cardiol* 6: 394–404.

Johnston, G.M., Eastment, J.K., Wood, J., and Taylor, P.M. (2002). The confidential enquiry into perioperative equine fatalities (CEPEF): mortality results of Phases 1 and 2. *Vet Anaesth Analg* 29: 159–170.

Johnston, G.M. and Steffey, E. (1995). Confidential enquiry into perioperative equine fatalities (CEPEF). *Vet Surg* 24: 518–519.

Johnston, G.M., Taylor, P.M., Holmes, M.A., and Wood, J.L. (1995). Confidential enquiry of perioperative equine fatalities (CEPEF-1): preliminary results. *Equine Vet J* 27: 193–200.

Jones, T., Bracamonte, J.L., Ambros, B., and Duke-Novakovski, T. (2019). Total intravenous anesthesia with alfaxalone, dexmedetomidine and remifentanil in healthy foals undergoing abdominal surgery. *Vet Anaesth Analg* 46: 315–324.

Joubert, K.E. (2007). Pre-anaesthetic screening of geriatric dogs. *J S Afr Vet Assoc* 78: 31–35.

Kienzle, E., Zentek, J., and Meyer, H. (1998). Body composition of puppies and young dogs. *J Nutrit* 128: 2680S–2683S.

Lombard, C.W., Evans, M., Martin, L., and Tehrani, J. (1984). Blood pressure, electrocardiogram and echocardiogram measurements in the growing pony foal. *Equine Vet J* 16: 342–347.

Ma, J., Smith, B.P., Smith, T.L. et al. (2002). Juvenile and adult rat neuromuscular junctions: density, distribution, and morphology. *Muscl Nerv* 26: 804–809.

Magrini, F. (1978). Haemodynamic determinants of the arterial blood pressure rise during growth in conscious puppies. *Cardiovasc Res* 12: 422–428.

Marr, C.M. (2015). The equine neonatal cardiovascular system in health and disease. *Vet Clin North Am Equine Pract* 31: 545–565.

Mazzatenta, A., Carluccio, A., Robbe, D. et al. (2017). The companion dog as a unique translational model for aging. *Semin Cell Develop Biol* 70: 141–153.

Mila, H., Feugier, A., Grellet, A. et al. (2015). Immunoglobulin G concentration in canine colostrum: evaluation and variability. *J Reprod Immunol* 112: 24–28.

O'Hagan, B., Pasloske, K., McKinnon, C. et al. (2012a). Clinical evaluation of alfaxalone as an anaesthetic induction agent in dogs less than 12 weeks of age. *Aust Vet J* 90: 346–350.

O'Hagan, B.J., Pasloske, K., McKinnon, C. et al. (2012b). Clinical evaluation of alfaxalone as an anaesthetic induction agent in cats less than 12 weeks of age. *Aust Vet J* 90: 395–401.

Pascoe, P.J. and Moon, P.F. (2001). Periparturient and neonatal anesthesia. *Vet Clin North Am Small Anim Pract* 31: 315–340.

Pereira, M., Valério-Bolas, A., Saraiva-Marques, C. et al. (2019). Development of dog immune system: from in uterus to elderly. *Vet Sci* 6 (83): 1–14.

Radakovich, L.B., Pannone, S.C., Treulove, M.P. et al. (2017). Hematology and biochemistry of aging-evidence of "anemia of the elderly" in old dogs. *Vet Clin Pathol* 46: 34–45.

Read, M.R., Read, E.K., Duke, T. et al. (2002). Cardiopulmonary effects and induction and recovery characteristics of isoflurane and sevoflurane in foals. *J Am Vet Med Assoc* 221: 393–398.

Schenk, H.C., Haastert-Talini, K., Jungnickel, J. et al. (2014). Morphometric parameters of peripheral nerves in calves correlated with conduction velocity. *J Vet Intern Med* 28: 646–655.

Schneider, M., Kuchta, A., Dron, F., and Woehrlé, F. (2015). Disposition of cimicoxib in plasma and milk of whelping bitches and in their puppies. *BMC Vet Res* 31 (11): 178.

Sideri, A.I., Galatos, A.D., Kazakos, G.M., and Gouletsou, P.G. (2009). Gastro-oesophageal reflux during anaesthesia in the kitten: comparison between use of a laryngeal mask airway or an endotracheal tube. *Vet Anaesth Analg* 36: 547–554.

Zaki, S., Ticehurst, K., and Miyaki, Y. (2009). Clinical evaluation of Alfaxan-CD(R) as an intravenous anaesthetic in young cats. *Aust Vet J* 87: 82–87.

16

Approach to a Patient in Shock

Benjamin M. Brainard, H. Nicole Trenholme, and Daniel Pang

Pathophysiology, Patient Evaluation, and Classification of Shock

Delivery of Oxygen

The majority of shock states in veterinary medicine occur due to disrupted tissue delivery of either oxygen (O_2) or substrate for metabolic energy generation (e.g., glucose). Shock may occur globally or regionally, depending on the etiology. The delivery of oxygen to tissues (DO_2) is described as the product of cardiac output (i.e., the volume of blood pumped by the heart per minute) and the O_2 content of that blood (i.e., mL oxygen/dL of blood, abbreviated as CaO_2 for arterial O_2 content) (Equation (1)). Oxygen delivery is the product of cardiac output (Q) and CaO_2, and shock results from deficiencies in either Q, CaO_2, or both. Cardiac output is the volume of blood pumped with each heartbeat multiplied by the number of heart beats/min. Therefore, it is calculated as the product of stroke volume (SV) and heart rate (HR) (Equation (2)). The stroke volume is in turn influenced by vascular tone (systemic vascular resistance, SVR), blood volume, and cardiac contractility (strength of cardiac contraction).

$$DO_2 = Q \bullet CaO_2 \tag{1}$$

$$Q^{\cdot} = HR \bullet SV \tag{2}$$

In order to calculate arterial O_2 content, the following equation applies:

$$CaO_2 = (1.34[Hb]SaO_2) + (0.003\,PaO_2) \tag{3}$$

Oxygen can be carried in the blood either attached to hemoglobin (Hb) or dissolved in the blood. In Equation (3), the first portion ($1.34 \cdot [Hb] \cdot SaO_2$) is the amount of O_2 in the blood that is bound to hemoglobin within red blood cells. Blood Hb concentration can be estimated as a third of the hematocrit (Hct; which is a similar value to the packed cell volume [PCV]). Considering saturation, each Hb molecule can hold up to four O_2 molecules, and saturation is a measure of the average bound O_2 in the blood (containing many individual Hb molecules). Oxygen attached to Hb is described as a combination of the concentration of Hb (in g/dL) and the saturation of Hb with O_2 (as a percent, commonly notated as SaO_2, for arterial saturation). The conversion factor (Hüfner's constant) varies by species but generally ranges from 1.31 to 1.39 mL O_2/g Hb. It serves to convert the saturation data to mL oxygen per dL of blood (i.e., 100 mL of blood). The second portion of the equation ($0.003 \cdot PaO_2$) accounts for the amount of O_2 that can be dissolved in a dL of blood, as related to the partial pressure of dissolved O_2 (PaO_2, for arterial partial pressure of O_2), multiplied by the conversion factor 0.003 vol%/mmHg. Notably, the hemoglobin-containing part of the equation contributes significantly more to CaO_2 than the dissolved component.

In the context of shock, disruption causing a decrease in delivery of either O_2 or cellular energy substrate will result in increased oxygen extraction (OE) in an attempt to support maintenance of oxygen consumption ($\dot{V}O_2$). An inadequate supply of O_2 and glucose to tissues impairs cellular ability to use aerobic respiration to create adenosine triphosphate (ATP). Cells can compensate to a degree (as long as adequate substrate is delivered) by using anerobic respiration. Anerobic respiration takes place in the cytosol (as opposed to the mitochondria, the site of aerobic respiration) and is less efficient than aerobic respiration, creating only a net 2 molecules of ATP (compared to a total of 36 ATP from aerobic respiration). Anerobic respiration also generates by-products, primarily lactate. The production of lactate generates a free hydrogen ion that is usually rapidly consumed in glycolysis, mitigating the development of acidosis. However, during moderate-to-severe anerobic conditions, lactate production increases and hydrogen ions produced during ATP hydrolysis begin to accumulate in

Fundamental Principles of Veterinary Anesthesia, First Edition. Edited by Gareth E. Zeiler and Daniel S. J. Pang.

Companion Website: www.wiley.com/go/VeterinaryAnesthesiaZeiler

the cytosol, resulting in acidosis. The by-products of aerobic respiration, carbon dioxide and water (CO_2 and H_2O, respectively), are easily excreted from the body, while lactate requires additional hepatic processing before excretion.

Concept Box 16.1
What is oxygen extraction?

Oxygen extraction (OE) refers to the ability of tissues to access arterial oxygen. Because all oxygen transport in the body is driven by diffusion, factors such as vascular density and CaO_2 are important contributors to ensure proper DO_2. To a point, and depending on oxygen supply and vessel density, as organ oxygen demand increases, more oxygen will be pulled from arterial blood by the tissues. In health, DO_2 generally exceeds tissue needs and only 20–30% of arterial oxygen that is delivered to tissues is used (with the remainder comprising venous oxygen content, CvO_2). The ratio between CaO_2 and CvO_2 describes the amount of oxygen removed by tissues from arterial blood and is referred to as the "oxygen extraction ratio" (OER). When the system is stressed, either due to physiologic demands such as increased muscle activity during exercise or due to conditions that decrease DO_2, more oxygen is taken from the arterial blood and the OER increases up to a theoretical maximum of around 65%.

Patient Evaluation and Indirect Markers of Shock

Understanding the pathophysiology of shock helps to describe the changes expected during physical examination. Physical examination findings can vary widely, depending on the primary pathology and stage of shock. When the primary cause of shock is due to decreases in CaO_2 (e.g., due to anemia or pulmonary disease), it is expected that the body will compensate to maintain oxygen delivery by increasing Q. In an effort to compensate for the reduced DO_2, patients will become tachycardic to improve Q and may have bounding pulses indicative of an increased SV. Capillary refill time (CRT) may also be shorter (e.g., less than one second) in patients with elevated Q. Under circumstances of increased Q, the patient may have normal to high blood pressure. If profound anemia is present, patients may also have pale mucous membranes, and if there is a component of hemolysis, icterus may be present (Figure 16.1). Patients with severe hypoxemia may have cyanotic mucous membranes, reflecting an elevated quantity (>5 g/dL) of deoxygenated Hb. If significant lactate is being generated, or if a patient has significant pulmonary disease, tachypnea is likely to be present. Tachypnea secondary to metabolic acidosis (e.g., a decrease in bicarbonate ion [HCO_3^-] concentration caused by exogenous acids such as keto acids or lactate production) facilitates exhalation of CO_2. Because CO_2 in the blood is

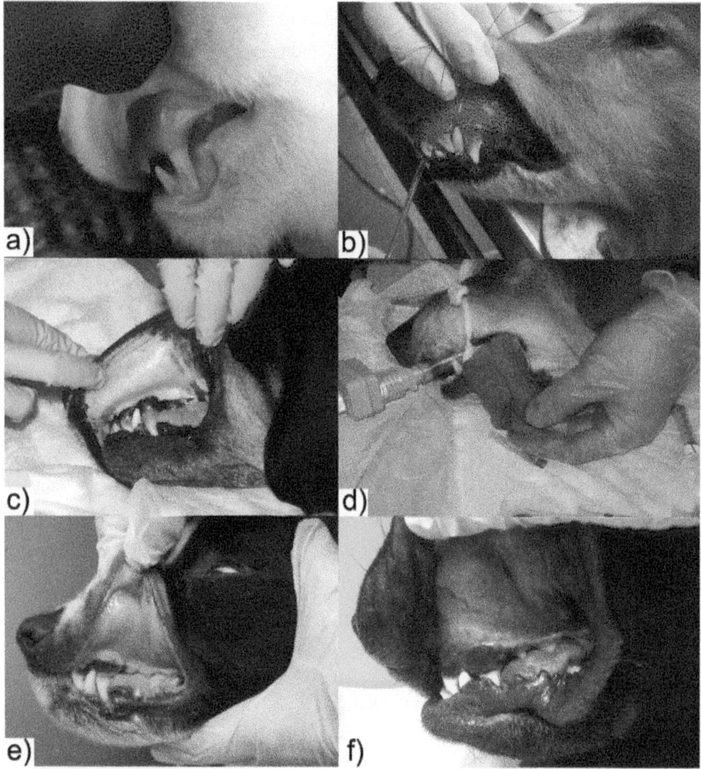

Figure 16.1 Variation in appearance of mucous membranes in small animals: (a) healthy with normal perfusion; (b) hyperemic; (c) pale due to vasoconstriction or anemia or both; (d) cyanotic; (e) icteric; (f) brown or muddy, in this case due to acetaminophen toxicosis.

effectively an acid (see Chapter 18), increased exhalation of CO_2 results in a respiratory alkalosis, compensating for acidemia (low blood pH). Tachypnea can also be a sign of hypoxemia, due to increased oxygen demand or decreased CaO_2, independent of blood pH. When the primary problem is reduced Q, clinical signs such as prolonged CRT, pallor of the mucous membranes, and tachycardia are expected. Pulses may be weak or thready in character, and the patient may have a depressed mentation (secondary to reduced cerebral perfusion). With hypovolemia, rectal temperature may be decreased due to poor perfusion as blood is shunted to the central circulation in an effort to protect perfusion of key organs (e.g., brain and kidneys). Systemic arterial blood pressure may be low and blood lactate concentration can be increased (increased lactate production from anerobic metabolism and reduced lactate metabolism secondary to decreased hepatic perfusion).

Shock can be broadly classified as "compensatory" or "decompensatory." The difference between compensatory and decompensatory shock is primarily related to the body's ability to make up for decreased oxygen delivery (DO_2). If the tissues can increase their oxygen extraction as DO_2 decreases, the tissues can delay the onset of anerobic metabolism while their oxygen (and substrate) requirements are met. At a certain point, however, the body is unable to compensate for the decreased DO_2, and oxygen consumption (VO_2) becomes dependent on supply (Figure 16.2). Means to maintain DO_2, which may eventually fail, include increased cardiac output (upper limit to tachycardia and contractility) and tachypnea (eventual respiratory muscle fatigue). When the body can no longer compensate, the patient enters decompensatory shock, leading to an increase in blood lactate concentrations. The effects of a systemic acidosis may become more profound

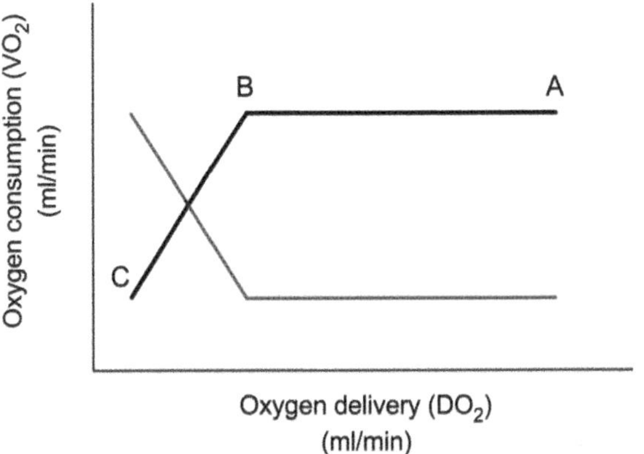

Figure 16.2 The relationship between oxygen consumption and oxygen delivery. (A, B) In healthy animals, oxygen delivery exceeds oxygen consumption. (B, C) Oxygen consumption is reduced as oxygen delivery decreases. Red line depicts blood lactate concentration, which increases as cellular metabolism shifts from aerobic to anerobic, as occurs during shock.

as the patient condition deteriorates. In the end stage of decompensatory shock, patients may become inappropriately bradycardic, hypotensive, and hypothermic. Cats in particular are prone to becoming bradycardic in shock states. Patients become profoundly hypotensive and may have extensive shunting of blood to the core organs and away from the periphery. This in turn causes the extremities to be cooler to the touch as compared to the core body temperature. Respiratory rates may decrease, resulting in hypoventilation, and other physiologic functions reflective of reduced organ perfusion can decline (e.g., urine production and mentation). If not corrected, this leads to complete cardiovascular collapse and death. The physical exam findings of patients with decompensatory shock include a change in mucous membrane color to purple or gray (sometimes termed "muddy"), reflecting poor perfusion. These patients often exhibit other evidence of systemic decompensation, such as hypoglycemia, progressive increases in anerobic metabolism (and subsequent increase in lactate), and acidosis.

In addition to physical examination, laboratory analysis can help to define the cause of decreased DO_2. Packed cell volume and total plasma protein (TPP) can confirm the presence of anemia with or without blood loss, and arterial blood gas analysis can confirm the presence of hypoxemia and acidosis. Pulse oximetry can also support a diagnosis of hypoxemia though it does not give any information regarding the presence of anemia (see Chapter 4). In a patient with a normal PCV and hypoxemia, cyanosis is noted when >5g/dL of Hb is deoxyhemoglobin (corresponding to an SaO_2 <85%). Additionally, if significant interruptions in tissue oxygen delivery are present, blood lactate concentration may be increased (generally, normal concentration is <2 mmol/L). With appropriate resuscitation from shock, the heart rate should move toward the normal range, and other signs of hypoperfusion (e.g., dull mentation and lack of urine production) should resolve. With increased perfusion, lactate will be transported to the liver for clearance, aerobic cellular respiration is restored, and the production of lactate is decreased. In animals with azotemia related to poor renal perfusion (pre-renal azotemia), the restoration of adequate circulating blood volume and renal perfusion should resolve the azotemia and restore urine production. Blood glucose may be variably affected due to the primary cause of the shock, but hypoglycemia should be treated to prevent continued negative energy balance from decreased energy substrate.

Classification of Shock

Types of shock are classified based on the underlying cause of decreased DO_2. The most common types of shock seen in veterinary medicine are hypovolemic shock and distributive shock. There are a number of different classification schemes for shock; the key aspect is to recognize the presence of shock and to discern the underlying cause. This allows the clinician to determine the best steps toward resuscitating the patient. Some patients may have more than one concurrent etiology of shock; an accurate and complete history and physical examination are critical to assess and treat these patients.

Hypovolemic Shock

Hypovolemic shock is caused by an absolute decrease in the amount of blood in the vasculature (absolute hypovolemia). Lower blood volume impairs the amount of blood the heart can pump (decreasing SV), and the animal with compensated hypovolemic shock should display significant tachycardia (to maintain Q despite a decreased SV). Other physical examination findings that can help to identify hypovolemic shock are weak pulses (sometimes described as "thready") and pale mucous membranes (in this case reflecting peripheral vasoconstriction), with a slow or even absent capillary refill time (Figure 16.1c). As hypovolemic shock progresses, in order to maintain perfusion to key organs (heart and brain), a compensatory vasoconstriction occurs. This serves to direct blood flow to the core organs and away from the periphery, which can result in a lower than expected rectal temperature and extremities that may be cold to the touch.

Common causes of hypovolemic shock include fluid losses from vomiting and diarrhea, uncontrolled urinary losses of fluid (e.g., due to diabetes mellitus, hypoadrenocorticism, or renal disease), hemorrhage (e.g., trauma, coagulopathy, or ruptured neoplastic mass), or third space losses (e.g., ascites, seromas, and pyometra). Therapy for hypovolemic shock is focused on restoring intravascular volume using intravenous fluid therapy, as well as stopping further loss of fluid from the body, as indicated.

> **Concept Box 16.2**
> **Hypovolemia versus dehydration.**
>
> It is important to distinguish between the terminology of hypovolemia (lack of fluid within blood vessels) and dehydration (lack of fluid within the cells and interstitial areas of the body). The two may occur concurrently, requiring both immediate intravascular volume resuscitation and more lengthy interstitial rehydration of the patient. However, animals with hypovolemic shock may be adequately hydrated (e.g., a healthy dog that is hit by a car and experiences hemorrhage), and dehydrated animals may not be hypovolemic (e.g., an animal with dehydration resulting from chronic renal disease).

Distributive Shock

Distributive shock is a condition of *relative* hypovolemia, which is defined as inadequate blood volume to fill the vasculature under specific conditions. Many of these conditions are characterized by inappropriate vasodilation. Similar to hypovolemic shock, less blood volume is returned to the heart, compromising Q, and the heart will attempt to compensate with tachycardia. Under normal circumstances, vascular tone (i.e., SVR) is tightly controlled so that blood flow, and thus oxygen delivery, can be appropriately directed to specific organs (e.g., muscles during exercise). Vasodilation is accomplished through local mechanisms, predominantly through the production and release of nitric oxide (NO) by endogenous nitric oxide synthase (NOS). A variant NOS that is inducible by various stimuli is termed "iNOS." In the context of the body's response to sepsis and septic shock, upregulation of iNOS results in production and release of NO in areas where increased blood flow is not needed. The consequence of this is widespread, inappropriate vasodilation. This results in a relative hypovolemia as the normal blood volume cannot adequately fill the abnormally increased intravascular space secondary to inappropriate vasodilation. Another cause of distributive shock is anaphylaxis, where widespread vasodilation follows the release of histamines and other inflammatory mediators. Additionally, in conditions of relative adrenal insufficiency (also sometimes termed "critical-illness-related corticosteroid insufficiency," CIRCI), patients may have a loss of vessel tone due to inadequate corticosteroid activity.

Physical exam findings for animals with compensatory distributive shock are consistent with inappropriate vasodilation and cardiac compensation. In septic shock, mucous membranes appear brick red from vasodilation with a rapid CRT that is a result of increased Q (Figure 16.1b). In decompensatory shock, mucous membrane color becomes purple or gray along with other signs of decompensatory shock. Animals with decompensatory distributive shock from sepsis have a poor to grave prognosis.

Obstructive Shock

Syndromes comprising obstructive shock are varied but have at their core a physical disruption of normal cardiovascular function or flow. In many ways, this category is a catchall and incorporates components of other categories of shock into the clinical presentations. One of the classic examples of obstructive shock is gastric dilatation-volvulus syndrome (GDV). Obstruction is caused by an enlarging gas-filled stomach, which increases intra-abdominal pressure, compromising perfusion to abdominal organs. The caudal vena cava is collapsed, resulting in decreased venous return to the heart and a subsequent decrease Q and pulmonary perfusion. An analogous presentation in a horse would be a large colon volvulus. Physical exam findings in patients with GDV include a large, tympanic abdomen, accompanied by tachycardia and weak femoral pulses. Tachypnea can be secondary to systemic acidosis or compromised diaphragm contraction (due to abdominal distension). Another important cause of obstructive shock is pericardial effusion. As fluid accumulates in the pericardial sac, and pressure increases within the pericardium and prevents complete diastolic filling of the right side of the heart (the right side of the heart has a thinner muscular wall and is more easily collapsed by pressure than the left). When effusion causes collapse of the right side of the heart, it is called "cardiac tamponade." Acute pericardial effusion results in clinical signs of collapse or exercise intolerance as a result of decreased Q. Animals with chronic pericardial effusions can have clinical signs of right-sided heart failure (e.g., ascites). Obstructive shock may also be caused by thromboembolic events. The alterations in perfusion caused by arterial thrombosis or thromboembolism are a good example of how the physical presence of obstruction results in differential effects across the body. Arterial thrombosis interrupts oxygen delivery to a part of the body while normal perfusion may be maintained to other areas. Physical exam findings of thrombosis are characterized by loss of function in the affected area, and may be manifested as pelvic limb paresis for aortic thrombosis, or dyspnea for patients with pulmonary thromboembolism. Muscles that are deprived of blood flow will exhibit swelling and pain (ischemic myopathy).

Other concerns related to obstructive events are the sequelae following resolution of the obstruction as blood flow returns to previously hypoperfused areas. Reperfusion injury occurs in the ischemic tissue and describes an inflammatory cascade initiated by superoxide and other free-radical molecules. These molecules are carried out by previously hypoperfused tissues as circulation is restored and may cause significant organ damage distinct from that of the initial obstructive event. In the context of anesthesia, obstructions that are resolved as part of a surgical procedure (e.g., large colon volvulus, GDV) may result in the release of vasoactive substances that cause vasodilation and other intracellular components (e.g., potassium) that may alter hemodynamic stability, resulting in hypotension and cardiac arrhythmias. Clear communication between the surgeon and anesthetist will allow the anesthetist to remain vigilant to anticipate and rapidly identify changes in blood pressure or cardiac rhythm and treat them appropriately.

Cardiogenic Shock

Any type of shock that results from a failure of the heart to generate adequate Q despite a normal or increased vascular volume is characterized as cardiogenic shock. Types of cardiac disease are diverse, but all manifest as a decreased Q, with the potential to cause tissue hypoperfusion. Cardiogenic shock may be worsened by the development of pulmonary edema from increased hydrostatic pressure in the pulmonary veins due to high left atrial pressures. This impairs the ability of the lungs to adequately oxygenate blood, compounding existing DO_2 deficiencies. Hypervolemia is a common occurrence in patients with chronic cardiac conditions due to the upregulation of the renin–angiotensin–aldosterone system. This causes retention of vascular volume. Cardiac diseases and anesthesia are covered in more depth in Chapter 17 but may be broadly characterized as diastolic failure or systolic failure.

Diseases associated with diastolic failure cause decreased SV due to inadequate cardiac filling during diastole. In general, animals with diastolic dysfunction benefit from therapies that make it easier for the heart to fill (e.g., extending diastole by decreasing heart rate) or easier for the heart to eject blood (e.g., by decreasing SVR through selective vasodilation). An example of a disease of diastolic function is feline hypertrophic cardiomyopathy. Anesthetic considerations include avoidance of medications that might cause tachycardia or severe vasoconstriction. Animals with systolic dysfunction have decreased SV due to an inability of the heart muscle to pump blood out of the heart into the aorta. An example of systolic dysfunction is dilated cardiomyopathy (where cardiac contractility is compromised).

In general, cardiogenic shock is a result of the progression of chronic heart disease as heart failure occurs. Additionally, as fluid volume increases in the pulmonary circulation secondary to hypervolemia (activation of the renin–angiotensin–aldosterone system) and/or compromised pulmonary circulation (secondary to cardiac dysfunction), there is a risk of pulmonary edema. This buildup of fluid is described as congestive heart failure. Should pulmonary edema occur, oxygenation may be compromised, further decreasing DO_2. Animals at risk of, or showing signs of, congestive heart failure should be treated before anesthesia (e.g., with diuretics to decrease vascular volume and/or positive inotropic drugs to increase the strength of cardiac contraction). Clinical signs of left-sided cardiogenic shock include pale mucous membranes with a slow CRT due to vasoconstriction and impaired filling, respectively. Animals are dyspneic and generally tachycardic (unless the cause of the shock is due to bradycardia such as might be caused by third-degree AV block) and will have a decreased rectal temperature due to hypoperfusion of the rectal mucosa. Cats with congestive heart failure may develop pleural effusion in addition to pulmonary edema, and thoracocentesis should be performed to resolve dyspnea before anesthesia. This can be a challenge as sedation may be required in order to perform this procedure.

Patients with arrhythmias may also develop cardiogenic shock. Arrhythmias may be bradyarrhythmias (causing a decrease in heart rate and therefore Q) or tachyarrhythmias (causing incomplete filling of the heart secondary to loss of time in diastole; Chapter 17).

Hypoxic Shock

"Hypoxic shock" or "hypoxemic shock" is a general term for conditions where impaired DO_2 to tissues is not caused by a problem with cardiac output, but rather it represents deficiencies in the CaO_2 portion of the oxygen delivery equation ([Equations (1) and (3)]; see also Chapter 18). Low blood O_2 concentration (hypoxemia) can result from pulmonary disease that prevents normal alveolar gas exchange, from airway obstruction or from the breathing of hypoxic gas mixtures. Pulmonary diseases that impair oxygenation of arterial blood include infectious disease (e.g., bacterial pneumonia) or noninfectious causes (e.g., neoplasia and pulmonary edema). In these patients, there may be limited clinical consequences if 100% O_2 is used as the fresh gas in the anesthetic circuit. By contrast, animals with pulmonary disease caused by fibrotic changes will have decreased pulmonary compliance that may impair ventilation or oxygenation, if severe. Hypoxic pulmonary vasoconstriction (HPV) is an endogenous protective mechanism whereby the lungs redirect blood flow away from alveoli with low O_2 tensions. This serves to route the majority of pulmonary blood flow to alveoli that can contribute to arterial oxygenation (as the alveoli with low O_2 tension would not contribute meaningfully to oxygenation). There is variation in the degree of HPV response among species. Certain volatile inhalant anesthetics (e.g., isoflurane and sevoflurane) when administered at a dose above 1 MAC (minimum alveolar concentration; see Chapter 8) can transiently impair the HPV response and may result in difficulty in the transition of patients from 100% O_2 to room air (21% O_2) following anesthetic procedures. This can be compounded by absorption atelectasis, pharmacologic effects of anesthetics on muscle strength and respiratory drive, and patient conformation (e.g., increased work of breathing in obese patients). In general, if anesthesia is necessary for a patient with significant impairment of oxygenation, a total intravenous anesthetic may be advantageous, especially for short procedures. However, if anesthesia can be delayed until pulmonary function is improved, this is preferable. Additionally, the utilization of 100% O_2 during the anesthetic episode causes adsorption atelectasis. In this process, the high inspired O_2 washes out the nitrogen gas that is usually present in the alveoli. Because nitrogen gas is poorly soluble in blood, it remains in the alveolus, helping to maintain open alveoli. Without this nitrogen present, there is greater collapse of alveoli, which may have an additive effect on patients that already have a compromised pulmonary system. This in turn may worsen recovery as the concentration of O_2 is changed from 100 to 21%. Animals with hypoxic shock are almost always tachypneic and may have pale or cyanotic mucous membranes if they are severely hypoxemic (Figure 16.1e). They are generally tachycardic and may have normal to slightly decreased body temperature. Pulse pressure is generally normal, and many have a normal blood lactate concentration.

Another critical cause of decreased CaO_2 is decreased red blood cell (RBC) concentration (anemia; as described by Equation (3)). Anemia should be corrected before anesthesia as it can affect the stability of anesthetized patients. Furthermore, anesthetic drugs that result in vasodilation (e.g., acepromazine and isoflurane) may result in sequestration of RBCs in the splenic vasculature and a critical drop in Hct. In general, transfusion of either packed red blood cells (pRBCs) or whole blood (WB) can be used to increase circulating RBC numbers before anesthesia (see the following text). In some cases (e.g., hemorrhage), anemia is accompanied by hypovolemia and therapy would include not only RBC replacement but also fluid therapy to replace lost vascular volume. Exposure to specific drugs (e.g., acetaminophen) or conditions (e.g., house fire) can cause hemoglobinopathies (resulting in methemoglobinemia and carboxyhemoglobinemia, respectively) that can impair the ability of Hb to bind O_2, effectively decreasing SO_2 and, consequently, DO_2. Anemic animals may require anesthesia for various emergent reasons. Animals with normovolemic anemia (e.g., due to hemolysis) generally have clinical signs reflective of elevated Q, including tachycardia, bounding pulses, and a CRT that is normal to fast. In animals with profound anemia, CRT may be difficult to assess as the mucous membranes appear pale or white due to lack of RBCs (Figure 16.1c). Cyanosis is also difficult to assess in anemic patients as they have a much lower Hb concentration than a patient with a normal Hct. Therefore, they will not appear cyanotic on physical examination until there is a much greater percentage drop in Hb bound to O_2. Patients with methemoglobinemia caused by acetaminophen (paracetamol) toxicity characteristically show facial swelling and brown mucous membranes (Figure 16.1f). Cats in particular are very sensitive to the oxidative damage caused by acetaminophen, and its use in cats is contraindicated.

Metabolic Shock

Metabolic shock denotes inadequate cellular energy in the presence of adequate perfusion and DO_2. Hypoglycemia is the most common cause of metabolic shock, where cellular ATP cannot be produced due to lack of substrate. This can occur with patients in septic shock as well as patients that have an insulinoma, synthetic liver failure, xylitol toxicity, or if they have been administered excessive exogenous insulin. Other causes of metabolic shock include scenarios where cellular DO_2 is not adequate for the cellular metabolic rate, as is seen with elevations in body temperature which causes a concomitant increase in energy demand (e.g., malignant hyperthermia and heat stroke) or scenarios where mitochondrial function is disturbed (e.g., cyanide or bromethalin poisoning, which disrupts the mitochondrial electron transport chain). Clinical signs in these patients are variable but are generally similar to other signs of shock such as tachycardia, pale mucous membranes, and tachypnea. Pulse pressure in these animals is generally normal to increase as they have normal vascular volume and an increased Q in the compensatory phase.

Concepts of Fluid Resuscitation

Intravenous fluid therapy plays an important role in resuscitation and fluid maintenance of patients with hypovolemia, dehydration, or both. Care should be taken when deciding the volume and type of fluids to administer during the pre-anesthetic resuscitation period as well as during the anesthesia and surgery period. Fluid administration can have negative sequelae, including volume overload, dilution of proteins within the blood (e.g., albumin and coagulation proteins), and alterations of plasma electrolytes.

Fluid choice is determined by the ultimate target of the administered fluids (i.e., intravascular, interstitial, or intracellular compartments). The compartments within the body allow variable movement of fluid and small molecules between them. Each compartment has different concentrations of electrolytes (e.g., sodium, potassium, and magnesium) and polar molecules (e.g., proteins and phosphate). The average animal is comprised of 3/5 total body water and 2/5 dry matter by weight. Total body water is either intracellular (2/3 of the total) or extracellular (1/3 of the total). There are some species and age-related variations, but this distribution of total body water is consistent across many mammalian species. Water that is outside of the cells is predominantly (75%) located in the interstitium with a small amount (25%) circulating in the plasma (Figure 16.3).

Fluid balance refers to the maintenance of water within the specific fluid compartments, and it can be represented by the balance between the oncotic and hydrostatic pressures within the vasculature and interstitium. This is best represented by Starling's law of the capillary:

$$J_v = K_f\left[(p_c - p_i) - s(p_p - p_i)\right] \quad (4)$$

where the fluid movement (flux) across the capillary (J_v) is the difference between hydrostatic pressure within the capillary (p_c) and interstitium (p_i) minus the oncotic pressure within the plasma (p_p) and the interstitium (p_i). This equation includes two coefficients: a filtration coefficient (K_f) and the osmotic reflection or Staverman's coefficient (s), which represents the contribution of plasma proteins. Over the past 20 years, the role of the glycocalyx in fluid balance has been further defined. The endothelial glycocalyx is rich in proteoglycans and glycoproteins and lines the vascular endothelium. Because the glycocalyx also contributes to fluid retention within the vascular space by opposing extravasation, Starling's law of the capillary may be reconsidered, replacing interstitial oncotic pressure with that of the glycocalyx (p_g), hence

$$J_v = K_f\left[(p_c - p_i) - s(p_p - p_g)\right] \quad (5)$$

We are still discovering new aspects of the glycocalyx and coming to an understanding of how its presence or destruction (e.g., from inflammatory diseases such as sepsis) may alter fluid balance and resuscitation choices.

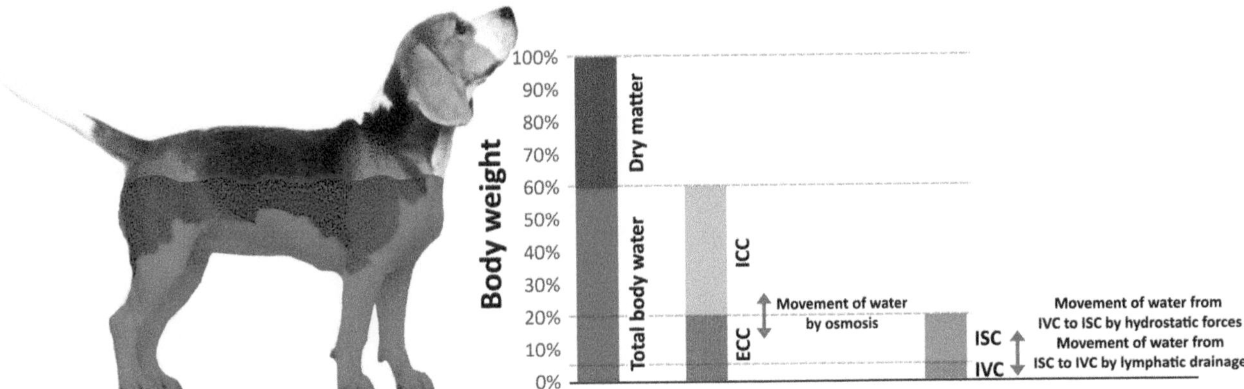

Figure 16.3 Total body water and fluid distribution in the body. ECC = extra-cellular component, ICC = intra-cellular component, ISC = interstital component, IVC = intravascular component.

Besides the effects of hydrostatic pressure, the osmotic pressure (tendency to attract water across semipermeable membranes) of a particular fluid compartment is highly dependent upon the concentration of sodium (Na), potassium (K), glucose (Glu), and urea nitrogen (BUN) in the compartment. The osmotic pressure in any given compartment can be calculated as

$$\begin{aligned}\text{Osm}(\text{mOsm}/\text{L}) \\ = 2[\text{Na}^+] + [\text{K}^+] + [\text{Glu}(\text{mg}/\text{dL})]/18 \\ + [\text{BUN}(\text{mg}/\text{dL})]/2.8\end{aligned} \tag{6a}$$

$$\begin{aligned}\text{Osm}(\text{mOsm}/\text{L}) \\ = 2[\text{Na}^+] + [\text{K}^+] + [\text{Glu}(\text{mmol}/\text{L})] \\ + [\text{BUN}(\text{mmol}/\text{L})]\end{aligned} \tag{6b}$$

Normal plasma osmolarity is approximately 300 mOsm/L with some variability between species. Isotonic fluids have a similar osmolarity to the plasma (i.e., about 300 mOsm/L), while hypertonic and hypotonic fluids have osmolarities that are relatively higher and lower than plasma, respectively. In general, isotonic fluids are the most appropriate fluid for intravascular volume resuscitation. In some circumstances, other fluid choices may be preferred. For example, in hypernatremia, it may be indicated to choose a fluid that is hypotonic (to replace free water loss), or a fluid that has a relatively higher sodium (to prevent rapid shifts of serum osmolarity). In fluids where the tonicity is primarily supported by dextrose (e.g., 5% dextrose in water; D5W), the fluids are essentially isotonic prior to administration, but once the dextrose is metabolized by the body, have delivered a hypotonic fluid (i.e., water). For this reason, these fluids are referred to as "hypotonic" even though a direct measure of osmolarity prior to administration would indicate that they are isotonic. These types of fluids (and other hypotonic fluids such as 0.45% saline) are contraindicated for use as a resuscitative fluid and are primarily used to treat dehydration (total body free water deficit) as opposed to hypovolemia, and are not covered in this chapter.

Isotonic Crystalloid Fluids

Before anesthesia, every effort should be made to improve the hemodynamic stability of the patient in shock, which may include volume resuscitation with isotonic crystalloids.

Isotonic fluids are frequently used in the resuscitation of patients with hypovolemic, obstructive, and distributive shock. In general, isotonic fluids are inexpensive and readily available. Sodium and chloride are the main electrolytes in isotonic fluids, and thus contribute the most to the tonicity of the fluid. Physiologic saline is comprised of a 0.9% solution of sodium chloride and is classified as an unbalanced isotonic crystalloid. Many isotonic fluids also contain small amounts of other electrolytes (e.g., potassium, magnesium, and calcium) and buffers (e.g., lactate and acetate), similar to plasma concentrations, and are classified as balanced isotonic crystalloids. Isotonic fluids are the first choice for rapid volume expansion; however, a large proportion (approximately 50%) of administered isotonic fluids redistribute between the body compartments within 20–40 min of administration. This concept

Concept Box 16.3
Fluid resuscitation for hypovolemia versus dehydration.

As previously described, the clinician must distinguish between hypovolemia and dehydration. The following section is mainly focused on addressing life-threatening hypovolemia in order to improve and maintain peri-anesthetic stability. However, in the post-operative period, the clinician must also consider correction of the patient's dehydration over a predetermined time period, which must be tailored to the individual. In most instances, once hypovolemia is corrected, dehydration can be safely corrected over 24–48 h. Some exceptions exist. In patients with a healthy heart and evidence of acute kidney injury, the clinician may elect to replace the volume of dehydration over a 12 h period. However, in the case of a patient that has advanced heart disease and is also profoundly dehydrated, the clinician may elect to replace that volume over 48 h or more. In order to calculate the volume of fluid to correct dehydration, the clinician should estimate percentage dehydration (usually detectable at ≥5–6%) and multiply this by the patient's body weight. This gives the volume of fluid in liters (iso- or hypotonic) necessary to replace in that patient. The calculated volume can be divided by the number of hours chosen over which to replace the fluid deficit. This volume is added to the hourly maintenance fluid requirement to give the overall rate of fluid administration. This formula gives the clinician a starting point, but the patient should be serially reassessed and the fluid plan should be adjusted based on the clinical picture.

of redistribution is especially important in hypovolemic patients, where an isotonic crystalloid bolus may initially improve perfusion parameters (e.g., heart rate, blood lactate concentration, and blood pressure), that worsen again following redistribution. This must be considered when planning the optimal time to induce anesthesia following fluid resuscitation.

A common approach to volume resuscitation with isotonic fluids is to administer boluses of 10–20 mL/kg IV over 5–10 min, followed by reassessment and monitoring. This can be repeated if deemed clinically appropriate; however, if more than one-third to one-half of the patient's blood volume (dog: 70–90 mL/kg; cat: 50–60 mL/kg; horse: 70–80 mL/kg) has been administered rapidly as isotonic crystalloid fluids, consideration should be given to other therapeutic options (vasopressors, blood products, etc.) to reduce the risk of a positive fluid balance and subsequent fluid overload, tissue edema, and ileus. If perfusion parameters improve after a bolus, the animal can receive continued crystalloid infusion at a lower rate (e.g., 2–5 mL/kg/h), anticipating the redistribution of the bolus as well as any ongoing losses (e.g., vomiting, diarrhea, and airway evaporation). If perfusion parameters worsen again, another bolus may be given. The theoretical maximum crystalloid dose is the circulating blood volume: 90 mL/kg in a dog and 60 mL/kg in a cat. Theoretical maximum infusion volumes in horses and ruminants vary with breed, but they are generally around 80 mL/kg. With larger infused amounts of crystalloid fluid, concern should be given for dilution of plasma proteins (albumin and coagulation factors), endothelial glycocalyx degradation, and hypothermia. Excessive administration of crystalloid fluids can also cause hypervolemia, resulting in volume overload and tissue edema, which can lead to hypoxemia and organ dysfunction. In patients where the anesthetist is concerned for the potential of volume overload, a rapid test fluid bolus of 3–5 mL/kg given over 5 min may pose less risk to the patient while also assessing response to therapy. If there is no change in physiologic parameters with that bolus, additional large volume fluid administration is unlikely to benefit the patient although each patient should be assessed individually to decide if the next step involves fluid therapy or another approach. If repeated large volume crystalloid boluses are administered with only a transient (20 min or less) response, then other interventions, such as colloid solutions, blood product transfusions, vasopressor therapy, and/or addressing the primary pathology, need to be considered (e.g., trocarization/derotation of stomach in GDV, pericardiocentesis for pericardial effusion, or removal of septic nidus). If patients show no improvement following fluid boluses, then continued large volume crystalloid fluid administration is not recommended and attention should be focused on aggressively treating the cause of shock.

Examples of resuscitative fluids and their components are available in Table 16.1. Isotonic crystalloids are generally interchangeable, and they include fluids such as Lactated Ringer's solution (LRS), Hartmann's solution, 0.9% saline, Normosol-R, and Plasma-Lyte-148. In general, the fluids with lower chloride (i.e., not 0.9% saline) are favored for resuscitation to avoid hyperchloremia, but all are suitable to achieve rapid intravascular volume expansion in animals. The presence of small amounts of potassium or calcium in these fluids is unlikely to impact circulating electrolyte concentrations. However, care should be taken if a simultaneous blood product transfusion is needed to not administer the transfusion in the same line as the fluids since these electrolyte solutions can cause precipitation of the citrate anticoagulant and clot formation.

Table 16.1 Intravenous fluids that can be used for resuscitation.

Fluid type	Osmolarity (mOsm/L)	pH	Buffer	Na^+ (mEq/L)	Cl^- (mEq/L)	K^+ (mEq/L)	Ca^{++} (mEq/L)	Mg^{++} (mEq/L)
Plasma-Lyte 148	296	5.5	Acetate	140	98	5	0	3
LRS	272	6.5	Lactate	130	109	4	3	0
Hartmann's solution	255	6.5	Lactate	131	112	5	2	0
Normosol-R	294	6.6	Acetate Gluconate	140	98	5	0	3
0.9% NaCl	308	5.0		154	154	0	0	0
7.5% NaCl	2567	5.5		1283	1283	0	0	0
6% Hetastarch	310	5.5		154	154	0	0	0
Plasma	300	7.4	Bicarbonate	145	105	5	5	1.5

Na^+: Sodium ion; Cl^-: Chloride ion; K^+: potassium ion; Ca^{++}: calcium ion; Mg^{++}: magnesium ion; LRS: lactated Ringer's solution.

Concept Box 16.4
Worked example of a fluid plan.

A two-year-old, 10 kg, female spayed Shih Tzu presents for evaluation of vomiting and inappetence for a duration of three days. She is quiet, alert, and responsive with a tender abdomen and has sunken eyes. Her vital parameters include heart rate of 150 beats per minute with strong synchronous femoral pulses, panting respiratory rate with pink but tacky mucus membranes, capillary refill time of two seconds, and a Doppler blood pressure of 140 mmHg. Laboratory work shows a PCV of 68% and total solids of 8.8 g/dL with a lactate concentration of 4 mmol/L and creatinine concentration of 2.3 mg/dL. She is diagnosed with a gastrointestinal obstruction and requires an exploratory laparotomy. Q1: What fluid resuscitation plan would you institute prior to induction of anesthesia? Q2: Assuming a dehydration of 5%, what volume of fluid, and rate of administration, would be required after surgery to rehydrate the patient over 36 h?

Answer: Q1: Balanced crystalloid administered IV to a total volume of 100–300 mL. Q2: Total fluid rate of 33 mL/h would be required. See end of chapter for detailed calculations.

Hypertonic Crystalloid Solutions

Hypertonic saline (HS) is the most commonly used hypertonic crystalloid solution, and it is typically used as 7.2% NaCl (23% NaCl is also available but must be diluted to 7% before use). There are many physiologic advantages of utilizing HS for resuscitation, especially in patients that are euhydrated but hypovolemic. Due to the high osmolality of HS (Osm = 2464 mOsm/L), it will initially improve preload by causing movement of fluid from the interstitial space into the intravascular compartment. This in turn can also reduce tissue edema, which may be of benefit in patients with traumatic brain injury or other parenchymal edema not secondary to cardiogenic shock. In addition to volume resuscitation, HS leads to an increase in cardiac contractility, improved rheology of red blood cells due to reduced viscosity (and therefore better microvascular circulation), and reduction of inappropriate vascular leaking of fluid into the interstitium. Hypertonic saline may also have some anti-inflammatory properties.

Hypertonic saline is typically administered at 2–4 mL/kg, IV, over 5–10 min in all species. HS has the potential to be administered more rapidly than isotonic crystalloids, and thus can more rapidly improve hemodynamic stability, especially in larger animals where it can be difficult to give large fluid volumes quickly. The improved intravascular volume from HS administration leads to normalization of heart rate and blood pressure in acutely hypovolemic animals. Because HS is a crystalloid fluid, the volume improvement will be transient as fluid redistributes (as described for isotonic fluids); however, the rapid stabilization achieved by being able to deliver a relatively small volume of HS will allow time for continued administration of resuscitative fluids or blood products, as indicated. In patients with dehydration, the degree of volume expansion may not be as profound because there is not as much interstitial fluid to translocate into the blood vessels.

In addition to direct volume resuscitation due to the hyperosmolar pull of the fluid, HS is also useful in the treatment of cerebral edema from traumatic brain injury or intracranial disease. If these, the patient may develop increased intracranial pressure. The autonomic nervous system attempts to maintain cerebral perfusion pressure (CPP), which represents the net blood flow supplying the brain with oxygen and nutrients. The CPP is the difference between the mean arterial pressure (MAP) and the intracranial pressure (ICP). In other words, the difference between the average pressure pushing blood into the brain (i.e., MAP) and that opposing blood inflow (i.e., ICP). This is represented by

$$CPP = MAP - ICP \tag{7}$$

ICP is determined by the contents within the skull, which is a fixed (nondistensible) vault/container. The intracranial components include the brain, cerebral spinal fluid, and blood within the vasculature. Cerebral edema describes a condition of increased brain interstitial water content. This edema increases the ICP because of the increase in volume within a fixed space. Hypertonic saline exerts an osmotic effect to reduce cerebral edema and thus decrease ICP and improve CPP. Although the hemodynamic effects of HS dissipate rapidly within 20–40 min post-infusion, as with other crystalloids, the reduction of intracranial hypertension may persist for two hours or more.

Hypertonic saline is relatively contraindicated in patients with severe dehydration or hypernatremia, as well as in patients that cannot tolerate acute volume expansion (e.g., those with heart disease and risk of congestive heart failure). Under anesthesia, an HS bolus should be administered slowly over 10–15 min to minimize vasodilation and subsequent hypotension that occurs as a renal response to elevated plasma sodium. Although this effect is transient, if the anesthetist is already battling hypotension in their patient, it may be undesirable.

Concept Box 16.5
Worked example of handling a patient in shock.

A 10-year-old, 30 kg, male neutered Golden Retriever presents to your clinic for acute collapse. On intake, he is quiet but minimally responsive and his heart rate is 180 beats per minute with fair pulse quality, respiratory rate is 60 breaths per minute, temperature is 97.5 °F (36.4 °C) with pale pink mucus membranes, and a capillary refill time of three seconds. He has a palpable fluid wave in his abdomen, which appears as blood when sampled (PCV 26% and total solids 4.0 g/dL). His peripheral PCV is 36% with a total solids of 4.8 g/dL and lactate concentration of 5.2 mmol/L. His Doppler blood pressure is 60 mmHg. What type of shock do you suspect that he is in? Is it compensated or decompensated? What would your initial fluid resuscitation plan be if you were to use hypertonic saline?

Answer: Compensated hypovolemic shock; administer hypertonic saline 60–120 mL IV over 10–20 min, followed by isotonic crystalloids at 20–30 mL/kg IV. It is likely that administration of blood products (red blood cells and plasma) will be needed to optimally stabilize the dog before surgery (to definitively stop the intra-abdominal hemorrhage). Surgery should not be delayed unnecessarily, and normotension is not the goal in this situation. In cases of ongoing hemorrhage, permissive hypotension (SAP > 80 mmHg) may be tolerated briefly until definitive therapy (i.e., surgery) can be instituted to stop the hemorrhage, after which full resuscitation can be completed.

Synthetic Colloids

Colloids are fluids designed to improve osmotic pressure within the vasculature and are isotonic solutions with larger-molecular-weight compounds added (usually carbohydrates) to increase the oncotic pressure of the fluid. Theoretically, intravascular retention of fluids is improved through increased osmotic pressure (Equation (5)). Colloid administration can lead to a sustained expansion of intravascular volume with slower redistribution of the fluids compared to crystalloids. Common compounds used in colloid solutions are hydroxyethyl starches (HES), gelatins, or dextrans of varying sizes. Fluids with HES are characterized by the concentration of HES listed as a percentage, molecular weight (MW) of the carbohydrate, degree of substitution, and the C2/C6 ratio (which refers to the preferential hydroxyethylation site at the glucose subunit carbon atoms). For example, 6% Hetastarch 650/0.7/13.4:1 indicates a 6% Hetastarch solution, with a starch MW of 650 kDa that is 70% substituted with a 13.4 to 1 ratio of C2:C6 substitutions. Colloid solutions are frequently made with 0.9% NaCl as a carrier solution although some use a modified Hartmann's solution.

Commercially available solutions are available as concentrations between 3 and 6%, with a greater colloidal osmotic potency at higher concentrations. The MW of the product reported on the bag is the average molecular weight, but the molecular weight can vary greatly, ranging between 10 and 10 000 kDa within a bag. In general, colloids with a higher average MW will have a longer plasma half-life due to delayed excretion and breakdown of the larger molecule by the kidneys and endogenous amylase. Importantly, products with slower degradation can also result in prolonged adverse effects, such as alterations in coagulation. Smaller and less complex colloids have an increased theoretical maximum volume of administration. Currently, a maximum daily volume of 20 mL/kg for higher MW HES (e.g., >600 kDa) and 40 mL/kg for lower MW HES (e.g., tetrastarch 130/0.4) is recommended. An overview of the properties of examples of synthetic colloids is included in Table 16.2. During anesthesia, synthetic colloids may be used to obtain a longer duration of action of volume expansion (4 mL/kg IV over 20 min) or for patients with panhypoproteinemia as a maintenance fluid (1–2 mL/kg/h) in place of isotonic crystalloids.

Table 16.2 Synthetic colloid fluids that can be used for resuscitation.

Fluid type	Concentration (%)	MW (kDa)	C2/C6 ratio	Degree of substitution	Recommended daily dose (volume or dose/kg)	Persistence in the body (days)
Tetrastarch	6–10	130	9:1	0.4	50 mL	2–3
Hetastarch	6	600–670	4–5:1	0.75	20 mL	5–6
Pentastarch	6–10	70–200	3–5:1	0.4–0.5	33 mL	5–6
Dextrans	6–10	40–70			1.5 g	28–42
Gelatins	3–5	30				2–7

C2/C6 ratio: the preferential hydroxyethylation site at the glucose subunit carbon atom binding of carbon 2 compared to carbon 6.

Following administration of HES, most of the colloid (70%) is processed by the kidneys and excreted in the urine. However, the remainder is either taken up by tissues or excreted in the bile. Dogs appear to have a more rapid elimination of some products (e.g., 7% HES 450/0.75) compared to humans due to elevated alpha-amylase activity, and the lower-molecular-weight HES products are excreted more rapidly. Hydroxyethyl starch administration may cause interference when using a refractometer to estimate total plasma protein, causing the value to approach 4.5 g/dL, but this does not appear to happen after short-term IV use. Additionally, urine specific gravity can be elevated for up to three hours after administration of an IV bolus of HES. Due to intravascular volume expansion, dogs may briefly have increases in heart rate and blood pressure following IV boluses of synthetic starches due to increased right atrial pressure and the Bainbridge reflex.

The use of synthetic colloids is not without risk. Two major areas of concern have been identified in human and veterinary patients. The administration of HES and other synthetic colloids has been associated with the development of coagulopathy as the molecule impairs primary hemostasis. The mechanism of platelet dysfunction may be a direct effect or through interference with normal function of von Willebrand factor (vWF) and coagulation factor VIII. Synthetic colloids may also be associated with accelerated fibrinolysis as integration into clots may weaken the final clot strength. Prolonged prothrombin and activated partial thromboplastin times have also been demonstrated following administration of HES, primarily demonstrated with in vitro experiments. Furthermore, if large doses are given, then as with crystalloids, a hypocoagulopathy can be caused by hemodilution of platelets and clotting factors. All of these effects resolve more rapidly when smaller MW HES solutions are used due to more rapid clearance.

The second concern with the use of synthetic colloids is the development of osmotic nephrosis, which is the accumulation of the carbohydrate molecule within the renal tubular cells. This has been associated with acute kidney injury (AKI) caused by tubular necrosis in human patients with sepsis treated with HES. In these cases, HES was used for resuscitation and for up to five days. These patients had a 1.5 times increased incidence of AKI compared to patients resuscitated with crystalloids. This evidence suggests that using HES during maintenance fluid therapy is not recommended. Low doses of HES (e.g., 2–6 mL/kg as IV bolus), such as would be used for volume expansion during anesthesia, have not been found to be associated with acute kidney injury, and the impacts in veterinary species are still unclear. In human medicine, a clear benefit to resuscitation with synthetic colloids as compared to crystalloids has not been shown, but this specific data is lacking for veterinary species. In addition, within the veterinary field, there are fewer options for colloid-based resuscitation (specifically in the use of species-specific albumin products; see the following section), and so the use of synthetic colloids remains relevant.

Natural Colloids

In addition to synthetic colloids, there are numerous natural colloids available (Table 16.3). For the purposes of pre-anesthesia and intra-operative stabilization, the most relevant products are albumin and fresh frozen or stored plasma. Historically, albumin was available as a human derived product. However, the use of human albumin in healthy dogs has been associated with severe life-threatening reactions. Although these reactions had not been definitively observed following administration of human albumin to critically ill veterinary patients, the commercial availability of canine albumin has decreased use of human albumin. Canine albumin is commercially available in the United States, with variable availability in other countries. Because the product is lyophilized, it may be reconstituted to different concentrations. Plasma in healthy animals (and thus in frozen plasma products) is approximately 5% albumin (0.05 g/mL [5 mg/dL] of albumin), and this concentration is preferred for administering canine albumin. Higher concentrations of albumin may be administered; however, the strong oncotic effect will result in fluid shifts into the vasculature and can cause significant intravascular volume expansion. The administration of 450 mg/kg of albumin is expected to result in an albumin increase of 0.5 g/dL, and most animals receive between 0.5 and 1.5 g/kg in a typical transfusion (the currently available canine product is supplied as a 5 g vial).

Alternatively, plasma (either as fresh frozen plasma [FFP] or stored plasma) may be considered for oncotic support. In general, plasma administration will not significantly change serum albumin concentrations. In order to increase serum albumin concentration by 1 g/dL, a patient would require 45 mL/kg of plasma. This is not practical and would lead to volume overload. However, there is some evidence that natural colloids have beneficial effects on the endothelial glycocalyx and for the treatment of vascular leak syndromes even without a significant increase in serum albumin concentration. Fresh frozen plasma administration is indicated in patients with coagulopathy due to the depletion or lack of production of soluble coagulation factors. Typically, doses of 10–20 mL/kg of plasma are administered to patients with coagulopathy, with reassessment of coagulation parameters following transfusion. Plasma products are type-specific for the dog erythrocyte antigen 1 (DEA 1) and should be thawed

Table 16.3 Natural colloids that can be used during resuscitation.

Natural colloid	Content	Indications	Contraindications	Risks
Fresh whole blood	RBCs, WBCs, platelet, coagulation factors, Ig, and albumin	Coagulopathy with anemia; active bleeding with thrombocytopenia	Volume overloaded and hemoconcentrated/ polycythemic	TRALI TACO NFHTR
pRBCs	RBCs and some plasma	Decreased oxygen-carrying capacity	Severe heart disease	
Fresh frozen plasma	Coagulation factors, albumin, alpha-2 macroglobulines, Ig, and ATIII	Liver failure, DIC, pancreatitis? Parvovirus?	Lack of coagulopathy Minor or major crossmatch reaction Previous transfusion reaction to that donor Concern for volume overload (severe RF or CHF)	NFHTR
Frozen plasma	FII, FVII, FVIII, FIX, FX, and vWF	Rodenticide toxicity for vitamin K antagonists		
Cryo-supernatant	Albumin, globulin, ATIII, protein C, protein S, FII, FVII, FIX, FX, FXI, and FXII			
Cryoprecipitate	FXIII, FVIII, fibrinogen, fibronectin, and vWF	vWF deficiency and hemophilia A		
Cryo-poor plasma	FII, FVII, FIX, and FX	Vitamin K–dependent coagulopathy		
Platelet-rich plasma	Platelets and some coagulation factors		1U/10kg	Questionable platelet efficacy NFHTR
Cryopreserved canine platelet concentrate	1U/10 kg increases platelets 20K	Thrombocytopenia with bleeding	Adequate platelets/no coagulopathy or high risk	NFHTR
Serum	Immunoglobulins	Failure of passive transfer	Immunogenic response	Ineffectiveness
Canine albumin	5%	Oncotic support		Volume overload
Human albumin	20% human albumin	Oncotic support	Competent immune response	Anaphylactoid reaction, hypersensitivity type II reactions, and death
IVIG	10% Human IVIG	ITP, IMHA? SARDS?	Non-immune-mediated disease	Very expensive

RBC: red blood cells; WBC: white blood cells; Ig: immunoglobulins; TRALI: transfusion-related acute lung injury; TACO: transfusion-associated circulatory overload; NFHTR: febrile nonhemolytic transfusion reactions; ATIII: antithrombin III; DIC: disseminated intravascular coagulation; F (roman number): coagulation factors; vWF: von Willebrand factor; IVIG: intravenous immunoglobulin; RF: renal failure; CHF: congestive heart failure; 1U: one unit (100–200 mL per bag).

slowly under controlled conditions before administration (excessive heat during thawing can denature the proteins). It is reasonable, if the blood type of the recipient is known, to administer type-matched plasma although the consequences of administration of mismatched plasma are not predicted to be severe. In horses, plasma is used in foals to treat failure of passive transfer, and specific hyperimmune plasma can be used to prevent rhodococcus pneumonia in susceptible foals. In adult horses, specific hyperimmune plasma can be administered as a component of treatment for Salmonellosis and acute diarrhea. In horses with enterocolitis, the use of plasma was associated with better outcome compared to treatment with hetastarch (HES 600/0.7). Plasma may also be used to support coagulation in horses with coagulopathy. Plasma may be used specifically to raise albumin in horses; however, this requires similar large volumes as in small animal therapy.

Cryoprecipitate is a product derived from FFP with high concentrations of von Willebrand factor, factors V and VII, and fibrinogen. Transfusion with cryoprecipitate is indicated for the treatment of von Willebrand disease and hypofibrinogenemia, and it should be given before surgery in patients with low circulating concentrations of vWF to prevent excessive hemorrhage during the procedure. Due to the low volumes typically administered, cryoprecipitate is not expected to result in significant oncotic effects.

While the production of blood and plasma products is outside the scope of this chapter, the following section reviews recommended monitoring associated with transfusions, which should be performed with administration of any blood product, whether they are plasma-based or contain RBCs.

Concept Box 16.6
Worked example of administering stored plasma.

A five-year-old, 10 kg, male neutered standard Dachshund presented three days after ingestion of a vitamin K antagonist rodenticide. At admission, he is tachycardic (HR 160 bpm), eupneic (20 rpm), normothermic (99.5 °F; 37.5 °C) with hyperdynamic pulse quality. Intake laboratory work shows that his PCV is 35%, TS 5.8 g/dL, and his PT and PTT are too high to read. How much stored plasma would you want to administer prior to rechecking his clotting times?

Answer: 150–200 mL plasma over four hours

Blood Products

Products containing red blood cells, including pRBC and WB, are indicated to increase blood Hb concentration and therefore DO_2. The use of blood products depends upon availability and demonstration of a need for the transfusion of RBCs to a patient. This requires identification of "transfusion triggers" and determining that the potential benefits of administration outweigh potential risks. In the typical patient, an Hct >20% is generally associated with adequate DO_2; however, this is not a strict rule. In reaching a decision to give a transfusion, it is more important to evaluate if the patient has clinical signs resulting from anemia. With acute, massive (>30–40% blood volume) hemorrhage, there is a loss of significant blood volume but the measured hematocrit can remain within the reference range, due to splenic contraction. Therefore, even in the presence of a normal Hct, if a patient has a history of hemorrhage that has not responded to other fluid resuscitation efforts (e.g., crystalloids, HS, etc.), then a transfusion may be an appropriate option. By contrast, a cat with chronic kidney disease and reduced erythropoietin production may have an Hct in the 15–20% range. Due to the chronicity and gradual onset of this type of anemia, these patients typically do not require a transfusion to achieve hemodynamic stability. These examples illustrate the limitations of applying a strict numerical transfusion trigger without considering clinical context and clinical signs. Appropriate clinical considerations include evidence of the impact of blood loss and compensatory changes (e.g., tachycardia and hypotension) and responses to fluid resuscitation. Additionally, critically ill patients may have a higher metabolic demand for oxygen and a correspondingly higher oxygen extraction ratio (OER) (see Concept Box 16.1). These patients may be more hemodynamically stable with a higher Hct that supports adequate tissue oxygenation (e.g., Hct of 25–30%). Finally, splenic vasodilation associated with anesthesia may sequester RBCs and cause an animal with compensated anemia to decompensate during anesthesia due to a sudden drop in Hct.

In patients that only need increased oxygen-carrying capacity, administration of pRBC should improve cardiovascular parameters with less risk of volume overload than with WB. However, patients with documented coagulopathy or hypovolemia can benefit from administration of WB (which contains RBC, plasma, and platelets, if fresh). Fresh WB (<24 h from donation), though it has no capacity to improve platelet number, has the added benefit of containing functional platelets that may aid in cessation of hemorrhage secondary to thrombocytopenia or platelet dysfunction. Consideration of concurrent pathologies in patients must also be considered, including the presence of cardiac or pulmonary pathology that may alter the ability of the patient to tolerate a transfusion of WB due to the volume transfused.

A general guideline for transfusion of pRBC is 10 mL/kg, and 20 mL/kg for WB transfusion. For a more accurate calculation:

$$Vol_T = BV \times BW(kg)(PCV_t - PCV_p) / PCV_D \tag{8}$$

where Vol_T is the volume in liters of whole blood or pRBC to be administered, BV is blood volume (90 mL/kg in dogs and 60 mL/kg in cats), PCV_t is the desired or target PCV, PCV_p is the PCV of the patient before transfusion, and PCV_D is the PCV of the donor animal or unit of blood. The PCV of an average unit of pRBC is 65%, which can be used as an estimate in this equation if an exact measure is not available.

Transfusion reactions are immunologic or other harmful reactions attributed to transfused blood products. Before administration of blood products, the donor and recipient should be blood typed and screened for transmissible diseases (see the American College of Veterinary Internal Medicine consensus guidelines for specific information for donor screening in your location). In addition, deficiencies in blood product storage (e.g., improper refrigeration) can result in adverse events.

Common blood types for veterinary species are listed in Table 16.4. Incompatible transfusions can be associated with mild to severe immunologic adverse reactions. While some clinics maintain a group of donor animals to provide blood for transfusion, commercial blood banks also provide blood and components for transfusion. A list of commercial blood banks is provided in Table 16.5.

To determine compatibility between donor and recipient, a crossmatch is performed. A major crossmatch combines serum from the recipient with the RBCs of the donor and tests for antibodies in the recipient's plasma against the donor cells. These antibodies may be present without previous exposure or can be induced by prior transfusions (patients usually develop antibodies three days following administration of the first transfusion). A minor crossmatch evaluates for antibodies in the donor's plasma directed against the recipient's RBCs. The latter is important when giving WB or plasma products. There are various commercially available kits that can be used in the clinic setting, or the components can be combined by the practitioner and observed for signs of RBC hemolysis or agglutination. A major crossmatch incompatibility dictates that the tested blood should not be transfused to the patient and an alternative donor tested. Minor crossmatch incompatibility can be addressed by using a more compatible donor or using washed pRBC.

In general, and if time allows, blood typing is recommended before administering blood products. Dogs can typically receive one transfusion without crossmatching or blood typing before encountering complications; however, canine patients are still at risk of developing a transfusion reaction with the first transfusion due to preexisting antigens (e.g., the *Dal* antigen). Horses can also typically receive a single blood transfusion before necessitating blood typing and crossmatching. In contrast, blood typing is mandatory for cats before blood product administration, and a crossmatch is strongly recommended, as administration of the inappropriate blood type to a cat may be fatal. Additionally, crossmatched compatible RBCs have a longer circulating half-life than those with minor incompatibilities. Blood typing in cats identifies A, B, and AB blood types; however, there is not currently a cage-side test that evaluates for the *Mik* antigen, so it is advisable to always perform a crossmatch in cats. Cats can receive a single xenotransfusion (i.e., blood from a dog) in their lifetime without repercussions. However, if they are exposed again to canine blood products, a transfusion reaction may be fatal. Similarly, compatibility of a horse to donkey blood would need to be confirmed with a crossmatch due to the potential of the presence of an antigen (donkey factor) in the donor. When choosing a blood donor for horses, it is advisable that they are Aa and Qa negative to reduce the risk of adverse events. Ruminants in theory can also typically receive a first transfusion without adverse effects; however, donors should be screened to be J negative. Crossmatching is not

Table 16.4 Blood types in domestic species. Blood types in bold are the ones of major focus.

Species	Blood types	Best donor	Miscellaneous
Dog	**DEA 1.1 and 1.2**, DEA 2–8, Dal, Kai-1, and Kai-2	DEA 1.1 neg	Most dogs can tolerate a single transfusion
Cat	**A, B, AB**, and *mik*	Having separate type A and B donors >5 kg Amenable to phlebotomy	Must be blood typed Never give A blood to B cat
Equine	**A**, C, D, K, P, **Q**, U, and T	Morgan gelding	30+ blood groups and these are major
Donkey	Donkey factor		
Bovine	A, B, C, F, **J** (lipid), L, M, R, S, T, and Z	Well conditioned and good temperament Not in mid- to late-term pregnancy	11 major acquire antigens in first 6 months of life
Goats	A, B, C, M, and J		
Sheep	A, **B (polymorphic)**, C, D, M, **R (soluble)**, and X		
Ferret	None		

Table 16.5 Commercial blood banks.

Resource	Website	Location	Email	Phone
The USA				
Blue Ridge Veterinary Blood Bank	https://www.brvbb.com	260 Shepherdstown Court Purcellville, VA 20132	BRVBBProducts@gmail.com	(540) 507-2940
HemoSolutions	https://www.hemosolutions.com	3890 Village Seven Road Colorado Springs, CO 80917	melissa@hemosolutions.com	(719) 380-1900 1 (800) 436-0219
Nine Lives Blood Services	https://www.catbloodbank.com	819 Brookside Lansing, MI 48912	aliceparr56@gmail.com	(517) 367-6050
The Veterinarians' Blood Bank	http://www.vetbloodbank.com	3849 South State Road 135 Vallonia, IN 47281	info@vetbloodbank.com	877-838-8533
Hemopet	https://www.hemopet.org	11561 Salinaz Avenue Garden Grove, CA 92843	info@hemopet.org	(714) 891-2022
Animal Blood Resources International	https://www.abrint.net	PO Box 609Stockbridge, MI 49285	customerservice@abrint.net	800-243-5759
PLASVACC USA	https://plasvaccusa.com	1535 Templeton Road Templeton, CA 93465	office@plasvaccusa.com	1-800-654-9743 (805) 434-0321
North American Veterinary Blood Bank	https://www.navbb.com	7951 Gainsford Ct #115B Bristow, VA 20136	donate@navbb.com	(703) 574-7417
Association of Veterinary Hematology and Transfusion Medicine	https://avhtm.org	PO Box 1234 Sahuarita, AZ 85629-1004	info@avhtm.org	(844) 430-4300
Northwest Veterinary Blood Bank	https://nwveterinarybloodbank.com	720 Virginia Street Bellingham, WA 98225		(360) 752-5554
Australia				
PLASVACC	http://plasvacc.com	6066 Cunningham Highway Kalbar Queensland 4309 Australia	plasmail@plasvacc.com	+61 7 5463 7600

recommended as there is a much less robust agglutinating antibody response in cattle. Small ruminants and camelids have a low frequency of adverse transfusion events; however, crossmatching could be considered to reduce the frequency of adverse events.

Blood products should be stored in dedicated refrigerators or freezers. Whole blood and pRBC should be stored at 1–6°C. These products should be gently mixed daily by rotating the bag, and the products evaluated daily for evidence of discoloration, breaks in the bag, and appropriate equipment function. With storage, blood products undergo biochemical and biomechanical changes that alter the longevity of the product following administration, including alterations of energy stores (ATP), decreased 2,3 DPG (2,3-diphosphoglycerate, important for oxygen offloading from Hb and delivery to tissues), oxidative damage to the cells, ammonia buildup as it is released from aged red blood cells, and alteration of cell shape. Together, these changes are referred to as "storage lesions." Plasma should be separated and frozen within eight hours of collection. When stored at −30°C, clotting factors (II, VII, VIII, IX, X, and vWF) remain active for a year. At −20°C, the proteins begin to degrade after six months. Certain coagulation factors (mainly the vitamin K–dependent factors II, VII, IX, and X) remain active in frozen plasma for four years (after the first year, it is no longer characterized as FFP but as stored plasma). Before administration, plasma products should be gently warmed to 37 °C (98.6 °F) using a recirculating warm water bath. This process may take 30 min or longer and should not be rushed as overheating of the product will denature the proteins and make the product ineffective. Plasma may occasionally be stored refrigerated in practices which have a frequent need. When refrigerated, plasma undergoes a significant decrease of coagulation protein activity within two weeks but remains useful for resuscitation.

Blood products should be administered through a filter via gravity filtration. Products that contain red blood cells should ideally never be passed through an electronic pump as the pressure within the pump mechanism can damage the cells. For small transfusion volumes, a syringe pump with 20 μm filter can be utilized. The filter is important to remove microthrombi that may be present. Blood products should be handled with aseptic technique to minimize the risk of bacterial contamination, and once the blood product bag is connected to an infusion set, the blood should ideally be administered within four hours. When smaller volumes are being administered (i.e., partial units of blood), an aliquot may be removed aseptically from the collection bag, administering that amount within four hours; the remainder of the unit may be used within 24 h as long as it is appropriately refrigerated between uses.

Patients should be monitored closely to observe for transfusion reactions. Blood products should initially be administered slowly (a common approach is an initial rate of 15–30% that of the final planned rate) with rectal temperature, physical examination, heart and respiratory rates, and blood pressure monitored every 15 min; if no reactions are noted with initial slow infusion (over 30–45 min), then the transfusion rate may be increased in order to complete it in four hours (or up to six hours in patients at risk of volume overload). The volume of the infusion is divided over the duration to obtain an hourly rate. The initial rate should be half the calculated hourly rate for the first 15 min. If there is no evidence of transfusion reactions, the infusion rate may be increased to the calculated rate.

The most common transfusion reactions are *febrile non-hemolytic transfusion reactions* (FNHTR), which are defined as an increase in body temperature by 1 °C. These reactions are typically self-limiting and are more common with blood products that have been stored longer (due to storage lesion) or are not leukoreduced (when white blood cells are removed in processing). If FNHTR occurs, the transfusion should be slowed, and the patient should continue to be monitored closely. Urticaria (cutaneous hives) may also be seen and are typically self-limiting. Hives may resolve with slowing of the transfusion, but should they persist, corticosteroids and/or antihistamines can be considered to treat the likely type I hypersensitivity reaction. Though uncommon with appropriate pre-transfusion screening, the more dangerous transfusion reaction is an acute immunologic transfusion reaction, which leads to rapid irreversible changes in the red blood cells and subsequent hemolysis of the transfused RBCs. It leads to a rapid progressive anemia and hyperbilirubinemia and may be fatal. If pigmenturia (indicating hemolysis) or signs of shock occur during the transfusion, it should be immediately discontinued and supportive care should be initiated. This should be tailored to the patient and may include administration of a different crossmatched blood product, fluid therapy, oxygen supplementation, or other measures as appropriate for the clinical scenario. Antihistamines or steroids are not indicated for prophylactic prevention of transfusion reactions.

Transfusion-associated circulatory overload (TACO) occurs in patients that develop hypervolemia during or as a result of a blood product transfusion and may require treatment with furosemide, oxygen supplementation, and in some instances mechanical ventilation. Additionally, some patients (~3%) receiving a transfusion can develop transfusion-related acute lung injury (TRALI), which is characterized clinically by development of a high-protein noncardiogenic pulmonary edema and clinical signs of dyspnea and hypoxemia. It develops within six hours of a transfusion, secondary to an antibody-mediated reaction causing complement mediated capillary leak within the pulmonary parenchyma. This type of edema is not responsive to diuretics, and patients typically require pulmonary support in the form of oxygen supplementation or mechanical ventilation.

Concept Box 16.7
Worked example of a blood transfusion in a dog.

A three-year-old, 4 kg, male neutered domestic shorthair cat presents to you after being attacked by a dog, sustaining numerous injuries. He initially went to his family veterinarian for stabilization, where he was found to be bradycardic (HR 100 bpm), tachypneic (RR 80 bpm), hypothermic (96 °F; 35.6 °C), with extensive wounds and a suspected femur fracture. He was resuscitated with 30 mL/kg LRS, which improved his vital parameters. He was administered methadone and his wounds were initially cleaned and bandaged prior to referral to your hospital. On presentation to you, his vital parameters included HR 240 bpm with weak pulses, RR 30 rpm, temperature 98.7 °F (37.1 °C), pale mucus membranes, and quiet to dull mentation. His Doppler blood pressure was 90 mmHg and intake laboratory work showed PCV 19% and TS 3.8 g/dL. In order to improve his stability for surgery the following day, you elect to give him a transfusion overnight. What volume of whole blood transfusion should be administered to improve his PCV to 25% and over how long? The donor PCV is 45%

Answer: $Vol_{WB} = (PCV_t - PCV_p)/PCV_D \times BV \times BW = (25 - 19)/45 \times 60 \times 4 = 32$ mL whole blood over four hours.

Hemoglobin-Based Oxygen-carrying Fluids (HBOCs)

There are a number of synthetic HBOCs that have been developed and studied. Oxyglobin is the only product to date that has been commercially available for the veterinary market (although it is currently unavailable). Oxyglobin is made from crosslinked bovine Hb molecules. It is unique in that it does not contain RBCs and can therefore be given without blood typing or crossmatching. It may also be given more than once. It is typically dosed at 10–20 mL/kg but has a strong oncotic effect and can cause vasoconstriction, which may predispose some patients to volume overload. Some of the volume effects can be mitigated through administration as a slow IV constant rate infusion rather than a bolus. Monitoring during and after administration is important although Hct measurement is no longer relevant (as the Hb is now free in the blood, as opposed to contained within RBCs). Hb concentration must be directly measured to evaluate CaO_2. Adverse effects of the HBOCs include discolored mucous membranes, increased central venous pressure and development of circulatory overload, pulmonary edema and pleural effusion, and difficulty interpreting some colorimetric serum chemistry analytes. Vomiting has also been noted in some patients. However, in patients that have received multiple transfusions and are difficult to crossmatch, those in more remote areas where appropriate storage of blood products is challenging, or in species without readily available blood products or donors, Oxyglobin or other HBOCs can be helpful for stabilizing anemic patients.

Considerations for Anesthesia

Pre-anesthetic Period

Every effort should be made to stabilize a patient with relative or absolute hypovolemia before induction of anesthesia. This process will be highly dependent on the type or types of shock present, previous therapies that have been instituted, and response of that patient to interventions. For patients that are in hypovolemic shock, restoration of intravascular volume can be performed using a single product or combinations of crystalloid, colloid, or blood products, as indicated. In some cases (e.g., uncontrolled [ongoing] intra-abdominal hemorrhage), surgery (and thus anesthesia) may be required to fully stabilize the patient. In these cases, the patient should be resuscitated to be as stable as possible before induction of general anesthesia, with the remainder of resuscitation occurring during the procedure. Resuscitation should be focused on discrete endpoints such as normalization (or improvement) in heart rate, blood pressure, mentation, respiratory rate, or blood lactate concentration. In cases of uncontrolled hemorrhage, such as with a bleeding splenic mass, the clinician may tolerate a less than ideal blood pressure (e.g., 80 mmHg systolic arterial blood pressure) until hemorrhage is controlled. This is termed "permissive hypotension" and minimizes the risk of clot dislodgement on tissue that has temporarily stopped bleeding. This transient measure can be considered to minimize ongoing blood loss until hemorrhage is definitively controlled (e.g., splenic vasculature ligated for a bleeding splenic neoplasia). Once hemostasis has been achieved, normalization of blood pressure may be pursued.

Patients with obstructive shock often also require fluid therapy in addition to definitive therapy in order to resolve the obstruction (e.g., decompression of the stomach for GDV or pericardiocentesis for patients with pericardial effusion). In obstructive shock caused by thrombosis, attention should be given to a possible cardiac etiology, and if there is a chance that an animal may have concurrent or borderline cardiogenic shock, IV fluids (and potentially anesthesia) are contraindicated. Cardiogenic shock is usually a condition of hypervolemia and, as such, therapy generally includes diuretic administration or positive inotropic therapy rather than IV fluids and vascular volume expansion (see Chapter 17). Stabilization for animals with hypoxic shock may involve the provision of supplemental oxygen (e.g., through an oxygen cage or nasal cannulae), or anesthesia and mechanical ventilation in severe cases. If shock is due to anemia, blood transfusion is indicated. If arrhythmias are present that are reducing Q, then anti-arrhythmic therapy is recommended before inducing anesthesia, if possible.

For patients with decompensated shock, once adequate volume resuscitation has occurred, the addition of vasopressors and/or inotropes to improve heart rate, SV, and SVR may be necessary. These drugs are given intravenously (ideally through a dedicated or central catheter) and generally as a constant rate infusion. Drugs that lead to improved contractility of the heart and increased heart rate generally exert their effect through agonism of the beta-1 adrenergic receptor, and those that cause peripheral vasoconstriction are agonists at the alpha-1 adrenergic receptor or V_1 receptor. Dobutamine causes dose-dependent beta agonism but can cause tachycardia at excessive doses. In dogs and cats, dopamine at moderate doses primarily provides beta stimulation while alpha agonism predominates at higher doses. Although norepinephrine is primarily used for vasoconstriction via alpha agonism, it can result in mild beta stimulation as well. Similarly, ephedrine, given as a bolus rather than an infusion, causes a release of endogenous norepinephrine stores and transiently results in alpha and beta agonism. Vasopressin has the unique ability to cause vasoconstriction through stimulation of the V_1 receptors in the vasculature regardless of systemic pH, making it the drug of choice for patients with acidosis and hypotension that is refractory to catecholamines. If bradycardia is contributing to hypotension through decreased heart rate caused by vagal tone, the use of anticholinergic drugs such as atropine or glycopyrrolate can be considered. Occasionally, patients may be unresponsive to adequate volume resuscitation and exogenous catecholamine administration as a result of low circulating cortisol concentrations. This condition, termed "relative adrenal insufficiency," requires supplementation with corticosteroids (usually hydrocortisone). Every effort should be made to stabilize a patient before anesthetic induction, as maintenance anesthetics typically depress cardiovascular function, leading to further compromise of DO_2. In patients that are difficult to stabilize, a decision must be made about the degree of urgency for surgical intervention balanced with the likelihood of adverse events that would occur without additional stabilization. An unstable and hypovolemic dog that requires anesthesia for removal of a nonperforating gastric foreign body merits more time for stabilization before anesthesia, while a patient with a GDV or septic peritonitis requires emergent surgery and is more likely to be anesthetized before full stabilization. A summary of vasoactive and inotropic drugs is provided in Table 16.6.

Induction Period

The induction of general anesthesia is the transition to loss of consciousness (anesthesia), and many reflexes are obtunded or lost during this transition. Respiratory rate and tidal volume usually decrease, and patients can be at risk of hypoxemia if an airway is not rapidly secured. Performing pre-oxygenation for three to five minutes by delivering an elevated fraction of inspired oxygen concentration with a facemask before inducing anesthesia can delay the development of hypoxemia for up to three minutes compared to induction without pre-oxygenation. This can provide a valuable safety margin in which to achieve endotracheal intubation in patients at risk of decompensation or at risk of delayed intubation (e.g., brachycephalic dog breeds).

Patients that are in, or have recently been in, a state of shock are more prone to gastrointestinal ileus, which can make them more likely to have nausea, vomiting, and regurgitation. This can increase the risk of aspiration pneumonia, which may compound other organ dysfunction or complicate recovery. Rapid endotracheal intubation and cuff inflation decreases the risk of aspiration. If regurgitation occurs during induction, suction can be used to aspirate contents and allow flushing and suctioning of the esophagus to reduce the chance of developing post-operative esophagitis. Placement of an orogastric tube following intubation may allow the anesthetist to further reduce the risk of aspiration by allowing complete gastric emptying. Post-operative vomiting, and perhaps nausea, may be decreased through the pre-anesthetic administration of an anti-emetic (e.g., maropitant and ondansetron).

Pre-emptive analgesia for surgery (e.g., opioids), aside from reducing the dose of volatile anesthetic necessary to maintain a patient under general anesthesia, also reduces the catecholamine surge associated with pain, which can result in diminished Q, arrhythmias, alterations in respiratory patterns, and increased oxygen consumption.

Table 16.6 Drugs used to support cardiovascular function that are vasopressors or positive inotropes.

Drug	Receptor agonism	Doses (IV)	Negative sequelae	Special notes
Dopamine	Dopaminergic Beta adrenergic Alpha adrenergic	0–5 mcg/kg/min 5–10 mcg/kg/min >10 mcg/kg/min	Can cause bradycardia (high dose)	May be associated with increased renal blood flow
Dobutamine	Beta adrenergic	0–20 mcg/kg/min	Can decrease SVR Tachycardia	At very high doses can have alpha stimulation Drug of choice with dilated cardiomyopathy
Norepinephrine	Alpha adrenergic (predominant) Beta adrenergic	0.1–2 mcg/kg/min	Can decrease DO_2 and increase lactate at high doses	First-line drug of choice with sepsis and relative adrenal insufficiency
Ephedrine	Alpha adrenergic (predominant) Beta adrenergic	0.04 mg/kg bolus	May have no effect in critically ill patients or with repeated dosing	Causes release of endogenous norepinephrine
Vasopressin	Vasopressin-1 (V_1)	0.01–0.08 U/kg/min IV	May cause bradycardia	Works well in acidic blood pH

SVR: systemic vascular resistance; DO_2: delivery of oxygen.

Monitoring the patient during anesthetic induction is important for recognition of alterations in cardiovascular status. Critically ill patients should have electrocardiogram (ECG) leads and a Doppler flow probe placed before inducing general anesthesia. In the absence of a Doppler probe (which is preferred because each heartbeat results in an audible pulse wave sound, providing continuous monitoring), serial oscillometric blood pressure readings can be obtained during induction. In patients that may require multiple infusions and/or may need a dedicated catheter lumen for a blood transfusion, having more than one IV catheter placed improves vascular access options. Multi-lumen catheters may be placed that allow concurrent administration of incompatible fluids. Blood products are anticoagulated with a citrate-containing solution that is prone to precipitation if mixed with calcium or other fluid additives. Therefore, any transfusion should be administered through a dedicated intravenous catheter with no other drugs or infusions delivered through that line.

Many anesthetic drugs alter the function of the cardiovascular system. Certain sedatives, such as a combination of butorphanol and midazolam, may be chosen as premedication or induction adjuncts in patients that are in shock because they produce a neuroleptanalgesic state with minimal systemic cardiovascular effects. Other opioids, such as hydromorphone or fentanyl, can be used instead of butorphanol to provide better analgesia and allow a greater reduction in inhalational anesthetic requirements. Some drug choices are more appropriate in certain species. For example, small ruminants and some pigs can be adequately sedated with benzodiazepine agonists alone, while dogs and cats given a benzodiazepine agonist alone may display paradoxical excitement (although this is less likely if they are very sick [>ASA IV]). Some drugs result in vasodilation (e.g., propofol or alfaxalone given as an IV induction bolus and inhalational anesthetics used during maintenance), while others do not (e.g., ketamine, opioids, propofol, and alfaxalone given as a lower dose constant rate infusion during maintenance). Alpha-2 adrenergic receptor agonist drugs are generally contraindicated in patients that are in shock as these drugs can reduce Q by up to 50%.

It is important to monitor patients after administration of any sedative or anesthetic medications, even more so when they are systemically ill, as applies to patients in shock and those with multiple comorbidities. For example, a patient with hypoproteinemia will have higher concentrations of unbound drug (for highly protein-bound drugs) in the plasma and therefore may require a dose reduction or show more profound adverse effects following administration (the unbound molecules are the molecules that exert the drug effect). These properties should be considered when choosing anesthetic protocols, recognizing that it may be impossible to avoid certain drugs, but the use of a multimodal balanced anesthetic technique (see Chapter 6) can decrease the required doses of individual drugs and ideally the side effects. Ketamine can result in an increase in sympathetic tone and tachycardia, which may be contraindicated in patients with cardiac dysfunction. However, in critically ill patients that no longer have the ability to respond with a sympathetic nervous system surge, ketamine may cause a reduced cardiac output due to a direct depressant effect on cardiac contractility. Thiopental is associated with ventricular bigeminy at higher doses and should be avoided in patients with cardiac disease. Although etomidate is an anesthetic induction drug that causes little cardiovascular depression, it impairs production of cortisol, which can compromise patients with compensatory shock and induce a relative adrenal insufficiency. More detailed discussions of indications and contraindications for specific anesthetic protocols are covered in specific chapters (see Chapters 17–19). Example sedation and anesthetic protocols for various species are provided in Tables 16.7 and 16.8, respectively. Importantly, there is no single protocol that can be utilized for every patient, and the drugs and approach chosen should be considered in the context of underlying pathology, patient demeanor, resuscitation status, and drug availability.

Anesthetic Maintenance

Anesthetic maintenance for patients with shock is directed toward maintaining adequate perfusion to tissues and appropriate analgesia while the primary cause of shock is addressed. In small animals and horses, this is generally abdominal surgery although diverse causes of shock may direct the surgeon elsewhere. Regardless of these factors, while maintenance of anesthesia in healthy animals can generally be accomplished using inhalant anesthetics alone (e.g., isoflurane or sevoflurane), the cardiovascular depressant effects of these drugs may necessitate an alternative approach in patients in shock in order to optimize cardiovascular function. The main cardiovascular side effects of isoflurane and sevoflurane are vasodilation, with some myocardial depression, which can be profound in some patients. Further vasodilation in patients with vasodilatory shock can lead to decompensation and cardiovascular collapse.

A useful approach in reducing the concentration of inhalational anesthetic needed to maintain general anesthesia is to give drugs that facilitate a reduction in inhalational anesthetic requirements ("MAC reduction/sparing"). This can be achieved using drugs with central nervous system (CNS) depressant properties, but without (or with fewer) adverse cardiovascular effects than inhalational

Table 16.7 Drugs used alone or in combination for sedation of animals in shock.

Species	Drug combination	Dose	Benefits	Things to watch for
Dogs/cats	Butorphanol	Up to 0.4 mg/kg IM or IV	Mild sedation and minimal CV effects	May be inadequate alone
	Midazolam	0.1–0.3 mg/kg IM or IV	Minimal CV effects	Possible paradoxical excitation
	± Alfaxalone	0.5–2 mg/kg IM	Predictable sedation	Myoclonus and apnea
Small ruminants	Midazolam	0.3 mg/kg IM or IV	Predictable sedation	Increases appetite
	± Butorphanol	0.2 mg/kg IM or IV	Mild-to-moderate sedation	Not a good single agent
	± Ketamine	0.5–1 mg/kg IV or 2–5 mg/kg IM	Immobilization and maintains oropharyngeal tone/respiratory drive	Tachyarrhythmias with higher doses and potential for hypotension with critically ill
Pigs	Midazolam	0.3 mg/kg IM or IN	Moderate sedation, minimal CV effects, and absorbed nasally	May be inadequate in more healthy pigs
	± Butorphanol	0.2 mg/kg IM	Synergistic with benzodiazepines	Not appropriate for stand-alone sedation
	± Ketamine	5–10 mg/kg IM	Typically makes intractable porcine able to be handled and IV catheter placed	Burned with administration and may be able to intubate with this drug addition
	± Xylazine	0.5–1 mg/kg IM	Synergistic sedation but try to avoid in patients with shock if possible	Decreases cardiac output and may make placement of IV catheters more challenging
Horses	± Acepromazine	10 mg total IM	Mild sedation for standing procedures	May cause vasodilation and hypotension if continuing to general anesthesia
	± Hydromorphone	0.04 mg/kg IM	Good adjunctive analgesia for standing procedures and lasts 8–12 h	May cause excitation if not painful
	Xylazine	0.2–0.7 mg/kg	Rapid onset, predictable sedation	Must titrate to effect in shock, can cause AV block.
	Detomidine	10–20 mcg/kg IV	Rapid onset, predictable sedation, and can continue CRI to effect to maintain standing sedation	Can over sedate and cause collapse, must titrate to effect, and can cause AV block
Small rodents	Butorphanol	2 mg/kg IM		
	Midazolam	2 mg/kg IM		
	± Ketamine	5 mg/kg IM		May facilitate intubation
	± Alfaxalone	1–2 mg/kg IM		May facilitate intubation and myoclonus

CV: cardiovascular; CRI: constant rate infusion; AV: atrioventricular.

anesthetics. A common approach to achieve this goal is with the administration of benzodiazepine agonists, either as a bolus or constant rate infusion (CRI). An alternative approach, or in combination with benzodiazepine agonists, is to give additional analgesic drugs. Potent opioids (e.g., fentanyl), given at higher doses in dogs (e.g., 10–20 mcg/kg/h, as a CRI), can reduce inhalant anesthetic requirements by up to 70%. In very sick dogs and cats, it is possible to maintain general anesthesia with just the combination of an opioid and benzodiazepine agonist. Drugs that may be administered as part of a multimodal anesthetic plan vary between species but include potent opioids, lidocaine (analgesia and CNS depression), ketamine (analgesia), and the intravenous anesthetic drugs (e.g., propofol and alfaxalone). These latter produce less cardiovascular depression when given by CRI but ventilation may need to be supported. Another excellent option to reduce inhalational anesthetic requirements and provide cardiovascular stability is through the use of locoregional analgesia, including epidural analgesia (this may be contraindicated in patients with coagulopathy, hypotension, infection, neoplasia, and local skeletal abnormalities), incisional line blocks, or fascial plane blocks. The substantial decreases in the dose of inhalant anesthetic gained through

Table 16.8 Drug options that can be used during the peri-anesthetic period for animals that have been treated for shock.

Species	Premedication	Induction	Maintenance	Special tips
Dogs	Opioid (choose one) • Fentanyl 2–5 mcg/kg IV • Methadone 0.3 mg/kg IV • Hydromorphone 0.1 mg/kg IV	Induction agent (choose one) • Ketamine 5 mg/kg IV • Propofol 6 mg/kg IV to effect • Etomidate 2 mg/kg IV (reserve for severe cardiac disease)	Volatile anesthetic (choose one) • Isoflurane • Sevoflurane	If intolerant of inhalants, transition to PIVA or TIVA • Propofol 0.05–0.4 mg/kg/min • Alfaxalone 0.05–0.25 mg/kg/min
	Lidocaine 2 mg/kg IV	± Midazolam 0.1 mg/kg	MAC or MIR reduction • Continue infusion of opioid (fentanyl 3–10 mcg/kg/h) or re-dose intermittent opioid (methadone 0.1 mg/kg or hydromorphone 0.05 mg/kg) • Lidocaine 3 mg/kg/h • Ketamine 0.5–1.5 mg/kg/h • Utilize local anesthetic techniques if possible	To maintain blood pressure • Complete volume resuscitation • Use of vasopressors (dopamine, dobutamine, or norepinephrine) • Maintenance crystalloids at 5 mL/kg/h
	Midazolam 0.2 mg/kg IV			
Cats	Opioid (choose one) • Fentanyl 2–5 mcg/kg IV • Methadone 0.3 mg/kg IV • Hydromorphone 0.1 mg/kg IV	Induction agent (choose one) • Ketamine 5 mg/kg IV (do not use with HCM) • Propofol 6 mg/kg IV to effect (if single procedure) • Alfaxalone 3 mg/kg IV to effect (no Heinz body anemia)	Volatile anesthetic (choose one) • Isoflurane • Sevoflurane	If intolerant of inhalants, transition to PIVA or TIVA • Propofol 0.05–0.4 mg/kg/min • Alfaxalone 0.05–0.15 mg/kg/min
	± Midazolam 0.2 mg/kg IV	± Midazolam 0.1 mg/kg	MAC or MIR reduction • Continue infusion of opioid (fentanyl 3–10 mcg/kg/h) or re-dose intermittent opioid (methadone 0.1 mg/kg or hydromorphone 0.05 mg/kg) • Ketamine 0.5–1.5 mg/kg/h (keep low doses with HCM) • Use local anesthetic techniques if possible	To maintain blood pressure • Complete volume resuscitation (smaller blood volume than dogs) • Utilization of vasopressors (dopamine or norepinephrine) • Maintenance crystalloids at 3 mL/kg/h
		Lidocaine 0.1–0.2 mL topically on arytenoids (reduce laryngeal spasm)		

Small ruminants	Midazolam 0.2 mg/kg IV or IM	Ketamine 5 mg/kg IV	Volatile anesthetic (choose one) ● Isoflurane ● Sevoflurane	Challenging intubation ● May need stylet to intubate ● Ensure that $ETCO_2$ produced on monitor corresponds with respiration – digestive gas can transiently produce capnograph reading
	Hydromorphone 0.1 mg/kg IV	± Midazolam 0.1 mg/kg IV	MAC reduction ● Re-dose hydromorphone 0.05 mg/kg or transition to fentanyl CRI 3–10 mcg/kg/h ● Lidocaine 2 mg/kg then 3 mg/kg/h ● Ketamine 0.5–1 mg/kg/h ● Local anesthesia if appropriate	To maintain blood pressure ● Complete volume resuscitation (tend to be more anemic than other species) ● Use of vasopressors (dopamine, dobutamine, or norepinephrine) ● Maintenance crystalloids at 5 mL/kg/h
	± Alfaxalone 1–2 mg/kg IM (if needed for further sedation to place IVC)	± Propofol 2–4 mg/kg IV to effect		Prone to regurgitation, so have suction and oral swab available – consider placement of an ororumenal tube post-intubation
Pigs	Unable to inject ● Detomidine gel 100 mcg/kg in edible substance (peanut butter and honey) until recumbent	May be able to intubate with drugs administered with injectable premeds	Volatile anesthetic (choose one) ● Isoflurane ● Sevoflurane	More difficult to intubate due to anatomy ● Sigmoid flexure ● Diverticulum ● Elongated snout with redundant tissue May need a stylet to intubate
	Able to inject ● Midazolam 0.3 mg/kg IM or IN ● Hydromorphone 0.1 mg/kg IM ● ± Ketamine 5–10 mg/kg IM ● ± Xylazine 0.5–1 mg/kg IM	If not, place IVC then ● Ketamine 5 mg/kg IV ● ± additional Midazolam 0.1 mg/kg IV ● ± Propofol 4 mg/kg IV to effect	MAC reduction ● Re-dose hydromorphone 0.05 mg/kg ● ± Lidocaine 2 mg/kg then 3 mg/kg/h ● ± Ketamine 0.5–1 mg/kg/h ● Local anesthesia if appropriate	Difficult to place IV catheter ● Can use ears and limbs ● Helpful to make nick in skin with needle at insertion point of catheter to reduce burring
	Can consider alfaxalone 1–2 mg/kg in place of ketamine (more useful for smaller pigs)	If unable to place IVC and unable to intubate: ● Administration of sevoflurane 5% in oxygen with a close-fitting mask until relaxation then intubate		To maintain blood pressure ● Complete volume resuscitation (tend to be more anemic than other species) ● Use of vasopressors (dopamine, dobutamine, or norepinephrine) Maintenance crystalloids at 5 mL/kg/h Consider antagonism of alpha-2 agonists (if used) and/or benzodiazepines if recovery is prolonged

(Continued)

Table 16.8 (Continued)

Species	Premedication	Induction	Maintenance	Special tips
Horses	Alpha 2 agonist (choose one) ● Detomidine 10–20 mcg/kg IV ● Xylazine 1.1 mg/kg IV	Ketamine 2.2 mg/kg IV	● Volatile anesthetic (choose one) ● Isoflurane ● Sevoflurane	Blind intubation ● All horses will have some degree of laryngeal trauma with intubation
	Opioid (choose one) ● Butorphanol 0.02–0.03 mg/kg IV ● Hydromorphone 0.04 mg/kg IV	Muscle relaxant (choose 1) ● Midazolam or diazepam 0.05–0.1 mg/kg IV ● Propofol 200 mg (1 bottle) IV per horse ● Guafenesin 50 mg/kg IV	● MAC reductionLidocaine 2 mg/kg bolus over 10 min then 3 mg/kg/h (discontinue 20 min prior to recovery) ● ± Ketamine 0.5–1 mg/kg/h ● ± Xylazine 0.25–0.5 mg/kg/h	Blood pressure maintenance ● Maintenance crystalloids 5 mL/kg/h ● ± Dobutamine 0.5–3 mcg/kg/min ● ± Hypertonic saline 1–2 L per horse ● ± Hydroxyethylstarch 4 mL/kg ● ± Ephedrine ● ± Norepinephrine
			As an alternative to inhalant, TIVA: ● Traditional triple drip (1300 mg ketamine + 650 mg xylazine in 1 L of 5% guaifenesin) given to effect (typically gives an hour of anesthesia) ● Alternative triple drip (1300 mg ketamine + 50 mg midazolam + 650 mg ketamine in 1 L 0.9% NaCl) titrated to effect	Recovery ● Sedation is important to allow time for metabolism of drugs and reduction of inhalant concentration (both inhalant and TIVA) ● Topical phenylephrine in nasal passages for edema (obligate nasal breathers)
Small rodents	Midazolam 1–2 mg/kg IM	If IVC in place: ● Ketamine 5 mg/kg IV ● ± Alfaxalone 2 mg/kg IV titrated to effect	Volatile anesthetic (choose one) ● Isoflurane ● Sevoflurane	Prone to bradycardia and arrest
	Opioid (choose one) ● Butorphanol 1–2 mg/kg IM ● Hydromorphone 0.2–0.3 mg/kg IM	If no IVC in place: ● Tight-fitting mask induction with Sevoflurane 5% in oxygen until relaxation ● Then can maintain with flow-by inhalant titrating to effect or attempt intubation	● MAC reductionLidocaine 2 mg/kg then 3–6 mg/kg/h ● Local anesthesia as appropriate (2–4 mg/kg lidocaine)	Intubation often extremely challenging ● May require scope assistance ● Stylet recommended ● May laryngospasm have topical lidocaine available ● Have very small ETT available ● Consider LMA for rabbits ● Prone to upper airway obstruction/mucus plug formation

± Ketamine 5 mg/kg IM ± Alfaxalone 3 mg/kg IM	Blood pressure maintenance • Maintenance crystalloids 10 mL/kg/h ± dextrose supplementation • If hemorrhage, consider hypertonic saline 2–4 mL/kg IV bolus • Maintain normal heart rate with anticholinergics ± norepinephrine 0.1–0.5 mcg/kg/min Rabbits: • Do not always respond to atropine and therefore can try treat bradycardia with glycopyrrolate • Norepinephrine is the vasopressor of choice May require antagonism to hasten recovery

PIVA: partial intravenous anesthesia; TIVA: total intravenous anesthesia; MAC: minimum alveolar concertation; MIR: minimum infusion rate; HCM: hypertrophic cardiomyopathy; $ETCO_2$: end-tidal carbon dioxide; ETT: endotracheal tube; LMA: laryngeal mask airway; alpha-2 agonist: alpha-2 adrenergic receptor agonists.

a multimodal approach can help to maintain arterial blood pressure and DO_2.

Total intravenous anesthesia (TIVA) refers to an anesthetic that is performed without the use of any inhalational anesthetic. Total intravenous anesthetic protocols are useful in specific circumstances where the usual anesthetic machines cannot be used (e.g., for magnetic resonance imaging, or field anesthesia in horses, or in patients with severe lung injury). Anesthesia is usually maintained with a constant rate infusion of an anesthetic drug (e.g., propofol), a neurolepanalgesic combination (e.g., fentanyl and midazolam), or a combination. In extremely ill canine patients where it is indicated to avoid inhalant anesthesia altogether, TIVA protocols provide a way to achieve adequate anesthesia, analgesia, and muscle relaxation to allow surgery.

As discussed in the preceding sections, blood pressure maintenance during anesthetic maintenance should be individually adjusted for the patient, procedure, and pathogenesis of shock but can include use of IV fluids (colloids, crystalloids, and blood products) to support vascular volume and DO_2. If an animal is receiving positive pressure ventilation during a procedure, the intermittent increases in intrathoracic pressure can impair venous return to the heart, causing variability in the blood pressure with each breath (pulse pressure variation). This phenomenon is more pronounced in hypovolemic animals and can indicate to the anesthetist that hypovolemia is present. Once the anesthetist is satisfied that intravascular volume is appropriate, if hypotension persists due to vasodilation (in the face of appropriate anesthetic depth) without decreasing anesthesia to an unacceptable level, vasopressors may be considered for cardiac output and arterial blood pressure support. If hypotension is secondary to decreased cardiac output, a positive inotrope can also be considered. The choice of vasopressors and inotropes varies with species and with anesthetist preference; some initial suggestions are listed in Table 16.6.

Damage Control Surgery

Damage control surgery refers to the concept of a brief anesthetic and surgery to rapidly stop hemorrhage and address other life-threatening injuries, with the plan to pursue more definitive treatment at a later time, when the patient is more stable. This concept is common in the human medical field for patient management following trauma or in the management of sepsis or other complex pathology, where the patient may not be able to tolerate the extensive intervention and lengthy anesthetic necessary for definitive therapy. However, in veterinary medicine, economics often play a role in necessitating a single surgical event. There may be a place for damage control surgery to aid in stabilization of a patient for transport to a referral hospital, when a prolonged period of travel is required, but its routine use in the veterinary space has not been fully defined.

Questions and Answers

There are more practice questions and answers available for this chapter on the website. Please visit http://www.wiley.com/go/VeterinaryAnesthesiaZeiler.

Questions

1) Total body water is ____________% of body weight, comprised of ____________% intracellular and ____________% extracellular.
   a) 60; 40; 20
   b) 20; 40; 60
   c) 60; 15; 5
   d) 20; 15; 5
2) True/False: Skin tent is a reliable marker of dehydration in all patients.
3) When administering intravenous fluids, we typically want to give fluid that is similar to the type of fluid loss that is occurring in a given patient. With a dog that has ingested playdough, they can develop salt toxicity and have hypotonic fluid (i.e., free water) loss. What type of fluid would be most appropriate for treating this?
   a) Lactated Ringer's solution
   b) Hypertonic saline 7.2%
   c) Synthetic colloid (e.g., Voluven)
   d) 5% dextrose in water

Answers

1) a
2) False
3) d

Further Reading

Blutinger, A.L., Zollo, A.M., Weltman, J., and Prittie, J. (2021). Prospective evaluation of plasma lactate parameters for prognosticating dogs with shock. *J Vet Emerg Crit Care* 31: 351–359.

Boysen, S.R. and Gommeren, K. (2021). Assessment of volume status and fluid responsiveness in small animals. *Front Vet Sci* 8: 630643.

Bruce, J.A., Kriese-Anderson, L., Bruce, A.M., and Pittman, J.R. (2015). Effect of premedication and other factors on the occurrence of acute transfusion reactions in dogs. *J Vet Emerg Crit Care* 25: 620–630.

Cohn, L.A., Kerl, M.E., Lenox, C.E. et al. (2007). Response of healthy dogs to infusions of human serum albumin. *Am J Vet Res* 68: 657–663.

Glover, P.A., Rudloff, E., and Kirby, R. (2014). Hydroxyethyl starch: a review of pharmacokinetics, pharmacodynamics, current products, and potential clinical risks, benefits, and use. *J Vet Emerg Crit Care* 24: 642–661.

Montealegre, F. and Lyons, B.M. (2021). Fluid therapy in dogs and cats with sepsis. *Front Vet Sci* 8: 622127.

Pascual, J.L., Khwaja, K.A., Chaudhury, P., and Christou, N.V. (2003). Hypertonic saline and the microcirculation. *J Trauma* 54: S133–S140.

Walton, R.A.L. and Hansen, B.D. (2018). Venous oxygen saturation in critical illness. *J Vet Emerg Crit Care* 28: 387–397.

Wardrop, K.J., Birkenheuer, A., Blais, M.C. et al. (2016). Update on canine and feline blood donor screening for blood-borne pathogens. *J Vet Intern Med* 30: 15–35.

Wardrop, K.J. and Brooks, M.B. (2001). Stability of hemostatic proteins in canine fresh frozen plasma units. *Vet Clin Pathol* 30: 91–95.

Woodcock, T.E. and Michel, C.C. (2021). Advances in the Starling principle and microvascular fluid exchange: consequences and implications for fluid therapy. *Front Vet Sci* 8: 623671.

Zollo, A.M., Ayoob, A.L., Prittie, J.E. et al. (2019). Utility of admission lactate concentration, lactate variables, and shock index in outcome assessment in dogs diagnosed with shock. *J Vet Emerg Crit Care* 29: 505–513.

17

Approach to a Patient with Cardiac Pathology

Jonathan Lichtenberger, Alicia Skelding, and Daniel Pang

Overview of Cardiac Anatomy and Physiology

The cardiovascular system is composed of two circulations operating in series: (1) the pulmonary circulation, which includes the right cardiac chambers and the lungs, and (2) the systemic circulation, which includes the left cardiac chambers and the other organs. Within each circulation, the ventricles are responsible for pumping blood forward, the arteries and arterioles distribute blood to other organs, the capillaries perfuse these organs and form an exchange system for gases and other substances, and the venules, veins, and atria act as a blood collection and reservoir system.

The key functions of the heart are (1) to provide adequate perfusion, oxygen supply, and other essential substances to all body tissues; (2) to drain blood from the venous system in order for target organs (mainly the lungs, kidneys, and liver) to remove waste products; and (3) to maintain adequate fluid distribution between different body compartments. These key functions are made possible by the electrical activity of the heart and the mechanical response that occurs within the heart. This excitation–contraction coupling allows the heart to contract during systole in order to eject blood into the great arterial vessels and to relax during diastole in order for the heart to fill with blood from the systemic and pulmonary veins. The anatomy of the mammalian heart ensures that blood is always moving forward thanks to the atrioventricular valves (i.e., the mitral and tricuspid valves) located between the ventricles and atria, and the semilunar valves (i.e., the aortic and pulmonic valves) located between the ventricles and great arteries. Figure 17.1 represents the normal cardiac anatomy.

Overview of Cardiac Pathophysiology

Definition of *Heart Disease*

Heart disease describes any condition that causes one of the fundamental functions of the heart to be impaired and can affect the myocardium, the valves, the vessels, the pericardium, the electrical system of the heart, or a combination of these. The term "heart failure" can be used when the patient demonstrates clinical signs of reduced cardiac output and failure of the heart to meet the oxygen and metabolic demands of the body (i.e., forward heart failure), or when the patient demonstrates clinical signs of congestion due to failure of the heart to maintain a balanced circulation (i.e., backward or congestive heart failure). Clinical signs of forward heart failure include lethargy, exercise intolerance, pallor, or syncope, whereas clinical signs of backward heart failure include dyspnea, tachypnea, coughing, abdominal distention, and subcutaneous edema.

Diagnosis of Heart Disease

Physical Examination

Diagnosing heart disease starts with obtaining a thorough history and a meticulous physical examination and cardiac auscultation (see Chapter 2). If possible, these should be performed in a calm environment before anesthesia. The examination should include palpation of the apex beat (i.e., the palpable heart beat on the chest surface), which will identify any potential thrill (i.e., palpable vibration of the chest wall) that would indicate the presence of at least a grade 5/6 heart murmur. While some conditions can be silent on auscultation, most heart conditions in dogs result in the presence of a heart murmur or an arrhythmia. The heart

Fundamental Principles of Veterinary Anesthesia, First Edition. Edited by Gareth E. Zeiler and Daniel S. J. Pang.

Companion Website: www.wiley.com/go/VeterinaryAnesthesiaZeiler

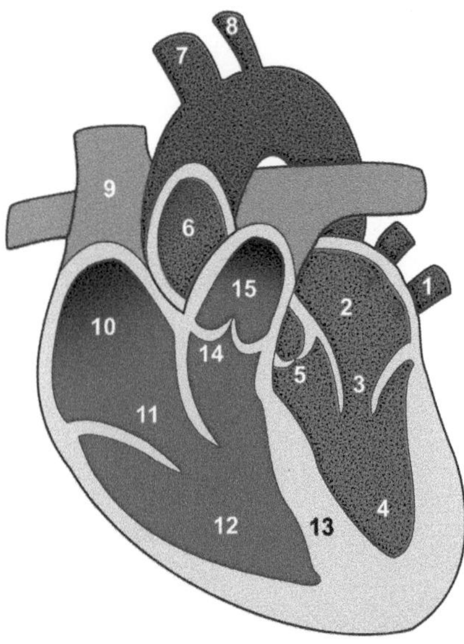

Figure 17.1 Normal cardiac anatomy: 1, pulmonary vein; 2, left atrium; 3, mitral valve; 4, left ventricle; 5, aortic valve; 6, aorta; 7, brachiocephalic trunk; 8, left subclavian artery; 9, cranial vena cava; 10, right atrium; 11, tricuspid valve; 12, right ventricle; 13, interventricular septum; 14, pulmonic valve; 15, main pulmonary artery. The left side of the heart carries oxygenated blood (red). The right side of the heart carries deoxygenated blood (blue).

rate and rhythm can provide useful information regarding the underlying disease process and should be documented. For example, knowing that a coughing dog has a respiratory sinus arrhythmia with a heart rate of 100 beats per minute is valuable information and an indication that the dog is likely not in active congestive heart failure. In contrast, dogs with active congestive heart failure are usually tachycardic due to increased sympathetic tone. Determination of the point of maximal intensity of a heart murmur (i.e., location at which the murmur is best heard), as well as its intensity (see Table 17.1), timing, and duration will help narrow down the differential diagnosis. It is important to note that the grade of a heart murmur does not always correlate with the severity of the underlying disease (online resource: Ettinger SJ (1970) Canine heart sounds. https://blog.wfmu.org/freeform/2007/04/365_days_93_ste.html).

Table 17.1 Grading of heart murmurs.

Grade	Descriptive characteristics
1/6	Very soft and localized heart murmur, and heard in a quiet environment only after careful auscultation
2/6	Soft and localized heart murmur but readily audible when the stethoscope is placed over the point of maximal intensity
3/6	Moderate-intensity heart murmur, usually regional (radiates over an entire area but remains mostly audible on one side of the chest only)
4/6	Loud heart murmur that can be auscultated over several areas (including both sides of the chest) without any palpable precordial thrill
5/6	Loud heart murmur with a precordial thrill
6/6	Very loud heart murmur with a precordial thrill still audible when the stethoscope is slightly lifted off the chest wall

Diagnosing heart disease in cats can be more challenging since some cats with severe heart disease have no auscultatory abnormalities and many cats with a heart murmur have no evidence of heart disease. The presence of a gallop sound (i.e., low-frequency diastolic sound best heard with the diaphragm of the stethoscope) or an arrhythmia is often indicative of myocardial disease in cats.

Heart murmurs are common in horses including both physiological flow murmurs and clinically relevant murmurs. Benign physiological flow murmurs tend to be soft (grade ≤ 3/6), short in duration (early to mid-systolic), crescendo–decrescendo, and best heard over the aortic and pulmonic valve (cranial and dorsal to the apex beat, i.e., forward under the triceps muscle mass). The intensity of physiological murmurs may change with exercise (they may disappear or become louder). Heart murmurs caused by valvular regurgitation are also common and may or may not be associated with valvular pathology. Arrhythmias are very common in horses and may be physiological or caused by a primary electrical disorder, structural heart disease, or systemic disturbances.

Diagnostic Tests

Echocardiography is the best tool to evaluate cardiac morphology and function and to provide a definitive diagnosis of the heart condition. It provides information regarding the dimensions of the cardiac chambers, thickness of the myocardium, valve morphology, as well as systolic and diastolic functions. This test is best performed by a skilled examiner who has a good understanding of cardiac conditions and their hemodynamic consequences. If a comprehensive echocardiogram is not feasible, point-of-care cardiac ultrasound by a trained veterinarian can provide useful information, especially regarding left atrial size and left ventricular contractility. For example, the presence of an enlarged left atrium may indicate that the patient is at high risk of fluid overload. Poor left ventricular contractility in a dog may indicate the presence of dilated cardiomyopathy (DCM).

Thoracic radiography is also useful as a pre-anesthetic test if the patient is experiencing respiratory symptoms or to assess cardiac disease severity if an echocardiogram is not feasible. For example, in a 12-year-old Cavalier King Charles Spaniel with a grade 3/6 left apical holosystolic heart murmur and presumed degenerative mitral valve disease (DMVD), thoracic radiographs can indicate the presence or absence of significant cardiomegaly, as well as signs of pulmonary venous congestion. The vertebral heart score (VHS) can be used to objectively assess cardiac size.

Breed variations in VHS have been documented and should be taken into consideration by the clinician. For example, small, brachycephalic, or chondrodystrophic breeds tend to have VHS ranges that are larger compared to other breeds (Jepsen-Grant et al., 2013).

Electrocardiography (ECG) is the best diagnostic test to evaluate cardiac arrhythmias. The following information can be obtained from a six-lead diagnostic ECG in small animals: heart rate, rhythm, mean electrical axis, and criteria indicating chamber enlargement. However, its sensitivity is poor to identify cardiac enlargement and the ECG should not be used for this purpose primarily. Ideally, a diagnostic ECG in small animals should be obtained in right lateral recumbency with the thoracic and pelvic limbs perpendicular to the trunk. It is important to place all limb leads properly to avoid misdiagnoses. During anesthesia, ECG monitors usually allow the visualization of one to three leads. Heart rate and rhythm are the main parameters assessed by the clinician since the patient's positioning is variable and the amplitude and duration of the different waves cannot be measured precisely. However, some obvious changes in the morphology of the QRS complex, S–T segment, and T wave can be relevant. For example, the development of an S–T segment deviation during a procedure should raise the concern of cardiac hypoxia (assuming that the S–T segment was normal at the beginning of the procedure and that the patient has remained in the same position) (Figure 17.2).

In some animals, ambulatory ECG (Holter monitoring) is necessary to identify intermittent arrhythmias. This is often used in the investigation of syncopal episodes or intermittent weakness for example. In horses, exercise testing often provides valuable information, including the effects of exercise on heart rate, rhythm, or murmur intensity. Some arrhythmias may only be apparent during or following exercise (such as ventricular tachyarrhythmias) or may disappear with exercise (such as second-degree atrioventricular block [AVB] due to high vagal tone).

Finally, cardiac biomarkers, such as N-terminal prohormone brain natriuretic peptide (NT-proBNP) in small animals, can be very useful during the pre-anesthetic assessment. NT-proBNP can be considered in patients for whom cardiac imaging is not possible, particularly if heart disease is suspected or if the breed is at high risk of heart disease. It is especially useful to distinguish cardiac versus respiratory causes of respiratory clinical signs (such as coughing, tachypnea, or dyspnea) (Ettinger et al., 2012; Fox et al., 2009). It can also be useful in asymptomatic cats with a heart murmur or with a genetic predisposition for hypertrophic cardiomyopathy (HCM; Fox et al. 2011). Due to its good negative predictive values, a normal NT-proBNP level indicates no heart disease or only mild heart disease in the majority of cases. Cats with elevated values still require an echocardiogram to obtain a definitive diagnosis. It is important to note that azotemia or hyperthyroidism can cause elevations in NT-proBNP in the absence of clinically significant cardiac disease.

Stages of Heart Disease

The following staging system was developed by the American College of Veterinary Internal Medicine (ACVIM) for the classification of DMVD in dogs (Keene et al., 2019). This system has since been used to describe other cardiac conditions such as dilated cardiomyopathy (DCM) in dogs or HCM in cats, with the aim of providing a framework for prognosis and therapeutic decision-making. It is also helpful to guide the assessment of anesthetic risk when assigning the American Society of Anesthesiologists (ASA) Physical Status Classification System (Figure 17.3). It is important to note that the ASA status is intended to reflect evaluation of the whole patient and is not limited to cardiac disease (see Chapter 2).

Stage A includes patients that are predisposed to heart disease but have no evidence of having developed such disease yet (for example an adult Cavalier King Charles

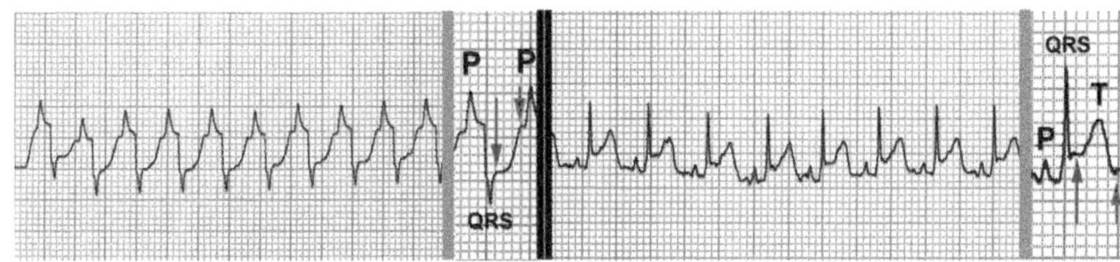

Figure 17.2 S–T segment changes. Left panel: Sinus tachycardia (heart rate, 220 beats per minute) with extreme S–T segment depression. The cat was under general anesthesia and had just received IV meperidine. Meperidine results in histamine release much more frequently than other opioids, and therefore the IV route of administration is typically avoided. The blue arrow indicates the J point (end of the QRS complex), which should be at the same vertical level as the tail of the T wave and baseline (red arrow). The changes resolved spontaneously: 25 mm/s; 1 cm = 1 mV. Right panel: Sinus rhythm (heart rate, 170 beats per minute) with moderate S–T segment elevation. The cat had mild, compensated hypertrophic cardiomyopathy: 25 mm/s; 1 cm = 1 mV. (Source: Reproduced with permission from Côté et al., 2011/John Wiley & Sons).

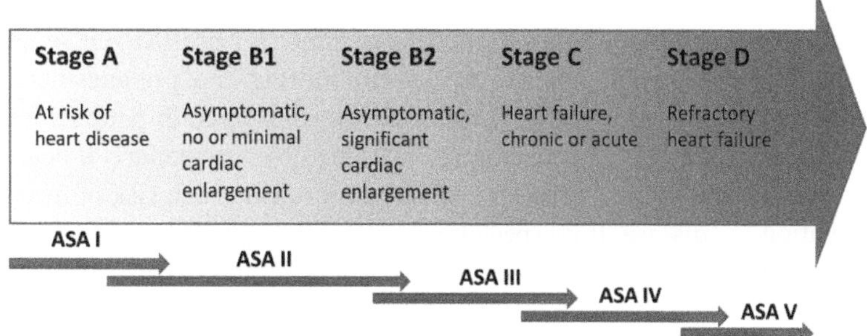

Figure 17.3 The American College of Internal Medicine classification of heart disease and the corresponding American Society of Anesthesiologists Physical Status Classification. Note: Determining ASA status should take into account the whole patient, including comorbidities.

Spaniel with a normal cardiac auscultation). These patients usually belong to the ASA I category, unless insufficient data is available (e.g., incomplete thoracic auscultation or high risk of occult disease such as DCM in Doberman Pinschers), in which case an ASA II category may be assumed.

Stage B includes asymptomatic patients with structural heart disease. This means they have never developed clinical signs of heart failure or other complications (such as aortic thromboembolism in cats). This stage can be further divided into substages. *Stage B1* includes patients with no or minimal echocardiographic or radiographic evidence of cardiac remodeling. These patients have a low risk of developing imminent congestive heart failure. *Stage B2* includes patients with evidence of significant cardiac enlargement. These patients have a higher risk of developing imminent congestive heart failure. Stage B1 patients usually belong to the ASA II category, while stage B2 patients usually belong to the ASA II–III categories (depending on the degree of cardiac changes).

Stage C includes patients with current or past signs of heart failure (and/or signs of aortic thromboembolism in cats). Those patients belong to the ASA III category when their heart failure has been stabilized well with cardiac medications and they have no evidence of other significant complicating factors, such as hemodynamically significant arrhythmias (ventricular tachycardia [VT], atrial fibrillation, and high-grade AVB) or marked pulmonary arterial hypertension. Patients with poorly controlled congestive heart failure or presenting with other complicating factors belong to the ASA IV category and should not be anesthetized until the cardiac disease has been stabilized.

Stage D includes patients with end-stage heart disease, with clinical signs of heart failure that have become refractory to standard treatment. Those patients often belong to the ASA IV–V categories and anesthesia should be avoided if possible.

Valvular Disease

Valvular Insufficiency

Mitral valve insufficiency or regurgitation is a condition in which a percentage of the left ventricular stroke volume is ejected backward, through the mitral valve, into the left atrium during systole (Figure 17.4). This can be caused by a primary valvular condition such as DMVD (also called "myxomatous mitral valve disease"), mitral valve dysplasia (congenital malformation of the valve), valvular endocarditis, or can occur secondary to distention of the mitral valve annulus due to DCM.

Degenerative Mitral Valve Disease in Dogs

Degenerative mitral valve disease is by far the most common cause of mitral valve insufficiency and is the most common heart condition in dogs, especially in aging small-breed dogs (e.g., Cavalier King Charles Spaniel, toy Poodle, etc.).

Degenerative mitral valve disease is usually suspected following auscultation of an adult-onset left apical systolic heart murmur (fifth intercostal space near the costochondral junction). In most cases, progression of the disease is slow and a heart murmur can be identified years before the onset of heart failure. Thus, most dogs with DMVD undergoing anesthesia are asymptomatic. An echocardiogram is necessary to obtain a definitive diagnosis of DMVD, but if the clinical suspicion is high based on historical and clinical data, thoracic radiographs can be adequate to determine disease severity before anesthesia if the dog is asymptomatic.

Anesthetic considerations should be based on the stage and hemodynamic consequences of the disease. Dogs with mild or stage B1 DMVD usually have a mild-to-moderate amount of mitral valve regurgitation and no-to-minimal enlargement of the left-sided cardiac chambers. The risk of fluid overload is considered low at this stage. However,

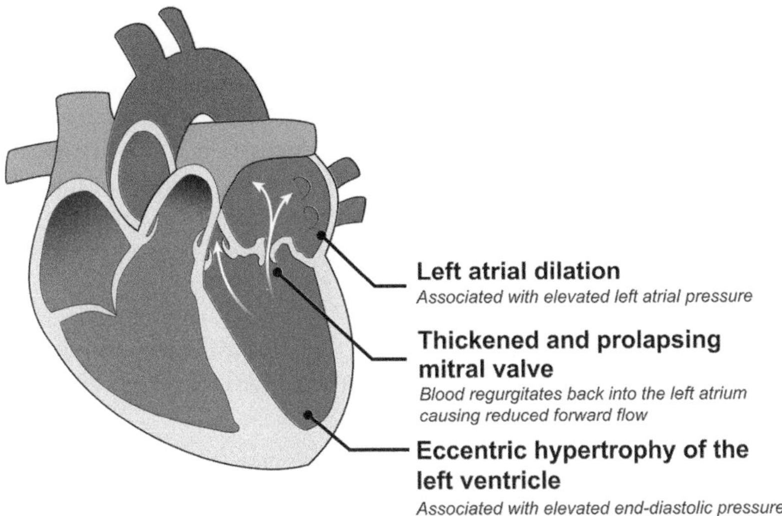

Figure 17.4 Pathophysiology of degenerative mitral valve disease (see the Figure 17.1 legend for anatomical descriptions).

care should be taken to avoid increasing the regurgitant fraction (i.e., the percentage of the total stroke volume that is regurgitating) during anesthesia, which can already be significant in some dogs.

Dogs with moderate or stage B2 DMVD usually have a moderate-to-severe regurgitant fraction (as high as 50–70% of the total stroke volume) leading to volume overload of the left atrium and ventricle. This volume overload results in eccentric hypertrophy (i.e., dilation) of the left cardiac chambers and increases in heart rate and systolic function. These consequences are compensatory mechanisms that help maintain adequate forward stroke volume. While systolic function is typically increased to improve cardiac output, large-breed dogs with DMVD are more prone to experiencing concurrent systolic dysfunction. Regardless of systolic function, myocardial wall stress and oxygen demand are usually minimally increased considering that the left ventricle is ejecting part of the blood into a low-pressure chamber, the left atrium, that offers little resistance to blood flow. The risk of fluid overload is considered increased at this stage and the anesthetic protocol should be adjusted to prevent this.

Anesthetic Management

Dogs presenting for anesthesia with stage B2 DMVD are commonly being treated with pimobendan (a positive inotrope and vasodilator) in order to delay the onset of congestive heart failure. If DMVD is diagnosed shortly before anesthesia and the procedure is not emergent, it is best to start pimobendan (if indicated) a few weeks before the procedure. This medication should be administered the morning of the procedure. Angiotensin-converting enzyme (ACE) inhibitors are sometimes used at this stage of DMVD. If this is the case, they should be withheld the day of the procedure as they have been found to result in greater hypotension that can be more difficult to correct in both dogs and cats (Coleman et al., 2016; Ishikawa et al., 2007).

Goals During Anesthesia

- Maintain left ventricular preload; avoid volume overload
- Maintain or increase heart rate
- Maintain or increase contractility
- Decrease afterload

Left ventricular preload should be maintained to ensure adequate forward flow. However, it is important to avoid volume overload; therefore, management is patient dependent based on volume status, coexisting disease, and volume loss during the procedure. A conservative fluid rate of 3 mL/kg/h of balanced crystalloid is usually adequate in most patients undergoing elective procedures that do not have signs of hypovolemia. A normal to high-normal heart rate is beneficial to maintain appropriate cardiac output. Bradycardia with mitral insufficiency is detrimental because it increases left ventricular volume. This increase in volume distends the mitral valve annulus, leading to increased mitral regurgitation. Similarly, adequate contractility will promote forward stroke volume and decrease the regurgitant fraction. Reduction in afterload improves forward stroke volume by decreasing the left ventricular pressures required for the ejection of blood into the aorta and by decreasing the regurgitant fraction.

The choice of anesthetic and analgesic protocol is typically dictated by the procedure and patient demeanor. Opioids are a good choice in this patient population as they have minimal cardiovascular effects. Mixed-agonist/

antagonist opioids (butorphanol and nalbuphine) are reasonable sedatives for noninvasive procedures. Full-*mu* agonist opioids provide excellent analgesia in dogs and cats, and are inhalant-sparing, more consistently in dogs. However, it is important to be aware that pure-*mu* agonist opioids can cause significant sinus bradycardia and bradyarrhythmias, which may require treatment (to optimize heart rate). If an additional sedative is needed, low-dose acepromazine (0.01–0.03 mg/kg, intramuscularly [IM]) can be used in dogs with mild (stage B1) DMVD because these patients tend to tolerate the decrease in afterload (Saponaro et al., 2013). Theoretically, any vasodilation resulting from acepromazine will also decrease preload (reduced venous return), which may not be tolerated in advanced stages of DMVD or hypovolemic animals. Alpha-2 adrenergic receptor agonists should be avoided because of the increase in afterload and subsequent bradycardia that they cause (Flacke et al., 1993; Saponaro et al., 2013), which can increase the regurgitant fraction and decrease forward stroke volume. An example premedication could be (1) butorphanol (0.2–0.4 mg/kg) + acepromazine (0.01–0.03 mg/kg, IM) for nonpainful procedures, and (2) hydromorphone (0.03–0.05 mg/kg, IM) or methadone (0.1–0.3 mg/kg, IM) + acepromazine (0.01–0.03 mg/kg, IM) for painful/surgical procedures in dogs with stage B1 DMVD (see Table 17.2).

Table 17.2 Summary table of anesthetic recommendations for dogs with degenerative mitral valve disease.

	Stage of degenerative mitral valve disease				
Anesthetic stage	**Stage A**	**Stage B1**	**Stage B2**	**Stage C**	**Stage D**
Premedication	Any, as long as appropriate patient evaluation has been completed	Opioid ± acepromazine	Opioid	Opioid, as dictated by patient	Opioid, as dictated by patient
Induction		Co-induction (e.g., alfaxalone/ propofol + midazolam)	Co-induction (e.g., alfaxalone/ propofol + midazolam)	Neuroleptic: opioid + benzodiazepine	Neuroleptic: opioid + benzodiazepine
Maintenance		Balanced approach (e.g., inhalant ± opioid CRI ± locoregional anesthesia)	Balanced approach (e.g., inhalant ± opioid CRI; ± lidocaine CRI in dogs ± locoregional anesthesia)	Balanced approach (e.g., inhalant + agents to decrease inhalant requirements)	Balanced approach (e.g., inhalant + agents to decrease inhalant requirements)
Support	Balanced crystalloid (5 mL/kg/h)	Balanced crystalloid (3–5 mL/kg/h) Heart rate (e.g., anticholinergic); contractility (e.g., sympathomimetic)	Balanced crystalloid (3 mL/kg/h) Heart rate (e.g., anticholinergic); contractility (e.g., sympathomimetic)	Balanced crystalloid (3 mL/kg/h) Sympathomimetic support Advanced anesthetic monitoring is recommended	Balanced crystalloid (3 mL/kg/h) Sympathomimetic support Advanced anesthetic monitoring is recommended
Monitoring	Anesthetic depth (eye position, palpebral reflex, jaw tone, and muscle relaxation) Body temperature ECG (HR + rhythm) NIBP (via Doppler or oscillometry) Pulse oximetry (SpO_2) Capnography ($PETCO_2$)	Anesthetic depth (eye position, palpebral reflex, jaw tone, and muscle relaxation) Body temperature ECG (HR + rhythm) NIBP (via Doppler or oscillometry) Pulse oximetry (SpO_2) Capnography ($PETCO_2$)	Anesthetic depth (eye position, palpebral reflex, jaw tone, and muscle relaxation) Body temperature ECG (HR + rhythm) NIBP (via Doppler or oscillometry) Pulse oximetry (SpO_2) Capnography ($PETCO_2$) ± ETInhalant	Anesthetic depth (eye position, palpebral reflex, jaw tone, and muscle relaxation) Body temperature ECG (HR + rhythm) IBP (via direct arterial catheter) Pulse oximetry (SpO_2) Capnography ($PETCO_2$) ± ETInhalant	Anesthetic depth (eye position, palpebral reflex, jaw tone, and muscle relaxation) Body temperature ECG (HR + rhythm) IBP (via direct arterial catheter) Pulse oximetry (SpO_2) Capnography ($PETCO_2$) ± ETInhalant

Table 17.2 (Continued)

	Stage of degenerative mitral valve disease				
Comments	Will tolerate most anesthetic protocols well if no evidence of cardiac disease	Support is dictated by animal's response to anesthesia	Support is dictated by response to anesthesia *Lidocaine*[a]	Animals should be instrumented with NIBP and ECG before induction of anesthesia Supervision by a board-certified anesthesiologist is recommended	Animals should be instrumented with NIBP and ECG before induction of anesthesia Should not be anesthetized without a board-certified anesthesiologist

CRI: constant rate infusion; ECG: electrocardiogram; HR: heart rate; NIBP: noninvasive arterial blood pressure; SpO_2: peripheral oxyhemoglobin saturation measured by pulse oximetry; $PETCO_2$: partial pressure of expired carbon dioxide; ETInhalant: end-tidal fraction of expired inhalation anesthetic concentration; IBP: invasive arterial blood pressure.

[a] *Lidocaine CRIs must only be used in canine patients.*

Induction of anesthesia can be performed using a co-induction technique to minimize the amount of induction drug required. Alfaxalone + midazolam or propofol + midazolam is well tolerated in this patient population. When using these combinations, it is advisable to start with a low dose of induction drug (alfaxalone or propofol, at one quarter of calculated total dose), immediately followed by the full calculated dose of midazolam (0.3–0.4 mg/kg) to avoid the paradoxical excitement that has been documented if midazolam is given first. Any reduction in cardiac output (bradycardia from opioids and more advanced stages of DMVD) will slow the delivery of injected drugs to the brain (site of action); therefore, additional time should be allowed for drugs to take effect (typically 30+ s longer than in healthy patients, but intubation should be attempted based on the animal's reflexes rather than the amount of time passed). Studies demonstrate that midazolam (0.4 mg/kg, IV) will result in a 24–62% decrease in induction drug dose, depending on premedication and speed of administration of induction drug.

General anesthesia can be maintained using a balanced anesthetic technique with inhalant anesthetics (isoflurane and sevoflurane) ± constant rate infusions of other drugs (such as an opioid ± lidocaine [in dogs] ± midazolam) ± locoregional anesthesia as dictated by the procedure. Continuous anesthetic monitoring is recommended in all patients undergoing general anesthesia and is especially important in animals with cardiac disease (see Table 17.2).

The clinician should be prepared to treat complications such as bradycardia and/or hypotension. Anticholinergic drugs are good choices to treat opioid-induced bradycardia and hypotension. Dobutamine has been demonstrated to attenuate inhalant-induced decreases in contractility in dogs with experimentally induced mitral valve insufficiency (Goya et al., 2018). Sympathomimetics with mixed adrenergic effects (dopamine and norepinephrine) are also appropriate choices for hypotension alone.

Dogs with severe DMVD along with current or previously documented clinical signs of heart failure belong to the stage C group. Left-sided congestive heart failure is characterized by the development of pulmonary edema. Only dogs with well-controlled congestive heart failure (free of pulmonary edema based on clinical signs and thoracic radiographs) should be considered for anesthesia. These patients are at high risk of further decompensation and are more likely to experience other complications during general anesthesia, such as arrhythmias (mostly supraventricular arrhythmias), systolic dysfunction, or pulmonary hypertension. These patients are commonly treated with a loop diuretic (furosemide or torasemide), pimobendan, an ACE inhibitor (benazepril or enalapril), and possibly other diuretics like spironolactone. Referral to a specialty center, or consulting an anesthesiologist (should referral not be possible), should be considered. It is strongly recommended to place monitoring devices (ECG and noninvasive blood pressure [NIBP]) before induction of anesthesia. These patients should be pre-oxygenated if they will tolerate it with minimal stress. These patients often benefit from a neuroleptanalgesic (opioid + benzodiazepine) induction to avoid the cardiovascular changes that can result from bolus doses of induction drugs (Table 17.2). Cardiovascular support (dopamine and dobutamine) should be prepared before induction of anesthesia and may need to be initiated before or immediately following anesthetic induction. Invasive arterial blood pressure (IBP) monitoring is advised. Doses of emergency drugs, and location of resuscitation equipment, should be prepared, and consent regarding cardiopulmonary resuscitation should be confirmed (see Chapter 20).

Finally, dogs with refractory heart failure (stage D) are not appropriate candidates for anesthesia (unless the procedure is necessary for their survival). These patients should be referred to a specialty center and closely monitored in the intensive care unit following the procedure.

Degenerative Valvular Disease in Horses

Valvular regurgitation is common in horses and can be physiological or due to valvular pathology (mostly degeneration causing thickening and prolapse of the valve). The aortic valve is most commonly affected, resulting in a holo-, pan-, or early diastolic murmur best heard over the aortic valve (deep under the triceps muscle in the standing horse). While many affected older horses have mild aortic regurgitation (AR) and remain asymptomatic, moderate-to-severe AR can lead to reduced performance, congestive heart failure, pulmonary hypertension, and arrhythmias. Significant AR is suspected when the heart murmur is loud (grade 3/6 or louder) and associated with hyperkinetic pulses. NIBP measurement is useful in assessing AR severity, and an elevated pulse pressure (>60 mmHg) tends to be associated with severe AR. An irregular cardiac rhythm should raise the suspicion of ventricular arrhythmias or atrial fibrillation, often associated with more advanced disease. Ventricular arrhythmias can lead to sudden cardiac death. An exercising ECG can demonstrate exercise-induced ventricular arrhythmias. If feasible, an echocardiogram will provide details about the pathological process affecting the valve and will be useful to determine the degree of left-sided volume overload.

Mitral valve regurgitation is also common in horses, and clinically significant regurgitation is often associated with a grade ≥3/6 holo- or pan-systolic heart murmur best heard over the left apex (behind the triceps muscle in the standing horse). Similarly to AR, a large volume of mitral regurgitation can lead to left-sided volume overload, pulmonary hypertension, congestive heart failure, and arrhythmias (including atrial fibrillation and ventricular arrhythmias).

Anesthetic Management

Routine anesthetic drugs used in horses are very different than in dogs and cats. Horses require premedication with an agent that provides reliable sedation to improve the quality of anesthetic induction and safer handling. Alpha-2 adrenergic agonists are the mainstay of premedication in adult horses. Horses with moderate-to-severe pathologic valvular disease should be referred to a facility with a board-certified anesthesiologist and the ability to perform advanced anesthetic monitoring (IBP, ECG, arterial blood gases, and end-tidal gases).

An example anesthetic protocol for these horses would be premedication with xylazine, induction with guaifenesin or benzodiazepine + ketamine, and maintenance with a balanced anesthetic technique using inhalant anesthetic (isoflurane and sevoflurane) + lidocaine and ketamine CRI. Sedation during recovery with a low-dose alpha-2 adrenergic agonist is helpful in promoting a smooth recovery (see Chapter 13).

Valvular Stenosis

Pulmonic Stenosis

Pulmonic stenosis (PS) is an obstructive malformation involving the pulmonic valve and/or the areas above or below the valve, impeding blood flow from the right ventricle to the main pulmonary artery (pulmonary trunk) (Figure 17.5). This leads to an elevated right ventricular pressure (i.e., pressure overload) and secondary concentric hypertrophy (i.e., thickening) of the right ventricle. In some cases, right atrial pressure can be increased as well.

Pulmonic stenosis is one of the most common congenital defects in dogs and is especially prevalent in some breeds, such as French and English Bulldogs. It is characterized by a systolic murmur best heard over the left heart base (third intercostal space at the sternal border and at the axilla). The degree of right-sided cardiac remodeling depends on the severity of the stenosis, which is determined by the pressure gradient between the right ventricle and the pulmonary artery (normal < 16 mmHg; mild = 16–50 mmHg; moderate = 50–80 mmHg; severe ≥ 80 mmHg). While dogs with mild PS are usually asymptomatic and have a good prognosis, dogs with moderate-to-severe stenosis are at risk of developing complications such as right-sided congestive heart failure (mostly ascites) or ventricular arrhythmias that can lead to sudden cardiac

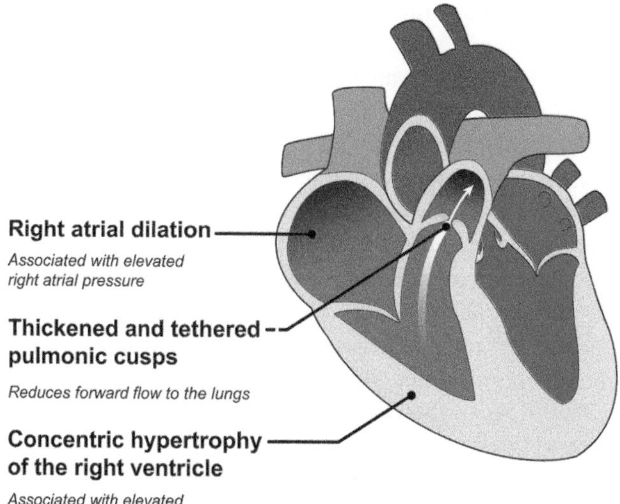

Figure 17.5 Pathophysiology of pulmonic stenosis (see the Figure 17.1 legend for anatomical descriptions).

arrest. Arrhythmias can develop due to ischemic lesions that can affect the hypertrophied myocardium.

Echocardiography is the best modality to determine the severity of PS, extent of ventricular hypertrophy, and identify any associated defects. Commonly associated defects include an atrial septal defect or *patent foramen ovale* (PFO), which are clinically relevant because right-to-left intra-cardiac shunting of blood can potentially lead to desaturation under anesthesia. A diagnostic six-lead ECG can be useful and can often indicate right ventricular hypertrophy (right deviation of the mean electrical axis and deep S waves in leads I, II, III, and aVF).

Anesthetic Management

Dogs with moderate or severe PS are often treated with a beta-blocker, such as atenolol, to prevent tachycardia and limit myocardial oxygen demand. In humans, these medications are continued the day of anesthesia and it is appropriate to do so in veterinary patients. If the patient's heart rate is relatively low at rest (less than 80 beats per minute), a half-dose may be given the morning of anesthesia.

Goals During Anesthesia

- Maintain or increase right ventricular preload
- Maintain low-normal heart rate and sinus rhythm
- Maintain contractility
- Maintain or increase systemic vascular resistance
- Avoid increases in pulmonary vascular resistance

In cases of PS, right ventricular compliance is decreased and therefore right ventricular stroke volume is dependent on maintenance of adequate preload (venous return). These patients are also dependent on atrial contraction ("atrial kick") for adequate right ventricular filling and, therefore, require maintenance of a normal sinus rhythm. Tachycardia, which decreases ventricular filling, should be avoided. Increases in pulmonary vascular resistance can further reduce forward blood flow and can be avoided by maintaining normocapnia and a high fraction of inspired oxygen (FiO_2).

Opioid premedication is beneficial as pre-emptive analgesia to alleviate stress and help prevent tachycardia during handling.

Induction of anesthesia can be performed using propofol or alfaxalone, with midazolam, as previously described.

Maintenance of anesthesia is best performed using a balanced anesthetic technique with inhalant anesthetic and constant rate infusions ± locoregional anesthesia, as dictated by the procedure (Table 17.3). These patients typically tolerate a balanced crystalloid at a rate of 5 mL/kg/h to maintain preload. The clinician should be prepared to treat hypotension with a conservative fluid bolus (5–7 mL/kg of a balanced crystalloid, delivered over 10–15 min, and repeated as needed) and support myocardial contractility by minimizing inhalant anesthetic concentration (e.g., with the use of inhalant-sparing techniques) and using mixed-agonist sympathomimetics (dopamine, ephedrine, and norepinephrine; beginning at a low dose and titrating

Table 17.3 Example protocols for anesthetic management of dogs and cats with degenerative mitral valve disease (DMVD), dilated cardiomyopathy (DCM), pulmonic stenosis (PS), subaortic stenosis (SAS), hypertrophic cardiomyopathy (HCM). Across columns indicates suitable suggestions for each listed cardiac condition.

	CARDIAC DISEASE				
	DMVD				
ANESTHETIC STAGE	Stage B1	Stage ≥ B2	DCM	PS/SAS	HCM
Premedication	Butorphanol	0.2 – 0.4 mg/kg; IM, IV			
	Fentanyl	2 – 4 mcg/kg; IM, IV			
	Hydromorphone	0.03 – 0.05 mg/kg; IM, IV			
	Methadone	0.1 – 0.3 mg/kg; IM, IV			
	Acepromazine 0.01 – 0.03 mg/kg; IM, IV			Dexmedetomidine IM, IV	3 – 5 mcg/kg;
	Premedication combinations can be used for sedation only ****Note: In fractious cats IM opioid + midazolam (0.2 mg/kg) + alfaxalone (1.5 – 2 mg/kg) can provide good sedation.*				

(Continued)

Table 17.3 (Continued)

	CARDIAC DISEASE				
	DMVD				
ANESTHETIC STAGE	Stage B1	Stage ≥ B2	DCM	PS/SAS	HCM
Induction	Alfaxalone 0.25 – 1 mg/kg; IV Propofol 0.5 – 1 mg/kg; IV *with* Midazolam 0.4 mg/kg; IV *Technique: midazolam immediately following alfaxalone or propofol and then induction agent titrated to effect to allow for endotracheal intubation* *In very sick or heavily sedated animals, midazolam + opioid may be enough for induction of anesthesia (neuroleptic induction).* *Example: fentanyl 3-10 mcg/kg, followed immediately by midazolam 0.4 mg/kg, IV*				
Maintenance	Inhalant (isoflurane, sevoflurane, desflurane) Technique for balanced anesthesia: — MAC Reduction: Fentanyl CRI: Canine 3 – 12 mcg/kg/h — 35 – 56% (isoflurane); Feline 3 – 12 mcg/kg/h — No studies in cats Hydromorphone CRI: Canine 0.01 – 0.02 mg/kg/h — After single dose, up to 50% (isoflurane); Feline 0.005 – 0.02 mg/kg/h — (a specific dosage has not been reported in cats) Methadone CRI: Canine 0.1 – 0.3 mg/kg/h — After single dose, 15 – 48% (isoflurane); Feline 0.1 – 0.3 mg/kg/h — After single dose, transient 25% (sevoflurane) Lidocaine CRI: Canine 50 – 200 mcg/kg/min — 18 – 40% (isoflurane, sevoflurane); Feline ** ***Not recommended due to more CV depression than equipotent doses of isoflurane alone*** Midazolam CRI: Canine 0.1 – 0.4 mg/kg/h — 10 – 30% (isoflurane); Feline 0.1 – 0.4 mg/kg/h — No CRI studies in cats *NOTE: All CRIs should be initiated following a loading dose (see premedication dosages)*				
Monitoring	*Advanced anesthetic monitoring is advised, ⊥indicates minimal monitoring equipment* Anesthetic depth: Eye position, palpebral reflex, jaw tone, muscle relaxation Cardiac rate and rhythm: ⊥ECG Arterial blood pressure: IBP or ⊥NIBP (Oscillometric, Doppler) *IBP advised in advanced cardiac disease* Oxygen saturation: ⊥SpO_2 End-tidal gas analysis: ⊥Capnography, Inhalant				
Fluid Therapy	Balanced crystalloid (Plasma-Lyte A, Normosol-R, Lactated Ringers) 3 mL/kg/h			Balanced crystalloid (Plasma-Lyte A, Normosol-R) 3 – 5 mL/kg/h	
CV Support	Anticholinergics Atropine 0.04 mg/kg, IV or Glycopyrrolate 0.005-0.01 mg/kg, IV Tx: bradycardia w/ hypotension Sympathomimetics α agonist (phenylephrine) to increase vascular resistance (and arterial blood pressure) β agonists (dobutamine) to increase HR and contractility or to primarily increase heart rate (isoproterenol) Mixed α & β agonists (dopamine, norepinephrine) to treat bradycardia and hypotension and contractility				

CRI: constant rate infusion; CV: cardiovascular; MAC: minimum alveolar concentration; HR: heart rate; ECG: electrocardiogram; IBP: invasive arterial blood pressure; NIBP: noninvasive arterial blood pressure; SpO_2: peripheral oxyhemoglobin saturation measured using pulse oximetry; Tx: treatment.

to effect). The latter are useful to increase vascular resistance and support contractility. Drugs that may result in tachycardia (anticholinergics) should be avoided. Hemodynamically significant arrhythmias should be treated immediately to maintain a sinus rhythm (see the section on cardiac arrhythmia in the following text). Recently, the use of a low-dose dexmedetomidine CRI (median dose of 0.5 mcg/kg/h) as part of a balanced anesthetic technique in dogs with PS has been described (Martin-Flores et al., 2021).

Subaortic Stenosis

Subaortic stenosis (SAS) is another common congenital defect affecting dogs, especially Golden Retriever, Newfoundland, and Boxer breeds. With SAS, a subvalvular ridge or ring of tissue causes blood flow obstruction through the left ventricular outflow tract, resulting in left ventricular pressure overload and concentric hypertrophy of the left ventricle. Dogs with mild-to-moderate SAS are usually asymptomatic. However, dogs with severe SAS can develop complications such as left-sided congestive heart failure and ventricular arrhythmias that can lead to sudden cardiac death. Physical examination usually reveals a systolic heart murmur best heard over the left heart base (third to fourth intercostal spaces just below the shoulder line), and femoral pulses are often weak and late rising.

Anesthetic Management

Chronic management of dogs with SAS includes similar therapy to PS, with the aim of preventing tachycardia and reducing myocardial oxygen demand.

Goals During Anesthesia

- Maintain or increase left ventricular preload
- Maintain low-normal heart rate and sinus rhythm
- Maintain contractility
- Maintain systemic vascular resistance

The anesthetic management is similar to patients affected by pulmonic stenosis (see the preceding section).

Myocardial Disease

Canine Myocardial Disease

Cardiomyopathies represent the second most common group of cardiac disorders in dogs and tend to primarily affect medium- to large-breed dogs. *Dilated cardiomyopathy* is the predominant form of canine cardiomyopathy and is defined as a primary myocardial disease characterized by reduced systolic function (poor contractility) and eccentric hypertrophy (dilation) of one or both ventricles. It is often associated with secondary mitral valve regurgitation due to distention of the mitral valve annulus.

DCM is often genetic in origin and is overrepresented in certain breeds, such as the Doberman Pinscher, Irish Wolfhound, and Great Dane. This disease is usually an adult-onset disease. The main possible complications of DCM are the development of congestive heart failure due to volume overload, which is predominantly left-sided (but can be right-sided in some dogs), and ventricular arrhythmias that can lead to sudden death, especially in the Doberman Pinscher. Giant-breed dogs with DCM are also likely to develop atrial fibrillation, which further reduces cardiac output due to the elevated heart rate and lack of functional atrial contraction.

DCM is usually insidious and its diagnosis is often established following the onset of clinical signs of forward or backward heart failure since physical examination findings in asymptomatic dogs can be more subtle than with valvular conditions. Cardiac auscultation may reveal a soft heart murmur (with a grade often lower than 3/6) and/or a gallop sound over the left apical area (fifth intercostal space near the costochondral junction). Arrhythmias may also be detected. While the presence of ventricular tachyarrhythmias is often characterized by intermittent premature contractions or "runs" of tachycardia on auscultation, atrial fibrillation is characterized by a very irregular rhythm (described as irregularly irregular) that sounds like "shoes tumbling in a dryer." Other signs, such as weak femoral pulses or pale mucous membranes, may also be observed. A definitive diagnosis of DCM is established with an echocardiogram. Thoracic radiographs are useful to identify cardiomegaly and evidence of congestive heart failure. ECG is used to characterize the arrhythmia, if present. Holter monitoring is often useful to further evaluate the frequency and severity of ventricular arrhythmias, especially considering their intermittent nature. Cardiac screening may be considered in some breeds and/or lines at high risk of DCM even in the absence of clinical signs or abnormal physical examination findings.

The incidence of diet-induced DCM in dogs has been increasing in some regions and is associated with feeding grain-free diets, which usually contain a high proportion of legumes. While the exact mechanism leading to DCM in dogs eating a grain-free diet has not been confirmed, some dogs may be deficient in the amino acid taurine. That being said, the majority of affected dogs have normal taurine blood levels. In cases of diet-induced DCM, cardiac morphology and function often improve with diet change and taurine supplementation, and cardiac medications can be progressively discontinued in some dogs.

Other possible diseases that can lead to a DCM phenotype include myocarditis (e.g., Chagas' disease in the southern part of North America and Leishmaniasis in the Mediterranean basin). Myocarditis is often associated with tachy- or bradyarrhythmias. Hypothyroidism can also be associated with myocardial dysfunction.

Finally, arrhythmogenic right ventricular cardiomyopathy (ARVC) predominantly affects Boxer dogs but is also seen with some frequency in English Bulldogs. It is characterized by ventricular arrhythmias, which can lead to syncope and sudden death. While most Boxer dogs with ARVC have a morphologically normal heart, some can exhibit a DCM phenotype (with systolic dysfunction and ventricular dilation). Most affected dogs have a normal physical examination, but arrhythmias may be identified during cardiac auscultation. Twenty-four hour Holter monitoring is the best diagnostic tool for dogs with suspected ARVC. It is important to note that Boxers often have a soft (grade ≤ 3/6), left basilar, systolic heart murmur that may be physiologic in origin (due to a benign elevation in aortic velocity or due to aortic stenosis). This type of heart murmur is not diagnostic for ARVC.

Anesthetic Management

Medical management of dogs with cardiomyopathies is complex and can vary dramatically from a case-to-case basis. It is important that the continuation or withholding of specific drugs perioperatively is made on a case-by-case basis.

Dogs with pre-clinical DCM may be treated with pimobendan with or without an ACE inhibitor. Pimobendan should be administered the morning of the procedure. However, ACE inhibitors should be withheld the day of the procedure due to a greater risk of hypotension under anesthesia that is more difficult to treat.

Chronic treatment of ventricular arrhythmias is usually achieved using drugs such as sotalol, mexiletine, or rarely amiodarone. Heart rate control in dogs with atrial fibrillation is achieved with drugs such as diltiazem, digoxin, and sometimes a beta-blocker. In most dogs these medications are continued on the day of anesthesia, but again this should be evaluated on a case-by-case basis. In humans with ARVC, it is recommended to continue beta-blockers and other anti-arrhythmic medications the morning of anesthesia, and this is likely a good recommendation for dogs as well (Alexoudis et al., 2009).

Dogs with congestive heart failure secondary to their myocardial disease are treated with diuretics, such as furosemide and spironolactone, and anesthesia is generally contraindicated unless the procedure is absolutely necessary.

Goals During Anesthesia

Maintain left ventricular preload
Maintain heart rate and sinus rhythm (or adequate rate control with atrial fibrillation)
Increase contractility
Decrease afterload

The management of cardiac performance during anesthesia in dogs with DCM is similar to that described for dogs with mitral valve regurgitation (see Table 17.3). Left ventricular preload should be optimized to ensure adequate ventricular filling and stroke volume; however, volume overload must be avoided. A conservative fluid rate (3 mL/kg/h) of balanced crystalloid is appropriate in normovolemic patients. A normal heart rate and sinus rhythm should be maintained to ensure adequate ventricular filling. These dogs are at higher risk for cardiac arrhythmias under general anesthesia, and arrhythmias should be treated if they are having a negative impact on cardiac output and arterial blood pressure. Due to the decreased systolic function, dogs with DCM benefit from inotropic drugs (dobutamine) to maintain or increase contractility during general anesthesia. Down-regulation of cardiac beta receptors may make these dogs resistant to beta-agonists such that higher doses are required.

Similar anesthetic protocols to those described for dogs with mitral valve regurgitation are also appropriate for dogs with DCM. Premedication with an opioid is suitable because this drug class (with the exception of morphine and meperidine [pethidine]) has minimal cardiovascular effects. Any drugs that alter cardiovascular performance (acepromazine and dexmedetomidine/medetomidine) should be avoided in this patient population. Pre-induction support of contractility with a beta-1 agonist (dobutamine) may be beneficial in these animals (Pagel et al., 1998). A co-induction technique, as described in the preceding text, is recommended and maintenance with a balanced anesthetic technique and advanced monitoring is appropriate. The use of a mixed-agonist sympathomimetic (dopamine and norepinephrine) can also be considered to provide both inotropic support and offset the vasodilatory effect of the inhalant anesthetic. Drugs that are likely to cause tachycardia (anticholinergics) should be avoided in dogs with atrial fibrillation or other tachyarrhythmias.

In dogs with ARVC, anesthetic procedures should be postponed until the arrhythmia can be well controlled with medication(s). Stress should be minimized on the day of anesthesia as significant stress can trigger or worsen any arrhythmias due to increased sympathetic tone (catecholamine release). There is limited veterinary literature on specific recommendations for the anesthetic management of these cases; however, similar recommendations as given in the preceding text are reasonable. Current human guidelines suggest caution in using positive inotropes or chronotropes due to the risk of precipitating tachyarrhythmias. Vasoconstrictors (e.g., phenylephrine) may be the preferred option to maintain arterial blood pressure. The performance of the cardiovascular system should be maintained as close to normal as possible in an effort to prevent triggering or worsening arrhythmias. Dogs with no risk for volume overload will tolerate 5 mL/kg/h of a balanced crystalloid. An opioid-based premedication without any drugs that alter cardiovascular performance (acepromazine and dexmedetomidine) is recommended. Maintenance with a balanced anesthetic technique and advanced anesthetic monitoring is appropriate. A lidocaine CRI may be beneficial in these dogs because it decreases inhalant requirement, provides analgesia, and has an anti-arrhythmic effect. It is important to note that lidocaine should be used with caution if the patient is already receiving mexiletine. Both drugs belong to the same class and their concurrent use could lead to toxic effects. Direct arterial blood pressure monitoring is ideal because it will allow for blood pressure measurement in the presence of arrhythmias, a situation in which noninvasive blood pressure measurement techniques generally perform poorly.

Feline Myocardial Disease

Feline cardiomyopathies are a heterogenous group of disorders affecting the myocardium. Cardiomyopathies represent the most common heart conditions in cats and are one of the most common causes of death in this species. The classification of feline cardiomyopathies is based on the structural and functional abnormalities that are affecting the myocardium although there is some degree of overlap between the different diseases (Luis Fuentes et al., 2020).

Hypertrophic cardiomyopathy is by far the most commonly encountered feline cardiomyopathy and is usually genetic in origin. It is characterized by a diffuse or regional increase in left ventricular wall thickness with a nondilated left ventricular cavity. These myocardial changes lead to diastolic dysfunction (impaired cardiac relaxation during diastole), which can progressively result in elevated left atrial pressure and left atrial enlargement (Figure 17.6). In the most severe cases, HCM can lead to the development of congestive heart failure (pulmonary edema or pleural effusion are both possible in cats with left-sided congestive heart failure), thrombus formation with a risk of aortic thromboembolism, or ventricular arrhythmias that can lead to sudden death. In some cats with HCM, left ventricular outflow tract obstruction (LVOT) can be present due to hypertrophy of the interventricular septum below the aortic valve or systolic anterior motion (SAM) of the mitral valve (present in approximately 30% of cats with HCM), a phenomenon during which the septal leaflet of the mitral valve is being pulled toward the LVOT. Other comorbidities such as systemic hypertension or hyperthyroidism can be associated with left ventricular hypertrophy and should be investigated when an HCM phenotype is identified.

The second most common feline cardiomyopathy is restrictive cardiomyopathy (RCM). RCM is characterized by diastolic dysfunction due the development of myocardial fibrosis without significant myocardial hypertrophy. With this disease, the left ventricle becomes very stiff (decreased compliance), leading to compromised ventricular filling during diastole and secondary atrial enlargement. Systolic dysfunction is often also seen in cats with severe RCM.

Dilated cardiomyopathy is extremely rare in cats and its pathophysiology is similar to DCM in dogs.

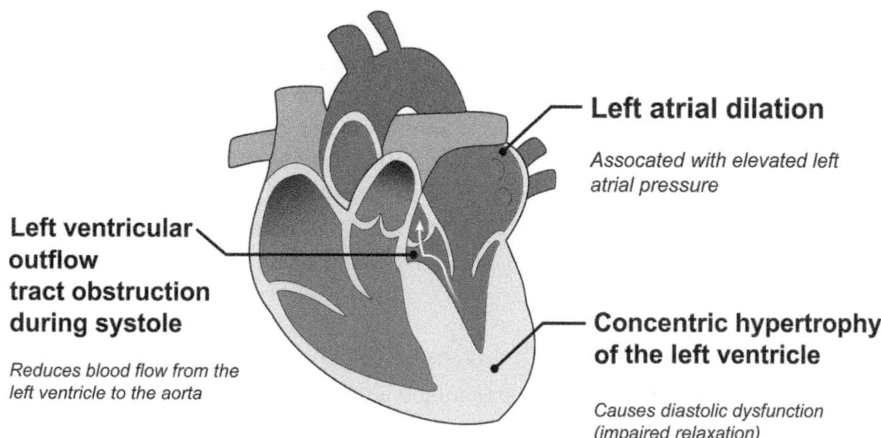

Figure 17.6 Pathophysiology of hypertrophic cardiomyopathy (see the Figure 17.1 legend for anatomical descriptions).

As described earlier, the detection and diagnosis of feline cardiomyopathies can be challenging. Many affected cats are asymptomatic and their heart disease remains unnoticed until they develop clinical signs of congestive heart failure or aortic thromboembolism. A preceding event that may have precipitated congestive heart failure can be identified in 14–30% of cases; anesthesia is one of the most commonly reported events. While the majority of cats with HCM have a heart murmur, some cats with underlying heart disease have a normal cardiac auscultation. However, the presence of a gallop sound or arrhythmia in some of these cats raises the suspicion of a heart condition and warrants further investigation before anesthesia.

Anesthetic Management

Long-term therapy in cats with myocardial disease can include a beta-blocker, such as atenolol, especially if LVOT obstruction is present. There is currently no existing veterinary literature, but based on the human literature the authors' preference is to continue the beta-blocker the morning of the anesthesia. In cats treated with an antiplatelet drug, such as clopidogrel or aspirin, these drugs should be withheld for at least seven days before elective surgical or dental procedures due to increased risk of bleeding. Similarly to dogs, ACE inhibitors should be withheld the day of the procedure as they result in greater risk of hypotension during anesthesia that is more difficult to treat. Pimobendan is used in select cases, especially cats with congestive heart failure characterized by ventricular systolic dysfunction and no LVOT obstruction based on an echocardiogram. These patients usually have advanced heart disease and should not be anesthetized unless absolutely necessary.

Goals During Anesthesia

- Maintain left ventricular preload, but avoid volume overload
- Maintain low–normal heart rate
- Avoid increases in contractility
- Maintain or increase afterload

In cats with HCM or RCM, the hypertrophied and/or fibrotic left ventricle is poorly compliant. Maintaining a relatively low heart rate and optimizing preload will help to optimize diastolic filling and improve stroke volume/cardiac output. Contractility is typically well maintained with HCM, and drugs that increase contractility should be avoided because they lead to increased myocardial oxygen demand, which may be poorly tolerated (causing the development of arrhythmias). A decrease in afterload is poorly tolerated in cats with LVOT obstruction because it worsens the pressure gradient that already exists.

Opioids are reasonable for premedication in this population of cats as they have minimal cardiovascular effects, and any vagally mediated bradycardia will likely be beneficial. In cats, butorphanol, buprenorphine, and methadone can provide acceptable sedation in combination with gentle handling and restraint. Acepromazine should be avoided as these cats are unlikely to tolerate the decrease in afterload (Saponaro et al., 2013). Alpha-2 adrenergic receptor agonists can be useful when greater levels of sedation are required. This drug class elicits vasoconstriction that causes an increase in systemic vascular resistance (afterload) and reflex bradycardia. In cats with hypertrophic obstructive cardiomyopathy, the use of alpha-2 adrenergic receptor agonists (such as dexmedetomidine/medetomidine) may reverse LVOT obstruction (Lamont et al., 2002). Due to depression of cardiac output by alpha-2 adrenergic receptor agonists, monitoring of arterial blood pressure is important when this drug class is used for premedication before general anesthesia. It is also important to note that alpha-2 adrenergic receptor agonists should not be used in cats with significant left atrial enlargement or cats already in congestive heart failure. An example sedation protocol for fractious cats could be butorphanol (0.2–0.4 mg/kg) + dexmedetomidine (0.005 mg/kg) or medetomidine (0.01 mg/kg), IM. An example premedication protocol before a surgical procedure could be methadone (0.1–0.3 mg/kg), IM.

Some cats may require more than just an IM opioid as a premedication due to their temperament and to alleviate stress during handling. In these cats, example premedication protocols could be (1) methadone (0.1–0.3 mg/kg) + midazolam (0.2–0.3 mg/kg) + alfaxalone (2–3 mg/kg), IM; or for more fractious cats, (2) methadone (0.1–0.3 mg/kg) + dexmedetomidine (0.003–0.008 mg/kg) or medetomidine (0.006–0.015 mg/kg) ± alfaxalone (1–2 mg/kg), IM.

For elective procedures and even routine veterinary visits, gabapentin has been shown to reduce stress and aggression in cats. The drug can be given orally by the owner 90 min before placing the cat into a carrier and transporting it to the veterinary hospital (Van Haaften et al., 2017). In cats pretreated with gabapentin, the lower end of IM sedation doses should be used.

Induction of anesthesia can be performed using a co-induction technique (alfaxalone + midazolam or propofol + midazolam) as described for dogs with DMVD. In cats with HCM or RCM, ketamine is generally avoided because it maintains sympathetic tone, leading to tachycardia, increased myocardial work, and myocardial oxygen demand.

General anesthesia can be maintained using a balanced anesthetic technique with inhalant anesthetics ± CRIs of other agents ± locoregional anesthesia as dictated by the procedure. A conservative fluid rate (3 mL/kg/h) of balanced crystalloids is appropriate in normovolemic patients. Advanced anesthetic monitoring is recommended (Table 17.3).

Treatment of bradycardia with anticholinergic drugs (atropine and glycopyrrolate) will increase heart rate, myocardial work, and myocardial oxygen demand, and therefore should be avoided unless bradycardia is severe and compromising arterial blood pressure. In cats, dopamine has been demonstrated to improve arterial blood pressure by increasing heart rate without causing tachycardia and is a good option in this patient population (Pascoe et al., 2006). In cats with HCM, dopamine was effective at increasing arterial blood pressure via increases in cardiac output following isoflurane-induced hypotension (Wiese et al., 2012).

Extra-cardiac and Intra-cardiac Shunts

Left-to-Right Shunting

Left-to-right shunting occurs when there is an abnormal communication between great vessels or chambers of the heart which allows blood to flow from the systemic (high-pressure [left]) circulation to the pulmonary (low-pressure [right]) circulation. The magnitude of blood flow across the shunting defect depends on the size of the communication and the pressure difference between the connected chambers or vessels. A left-to-right shunt leads to volume overload and subsequent enlargement of the cardiac chambers and vessels that receive the shunted blood.

The *ductus arteriosus* is a normal fetal blood vessel that connects the main pulmonary artery to the aorta in order to bypass the lungs, which are nonfunctional in the fetus. This vessel normally closes soon after birth but can persist for a few weeks in some species (e.g., horses). A *patent ductus arteriosus* (PDA) is an abnormal persistence of this vessel, which usually results in abnormal shunting of blood from the aorta to the pulmonary artery (left-to-right PDA). This defect is more common in female dogs and some breed predispositions are recognized, such as the Poodle, Shetland Sheepdog, Welsh Corgi, Collie, Pomeranian, and German Shepherd. A characteristic continuous "machinery" murmur (i.e., present continuously during systole and diastole) is best heard over the left heart base (left thorax, third to fourth intercostal spaces) and is often associated with a palpable thrill. Femoral pulses are usually bounding due to the greater pulse pressure (i.e., the difference between systolic and diastolic blood pressures). The diastolic systemic pressure is usually low due to the shunting of blood volume to the lower resistance pulmonary circulatory system. The PDA leads to volume overload of the pulmonary arteries and veins (pulmonary overcirculation), left atrium, left ventricle, and aortic arch. Therefore, the primary complication of a PDA is left-sided congestive heart failure.

In rare cases, and particularly in dogs with a large PDA, pulmonary hypertension may be present from birth or may develop over time as a result of pulmonary vascular remodeling, causing right-to-left or bidirectional shunting (see the next section). Notably, these animals will not have the characteristic continuous heart murmur.

A ventricular septal defect (VSD) is a communication between the two ventricles. Most VSDs are small and occur in the membranous portion of the interventricular septum, just below the aortic valve. In these cases, the normal pressure difference between the left and right ventricle is maintained, and although the amount of blood shunting from the left ventricle to the right ventricle may be small, the blood flow velocity is high, which results in a loud systolic heart murmur best heard over the right mid-thoracic area. Small VSDs have little hemodynamic consequence, but larger defects can lead to enlargement of the left atrium, left and right ventricles, as well as pulmonary overcirculation. VSDs are the most common congenital defects in horses and cats; similar to dogs, the prognosis depends on the size and location of the defect.

A combination of thoracic radiographs and echocardiogram is indicated in these cases to obtain a definitive diagnosis, evaluate the consequences of the shunt on cardiac dimensions and function, and determine if pulmonary hypertension or other associated defects are present.

Anesthetic Management

If the defect leading to left-to-right shunting can be surgically corrected, this should be performed before general anesthesia for an elective procedure.

Goals During Anesthesia

- Maintain left ventricular preload
- Maintain heart rate
- Maintain contractility
- Maintain systemic vascular resistance
- Maintain pulmonary vascular resistance

In patients with a small left-to-right shunt without evidence of volume overload (i.e., without significant enlargement of the left-sided cardiac chambers), ventricular preload, heart rate, and contractility should all be maintained as close to normal as possible. In patients with a large left-to-right shunt and therefore a higher risk of developing congestive heart failure, goals of anesthesia are similar to those in patients with left-sided volume overload. Systemic vascular resistance should be maintained and any anesthetics that dramatically increase or decrease vascular resistance should be avoided (e.g., acepromazine and dexmedetomidine/medetomidine). Increases in systemic vascular resistance and/or decreases in pulmonary vascular resistance may increase pulmonary blood flow and the magnitude of left-to-right shunting.

Premedication with an opioid is appropriate in these cases. Acepromazine can decrease systemic vascular resistance and should be avoided, especially in patients with preexisting pulmonary hypertension in which a significant decrease in systemic vascular resistance may reverse shunt flow. Alpha-2 adrenergic agonists (e.g., dexmedetomidine/medetomidine) significantly increase systemic vascular resistance and are contraindicated.

A co-induction technique using alfaxalone or propofol, and midazolam, as previously described, is ideal to lower the dose of induction agent. High doses of alfaxalone or propofol can transiently decrease systemic vascular resistance and may be poorly tolerated.

Anesthesia can be maintained with an inhalant anesthetic (isoflurane and sevoflurane). Strategies to decrease inhalant requirements are recommended, such as CRIs of other agents and locoregional anesthesia, as dictated by the procedure. A conservative fluid rate (3 mL/kg/h) of a balanced crystalloid is appropriate to maintain left ventricular preload but avoid volume overload in normovolemic patients. These patients may benefit from support with a mixed-agonist sympathomimetic (dopamine and norepinephrine) to maintain cardiac contractility, heart rate, and also systemic vascular resistance in the face of inhalant anesthetics. Advanced anesthetic monitoring is warranted (Table 17.3).

Right-to-Left Shunting

Right-to-left shunting occurs when an abnormal communication between chambers of the heart or great vessels allows blood from the venous side to bypass the lungs and to directly enter the systemic circulation. This only occurs in cases of elevated right-sided pressures due to the presence of pulmonary hypertension or the presence of an obstructive lesion distal to the communication. Examples of defects causing right-to-left shunting include an atrial septal defect with pulmonic stenosis, a VSD with pulmonic stenosis (this is called "tetralogy of Fallot" if dextroposition of the aorta is also present), or a PDA with severe pulmonary hypertension (reverse PDA). Cyanosis is often present in these patients because of shunting of deoxygenated blood into the systemic circulation, which can be symmetrical (i.e., affecting the cranial and caudal potions of the body) or asymmetrical (i.e., when cyanosis only involves the caudal portion of the body). Asymmetrical cyanosis is also known as "differential cyanosis." Differential cyanosis is often present with reverse PDA. Chronic hypoxemia stimulates red blood cell production, and erythrocytosis is often present if there is significant right-to-left shunting of blood.

Severe erythrocytosis can result in blood hyperviscosity and therefore therapeutic phlebotomy is often performed to keep the hematocrit <70–75%.

Anesthetic Management

Elective procedures should be avoided in these patients and referral to a specialty center with a board-certified anesthesiologist is highly recommended. Some patients may be treated with a nonselective beta-blocker such as propranolol to limit vasodilation.

Ideally, hematocrit should be <60% before induction of anesthesia.

Goals During Anesthesia

Maintain preload
Maintain heart rate and rhythm
Maintain systemic vascular resistance
Decrease pulmonary vascular resistance

Premedication with an opioid is important to minimize stress and encourage the patient to tolerate pre-oxygenation. Drugs that decrease vascular resistance (e.g., acepromazine) must be avoided. Proper pre-oxygenation is critical in these animals as they become hypoxemic very quickly due to their preexisting physiology.

Either a neuroleptic induction technique (e.g., opioid + midazolam) or a co-induction technique (e.g., propofol/alfaxalone + midazolam) can be used depending on the ASA status of the animal.

Maintenance of anesthesia using a balanced anesthetic technique and advanced anesthetic monitoring is appropriate. Animals not at risk for volume overload will tolerate a fluid rate of 5 mL/kg/h of a balanced crystalloid. Mechanical ventilation is recommended to maintain a relative hypocapnia, which will help decrease pulmonary vascular resistance. Hypercapnia must be avoided because it will stimulate pulmonary vasoconstriction and worsen right-to-left shunting of blood. Similarly, anesthesia with 100% FiO_2 is recommended to avoid hypoxic pulmonary vasoconstriction. Systemic hypotension will also worsen right-to-left shunting and should be treated quickly with vasoconstrictors (e.g., phenylephrine and norepinephrine).

Cardiac Arrhythmias

Heart rate and rhythm have a crucial impact on cardiac output. Animals routinely experience bradycardia or tachycardia during anesthesia and there is no consensus on when these should be treated; therefore, adequate

Table 17.4 Normal resting heart rates (beats per minute) in cats, dogs, and horses.

Species	Heart rate
Cats	140–240 in hospital setting, as low as 100–120 at home or during sleep
Kittens	220–260
Small dogs	80–160
Large dogs	60–140
Puppies	Up to 220
Horses	28–44
Foals	80–100

understanding of normal heart rate and rhythm and how to evaluate the consequences of change to the animal is important. Normal heart rate varies with age, between species and breeds, and depends on the temperament of the animal (Table 17.4).

Cardiac arrhythmias are defined as disturbances of the cardiac rhythm as compared to a normal sinus rhythm. A sinus rhythm is present when the electrical impulses originate in the sinus node and the following ECG characteristics are present: the heart rate is within the reference range and adapted to the situation, the R–R interval is regular, P waves have a normal and relatively constant morphology, every P wave is followed by a QRS complex, and every QRS complex is preceded by a P wave with a constant P–R interval.

Arrhythmias can be classified as disturbances of impulse formation (cardiac excitability), disturbances of impulse conduction, or a combination of both. For the purpose of anesthesia, it is important to identify arrhythmias that lead to an elevated heart rate (tachyarrhythmia) and arrhythmias that lead to a slow heart rate (bradyarrhythmia). Arrhythmias may be preexisting as a result of primary heart disease or metabolic disturbances, or can occur secondary to the effects of certain anesthetic drugs on the electrical properties of the heart. Some arrhythmias, such as a respiratory sinus arrhythmia, are normal and common in dogs and horses, and do not require specific treatment.

When an arrhythmia is detected on physical examination before general anesthesia, an ECG should be performed to determine the exact nature of the arrhythmia. Other diagnostic tests may be indicated on a case-by-case basis, including 24-h Holter monitoring (especially useful for intermittent arrhythmias), echocardiography to determine if underlying structural heart disease is present, complete bloodwork including electrolytes, or an abdominal ultrasound to determine if extra-cardiac disease is causing the arrhythmia. In cases of bradyarrhythmias (marked sinus bradycardia, sinus node dysfunction, and atrioventricular block), an atropine response test may be indicated to determine if the arrhythmia is vagally mediated and to determine if the animal will respond to an anticholinergic drug before anesthesia is planned.

Table 17.5 summarizes the most common arrhythmias and recommendations for how they can be managed under anesthesia.

Tachyarrhythmias

It is important to distinguish between sinus tachycardia and other tachyarrhythmias. Sinus tachycardia is a sinus rhythm with an abnormally elevated heart rate. This is a normal physiologic response to increased sympathetic tone and can result from a light plane of anesthesia, pain, certain anesthetic drugs (e.g., ketamine, sympathomimetics, and parasympatholytics), metabolic disturbances, and heart disease. Sinus tachycardia during anesthesia is managed by treating the underlying cause rather than attempting to directly slow the heart rate.

Tachyarrhythmias are characterized by the presence of ectopic beats that can be supraventricular or ventricular in origin. They can be associated with certain cardiac diseases or can occur secondary to an extra-cardiac condition. Generally, primary tachyarrhythmias should be treated when they are associated with frequent pulse deficits, indicators of poor perfusion (pale mucous membranes, prolonged capillary refill time [CRT], and cold extremities), hypotension, or associated with a risk of sudden death. Physiologic abnormalities resulting in tachycardia and/or tachyarrhythmias should ideally be corrected before induction of anesthesia.

During anesthesia, sinus tachycardia and tachyarrhythmias limit diastolic filling and can therefore have a detrimental impact on cardiac output and arterial blood pressure. In animals with specific types of heart disease, this may be poorly tolerated (see discussion in the preceding text).

Supraventricular Tachyarrhythmias

Supraventricular tachyarrhythmias represent a heterogenous group of arrhythmias including atrial premature contractions (APCs), focal atrial tachycardia (when more than three APCs are present in succession), atrial fibrillation (typically secondary to marked atrial dilation or associated with a structurally normal heart in giant-breed dogs), atrial flutter, or accessory pathway-mediated supraventricular tachycardia. These arrhythmias are usually characterized by a narrow QRS complex. A preceding ectopic P′ wave is present in the case of APCs or focal atrial tachycardia, while atrial fibrillation is characterized by an irregular R–R interval with an undulating baseline. While rapid supraventricular tachyarrhythmias can impair cardiac output

Table 17.5 Common arrhythmias and management during anesthesia.

	Type of arrhythmia	Arrhythmia characteristics	Causes	Management during anesthesia
	Respiratory sinus arrhythmia	Sinus rhythm with a cyclical variation in R–R interval.	Very common and physiologic in dogs, usually due to changes in vagal tone during respiration.	None, unless associated with profound bradycardia. Usually eliminated by increased sympathetic tone. In the case of profound bradycardia associated with hypotension, an anticholinergic can be used in dogs and cats. Atropine 0.02–0.04 mg/kg, IV, or glycopyrrolate 0.01 mg/kg, IV.
P′	Atrial premature contraction	Normal narrow QRS morphology. The P wave associated with the APC can be altered in morphology (P′ wave) and may blend with the preceding T wave.	Most commonly, atrial dilation or myocardial disease. Can sometimes be seen without any structural heart disease.	None when isolated in any species. Ensure adequate perfusion (capillary refill time and mucous membrane color), oxyhemoglobin saturation (SpO_2), and arterial blood pressure. Anticholinergics are usually avoided.
	Atrial tachycardia	Normal narrow QRS morphology. Rapid series of P′–QRS–T. The onset and termination may be abrupt.	Most commonly, atrial dilation or myocardial disease. Can sometimes be seen without any structural heart disease.	If preexisting, it should be controlled before considering anesthesia. Commonly used drugs in dogs are diltiazem or sotalol. In horses, diltiazem and digoxin are often used. During anesthesia, if excessive heart rate is having a negative impact on arterial blood pressure and/or peripheral perfusion, opioid administration may decrease atrial rate. If not, a calcium channel blocker (diltiazem) or a beta-adrenergic receptor blocker may be required. Drugs that cause tachycardia should be avoided (anticholinergics) or used with caution (sympathomimetics).
	Atrial fibrillation	Normal narrow QRS morphology Nonvisible P waves, undulating baseline Irregularly irregular R–R interval.	Most commonly, primary heart disease causing severe atrial dilation. Lone atrial fibrillation is seen in giant-breed dogs and horses.	If preexisting, heart rate should be controlled before considering anesthesia. Commonly used drugs are diltiazem and digoxin. If associated with hypotension, support with dobutamine. Anticholinergic agents are typically avoided. In horses, pharmacologic conversion with quinidine or transvenous electrical cardioversion may be considered (requires general anesthesia).

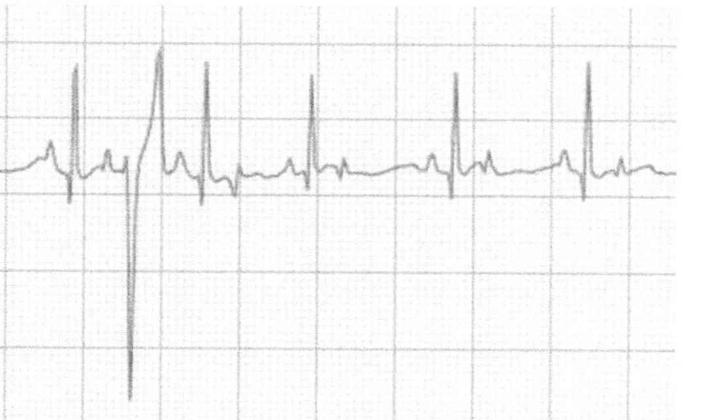	Ventricular premature contractions (isolated)	Wide QRS complex with large T wave of opposite polarity. Not associated with P waves. Occur at a faster rate that the underlying sinus rate.	Primary heart disease (cardiomyopathy, myocarditis, severe valvular disease, and severe ventricular hypertrophy). Associated with certain extra-cardiac diseases (gastric dilation-volvulus, splenic disease, abdominal mass, pheochromocytoma, endotoxemia, polytrauma, hypoxemia, pain, anemia, hypokalemia, high sympathetic tone, etc.).	Treatment of the underlying cause, if possible Ensure adequate perfusion (capillary refill time and mucous membrane color), oxyhemoglobin saturation (SpO_2), and arterial blood pressure. Consider measuring blood gases and electrolytes. If frequent and associated with indices of poor cardiac output: Lidocaine: Dogs 2 mg/kg, IV, then 50–75 mcg/kg/min CRI (rates of up to 200 mcg/kg/min can be used during general anesthesia in dogs; Moran-Muñoz et al., 2017; Vlaverde et al., 2004). Horses 0.5–2 mg/kg, IV, then 25–50 mcg/kg/min CRI. Procainamide: If resistant to lidocaine Dogs 2–10 mg/kg, IV, over 10 min then 20–40 mcg/kg/min.
	Ventricular tachycardia	More than three VPCs in succession.	When ventricular tachycardia is fast (>200 beats/min), it is often associated with a primary cardiac disease. Extra-cardiac causes of ventricular tachycardia are often associated with a slower heart rate. When slower than 160 beats/min, the rhythm is usually called "accelerated idioventricular rhythm." In horses, treatment should be initiated if HR > 100 beats/min.	Treatment of the underlying cause, if possible Ensure adequate perfusion (capillary refill time and mucous membrane color), oxyhemoglobin saturation (SpO_2), and arterial blood pressure. Consider testing blood gases and electrolytes. Lidocaine: Dogs 2 mg/kg, IV, then 50–75 mcg/kg/min CRI (rates of up to 200 mcg/kg/min can be used during general anesthesia in dogs; Moran-Muñoz et al., 2017; Vlaverde et al., 2004). Horses 0.5–2 mg/kg, IV, then 25–50 mcg/kg/min CRI Cats 0.25–0.75 mg/kg, IV, slowly over 5 min if absolutely necessary, then 10–15 mcg/kg/min CRI (use with extreme caution in cats). Procainamide: If resistant to lidocaine Dogs 5–10 mg/kg, IV, over 10 min then 20–40 mcg/kg/min Cats 1–2 mg/kg, IV, over 10 min, then 10–20 mcg/kg/min (poorly studied in cats and monitor for hypotension).

(Continued)

Table 17.5 (Continued)

	Type of arrhythmia	Arrhythmia characteristics	Causes	Management during anesthesia
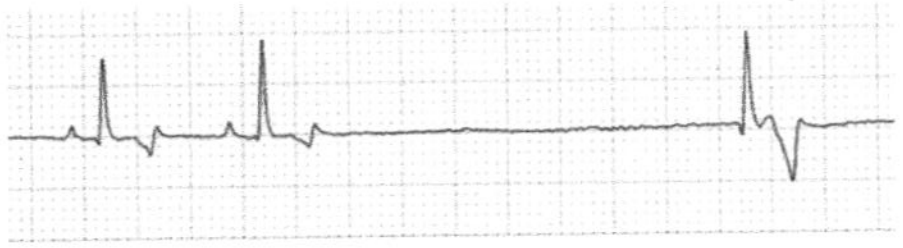 P	Sinus pause with escape beat	No P wave for at least two R–R intervals. A junctional (narrow QRS complex) or ventricular (wide QRS complex) escape beat may terminate the pause.	Sinus node dysfunction or sick sinus syndrome. High vagal tone. Drug induced (high-dose opioids, alpha-2 adrenergic receptor agonists, and temporary with parasympatholytics).	Anticholinergics (atropine and glycopyrrolate) if vagally induced or secondary to opioids. If caused by primary sinus node dysfunction, anticholinergics are often administered as part of premedication. If not responsive to anticholinergics and the pauses are severe, temporary electrical pacing may be considered or the patient should be recovered from anesthesia.
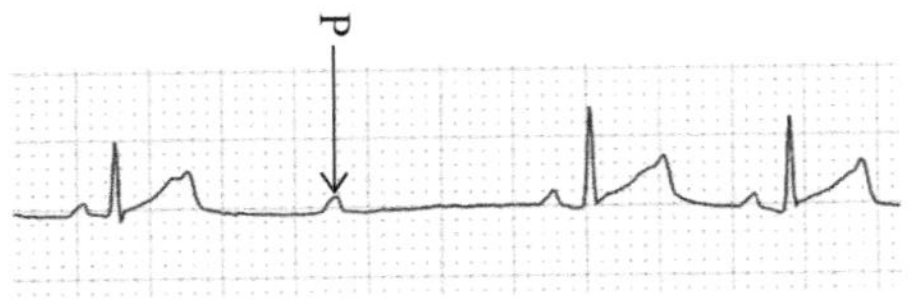	Second-degree atrioventricular block (2° AVB)	P waves intermittently not associated with a QRS complex. Mobitz Type I (Wenckebach): progressive prolongation of PR interval Most common type in horses Mobitz Type II (Hay): uniform PR intervals.	High vagal tone. Drug induced (high-dose opioids, alpha-2 adrenergic receptor agonists, and temporary with parasympatholytics). Atrioventricular nodal disease (degenerative, neoplastic, and inflammatory).	Anticholinergics (atropine and glycopyrrolate) if vagally induced or secondary to opioids. If caused by primary cardiac disease, anticholinergics are often administered as part of premedication. Note: Anticholinergics contraindicated if 2° AVB is secondary to hypertension associated with alpha-2 adrenergic receptor agonist administration. Isoproterenol (beta-adrenergic receptor agonist) may be used for high-grade 2° AVB. If not responsive to anticholinergics and the ventricular rate is slow, temporary electrical pacing may be considered or the patient should be recovered from anesthesia. In horses, exercising the horse to increase sympathetic tone should eliminate the arrhythmia unless it is pathologic.Routine use of anticholinergic in horses is not recommended (risk of colic).
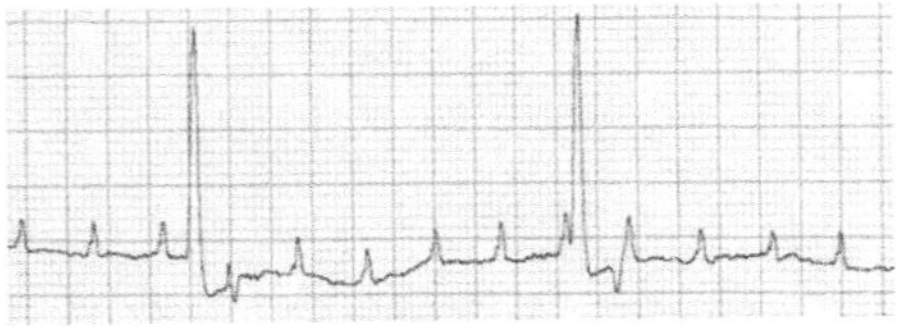	Third-degree atrioventricular block (3° AVB)	No association between P waves and QRS complexes. A junctional (narrow QRS complex) or ventricular (wide QRS complex) escape rhythm is present (rate usually 30–60 beats/min).	Atrioventricular nodal disease (degenerative, neoplastic, and inflammatory).	Elective anesthesia is contraindicated. Isoproterenol (beta-adrenergic receptor agonist) may be used for 3° AVB. Electrical pacing (transvenous lead or external patches).

and cause myocardial hypoxia, the risk of sudden death is low compared to ventricular tachyarrhythmias.

Horses are especially prone to atrial fibrillation, which is usually associated with little or no cardiac morphological changes (lone atrial fibrillation) or can be secondary to atrial enlargement due to congenital or acquired heart disease. Transient potassium depletion (due to furosemide administration or sweating during exercise) has also been reported as a predisposing cause of atrial fibrillation. In this species, paroxysmal atrial fibrillation is not uncommon and tends to return to a normal sinus rhythm within 24–48 h after its onset.

Ventricular Tachyarrhythmias

Ectopic beats originating from the ventricles are called "ventricular premature contractions" (VPCs) or ventricular tachycardia (when more than three VPCs are present in succession). These ectopic beats are characterized by an abnormally wide QRS complex with a large T wave of opposite polarity, are not associated with a preceding P wave, and occur at a faster heart rate than the sinus rate.

Ventricular arrhythmias can be caused by a primary cardiac disease or can occur secondary to another systemic illness. When underlying cardiac disease is present, such as cardiomyopathy, severe valvular disease, or myocarditis, VT is more likely to occur at a fast rate (greater than 200 beats per minute). In this case, cardiac output can be significantly reduced, and the risk of developing ventricular fibrillation and cardiac arrest is significant. The following genetic conditions are particularly associated with a high risk of VT and sudden death: ARVC in Boxers and English Bulldogs, DCM in Doberman Pinschers, and inherited ventricular arrhythmias in German Shepherds Dogs and Rhodesian Ridgebacks. Ventricular arrhythmias can also be present in conditions causing myocardial hypoxia such as HCM, subaortic stenosis, and pulmonic stenosis.

Isolated VPCs and "slow" VT (rate lower than 160 beats per minute, also called "accelerated idioventricular rhythm") are often seen with extra-cardiac conditions such as splenic disease or other abdominal diseases, trauma, hypoxia, conditions causing systemic inflammation, anemia, or electrolyte disturbances such as hypokalemia. When the heart rate is relatively low, ventricular arrhythmias usually do not affect cardiac output and the risk of sudden death is low. In cats, the presence of ventricular arrhythmias is associated with an underlying myocardial disease in the majority of cases (Côté and Jaeger, 2008). In horses, occasional isolated VPCs can be detected at rest or following exercise in normal individuals. However, frequent and polymorphic VPCs and VT are considered to be abnormal and can be associated with cardiac or extra-cardiac conditions.

Ventricular tachyarrhythmias should be treated if there is evidence of impaired perfusion and/or if there is concern that the ventricular rhythm may result in ventricular fibrillation (e.g., rapid ventricular tachycardia and presence of R-on-T phenomenon). During anesthesia, an attempt should be made to control hemodynamically significant ventricular tachyarrhythmias because of the impact that anesthetic drugs already have on the cardiovascular system.

Bradyarrhythmia

Sinus bradycardia is a sinus rhythm with an abnormally low heart rate. Sinus bradycardia can result from peri-operative drugs (e.g., alpha-2 adrenergic agonists and opioids), enhanced vagal tone, metabolic disturbances (e.g., hypothermia and hyperkalemia), and primary cardiac disease, and there is no consensus to when it should be treated. In general, bradycardia should be treated when it is associated with indicators of poor perfusion, hypotension, or a concern that it may result in sinus arrest. Bradycardia associated with severe hypothermia is dangerous as it will not respond to pharmacologic intervention.

The two most common pathologic bradyarrhythmias in dogs are sinus node dysfunction and atrioventricular block (including second- and third-degree AVB). Sinus node dysfunction is characterized by periods during which the sinus node fails to discharge leading to a pause. Sinus node dysfunction can lead to the clinical syndrome of sick sinus syndrome (SSS). Dogs with SSS often show signs of lethargy, pre-syncope (episodes of dizziness for example), or syncope. Certain breeds such as miniature Schnauzers and West Highland White Terriers are predisposed to SSS. Second-degree AVB is characterized by an intermittent lack of atrioventricular conduction (P waves intermittently not followed by QRS complexes on ECG), while third-degree AVB is characterized by a complete failure of atrioventricular conduction with the presence of a ventricular or junctional escape rhythm. In cases of third-degree AVB, the ECG shows a normal or elevated atrial rate (P waves) and independent QRS complexes (often wide, similar morphology to VPCs) with a slow rate of 30–60 beats per minute. There are multiple possible causes of bradyarrhythmias including drugs (e.g., alpha-2 adrenergic agonists and opioids), degeneration of the conduction system (most common in older dogs), infiltrative disease (i.e., neoplastic), ischemia, metabolic disease, endocarditis, or trauma. Second-degree AVB can be physiologic due to a high vagal tone. This is especially true in brachycephalic dog breeds and horses.

Pharmacologically Induced Arrhythmias

Anesthetic drugs can result in tachycardia/tachyarrhythmias and bradycardia/bradyarrhythmias. It is important to understand the pharmacodynamic effect of anesthetic drugs on the cardiovascular system.

Pure-*mu* agonist opioids cause vagally mediated bradycardia and have recently been confirmed to prolong PR and QT intervals in dogs (Keating et al., 2020). This can predispose dogs to the development of bradyarrhythmias, such as second-degree AVB, especially in combination with general anesthesia. Opioid-induced bradycardia or bradyarrhythmias typically respond well to administration of anticholinergics (0.01 mg/kg glycopyrrolate, IV; or 0.02–0.04 mg/kg atropine, IV). Note that anticholinergics can cause transient worsening of bradycardia and/or second-degree AVB (for up to three minutes with glycopyrrolate), especially at lower doses (Chin and Seow, 2005); this is usually resolved by repeating the dose.

Alpha-2 adrenergic receptor agonists are commonly used in veterinary species. One of their adverse effects is an increase in vascular resistance that triggers a reflex bradycardia. Some animals that are administered this class of drug will exhibit profound sinus bradycardia, sinus pauses, and second-degree AVB. Treatment of this bradycardia with anticholinergics is not recommended as the associated increase in myocardial work (increased heart rate in the presence of increased afterload) can induce malignant arrhythmias. In healthy dogs that received medetomidine and glycopyrrolate followed by isoflurane anesthesia, the combination of these drugs resulted in reduced left ventricular systolic function, increased vascular resistance (and therefore, arterial blood pressure), and no improvement in cardiac output or oxygen delivery compared to dogs that had only received medetomidine (Moraes et al., 2004a; Moraes et al., 2004b). A 2021 study demonstrated that high doses of dexmedetomidine 10 min after the administration of atropine followed by inhalant anesthesia increased cardiac troponin I levels, indicating subclinical myocardial damage (Huang et al., 2021). Recently, a study in dogs demonstrated that dexmedetomidine-induced bradycardia and second-degree AVB can be successfully treated with intravenous lidocaine (Tisotti et al., 2021). This treatment should not be used in cats because intravenous lidocaine has been found to increase systemic vascular resistance and has not been evaluated in combination with dexmedetomidine, whereas in dogs intravenous lidocaine in combination with dexmedetomidine decreases systemic vascular resistance. Some texts advocate the use of anticholinergics to treat alpha-2 adrenergic receptor agonist-associated bradycardia and concurrent hypotension during inhalant anesthesia, once the inhalational anesthetic is likely to be causing some systemic vasodilation. The cardiovascular impact of this is poorly studied. Before treatment, it is important to ensure that the animal is truly hypotensive, that is, the arterial BP reading is accurate.

When used as induction drugs, alfaxalone and propofol result in a transient, dose-dependent decrease in systemic vascular resistance, which may result in a compensatory increase in heart rate. This increased heart rate at induction can be marked and result in a tachycardia but is usually well tolerated in healthy patients. Premedication with an opioid may prevent tachycardia after induction although it is still a common phenomenon for which the clinician should be prepared. In patients that are unlikely to tolerate tachycardia, a neuroleptic induction is recommended though this approach is most effective in patients with a high ASA status. Ketamine enhances sympathetic tone and results in increases in heart rate that can persist for 20 min after a single bolus and should be avoided in patients with preexisting tachyarrhythmias or that are unlikely to tolerate tachycardia.

Pericardial Effusion

Pericardial effusion (PE) is the most common pericardial disorder in the dog and is defined by an abnormal accumulation of fluid between the epicardial surface of the heart and the parietal pericardium. PE in dogs most commonly occurs secondary to neoplasia including hemangiosarcoma, heart base tumors (such as chemodectoma), or mesothelioma. Idiopathic pericarditis is the second most common cause of PE.

The most important pathophysiologic effect of PE is impairment of the diastolic filling of the heart (i.e., cardiac tamponade) leading to decreased cardiac output and, in severe cases, cardiogenic shock. Animals with cardiac tamponade often exhibit clinical signs including weakness, collapse, pallor, muffled heart sounds, hypotension, tachycardia, right-sided heart failure (including ascites and pleural effusion), weak femoral pulses, or jugular distention. The onset of clinical signs depends on the rate and volume of PE and distensibility of the pericardium. Acute pericardial effusion can lead to cardiac tamponade rapidly, even with a small volume of effusion. In contrast, chronic, slow-accumulating PE allows the pericardium to stretch delaying the onset of cardiac tamponade. The ECG may reveal low-amplitude QRS complexes, with electrical alternans (beat-to-beat alternating amplitude of the QRS complexes). Thoracic radiographs may reveal a large globoid cardiac silhouette, but cardiac ultrasound is the most accurate noninvasive method of detecting PE.

Anesthetic Management

Animals with severe PE often respond well to very low doses of sedatives. Sedation is useful to calm the animal and allow for intravenous catheter placement and pericardiocentesis. A combination of IM butorphanol (0.1–0.4 mg/

kg) ± midazolam (0.1–0.2 mg/kg) is useful in this patient group.

Animals with less severe PE may require general anesthesia for thoracotomy or pericardiectomy, but these patients are rarely in circulatory distress, and if so, they should be stabilized before induction of anesthesia. These patients should be referred to a specialty center with an anesthesiologist.

Goals During Anesthesia

Optimize preload
Maintain heart rate
Maintain contractility
Maintain systemic vascular resistance

Before inducing anesthesia, animals should be volume resuscitated to ensure they have adequate preload to maintain ventricular filling. Providing adequate preload is important as PE can restrict cardiac filling.

An opioid can be used for premedication. Drugs that decrease systemic vascular resistance (acepromazine) should be avoided. Alpha-2 adrenergic receptor agonists are also a poor choice in this patient population because of the resulting reflex bradycardia and decrease in cardiac output.

Induction of anesthesia can be achieved using a co-induction technique as previously described. Anesthesia can be maintained using a balanced approach (inhalant anesthesia ± CRIs ± locoregional anesthesia) and advanced anesthetic monitoring (invasive arterial blood pressure is indicated). A balanced crystalloid at a rate of 5 mL/kg/h is appropriate, if normovolaemic.

Questions and Answers

There are more practice questions and answers available for this chapter on the website. Please visit http://www.wiley.com/go/VeterinaryAnesthesiaZeiler.

Questions

1) Degenerative mitral valve disease (DMVD) is the most common cardiac condition in dogs. Which of the following goals is appropriate during anesthesia of a dog with stage B2 DMVD?
   a) Decrease heart rate
   b) Decrease afterload
   c) Maintain left ventricular preload with a generous fluid bolus
   d) Decrease contractility
2) Which of the following findings can indicate significant aortic regurgitation in horses?
   a) A soft heart murmur (grade < 3/6) over the aortic valve region
   b) Hypokinetic pulses
   c) An elevated pulse pressure (>60 mmHg)
   d) A low heart rate
3) Which of the following approach is not appropriate when anesthetizing a one-year-old dog with compensated but severe pulmonic stenosis?
   a) Maintain preload with a balanced crystalloid at a rate of 5 mL/kg/h
   b) Alleviate stress with opioid premedication
   c) Maintain a high heart rate by administration of an anticholinergic during premedication
   d) Maintain a normal pulmonary vascular resistance by maintaining normocapnia and a high fraction of inspired oxygen

Answers

1) b
2) c
3) c

Further Reading

Alexoudis, A.K., Spyridonidou, A.G., Vogiatzaki, T.D., and Iatrou, C.A. (2009). Anaesthetic implications of arrhythmogenic right ventricular dysplasia/cardiomyopathy. *Anaesth* 64: 73–78.

Chin, K.J. and Seow, S.C. (2005). Atrioventricular conduction block induced by low-dose atropine. *Anaesth* 60: 935–936.

Coleman, A.E., Shepard, M.K., Schmiedt, C.W. et al. (2016). Effects of orally administered enalapril on blood pressure and hemodynamic response to vasopressors during isoflurane anesthesia in healthy dogs. *Vet Anaesth Analg* 43: 482–494.

Côté, E., Edwards, N.J., Ettinger, S.J. et al. (2015). Management of incidentally detected heart murmurs in dogs and cats. *J Am Vet Med Assoc* 246: 1076–1088.

Côté, E. and Jaeger, R. (2008). Ventricular tachyarrhythmias in 106 cats: associated structural cardiac disorders. *J Vet Intern Med* 22: 1444–1446.

Ettinger, S.J., Farace, G., Forney, S.D. et al. (2012). Evaluation of plasma N-terminal pro-B-type natriuretic peptide concentrations in dogs with and without cardiac disease. *J Am Vet Med Assoc* 240: 171–180.

Flacke, W.E., Flacke, J.W., Bloor, B.C. et al. (1993). Effects of dexmedetomidine on systemic and coronary hemodynamics in the anesthetized dog. *J Cardiothor Vascul Anesth* 7: 41–49.

Fox, P.R., Oyama, M.A., Reynolds, C. et al. (2009). Utility of plasma N-terminal pro-brain natriuretic peptide (NT-proBNP) to distinguish between congestive heart failure and non-cardiac causes of acute dyspnea in cats. *J Vet Cardiol* 11 (Suppl 1): S51–S61.

Fox, P.R., Rush, J.E., Reynolds, C.A. et al (2011). Multicenter evaluation of plasma N-terminal probrain natriuretic peptide (NT-pro BNP) as a biochemical screening test for asymptomatic (occult) cardiomyopathy in cats. *J Vet Intern Med* 25: 1010–1016.

Goya, S., Wada, T., Shimada, K. et al. (2018). Dose-dependent effects of isoflurane and dobutamine on cardiovascular function in dogs with experimental mitral regurgitation. *Vet Anaesth Analg* 45: 432–442.

Huang, H.Y., Liao, K.Y., Shia, W.Y. et al. (2021). Effect of administering dexmedetomidine with or without atropine on cardiac troponin I level in isoflurane-anesthetized dogs. *J Vet Med Sci* 83: 1869–1876.

Ishikawa, Y., Uechi, M., Ishikawa, R. et al. (2007). Effect of isoflurane anesthesia on hemodynamics following the administration of an angiotensin-converting enzyme inhibitor in cats. *J Vet Med Sci* 69: 869–871.

Jepsen-Grant, K., Pollard, R.E., and Johnson, L.R. (2013). Vertebral heart scores in eight dog breeds. *Vet Rad Ultraso* 54: 3–8.

Keating, S., Fries, R., Kling, K. et al. (2020). Effect of methadone or hydromorphone on cardiac conductivity in dogs before and during sevoflurane anesthesia. *Front Vet Sci* 7: 573706.

Keene, B.W., Atkins, C.E., Bonagura, J.D. et al. (2019). ACVIM consensus guidelines for the diagnosis and treatment of myxomatous mitral valve disease in dogs. *J Vet Intern Med* 33: 1127–1140.

Lamont, L.A., Bulmer, B.J., Sisson, D.D. et al. (2002). Doppler echocardiographic effects of medetomidine on dynamic left ventricular outflow tract obstruction in cats. *J Am Vet Med Assoc* 221: 1276–1281.

Luis Fuentes, V., Abbott, J., Chetboul, V. et al. (2020). ACVIM consensus statement guidelines for the classification, diagnosis, and management of cardiomyopathies in cats. *J Vet Intern Med* 34: 1062–1077.

Martin-Flores, M., Moy-Trigilio, K.E., Campoy, L., and Araos, J. (2021). The use of dexmedetomidine during pulmonic balloon valvuloplasty in dogs. *Vet Rec* 188: e75.

Moraes, A.N., Mirakhur, K., McDonell, W. et al. (2004a). Modification of the cardiopulmonary response to medetomidine in isoflurane anesthetized dogs following treatment with glycopyrrolate. *Vet Anaesth Analg* 31: 13–14.

Moraes, A.N., O'Grady, M., McDonell, W. et al. (2004b). The echocardiographic effects of glycopyrrolate pretreatment in the response to medetomidine in dogs anesthetized with isoflurane. *Vet Anaesth Analg* 31: 14.

Moran-Muñoz, R., Valverde, A., Ibancovichi, J.A. et al. (2017). Cardiovascular effects of constant rate infusions of lidocaine, lidocaine and dexmedetomidine, and dexmedetomidine in dogs anesthetized at equipotent doses of sevoflurane. *Can Vet J* 58: 729–734.

Pagel, P.S., Hettrick, D.A., Kersten, J.R. et al. (1998). Cardiovascular effects of propofol in dogs with dilated cardiomyopathy. *Anesthes* 88: 180–189.

Pascoe, P.J., Ilkiw, J.E., and Pypendop, B.H. (2006). Effects of increasing infusion rates of dopamine, dobutamine, epinephrine, and phenylephrine in healthy anesthetized cats. *Am J Vet Res* 67: 1491–1499.

Reef, V.B., Bonagura, J., Buhl, R. et al. (2014). Recommendations for management of equine athletes with cardiovascular abnormalities. *J Vet Intern Med* 28: 749–761.

Saponaro, V., Crovace, A., De Marzo, L. et al. (2013). Echocardiographic evaluation of the cardiovascular effects of medetomidine, acepromazine and their combination in healthy dogs. *Res Vet Sci* 95: 687–692.

Skelding, A.M. and Valverde, A. (2020). Sympathomimetics in veterinary species under anesthesia. *Vet J* 258: 105455.

Tisotti, T., Valverde, A., Hopkins, A. et al. (2021). Use of intravenous lidocaine to treat dexmedetomidine-induced bradycardia in sedated and anesthetized dogs. *Vet Anaesth Analg* 48: 174–186.

Valverde, A., Doherty, T.J., Hernández, J. et al. (2004). Effect of lidocaine on the minimum alveolar concentration of isoflurane in dogs. *Vet Anaesth Analg* 31: 264–271.

van Haaften, K.A., Forsythe, L., Stelow, E.A., and Bain, M.J. (2017). Effects of a single preappointment dose of gabapentin on signs of stress in cats during transportation and veterinary examination. *J Am Vet Med Assoc* 251: 1175–1181.

Wess, G., Domenech, O., Dukes-mcewan, J. et al. (2017). European Society of Veterinary Cardiology screening guidelines for dilated cardiomyopathy in Doberman Pinschers. *J Vet Cardiol* 19: 405–415.

18

Approach to a Patient with Respiratory Pathology

Carolyn Kerr and Gareth Zeiler

Overview of Airway, Thoracic, and Lung Pathology

1) Patients with underlying respiratory disease may require anesthesia for diagnostic or therapeutic procedures that may or may not include interventions directed at resolving or alleviating symptoms associated with their respiratory condition.
2) In some instances, patients may be asymptomatic at rest; however, a thorough history and physical examination may reveal clinical signs supporting the presence of underlying disease affecting the respiratory system. Diagnostic tests should be performed to characterize the primary disease and any concurrent conditions.
3) Sedation, general anesthesia and the associated change in body position alter a patient's work of breathing and can impair the ability of the respiratory system to achieve adequate carbon dioxide removal and oxygen uptake. In patients with underlying respiratory disease, the risk of complications and mortality associated with anesthesia is increased.
4) Respiratory diseases commonly encountered in veterinary medicine can be divided into those affecting the upper airways, lower airways, the thorax (including the intrathoracic space), and the lung parenchyma.
5) Providing medical or surgical care to animals with advanced respiratory pathology can become complex and require expertise and specialized equipment. Early referral to a hospital capable of handling these cases should be strongly considered.

Emergency Management of Patients in Respiratory Distress

Management of patients in respiratory distress often requires rapid intervention, including endotracheal intubation to secure an airway. Therefore, it is helpful to prepare an emergency equipment kit ready for use. A kit should include a range of facemasks, orotracheal tubes (a size range from 3.0 mm to 10.0 mm should be available), means to secure the orotracheal tube, gauze swabs (to remove excessive saliva), laryngoscope, monitoring equipment including a pulse oximeter, electrocardiogram and blood pressure monitor, system to permit suctioning the airway, intravenous (IV) anesthetics suitable for induction of anesthesia, and intravenous catheterization supplies. A range of endotracheal tubes with embedded radiopaque marking should be available for patients with tracheal collapse.

Respiratory distress is caused by severe alterations in pulmonary gas exchange resulting from abnormalities in any part of the respiratory system. A patient may present to the veterinarian in respiratory distress or it may develop at any point in the peri-anesthetic period. Figure 18.1 outlines typical clinical signs and an approach to the initial management of a patient in respiratory distress.

Administration of sedative and/or analgesic drugs is recommended in animals exhibiting signs of anxiety, pain, or discomfort. The choice of drug will vary with the species; however, it is generally recommended that drugs are administered intravenously and titrated to effect through an intravenous catheter. Recommended drugs and doses in different species are outlined in Table 18.1. Unfortunately, sedation has the potential to worsen a patient's clinical signs, particularly if upper airway obstruction is contributing to respiratory distress. Therefore, animals that have received a sedative should be closely observed and material available for intervention (e.g., induction of general anesthesia and endotracheal intubation). If acute inflammation or edema of the upper airways is contributing to the patient's condition, anti-inflammatories will reduce the severity of airflow obstruction. If the inflammation and edema is caused by an insect envenomation (e.g., African

Fundamental Principles of Veterinary Anesthesia, First Edition. Edited by Gareth E. Zeiler and Daniel S. J. Pang.

Companion Website: www.wiley.com/go/VeterinaryAnesthesiaZeiler

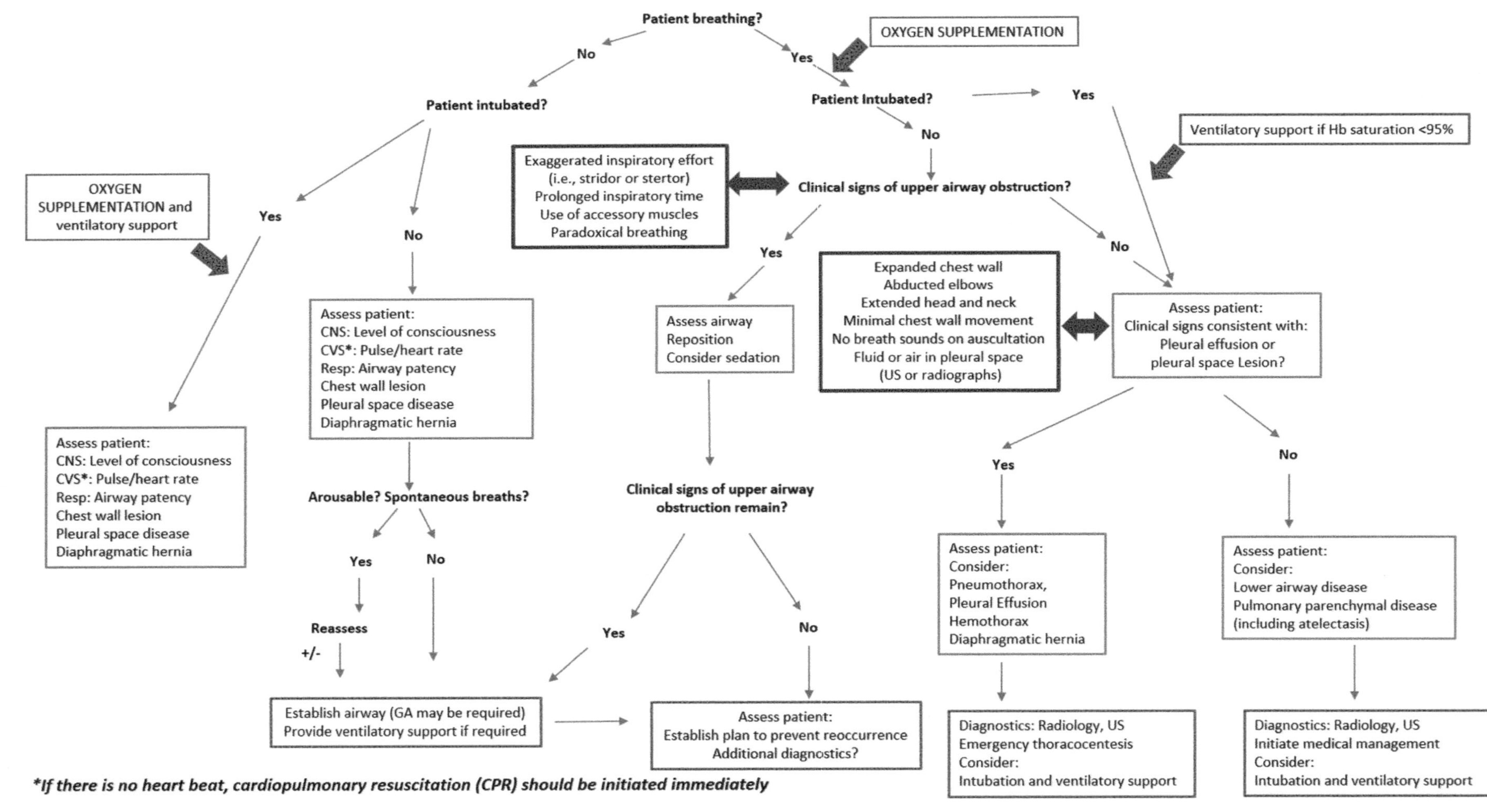

Figure 18.1 A decision flow diagram that can be used to manage a patient in respiratory distress. CVS: cardiovascular system; CNS: central nervous system; Resp: respiratory system; US: ultrasound; GA: general anesthesia; Hb: hemoglobin.

Table 18.1 Drugs commonly used in the immediate peri-anesthetic period in patients with respiratory disease.

Drug	Dose (mg/kg unless otherwise stated)	Mode of administration	Potential acute adverse effects
Sedative and analgesic drugs			
Canine and feline			
Acepromazine	0.01–0.02	IM, IV	Oversedation and upper airway muscle relaxation
Dexmedetomidine	0.25–1.00 mcg/kg	IM, IV	As above
Medetomidine	1–4 mcg/kg	IM, IV	As above
Alfaxalone	1–2	IM, IV	As above
Midazolam	0.1–0.2	IM, IV	As above
Butorphanol	0.2–0.4	IM, IV	As above
Methadone	0.2–0.4	IM, IV (slowly)	As above
Equine			
Xylazine	0.2–.5	IM, IV	Oversedation and upper airway muscle relaxation
Romifidine	20–50 mcg/kg	IM, IV	As above
Detomidine	2–10 mcg/kg	IM, IV	As above
Butorphanol	0.02–0.04	IM, IV	As above
Morphine	0.1–0.2	IM, IV (slowly)	Histamine-mediated hypotension (not common)
Respiratory drugs			
Canine and feline			
Bronchodilators			
Terbutaline	0.01	SC, IV, and IM	Tachycardia and muscle tremors
Salbutamol (Albuterol)	100 mcg (one puff of metered dose puffer)	Via metered dose inhaler and chamber	Tachycardia and muscle tremors
	0.005–0.01	IV, IM	
Atropine	0.02	IV	Tachycardia, arrhythmias, and drying (thickening) of airway secretions
Anti-inflammatories			
Dexamethasone sodium phosphate	0.5–1	IV	
Prednisolone sodium succinate	2	IV	
Equine			
Bronchodilators			
Salbutamol (Albuterol)	1–2 mcg/kg (1–2 puffs per 100 kg)	Via metered dose inhaler and chamber	Tachycardia, muscle tremors, and sweating
Atropine	0.01–0.02	IV	Tachycardia, arrhythmias, and drying of airway secretions
Gastrointestinal drugs			
Canine and feline			
Anti-emetics			
Maropitant	1.0	SC, IV (slowly)	Pain at injection site (SC)
	2.0	PO	

(Continued)

Table 18.1 (Continued)

Drug	Dose (mg/kg unless otherwise stated)	Mode of administration	Potential acute adverse effects
Ondansetron	0.5–1	IV	
Proton Pump Inhibitors			
Omeprazole	1	PO	
Pantoprazole	1	IV slowly	
Prokinetics			
Cisapride	1	IV at a rate of 0.5 mg/kg/h	Arrhythmias
Metoclopramide	1 1–2	SC IV as CRI over 24 h	Neurological signs (extrapyramidal)
Histamine Type-2 antagonists			
Famotidine	0.5–1.0	PO, IV, or SC	Drug interactions; do not use with omeprazole
Antacids			
Sucralfate (Suspension)	0.5–1.0 g per dog 0.25–0.5 g per cat	PO PO	Ptyalism

mcg: micrograms; g: grams; IM: intramuscular; IV: intravenous; SC: subcutaneous; PO: per *os*; CRI: constant rate infusion.

honey bees), then the addition of a low dose of adrenaline (0.001–0.003 mg/kg IV) is effective to reduce swelling.

Although the underlying etiology of respiratory distress will vary, if a patient has a patent airway, oxygen supplementation is warranted. Different methods of supplementing a patient's inspired oxygen are outlined in Table 18.2. Patients with acute respiratory distress may have altered body temperature and addressing this can help alleviate symptoms. Oxygen support is strongly recommended in hyperthermic patients.

Marked partial or complete upper airway obstruction requires immediate intervention. In some instances, simply repositioning the animal, examining the oropharynx, and/or exteriorizing the tongue may relieve the airway obstruction. Depending on the species and location of the obstruction, an orotracheal tube may be required to permit adequate gas flow. If orotracheal intubation is not possible, then a tracheostomy tube or nasotracheal tube may be required. Various strategies used to secure an airway are outlined in Table 18.3.

In conscious small animal patients, general anesthesia is required to establish either an orotracheal or an alternative airway, such as a tracheostomy. Horses, as obligate nasal breathers, are particularly vulnerable to upper airway obstruction; however, if the obstruction is due to soft-tissue or laryngeal abnormalities, it may be possible to place a nasal or nasotracheal tube until a more permanent solution can be established. Placement of a tracheostomy tube in large animals can generally be achieved using local anesthesia.

Clinical signs indicative of significant pleural space disease include minimal to absent chest movement on inspiration, chest wall distension, and the absence of air sounds on thoracic auscultation. In severe cases, the patient may be gasping, have cyanotic mucus membranes, and have pulses that are either nonpalpable or weak. In dogs with short hair coats, distended jugular veins may be visible. Thoracocentesis should be performed in patients with respiratory distress and signs consistent with pleural effusion or pneumothorax. Ideally, interventions aimed at removing air or fluid from the pleural space are performed after survey thoracic radiographs or ultrasonography; however, in urgent situations when the patient is not responding to oxygen therapy, this may not be feasible. Thoracocentesis can be performed using an over-the-needle catheter or butterfly catheter (for smaller patients) placed in the seventh intercostal space. When air is suspected, the catheter should be placed at the junction of the upper and middle thirds of the chest when the patient is in sternal recumbency or at the highest point when the animal is in lateral recumbency. If fluid is suspected to be present, the catheter should be placed closer to the costochondral junction. If a chest tube is already in place but there is a pneumothorax, then it should be carefully examined as a potential source of air leak. Placing a chest drain is useful for patient management because it can be used to evacuate air or fluid from the thorax without the stress of repeated thoracocenteses.

In companion animals with respiratory distress resulting from pulmonary parenchymal disease, if oxygen

Table 18.2 Strategies used to supplement inspired oxygen content in veterinary species.

Technique	Description	Species typically employed	Typical oxygen flow rates[a]	Approximate inspired oxygen (%)
Flow-by	Oxygen provided to patient via either breathing circuit or tubing directly from oxygen source. Source held within 2 cm patient's nose/mouth.	Canine, feline	100–200 mL/kg/min	25–35
Face mask	Clear face mask attached to anesthetic breathing circuit placed over patient's muzzle. Higher FiO_2 will be achieved if a seal can be created to minimize entraining room air into mask.	Canine, feline, neonatal equine, or bovine	100 mL/kg/min	30–95
Nasal catheter	Nasal catheter (soft rubber catheter) with multiple fenestrations placed in ventral nasal meatus and connected to oxygen supply. Catheter generally placed to level of medial canthus of the eye. Unilateral or bilateral.	Canine, feline, foals, and calves	50–100 mL/kg/min up to 5 L per nostril	30–70
Traditional nasal cannulas	Prongs that extend approximately 1 cm into each nostril, are connected to oxygen supply.	Canine, feline	50–100 mL/kg/min	30–60
High-flow nasal cannulas (HFNC)	Specifically designed nasal cannulae that are connected to an HFNC ventilator.	Canine and feline	0.5–2 L/kg/min (can go to 60 L/min)	21–100
Transtracheal	Oxygen delivered through a tracheostomy or transtracheal catheter.	Canine, neonatal equine, or bovine	10–20 mL/kg/min	50–95
Oxygen hood	Oxygen is supplied into an enclosure that is either a commercial clear plexiglass structure that at least the animals head and thorax can be placed in or a hood created using an Elizabethan collar and plastic wrap.	Canine and feline	Up to 300 mL/kg/min depending on size and nature of hood and oxygen supply capabilities.	40–95
Oxygen cage	Commercial cage that is sealed and permits regulation of O_2, CO_2, and humidity.	Canine and feline	Variable depending on system. Typically, 2–10 L/min	50–60
Mechanical ventilation	Traditional positive pressure ventilation in a patient with a sealed airway.	Canine and feline	Variable depending on system. Typically, 2–10 L/min	21–100

a) Note: Most small animal anesthetic machines are equipped with flow meters with a maximum flow rate of 5–8 L/min while large animal machines typically have a maximum flow rate of 10–15 L/min.
FiO_2: fraction of inspired oxygen; CO_2: carbon dioxide; O_2: oxygen.

supplementation does not improve symptoms, inducing anesthesia, establishing a secure airway, and instituting positive pressure ventilation using a ventilator capable of providing positive end expiratory pressure (PEEP) and variable fraction of inspired oxygen (FiO_2) are indicated. Under such circumstances, the level of supportive care and intensive monitoring required is best provided by tertiary referral hospitals. In large animal patients with acute pulmonary edema following upper airway obstruction, diuretics, anti-inflammatory drugs, and oxygen supplementation are recommended.

History and Diagnostic Workup of Patients with Respiratory Disease Before Anesthesia

History

Obtaining a thorough history and pre-anesthetic workup will provide essential information regarding the severity of a patient's airway disease, permit optimizing the patient's status before anesthesia, forewarn the anesthesia and surgical teams of likely complications, and allow owners to be informed regarding the risk of peri-anesthetic complications (see Chapter 2).

Table 18.3 Strategies used to secure a patient's airway and permit connection to an anesthetic machine.

Technique	Description	Advantages	Limitations
Supraglottic airway device	Placement of a device that covers the opening of the larynx and epiglottis via the oropharynx. Reported use in dogs, cats, and rabbits.	Reduces risk of trauma to larynx and provocation of laryngospasm.	Does not protect the airway from aspiration to the same degree as a cuffed endotracheal tube.
Direct orotracheal intubation	Placement of an endotracheal tube into the trachea via the oropharynx by visualizing the larynx. Use of a laryngoscope recommended. Routinely performed in canine, feline, and small ruminants.	Permits examination of oropharynx, arytenoids, epiglottis, and vocal folds. Low probability of trauma if patient at appropriate depth of anesthesia while procedure performed. Permits creation of a sealed airway and decreases risk of aspiration.	Requires adequate relaxation of masticatory muscles and temporomandibular joint to permit visualization of larynx.
Blind orotracheal intubation	Placement of an endotracheal tube into the trachea via the oropharynx without visualization. Insertion is timed with inspiration. Routinely performed in equine. Can be performed in rabbits; however, it requires practice and can result in trauma to larynx with improper technique.	Ease of technique and low risk of complications in equine. Permits creation of a sealed airway and decreases risk of aspiration.	In horses with laryngeal paralysis, a smaller orotracheal tube is required to bypass the larynx.
Orotracheal intubation with direct palpation	Manual placement of an endotracheal tube into the trachea via the oropharynx. Performed in mature bovine.	Method permits securing airway rapidly in a large animal predisposed to regurgitation. Permits creation of a sealed airway and decreases risk of aspiration.	Patient must be large enough to permit arm placement into oral cavity.
Orotracheal intubation using a stylet	Placement of a stylet into the trachea using direct observation. Stylet used as a guide for endotracheal tube. Routinely performed in goats and sheep when direct orotracheal tube placement via direct observation challenging in dogs and cats.	Suitable technique when visualization of larynx is challenging with orotracheal tube in oropharynx. Permits creation of a sealed airway and decreases risk of aspiration. Permits creation of a sealed airway and decreases risk of aspiration.	Tube tip can get caught on arytenoid cartilages as it is passed from oropharynx into trachea blindly.
Flexible fiberoptic intubation	Placement of a flexible fiberoptic endoscope inside the orotracheal tube with subsequent advancement of endoscope into trachea via the oropharynx. Technique commonly used in rabbits. Suitable in any species with potentially challenging airway.	Excellent technique that can be used in any species in which a challenging orotracheal intubation is anticipated. Permits creation of a sealed airway and decreases risk of aspiration.	Requires specialized equipment.
Nasotracheal intubation	Placement of tube into the trachea via the nasal passage.	Easily performed in the sedated equine. Permits creation of a sealed airway and decreases risk of aspiration.	Smaller tube required than when orotracheal intubation performed, and therefore resistance to breathing is increased.
Tracheotomy ± tracheostomy	Creation of an incision over the trachea in the mid-cervical region to create space (a tracheostomy) to allow placement of a tube into the trachea directly.	Suitable means to secure an airway when other techniques have failed or are anticipated to fail based on examination of the airway. Can be performed with local anesthesia infiltration in large animals in small animals generally performed under general anesthesia. Permits creation of a sealed airway and decreases risk of aspiration.	In conscious small animal patients best performed under general in combination with local anesthesia.

Physical Examination

The discussion in the following text specifically focuses on evaluating the respiratory system; however, a complete physical examination is required for all patients before nonurgent or nonemergent sedation or general anesthesia.

Carefully observing a patient at rest, before any interventions, can provide important information regarding the respiratory system. Respiratory frequency and effort should be noted with the degree of accessory muscle involvement during inspiration and expiration. Body position, restlessness, and facial expressions may signal excessive work of breathing or inadequacies in gas exchange (Figure 18.2).

The normal breathing cycle involves an active inspiratory phase, a passive expiratory phase (with the exception of the horse, in which it is active), and an end expiratory pause. The presence of audible respiratory noise on inspiration or expiration is indicative of an obstructive abnormality in the major airways. Stridor, a high-pitched sound, is most commonly associated with laryngeal or tracheal disease. If stridor is most noticeable on inspiration, it typically involves the extrathoracic airways, while stridor on exhalation indicates an obstruction in the intrathoracic airways. Stertor, a snoring like sound, on inspiration or expiration, originates from structures above the larynx.

An increased respiratory muscular effort signals an increase in energy (work) required to inspire or expire respiratory gases. In normal patients at rest, contraction of the inspiratory muscles leads to an increase in intrathoracic volume which decreases the pressure in the alveoli, resulting in a pressure gradient (gases always flow down a pressure gradient from a higher pressure to a lower pressure; during inspiration the alveolar pressure is less than atmospheric pressure) and subsequent airflow from the upper to the lower airways. Conversely, during expiration, the inspiratory muscles relax and return to their pre-inspiratory resting state which causes a decrease in intrathoracic volume and increase in alveoli pressure. Thus, gas flow from the lower to the upper airways (atmospheric pressure lower than alveolar pressure).

At rest, the work of breathing is primarily due to overcoming the elastic resistance (intrinsic recoil characteristics of lung parenchyma and chest wall after expansion) of the lung and chest wall during inspiration, properties that determine the pulmonary compliance (i.e., elastic resistance is the inverse of compliance). In the conscious animal,

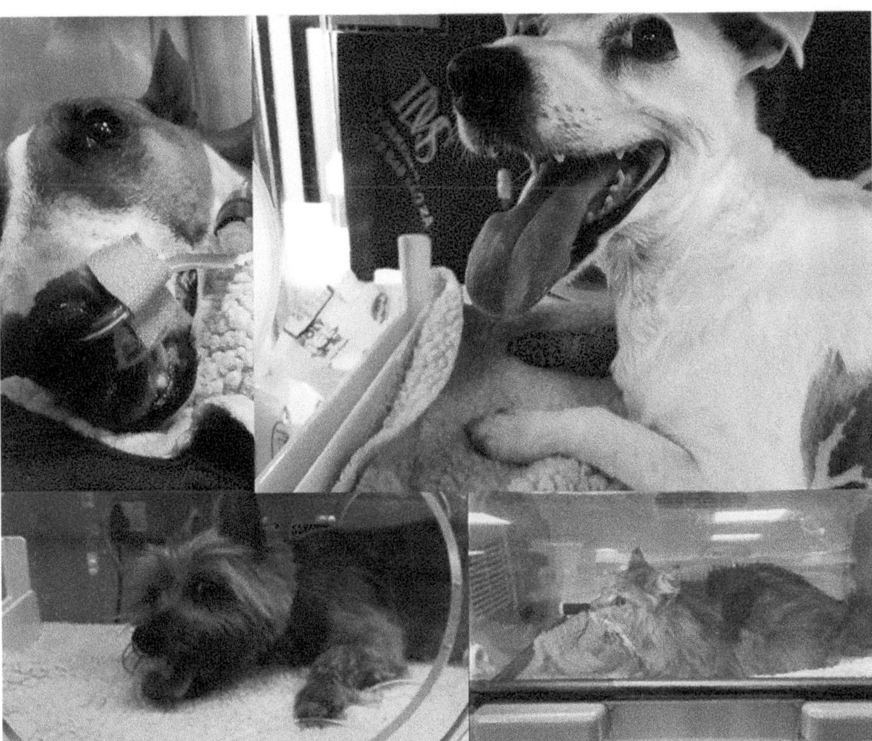

Figure 18.2 Examples of dogs and a cat in respiratory distress. Appearance can include cyanotic mucous membranes and tongue, open mouth breathing, tightened lip muscles (grimacing), vacant staring into the distance or an intense focused expression, and open mouth gasping. All animals pictured had oxygen supplementation, but their tongues remain cyanotic indicating ongoing hypoxemia/ hypoxia. Further steps could include increasing oxygen concentration delivered, and identifying and treating underlying cause or considering ventilation support. (*Source:* Courtesy of Valley Farm Animal Hospital.)

a decrease in lung or thoracic compliance, associated with pulmonary parenchymal or intrathoracic disease, typically results in an increase in respiratory frequency (not to be mistaken for panting) and reduction in tidal volume as the animal tries to minimize their work of breathing.

While the flow of gases in and out of the airways does not contribute to the majority of the work of breathing in a normal animal at rest, if airways are reduced in diameter, the contribution of airway gas flow resistance to the total work of breathing can increase dramatically. While the airways are not linear tubes, the Hagen–Poiseuille law provides a useful means to estimate the impact of changes in airway radius on the resistance to laminar airflow. As illustrated in Figure 18.3, if the radius of an airway is reduced by 50%, the resistance to gas flow will increase 16-fold. A reduction in airway radius can occur with increased airway secretions, edema, mucoid plug formation, and if a small diameter endotracheal tube is used. The reduced diameter of the airway can create significant increases in the work of breathing. Turbulent gas flow patterns, high gas flow rates, and a reduction in lung volume can also lead to further increases in airway resistance and work of breathing.

The relative time spent during, and effort associated with, inspiration versus expiration also provides important information to the clinician regarding the location of the patient's disease. Animals with conditions characterized by upper airway obstruction generally have an increase in inspiratory time and effort (in addition to noise) relative to expiratory time while animals with obstructive lower airway disease exhibit a prolonged expiratory time and effort. Open-mouthed breathing combined with an increase in respiratory effort in a companion animal at rest is often indicative of a partial or complete upper airway obstruction.

Visual examination of the upper airways and palpation of the pharynx, larynx, guttural pouches (equine), trachea and thorax, as well as thorough auscultation of upper and lower airways are recommended during a pre-anesthetic clinical examination. The presence and nature of any nasal discharge can provide valuable information regarding upper (often, but not exclusively, unilateral discharge) or lower (often bilateral discharge) airway disease. Patients with tracheal disease typically have a harsh dry cough, described as a goose honking sound that may be elicited with tracheal palpation. When pleural space disease is present, thoracic auscultation will result in a decrease in breath sounds while pulmonary parenchymal disease may result in an increase in breath sounds, crackles, and/or wheezes. Lung percussion in large animal patients can also provide further information regarding the presence of pleural effusion.

In some cases, body condition may provide an indicator as to the severity and chronicity of the disorder. For instance, animals with pleural space or parenchymal lung disease frequently have a history of weight loss due to inappetence and/or increased metabolic demand. Alternatively, limitations in exercise capacity due to upper airway obstruction

Resistance to laminar flow of a fluid (gas, liquid) in an straight unbranched tube can be explained by Poiseuille's Law.

Poiseuille's Law is

$$Q = \frac{\Delta P \pi r^4}{8 n l}$$

This equation can be separated into a change in pressure (ΔP) component and a resistance ($\frac{\pi r^4}{8nl}$) component

$$Q = \frac{\Delta P}{1} \times \frac{\pi r^4}{8 n l}$$

This equation can be re-written to focus on resistance (R) to flow as follows: Q = ΔP/R (which is Q = ΔP/1 x 1/R) and if resistance is considered alone

$$R = \frac{8nl}{\pi r^4}$$

Simplifying this equation to illustrate the impact of changes in radius, by using values of 1 for n and l, shows that halving the radius of a tube results in a 16-fold increase in resistance (from 0.16 to 2.5 in the example below).

$$R = \frac{8 \times 1 \times 1}{3.14 \times 2^4} = 0.16$$

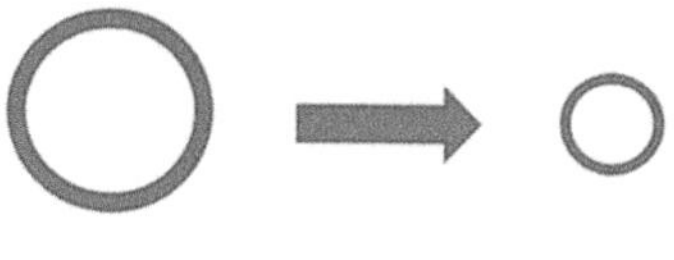

$$R = \frac{8 \times 1 \times 1}{3.14 \times 1^4} = 2.5$$

Figure 18.3 The Hagen–Poiseuille law (also known as "Poiseuille's law") can be used to hypothetically explain gas flow characteristics in a straight unbranched tube, such as the trachea, bronchus, or bronchiole. The figure resolved the equations for resistance to demonstrate what the effect of resistance is when the airway is narrowed. *Q*: flow; ΔP: pressure difference; *r*: radius; *n*: viscosity; *l*: length.

may lead some patients to gain weight, which may impact the decision on timing of planned interventions and/or the prognosis associated with an intervention.

The color of a patient's mucus membranes or tissues can in some instances give an indication of the adequacy of a patient's oxygenation. In general, if cyanosis, a bluish to purple color is observed, the patient has >5 g/dL of deoxygenated hemoglobin (Figure 18.4). In a patient with a normal hematocrit, this quantity of deoxygenated hemoglobin occurs when the oxygen partial pressure is approximately 40 mmHg. In addition to being a very late indicator of poor oxygenation, anemia, profound vasoconstriction, ambient lighting conditions, and pigmentation can alter the ability to detect cyanosis. Therefore, the absence of cyanosis is not a sensitive indicator of adequate oxygenation. Further discussion of hypoxemia is provided in the following text.

Arterial Blood Gas Analysis, Oxyhemoglobin Saturation, and Capnography

Arterial blood gas analysis provides the most reliable and accurate information regarding the adequacy of a patient's oxygenation (investigation of oxygen; O_2) and ventilation (investigation of carbon dioxide; CO_2). Jugular or mixed venous CO_2 partial pressures can be a reasonable estimate of arterial CO_2 in normal animals; however, in hemodynamically unstable patients, the use of peripheral venous blood samples to determine adequacy of ventilation is not recommended.

Noninvasive measurement of arterial hemoglobin saturation of O_2 using pulse oximetry is a valuable tool to assess oxygenation, particularly in companion animals. The relationship between arterial oxyhemoglobin saturation, O_2 partial pressure, O_2 content, and O_2 available to tissues is outlined in Figure 18.5. It is important to note the dramatic decrease in O_2 content and availability once O_2 partial pressures and oxyhemoglobin saturation fall below 60 mmHg and 90%, respectively. There are a number of practical considerations that need to be followed to obtain an accurate pulse oximeter reading (Chapter 4). For example, in a conscious patient that is moving (i.e., rhythmic movement during panting), an erroneous reading can occur.

Accurately determining the ventilatory status, with arterial CO_2 partial pressure, of an awake nonintubated patient is challenging. In hemodynamically stable patients at rest, central venous blood CO_2 partial pressures are generally 4–6 mmHg above arterial values. In unstable patients, this relationship is unpredictable. A convenient alternative to blood gas analysis is to use a capnograph (or capnometer), which continuously measures the end-tidal carbon dioxide partial pressure ($PE'CO_2$). Assessing ventilatory status noninvasively using a sidestream capnometer can be performed (e.g., via nasal cannulae/prongs); however, the accuracy is limited if the sampling site is not from within the airways and if the respiratory rate is rapid (i.e., >25 breaths per minute) or if there is open mouth breathing. Oxygen supplementation, with O_2 inflow adjacent to the capnograph sampling site, may also alter the accuracy of capnograph measurements and should be considered when interpreting the results.

Hypoxemia

Hypoxemia refers to inadequate arterial blood O_2 content and is considered to be present when arterial O_2 partial pressure is at or below 60 mmHg in animals with normal hemoglobin levels. As illustrated in Figure 18.5, oxyhemoglobin saturation and the O_2 content of blood begin to fall precipitously below this O_2 partial pressure. The major mechanisms leading to hypoxemia are outlined in Table 18.4 and Figure 18.6.

When hypoventilation, but not apnea, is the primary etiology of a patient's hypoxemia, the patient's alveolar O_2 partial pressure can be increased with O_2 supplementation and the patient's oxygenation status will improve. The relationship between alveolar O_2 partial pressure (PAO_2; note

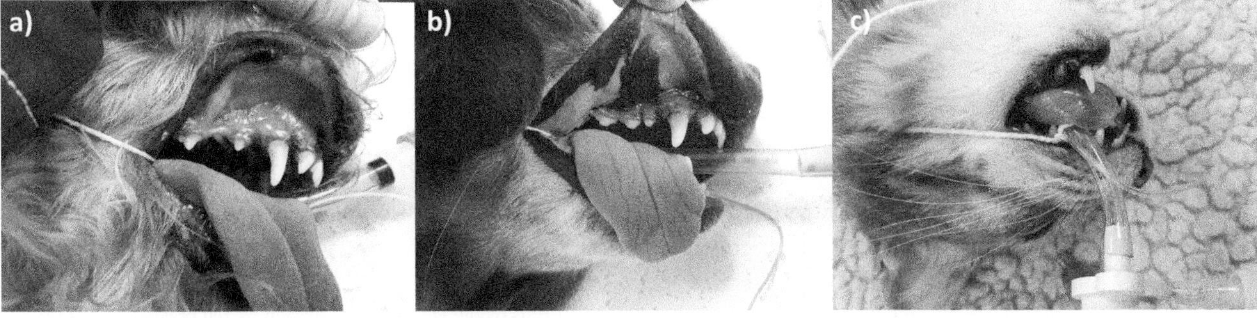

Figure 18.4 Photos of the tongue and mucous membranes in (a) a normal dog with no cyanosis, (b) a dog with cyanosis, and (c) a cat with cyanosis. (*Source:* Courtesy of Valley Farm Animal Hospital.)

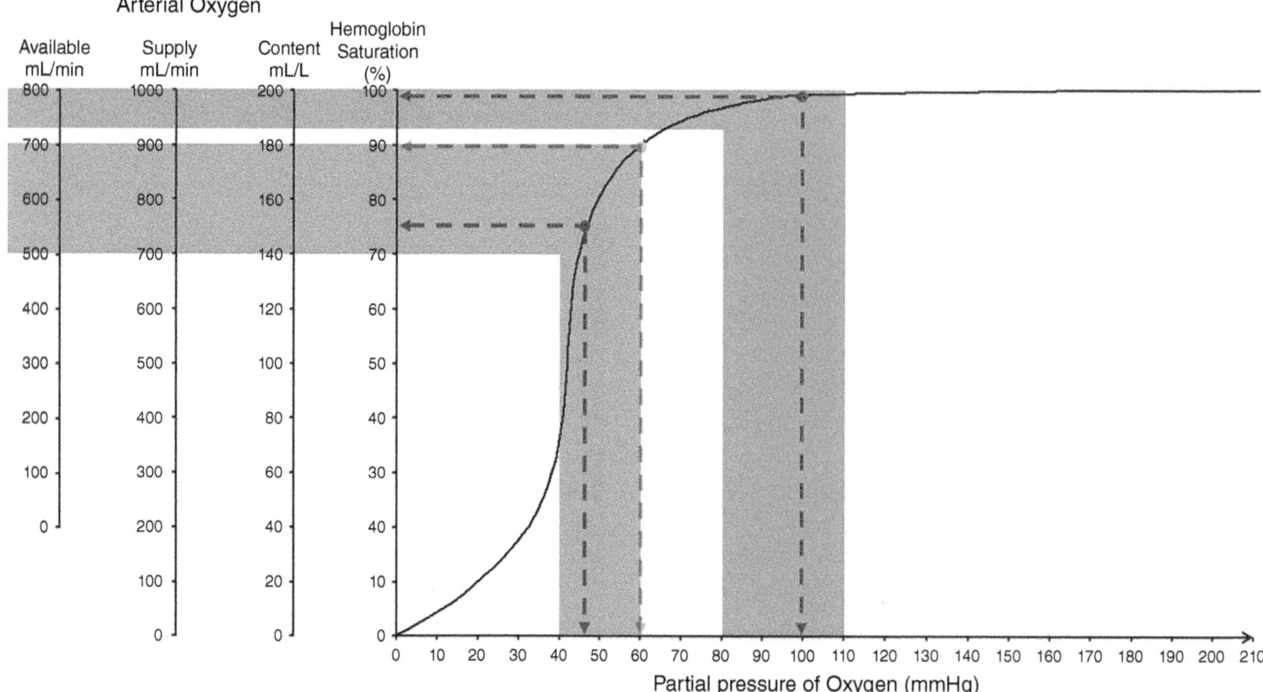

Figure 18.5 The oxygen–hemoglobin dissociation curve, demonstrating the relationship between hemoglobin saturation, partial pressure of oxygen, oxygen supply and content, and oxygen available to tissues. (*Source:* Adapted from Benumof (1994).)

Table 18.4 Causes of hypoxemia in patients with normal hemoglobin concentrations.

Causes of hypoxemia	Explanation	Clinical scenario's	Response to oxygen
Low FiO_2	Decreased PAO_2	Altitude Low FiO_2 associated with N_2O administration (or other gases in a fresh gas mixture)	PaO_2 increases
Hypoventilation	Increased $PACO_2$ resulting in decreased PAO_2	Respiratory depressant drugs such as opioids and/or anesthetics Neurological disease (central to peripheral) Upper airway obstruction Severe pulmonary disease Intrathoracic or chest wall disease	PaO_2 increases
Diffusion barrier	Thickened alveolar capillary membrane resulting in barrier to gas diffusion across alveolar capillary membrane[a]	Pulmonary edema Pulmonary disease	PaO_2 increases
Ventilation/ perfusion mismatch	Poor ventilation in some regions of lung resulting in low PAO_2. Pulmonary arterial blood suppling pulmonary capillaries in latter regions will have a reduced PaO_2	Pulmonary disease Pleural space disease	PaO_2 increases
Intrapulmonary shunt (right-to-left shunt)	Portion of pulmonary arterial blood (deoxygenated) is not in proximity to ventilated alveoli when traversing pulmonary capillaries therefore gas exchange does not occur. The poorly oxygenated blood mixes with oxygenated blood and returns to left side of heart.	Pulmonary disease Pleural space disease Atelectasis (common in large species under general anesthesia)	No response
Extrapulmonary shunt (right-to-left shunt)	Portion of pulmonary artery blood (deoxygenated) bypasses lung and returns to left side of heart	Cardiac defect Patent ductus arteriosus	No response

PAO_2: alveolar oxygen partial pressure; FiO_2: fraction of inspired oxygen; N_2O: nitrous oxide; PaO_2: arterial oxygen partial pressure; $PACO_2$: Alveolar carbon dioxide partial pressure.

[a] As described by the Fick equation, the diffusion of gas across a membrane is inversely proportional to the thickness of the membrane ($V_{gas} = A/T \times D\,[P1 - P2]$, where A is the surface area of membrane for diffusion, T is the thickness of membrane for diffusion, D is the diffusion coefficient, and $[P1 - P2]$ is the partial pressure difference).

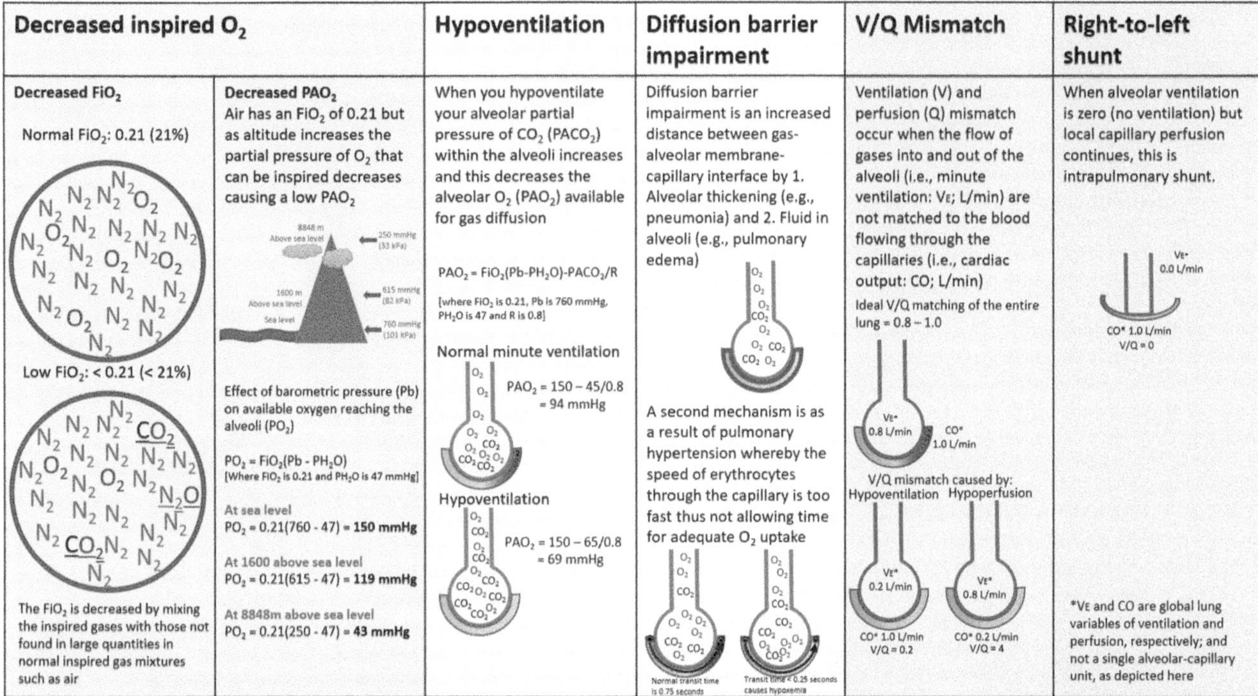

Figure 18.6 The five causes of hypoxemia.

the uppercase "A" indicating alveolar whereas a lowercase "a" indicates arterial) and alveolar ventilation, reflected by partial pressure of CO_2 ($PaCO_2$ is used because it approximates PACO2 in most clinical presentations), is best described by the alveolar gas equation:

$$PAO_2 = FiO_2(Pb - PH_2O) - PaCO_2/R$$

where FiO_2 is the fraction of inspired oxygen, Pb is the barometric pressure (760 mmHg at sea level), PH_2O is the water partial pressure in inspired air (47 mmHg at normal body temperature), $PaCO_2$ is arterial carbon dioxide partial pressures, and R is the respiratory quotient or respiratory exchange ratio, a measure of CO_2 produced relative to O_2 consumed, which is generally considered to be 0.8–0.9 for most mammals.

As outlined in Figure 18.7, in a healthy animal breathing room air, the PAO_2 is generally 100–110 mmHg. If a period of apnea or marked hypoventilation occurs, this can result in a significant reduction of PAO_2 and fall in arterial partial pressure of oxygen (PaO_2). If the FiO_2 is increased, by providing O_2 via face mask, the impact of a period of apnea or hypoventilation on arterial oxygenation is negligible.

Increasing the PAO_2 may also improve oxygenation when gas diffusion across the alveolar capillary membrane is impaired or when there is ventilation–perfusion mismatch in the lung. However, an increase in PAO_2 will not improve PaO_2 when blood does not come into contact with alveoli, as occurs with intrapulmonary and extrapulmonary shunting of blood.

The impact of the degree of intrapulmonary shunting (alveolar capillaries are perfused, but there is no ventilation of the alveoli) on the response to O_2 therapy is illustrated in Figure 18.8. As illustrated, the response to O_2 supplementation is dependent on the degree of shunt. Unfortunately, patients with large intrapulmonary or extrapulmonary shunt (>30%) will not have an increase in PaO_2 in response to O_2 supplementation. This scenario is frequently observed in horses anesthetized for colic surgery, during which significant intrapulmonary shunt occurs due to body position (dorsal recumbency), general anesthesia (muscle relaxation and cranial migration of diaphragm), and increased intra-abdominal pressure (impairing diaphragm excursion).

Hypercapnia and Hypocapnia

Arterial partial pressure of CO_2 is directly proportional to CO_2 production and inversely proportional to alveolar ventilation. During general anesthesia, CO_2 production is generally stable (with the rare exception of malignant hyperthermia or occasional case of hyperkalemic periodic paralysis or hyperthermia); therefore, hypercapnia (higher $PaCO_2$, above a normal reference interval for the species) and hypocapnia (lower $PaCO_2$, below a normal reference interval for the species) reflect decreases and increases in alveolar ventilation, respectively. The major causes of hypercapnia and hypocapnia in both a conscious and an anesthetized patient are outlined in Table 18.5.

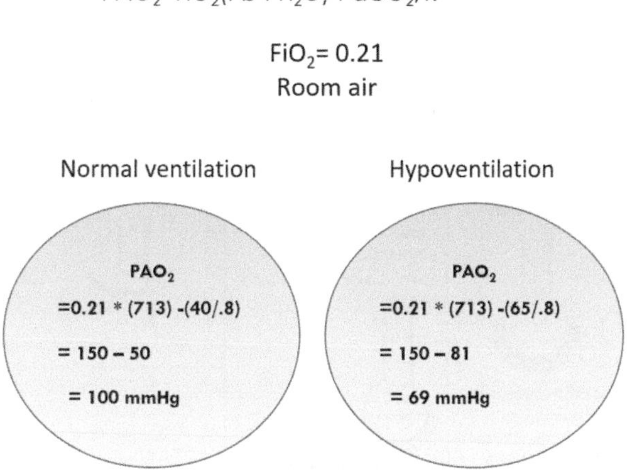

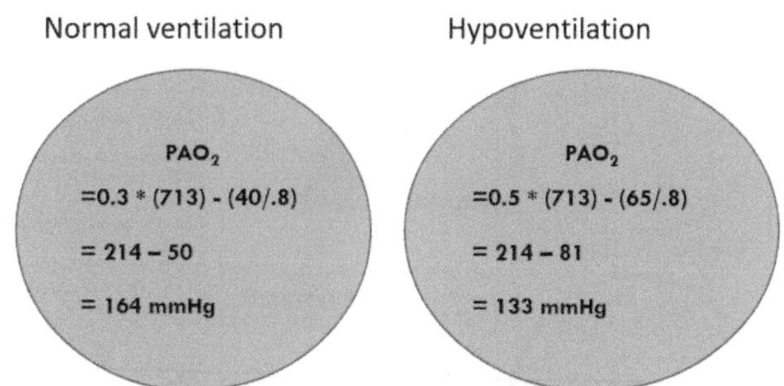

with where: PAO_2: alveolar oxygen partial pressure; FiO_2: fraction of inspired oxygen; Pb: barometric pressure (760 mmHg at sea level); PH_2O: water partial pressure in inspired air (47 mmHg); $PaCO_2$: arterial carbon dioxide partial pressure; R: respiratory quotient or respiratory exchange ratio (considered to be 0.8 – 0.9 for most mammals).

Figure 18.7 The effect of hypoventilation on alveolar partial pressure of oxygen and why hypoventilation causes hypoxemia that is responsive to oxygen supplementation.

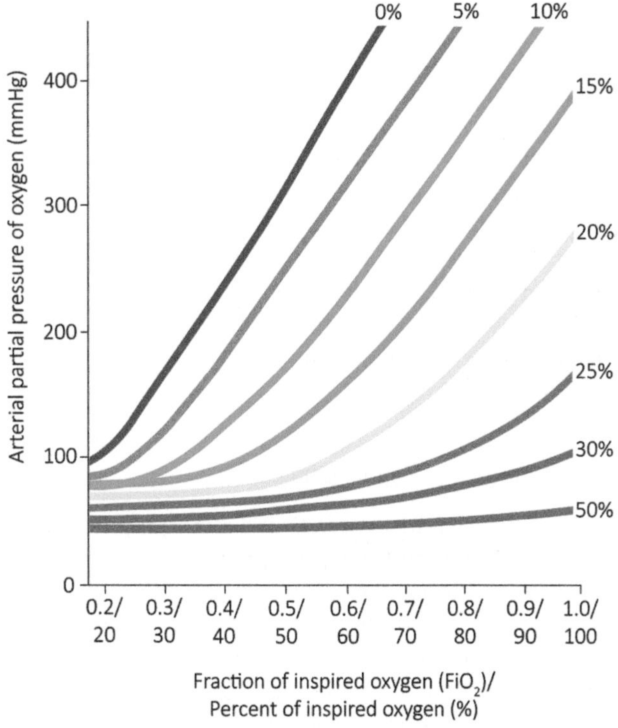

Figure 18.8 The effect of different magnitudes of right-to-left intrapulmonary shunt (curves on graphs indicate % shunt) on the arterial partial pressure of oxygen at different fractions of inspired oxygen. As shunt fraction increases above 25%, increasing the percentage of inspired oxygen has a minimal effect on increasing arterial partial pressure of oxygen. (*Source:* With permission from Benatar et al. (1973).)

Table 18.5 Causes of altered ventilation.

Hypoventilation	Common clinical scenarios
Decreased central drive to ventilate	Sedatives Opioid analgesics Anesthetics Pathology of the central nervous system (secondary to trauma, inflammation, or mass)
Decreased ability to ventilate[a]	Airway obstruction Increased dead space ventilation Respiratory muscle fatigue Neuromuscular disease Thoracic wall or diaphragmatic disease Pleural space disease
Hyperventilation	**Common clinical scenarios**
Respiratory center stimulation	Hypoxemia and hyperthermia
Metabolic (nonrespiratory) acidosis	Lactic acidosis (shock and sepsis), uremic acidosis (renal failure), and diabetic ketoacidosis
Iatrogenic	Excessive tidal volume or respiratory rate with positive pressure ventilation (manual or mechanical)

a) Most conscious patients will compensate for a decreased ability to achieve alveolar ventilation by increasing minute ventilation (respiratory frequency) to achieve normal arterial carbon dioxide partial pressure. However, if there is a combination of a decreased ability to ventilate and decreased central drive to ventilate, arterial carbon dioxide partial pressure will rise.

Importantly, the relative fraction of a tidal volume breath that contributes to alveolar ventilation can vary tremendously among species as well as within individual animals based on their pattern of breathing. The relationship between $PaCO_2$, dead space, tidal volume, and alveolar ventilation is further outlined in Figure 18.9.

Patients with respiratory disease often have an increase in dead space (alveolar or mechanical dead space); therefore, the relative amount of a tidal volume that ventilates the alveoli is reduced. The volume of dead space has implications for both the spontaneously breathing patient and the mechanically ventilated patient, whereby when dead space is increased, minute ventilation will have to be increased (Figure 18.10). Spontaneous breathing animals are likely to tire because of the increased energy requirement required to support the increased minute volume.

Diagnostic Imaging

Radiographic examination of both upper and lower airways and lungs are routine adjuncts to the physical exam for patients with respiratory disease. For equine patients with upper airway disease, ultrasound of the upper airways to assess laryngeal structure and function may also be used to assess soft-tissue structures. Thoracic ultrasound is

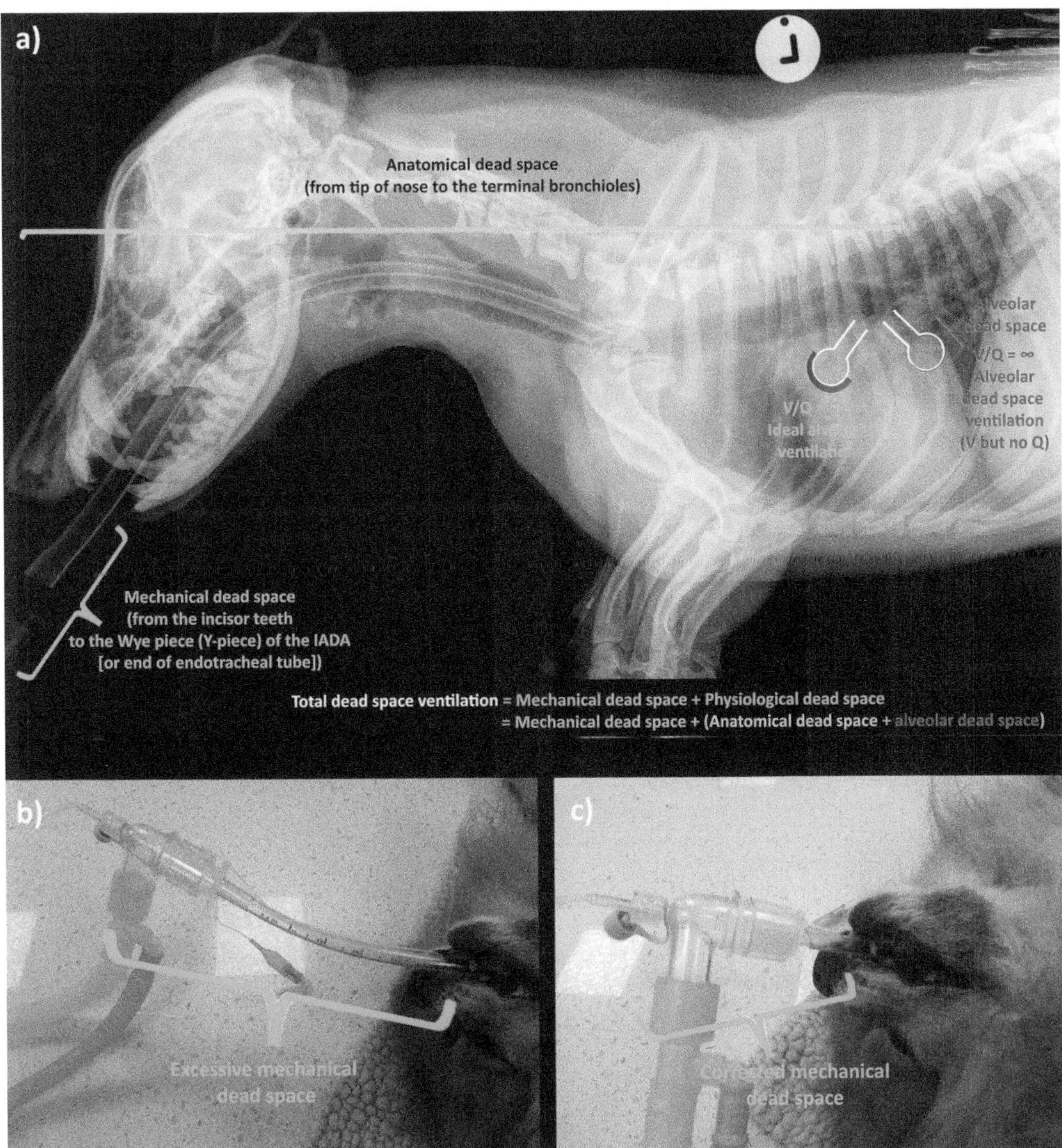

Figure 18.9 Different types of dead space (a). Mechanical dead space is the volume between the entrance to the upper airway (usually taken as the nostrils or incisors) and site where fresh gas enters the breathing system. It is common for endotracheal tubes to create mechanical dead space (portion of tube extending between incisors). Mechanical dead space is easily increased further with the addition of connectors, gas sampling chambers, and elbows (b, c). Mechanical dead space can be reduced by trimming endotracheal tubes (c), minimizing the number and volume of connectors, and using pediatric sampling chambers (when appropriate). IADA: inhalation anesthetic delivery apparatus. (*Source:* Courtesy of Valley Farm Animal Hospital).

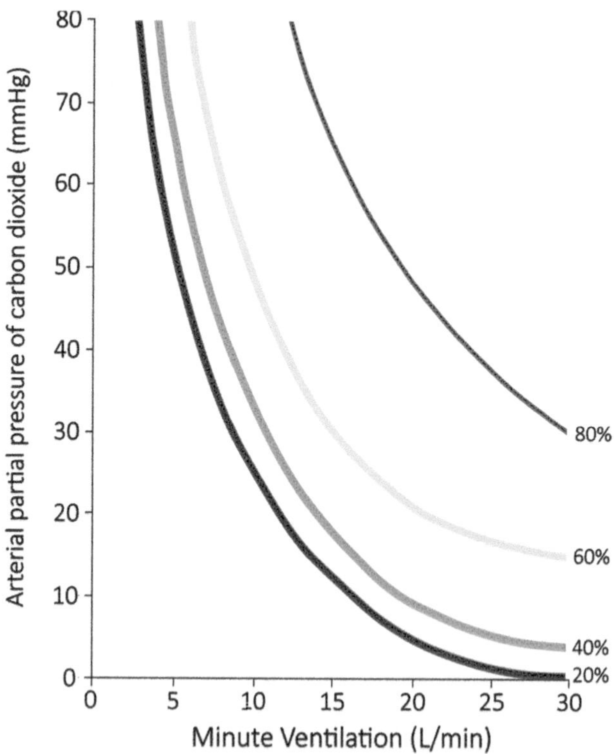

Figure 18.10 Relationship between arterial partial pressure of carbon dioxide and minute ventilation at different percentages of dead space (% lines) in spontaneous or mechanically ventilated animals. As dead space percentage increases, minute ventilation (i.e., tidal volume or respiratory rate or both) must be increased to maintain arterial partial pressure of carbon dioxide. (*Source:* With permission from Kerr and McDonell (2009).)

optimally added to the diagnostic workup in any species in which pleural space disease (e.g., effusion, diaphragmatic hernia) is suspected. Fluoroscopy is particularly useful and commonly used in companion animals with dynamic airway obstruction such as pharyngeal or tracheal collapse. In most cases, general anesthesia is required to obtain diagnostic computed tomography (CT) or magnetic resonance imaging (MRI) images to further characterize the pathology affecting the respiratory tract.

Endoscopy, Bronchoscopy, and Bronchoalveolar Lavage

In large animals, endoscopy is routinely performed for airway examination and bronchoalveolar lavage (BAL) with patients awake (usually sedated) and standing. In small animals, general anesthesia is required to permit airway examination and perform BAL. The information obtained from these diagnostic procedures can assist with both the diagnosis of the underlying disease and monitoring the response to therapy.

Principles of Anesthetic Management of Patients with Respiratory Disease

Sedation and general anesthesia can result in a decrease in respiratory function, as indicated by a decreased alveolar ventilation, reduced arterial oxygen partial pressure, and increased work of breathing. The degree of change is dependent on the species, the presence of underlying disease, patient positioning, anesthetic drugs, anesthetic equipment, and supportive therapies employed, such as O_2 supplementation and positive pressure ventilation (Concept Box 18.1). Expected changes in healthy patients in different veterinary species with different anesthetic protocols have been described elsewhere (see Further Reading). Unfortunately, patients with respiratory disease are at increased risk of worsening respiratory function compared to healthy patients, and the severity of change can be difficult to predict so that close monitoring throughout the peri-anesthetic period is important. In addition to standard practices such as a thorough pre-anesthetic assessment, additional principles that should guide the anesthetic management of a patient with respiratory disease are outlined in Table 18.6.

Critical times, during which morbidity and mortality are increased, include periods following premedication until a secure airway is established, and following tracheal extubation.

Concept Box 18.1

Ventilatory support

What are the indications for providing ventilatory support during anesthesia?

1. Impaired gas exchange
   a. Inadequate carbon dioxide removal (hypoventilation): If $PaCO_2$ is above 55 mmHg or $PE'CO_2$ is above 50 mmHg, ventilatory support is recommended.
   b. Inadequate oxygen uptake (hypoxemia): If PaO_2 is below 80 mmHg while the patient is receiving oxygen supplementation, positive pressure ventilation is recommended.
2. Excessive work of breathing: Many conditions can lead to an increase in the work of breathing for a patient. In general, they can be considered to be a result of:
   a. An increase in airway resistance: The radius of the airway has a dramatic impact on the resistance to airflow. Common causes of an increase in airway resistance include secretions, soft-tissue swelling or masses, and bronchoconstriction.
   b. Reduced thoracic compliance: Patient factors such as pleural effusion or gastric detention can dramatically reduce thoracic compliance.

Concept Box 18.1 (Continued)

c. Reduced lung compliance: Pneumonia, pulmonary masses, and pulmonary edema can reduce pulmonary compliance.

3. Inability to ventilate – due to patient or procedure being performed:
   a. Airway obstruction
   b. Thoracotomy
   c. Disruption in thoracic structure such as diaphragmatic hernia, pneumothorax, and pleural effusion
   d. Muscle paralysis (intentional) or secondary to neuromuscular disease

How can ventilatory support be provided?

1. Manually
2. Using a mechanical ventilator

What are the typical goals when providing ventilatory support?

1. Achieving adequate gas exchange. Targets include
   a. $PaCO_2$ range of 35–55 mmHg ($PE'CO_2$ = 40–60 mmHg)
   b. PaO_2 > 100 mmHg (Hemoglobin saturation > 98%)
2. Minimizing cardiovascular and respiratory adverse effects of positive pressure ventilation. This is achieved through using tidal volumes less than or equal to 15 mL/kg and minimizing the mean and peak airway pressures.

What is the appropriate strategy to provide manual ventilatory support in a patient?

1. Establish a secure sealed airway in the patient.
2. If available, connect capnograph monitor into breathing circuit and place pulse oximeter probe on the patient.
3. While the patient is connected to the anesthetic breathing circuit, close the pressure relief valve (pop-off valve), wait for the rebreathing bag to partially fill, and then squeeze the partially filled rebreathing bag.
4. Stop squeezing the rebreathing bag once the patient chest rises to the normal end inspiratory position or the airway pressure (as measured on the manometer of the breathing system) reads 10–15 cmH_2O.
5. Open the pressure relief valve.
6. Observe the $PE'CO_2$ and pulse oximeter.
7. Repeat at normal respiratory frequency with adjustments made based on $PE'CO_2$.

Further details are provided in the following text for commonly encountered respiratory conditions in companion and equine patients. In many cases, the patient is scheduled to undergo surgery to reduce the impact of the primary condition; however, in some cases, patients may be undergoing procedures unrelated to the respiratory condition on an urgent or elective basis. Further information regarding specific conditions is provided in Further Reading.

Upper Airway Disease

Despite different etiologies and characteristics, conditions affecting the upper airways generally result in similar consequences and clinical signs. Most notably, upper airway abnormalities lead to a reduced airway diameter and increased upper airway resistance to airway gas flow. As noted earlier, the change in intrathoracic pressure is proportional to airway resistance (see Figure 18.3). Therefore, as a result of increased airway resistance, a patient must create a greater negative intrathoracic pressure on inspiration to achieve adequate alveolar ventilation. This is evident as an increase in inspiratory muscle effort. In mildly affected animals, this may only be evident during exercise when high airway gas flow occurs, while severely affected animals may have respiratory distress at rest. In patients with severe upper airway pathology, complete respiratory obstruction can occur with mild changes in muscle tone (e.g., following sedation) or soft-tissue swelling.

Canine Brachycephalic Obstructive Airway Syndrome

Brachycephalic obstructive airway syndrome (BOAS), also referred to as "brachycephalic syndrome" or "brachycephalic airway syndrome," is a condition of brachycephalic breeds characterized by a combination of both primary and secondary abnormalities of the respiratory tract that result in reduced airway diameter, an increased work of breathing, and partial to complete upper airway obstruction. Breeds most reported to have BOAS include English and French Bulldogs, Pugs, and Boston Terriers.

There are several excellent reviews discussing the major abnormalities, pathology, and clinical signs in patients with BOAS, and readers can consult them for further details (see Further Reading). Characteristic clinical signs associated with BOAS include snoring, stridor during sleep and/or exercise, an increase in inspiratory effort, exercise intolerance, syncope, cyanosis, and collapse. In some patients, complete airway obstruction may occur when O_2 demand and minute ventilation are increased, as occurs during exercise, hyperthermia, or when the patient is placed in stressful circumstances. Alternatively, airway obstruction

Table 18.6 Principles of anesthetic management of patients with respiratory disease.

Principle	Clinical application
1. Determining patient history and current medication	Previous anesthesia history Disease progression Current medication (nonsteroidal anti-inflammatory drugs and steroids)
2. Clinical examination and diagnostic workup	Diagnostic imagining for concurrent disease like aspiration pneumonia Thermoregulation, and identifying hyperthermia is a common observation Hematology and serum chemistry tests are routinely recommended to detect underlying disease and to serve as baseline values in the event of post-operative complications.
3. Improve the patient's respiratory status before anesthesia	i. For elective procedures: initiate and continue medical management of respiratory condition until anticipated level of improvement is observed ii. Emergency: provide oxygen supplementation and stabilize patient if possible, including removing pleural fluid, providing hemodynamic support, and treating bronchospasm iii. Manage concurrent disorders. Patient hydration should be normalized if possible, before anesthesia. Obese patients should receive nutritional consultation and weight loss before elective procedures.
4. Establish plan including emergency management of situations that are likely to occur based on patient's pre-operative condition	i. Appropriate anesthetic equipment should be prepared and readily available, which includes appropriate breathing systems, face masks, and equipment for tracheal intubation or temporary tracheostomy. ii. Trained staff are required in the event of a challenging airway. iii. Strategies to manage emergencies should be discussed with veterinary team.
5. Maintain hemoglobin oxygen saturation throughout the anesthetic period	i. Preoxygenate patients before induction of anesthesia if possible. Administration of O_2 by sealed close-fitting face mask can increase a patient's inspired oxygen fraction from 0.21 to over 0.80 (with an oxygen flow rate of approximately 100 mL/kg/min). Intranasal administration of oxygen through nasal cannulae or nasal prongs is also effective and can be used as an alternative if the patient does not tolerate a face mask. ii. Strategy for oxygen supplementation and ventilatory support in recovery in place if appropriate.
6. Ensure a secure airway is established whenever feasible	i. Placement of a cuffed endotracheal tube in trachea will permit positive pressure ventilation if required.
7. Minimize the patient's work of breathing	i. Consider patient positioning, thoracic cage function and airway resistance.
8. Be prepared to support ventilation with manual or mechanical ventilator	i. Manual technique reviewed with veterinary team members ii. If available, ventilator should be prepared for use on individual patient (appropriate bellows and settings)
9. Monitor oxygenation and ventilation throughout anesthesia	i. Utilize pulse oximeter, blood gas analysis, and capnometry when available.
10. Practice environmentally safe anesthetic techniques	i. Avoid inhalant anesthetic administration when a secure airway is not in place and scavenging cannot be performed.
11. Optimize recovery	i. While important in all patients, achieving normothermia before anesthesia recovery is regarded as critical in patients with upper airway disease. Hypothermia leads to shivering, which increases oxygen demand, while hyperthermia triggers panting. Either situation alters normal respiratory pattern and effort during anesthetic recovery, which could lead to further compromise of the patient's airway. The patient's temperature should be close to normal before anesthetic drugs are discontinued and recovery initiated. ii. Oxygen support

may also occur when a brachycephalic patient is asleep, and pharyngeal muscles relax. Even when not exhibiting signs of distress, $PaCO_2$ has been reported to be higher, and PaO_2 lower, in a sample of brachycephalic dogs compared to control mesocephalic or dolichocephalic dogs. This suggests some degree of habituation to chronic hypoventilation.

In addition to respiratory abnormalities associated with BOAS, brachycephalic breeds may have concurrent conditions that can impact anesthetic management and outcomes. Relevant to anesthesia is the high frequency and severity of gastrointestinal signs, including regurgitation and vomiting. Dogs with BOAS have a high prevalence of

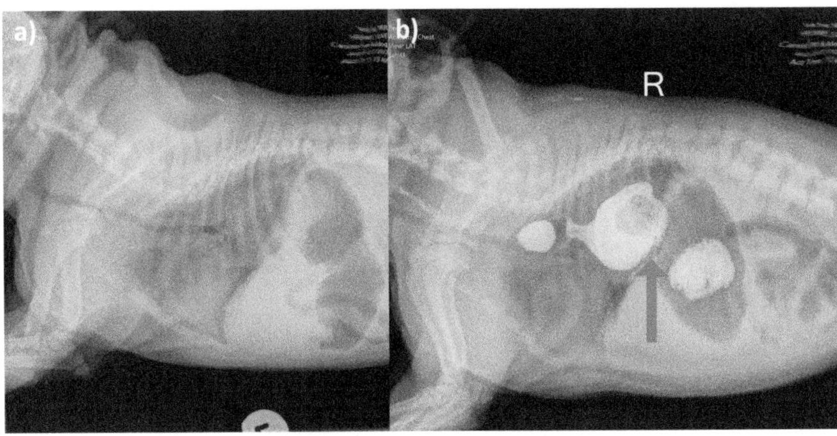

Figure 18.11 Right lateral thoracic radiographs of a French Bulldog with brachycephalic obstructive airway syndrome (BOAS) before (a) and after (b) ingesting a bolus of food dyed with barium. The passage of food into the stomach is hindered by a sliding hiatal hernia, indicated by the blue arrow. (*Source:* Courtesy of Valley Farm Animal Hospital.)

(sliding) hiatal hernia, gastroesophageal reflux, gastritis, and pyloric obstruction (Figure 18.11). A history of gastrointestinal disease is associated with the development of aspiration pneumonia.

In terms of the cardiovascular system, dogs with BOAS are reported to have a higher packed cell volume (PCV), may be hypercoagulable, have higher systolic arterial blood pressure, and higher vagal tone (predisposing them to bradycardia). While the underlying mechanism for these cardiovascular changes is unknown, they may reflect lower PaO_2, inflammation, endothelial damage, and greater negative inspiratory intrathoracic pressures. Some brachycephalic breeds also have an increased incidence of cardiac abnormalities (see Chapter 17) and most have abnormal ocular conformation. The latter characteristics have implications for patient management before and during anesthesia.

Soft palate resection (staphylectomy) to shorten the excessively long soft palate, enlargement of the nares (rhinoplasty), and resection of everted laryngeal saccules and tonsils are the common surgical procedures performed in patients with clinical signs attributed to obstructive airway syndrome (Figure 18.12). More recently, laser-assisted turbinectomy has been added to potential surgical interventions aimed at reducing the severity of airway obstruction in brachycephalic patients. While these procedures have been reported to improve both the respiratory and gastrointestinal status of patients post-operatively, unfortunately, the peri-operative complication and mortality rate in this patient population are high, with rates of 6–26% and 2.4–3.3% being reported, respectively.

In general, brachycephalic dogs with higher ASA status and/or those having invasive versus noninvasive procedures have a higher risk of peri-anesthetic complications. Consideration of a brachycephalic patient's current physical condition and potential strategies to optimize a patient's condition pre-operatively, intra-operatively, and post-operatively will help prepare for complications and may improve patient outcomes irrespective of the procedure for which they require anesthesia.

Canine Laryngeal Paralysis

Normally, contraction of the paired *cricoarytenoideus dorsalis* muscles during inspiration abducts the arytenoids and vocal folds, widening the *rima glottidis*, which minimizes the resistance to gas flow. Laryngeal paralysis occurs secondary to the disruption of the innervation of the intrinsic laryngeal muscles, resulting in abnormal abduction and adduction of the arytenoid cartilages and vocal folds. While there is a congenital form of laryngeal paralysis, which manifests in the first few weeks of a dog's life and is often associated with a central lesion, the acquired form of the disease is more common and is typically observed later in life. There are numerous potential etiologies leading to laryngeal dysfunction. Idiopathic polyneuropathy is the most common cause. Dysfunction of the caudal laryngeal nerve, a terminal branch of the recurrent laryngeal nerve, generally leads to the first significant signs of the polyneuropathy. Affected breeds (acquired form) include Labrador Retrievers, Golden Retrievers, Irish Setters, St-Bernards, Newfoundlands, Afghan Hounds, and Brittany Spaniels. Other potential causes of laryngeal paralysis secondary to a peripheral neuropathy include trauma, masses, or surgical trauma in the neck or cranial mediastinum.

Clinical signs of laryngeal paralysis range from a change in phonation (bark), coughing, dysphagia or gagging, increased inspiratory sounds, decreased exercise tolerance, respiratory distress, cyanosis, hyperthermia, and collapse. Dogs are generally more severely affected in hot weather and during exercise.

Diagnosis is made based on laryngeal examination performed under heavy sedation or a light plane of general anesthesia. A lack of abduction of arytenoid cartilages during inspiration, laxity of the vocal cords, and edema of the corniculate processes is supportive of the diagnosis.

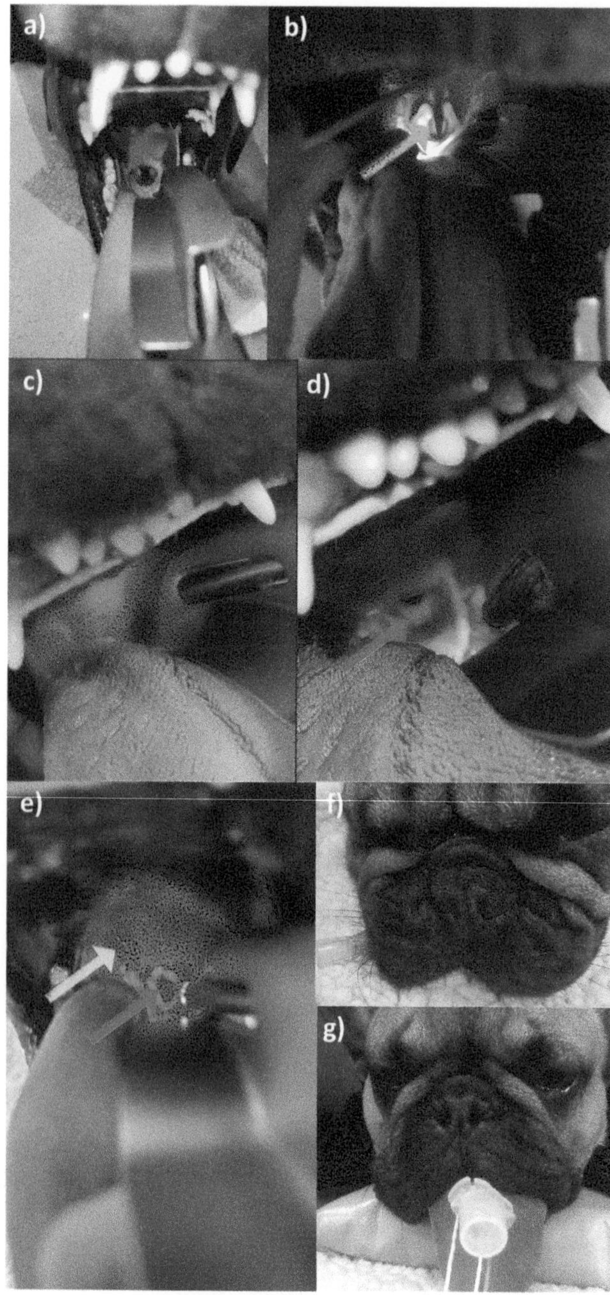

Figure 18.12 (a, b) Normal oropharynx and *rima glottides* in a dog, the vocal cords (green arrow) are visible and no everted laryngeal saccules are seen, (c) an elongated soft palate preventing ventroflexion of the epiglottis, (d) everted laryngeal saccules (blue arrow) and elongated soft palate partially occluding the *rima glottides*, and (e) collapsed larynx, everted saccules (blue arrow), and inflamed and enlarged tonsillar lymph nodes (yellow arrow), and stenotic nares (f) before and (g) after rhinoplasty (naroplasty). (*Source:* Courtesy of Valley Farm Animal Hospital.)

Medical management focused on patient weight loss, anti-inflammatory medication, and exercise restriction may be recommended for patients with unilateral laryngeal paralysis; however, when laryngeal paralysis is bilateral, the severity of the patient's condition may be inadequately improved with medical therapy. Surgical correction aimed at unilateral arytenoid cartilage lateralization generally reduces airway obstruction and improves quality of life. Some patients may be scheduled for permanent tracheostomy.

Concurrent conditions that are relatively common in dogs with laryngeal paralysis with relevance to anesthesia include gastroesophageal regurgitation and aspiration pneumonia. The presence of systemic disease such as myasthenia gravis, hypothyroidism or neoplasia also needs to be investigated.

Canine Tracheal Collapse

Tracheal collapse, resulting from progressive degeneration of the tracheal cartilage, malformation of tracheal rings, and/or laxity of the *trachealis dorsalis* muscle, is a condition leading to airway obstruction in toy and small-breed dogs. Most patients are middle-aged; however, symptoms have been reported in dogs as early as six months of age. Yorkshire Terriers represent the most common breed of dogs presenting for symptoms related to tracheal collapse, but Miniature Poodles, Pugs, Maltese, Chihuahua, and Pomeranians are also commonly affected. Bronchomalacia, a condition characterized by collapse of the bronchi and bronchioles, is common in dogs with tracheal collapse but it can also occur as an isolated syndrome in dogs of all sizes and breeds. Laryngeal dysfunction has also been reported in a significant number of dogs with tracheal collapse. The underlying cause of the tracheal or tracheobronchial cartilage degeneration is unknown. It is proposed that it may be primary (congenital) or secondary to chronic inflammation. In primary cases, pathophysiology is likely to be multifactorial, associated with chronic inflammatory changes due to coughing, impaired mucociliary clearance within the airways, and, in severe cases, repeated collapse of airways. Factors known to precipitate clinical signs include airway irritants, chronic bronchitis, laryngeal paralysis, respiratory tract infections, obesity, and tracheal intubation.

Common presenting signs of tracheal collapse are a persistent dry, paroxysmal (i.e., a sudden recurrence or intensification of coughing) "goose-honk" cough, tracheal sensitivity, and varying degrees of respiratory difficulty. In some cases, patients may present in severe respiratory distress with cyanosis. On physical examination, the patient's respiratory pattern may indicate the location of the collapse. Extrathoracic tracheal collapse results in increased inspiratory respiratory effort while intrathoracic airway collapse results in increased expiratory respiratory effort. Gentle tracheal palpation may elicit a dry harsh cough and auscultation may reveal inspiratory and/or expiratory stridor. Thorough auscultation of the lower airways should also be performed to detect the presence of lower airway and/or concurrent pulmonary parenchymal disease. Although not definitively linked, cardiovascular disease, specifically mitral valve disease, with left atrial enlargement is common in the breeds affected by tracheal collapse and should be considered during auscultation and further workup.

Where available, fluoroscopic evaluation of airways of the conscious patient is preferred over radiographic examination to characterize the extent and location of the airway collapse. When unavailable, thoracic radiographs taken during inspiratory and expiratory phases of respiration are recommended, but false positives and false negatives are common (Figure 18.13).

Radiographs of the lower airways and lung parenchyma should also be included to evaluate the presence of concurrent respiratory disease. Computed tomography, bronchoscopy, and BAL are generally reserved for patients that are undergoing interventions to correct the condition and will be discussed in the following text.

In patients that are not in respiratory distress, medical management with antitussives, bronchodilators, anti-inflammatories, and antimicrobials are generally initiated and are reported to improve symptoms in a large percentage of dogs.

Surgical and minimally invasive treatments currently recommended for patients with tracheal collapse include the placement of tracheal ring prostheses or endoluminal stents. In dogs with severe tracheal collapse, these interventions may dramatically improve quality of life and survival time. Extraluminal stent placement is associated with a high incidence of post-operative laryngeal paralysis (approximately 50%); therefore prophylactic laryngeal lateralization is ideally performed during the same anesthetic. Complications that occur immediately following intraluminal stent placement include stent fracture or migration and the development of pneumothorax. Mishaps, including stent placement in the larynx or endotracheal tube, will require stent removal and replacement before anesthetic recovery.

Following extraluminal prosthesis or endoluminal stent placement, patients will require continued (i.e., lifelong therapy) medical management post-operatively with only gradual reductions in dose or number of medications to prevent recurrence of clinical signs.

Feline Brachycephalic Disease

Persian, Himalayan, and British Shorthair cats have stenotic nares and abnormal nasal turbinates that result in an increased work of breathing. Anesthetic management practices should follow the same principles as discussed in the preceding text with canine patients with BOAS.

Feline Laryngeal Paralysis

Overall, laryngeal disease is much less commonly reported in cats relative to dogs. Middle-aged to older cats represent most feline patients presenting with clinical signs. Reported causes of laryngeal dysfunction include neoplasia, trauma, and iatrogenic, but the cause often is unknown. Cats can be affected with unilateral or bilateral laryngeal dysfunction, with clinical signs similar to those reported in dogs.

Equine Recurrent Laryngeal Neuropathy (Roarers)

One of the most common causes of upper airway obstruction in the equid occurs as a result of neurogenic atrophy of the intrinsic laryngeal musculature leading to progressive

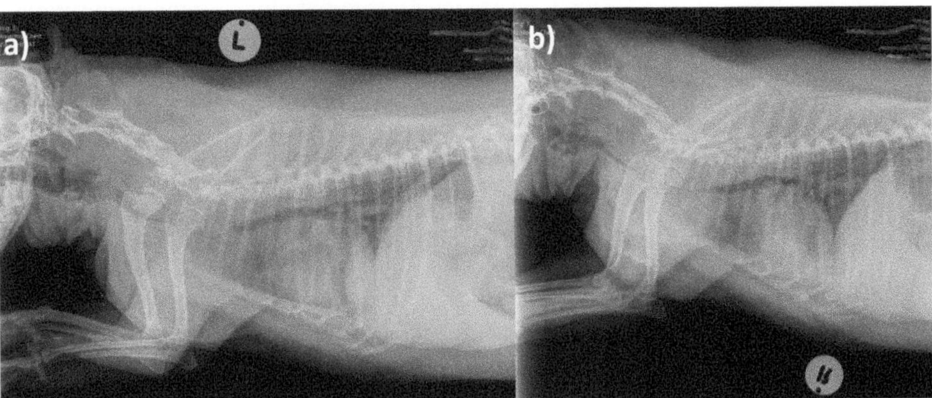

Figure 18.13 Left (a) and right (b) lateral thoracic radiographs of a dog with a collapsing trachea. Radiographs were taken at different stages in the respiratory cycle, and variable appearance of trachea reflects dynamic nature of this disease. Trachea is narrowed at the level of the cervical spine and thoracic inlet (a, b). (*Source:* Courtesy of Valley Farm Animal Hospital.)

loss of both abductor and adductor arytenoid function. While the adductor muscles may be affected, it is the dysfunction of the *cricoarytenoideus dorsalis* muscles, the principal abductor in the larynx that leads to clinical signs. Large-breed horses, such as Thoroughbreds, warmbloods, and draft horses, are more commonly affected than small-breed horses or ponies. Generally, the condition is unilateral, with the left side most commonly affected; however, in some horses the disease is bilateral. Etiology is considered idiopathic in most cases though perivascular jugular vein injections, guttural pouch mycosis, abscessation, or neoplasms within the head and neck can damage the recurrent laryngeal nerve.

Horses can be as young as a few months of age when clinical signs become evident, but the condition generally manifests during training. Horses may present for poor performance, which is generally associated with an increase in inspiratory noise. The sound may vary from a soft whistle to a roaring sound, which is louder at higher speeds.

Several different surgical procedures are used to improve clinical signs associated with a lack of arytenoid cartilage abduction. Most commonly, laryngoplasty is performed by placing sutures on the dorsal aspect of the larynx between the cricoid cartilage and the muscular process of the arytenoid on the most severely affected side (tie-back procedure). Unilateral or bilateral ventriculocordectomy, removal of the vocal cord and laryngeal saccule, is also commonly performed.

Techniques and Specific Principles of Anesthetic Management of a Canine or Feline Patient with Upper Airway Disease

Major concerns when anesthetizing companion animal patients with upper respiratory disease include the following:

- Potential for upper airway obstruction at any time during the peri-anesthetic period
- Difficult orotracheal intubation
- Need for further airway assessment following induction of anesthesia before securing the airway
- Impact of different drugs on the assessment of upper airway function and risk of compromising respiratory function
- Impact of surgical location on patient monitoring and management during anesthesia
- Potential need for extubation during the maintenance phase of anesthesia
- Patient predisposition to regurgitation and aspiration

Pre-anesthetic Period

In addition to a general history, specific information regarding respiratory noise, heat tolerance (canine), previous anesthesia, and surgery, including airway surgery, and the presence of cardiac disease should be obtained. In companion animals, inquiries regarding sleeping patterns, the presence of snoring, exercise tolerance, and syncopal episodes should also be included.

Whole body barometric plethysmography is a validated noninvasive objective method of quantifying the severity of airway obstruction in brachycephalic dogs; however, the latter tool is not readily available. At present, laryngeal as well as thoracic auscultation and the use of a three-minute trot test are recommended to improve the sensitivity of clinical examination for BOAS diagnosis (see Further Reading). Dogs with BOAS should also be graded using breed-specific functional grading systems (http://www.vet.cam.ac.uk/boas). Dogs that are graded as II or III are at increased risk of airway obstruction during sedation and peri-anesthetic period.

Due to the possibility of a general polyneuropathy, dogs with laryngeal paralysis should have a full neurological examination before anesthesia. Hindlimb weakness with neurological deficits is not uncommon in Labrador Retrievers with laryngeal paralysis and may impact anesthetic recovery time.

In dogs with laryngeal paralysis, thyroid function screening is recommended, and in select cases, acetylcholine antibody testing (for myasthenia gravis) may be indicated based on the patient physical examination findings. In cats with laryngeal paralysis, the presence of concurrent disease should be investigated with an in-depth diagnostic investigation before anesthesia.

Due to the high prevalence of esophageal and gastric disease in dogs with BOAS, owners should be questioned on the presence of ptyalism, choking, regurgitation, and vomiting. Owners of dogs with laryngeal paralysis or tracheal collapse should also be questioned for signs of dysphagia in their dogs, such as gagging or coughing. Dogs with concurrent gastric and esophageal disease are routinely given omeprazole (or other proton pump inhibitors) before surgery (see Further Reading). Anti-emetic medications, such as maropitant, should also be included in the peri-operative period in patients with a history of vomiting. Metoclopramide, administered pre-operatively, has been associated with variable outcomes in several retrospective studies and seems to be a limited benefit. Doses of the commonly administered gastrointestinal medications are outlined in Table 18.1. A small retrospective study assessing cisapride, a prokinetic, as a constant rate infusion before induction of anesthesia showed potential benefits of a decrease in post-operative frequency of aspiration pneumonia in dogs with laryngeal paralysis; however, this drug may not be readily available and, to date, large clinical trials have not been published.

Anesthetic Period

As with patients in respiratory distress, equipment and team preparation before premedication are important when dealing with these patients. A range of facemasks, orotracheal tubes (a wide range of sizes should be prepared, especially for brachycephalic breeds because of the potential for a hypoplastic trachea), means to secure the orotracheal tube, gauze swabs (to remove excessive saliva), laryngoscope, monitoring equipment including a pulse oximeter, ECG and blood pressure monitor, system to permit suctioning the airway, intravenous anesthetics suitable for induction of anesthesia, and IV catheterization supplies should be prepared. If available, in-circuit manometry to permit monitoring of airway pressures during positive pressure ventilation is highly recommended. For patients undergoing bronchoscopy, a bronchoscope adaptor, which can be placed between the endotracheal tube and breathing circuit, will permit oxygen supplementation during bronchoscopy. In very small patients, where endoscope passage through the endotracheal tube is not possible, extubation will be required and oxygen can be delivered through the endoscope sleeve or via a urinary catheter attached to the anesthetic breathing circuit and inserted into the oropharynx. It is advised that the anesthetist should be prepared to assist with ventilation, either manually or with a ventilator, if available.

To date, no single premedication drug protocol has been shown to be superior for use in patients with upper airway disease. If sedative drugs, such as dexmedetomidine, medetomidine, or acepromazine, are included in the premedication protocol, beginning with low doses is strongly recommended as the response to sedation, in terms of respiratory function, is difficult to predict. In mature, quiet dogs with upper airway disease, adequate sedation may be achieved with an opioid drug alone. The intended procedure requiring general anesthesia plays a major role in determining which opioid analgesic is an appropriate addition to the premedication drug protocol. For noninvasive procedures, avoiding *mu* agonist opioid drugs is recommended due to their known association with delayed gastric emptying, vomiting, regurgitation, and gastroesophageal reflux. If a pure-*mu* agonist is required for intra- or post-operative analgesia, methadone or meperidine (pethidine) are preferred over morphine or hydromorphone due to the lower incidence of vomiting associated with their administration. Additionally, meperidine is associated with less panting than methadone (or hydromorphone).

If diagnostic or minimally invasive procedures are planned, butorphanol is a suitable opioid drug, particularly if a multimodal approach to analgesia can be applied through concurrent use of local anesthetics and/or nonsteroidal anti-inflammatory drugs (NSAIDs). It has the advantage of not usually causing panting or vomiting.

In patients with suspected laryngeal paralysis, numerous drug protocols have been assessed for the purpose of determining the drug or drug combination that permits the best laryngeal examination while minimizing the effects on laryngeal function. Overall, premedication to achieve light sedation is recommended. This may include acepromazine or dexmedetomidine (low dose), combined with butorphanol (IM or IV). However, further analgesia may be required for surgery (if performed) following butorphanol premedication. In some cases, laryngeal examination may be possible in dogs that have received an alpha-2 adrenergic receptor agonist in combination with an opioid analgesic.

Pre-oxygenation is recommended before a rapid and smooth induction of general anesthesia using propofol or alfaxalone. In many cases, time to assess airway function is required after induction of anesthesia and before orotracheal intubation. Pre-oxygenation reduces the risk of hypoxemia during the airway examination. Additionally, the anesthetist must be prepared to either use additional bolus doses or initiate an intravenous infusion of propofol or alfaxalone to maintain general anesthesia. During such examinations, pulse oximetry can be invaluable in monitoring oxygenation (in combination with assessment of ventilation quality: noise and effort). Doxapram, a nonspecific central respiratory stimulant, is effective at stimulating the rate and depth of breathing and is administered at a dose of 0.5–1.5 mg/kg IV to facilitate laryngeal examination in dogs suspected of having laryngeal paralysis.

Maintenance of anesthesia can be accomplished with inhalational or injectable drugs, or a combination of these. If the use of inhalant anesthetics is contraindicated, administration of an injectable drug as an infusion is a feasible alternative (see Chapter 7). When bronchoscopy, BAL, and/or endoluminal stenting are planned, the use of injectable agents is preferred to minimize room contamination and exposure of personnel to inhalational anesthetics.

Depending on the scheduled procedure, additional techniques to optimize analgesia may be needed, such as systemic opioid or lidocaine infusions and local or regional anesthetic techniques. NSAIDs may also be included preemptively if there are no contraindications. If airway disease is judged to be severe, and/or the probability of steroid administration is high during post-operative recovery, it is recommended that NSAIDs only be given following anesthetic recovery.

Intra-operative monitoring should be tailored to the patient's condition. It is strongly recommended that at minimum, SpO_2, $PE'CO_2$, heart rate and rhythm (ECG), blood pressure, and temperature are monitored throughout anesthesia. During recovery, the animal should be observed for signs of regurgitation and significant tissue swelling (associated with risk of airway obstruction).

Anesthetic Recovery and Post-anesthetic Period

Irrespective of surgical intervention, respiratory distress, regurgitation, aspiration pneumonia, and death occur at a higher frequency in dogs with upper airway disease. Brachycephalic breeds have a high incidence of complications during anesthetic recovery compared to nonbrachycephalic controls. Post-anesthetic complications most commonly reported following brachycephalic airway surgery include respiratory distress or dyspnea, excitement, pharyngeal edema, post-operative hemorrhage, regurgitation, aspiration pneumonia, and death. Importantly, dogs should be considered at risk of developing post-operative complications for 24–48 h following airway surgery.

In general, brachycephalic dogs tolerate an orotracheal tube during anesthetic recovery for a longer period of time relative to nonbrachycephalic breeds (Figure 18.14). If they remain calm, extubation can be delayed until the patient objects to the presence of the orotracheal tube, as indicated by coughing, pawing directed at the face, or being capable of maintaining their head in an elevated position (indicating reasonable muscle tone). Doing this reduces the risk of partial or complete airway obstruction following extubation in these breeds. In cats, extubation is not delayed, to avoid triggering laryngospasm. Before extubation, a thorough evaluation and gentle suctioning or swabbing of the airway should be performed to ensure that the airway and oropharyngeal area is clear of debris and fluid.

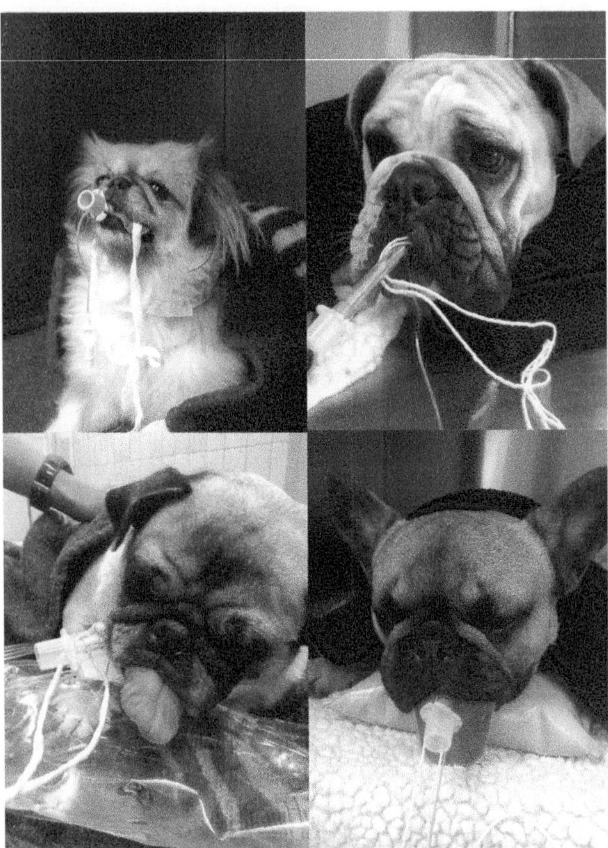

Figure 18.14 Examples of brachycephalic dogs recovering from general anesthesia. Brachycephalic dog breeds often tolerate an endotracheal tube in place until they are fully conscious and alert. (*Source:* Courtesy of Valley Farm Animal Hospital.)

Positioning of patients with upper airway disease for recovery from anesthesia should also be considered. Unless contraindicated, the brachycephalic patient should be placed in sternal recumbency. Dogs with laryngeal paralysis are generally larger and therefore they are generally recovered in lateral recumbency with their head elevated.

Considering the high risk associated with anesthetic recovery, noninvasive monitoring equipment should be maintained in place if possible (particularly a pulse oximeter). Drugs and supplies to induce anesthesia and re-intubate the patient should be available in case respiratory distress or airway obstruction occurs during recovery. Control of the airway may require providing an alternative airway, such as tracheostomy.

Sedation may be required if the patient exhibits dysphoria during recovery. Low doses of an alpha-2 adrenergic receptor agonist (for example, dexmedetomidine at 0.5–1 mcg/kg) have the advantage of being relatively short acting and reversible. If IV acepromazine is used, it should be given before extubation so there is sufficient time for it to take effect (at least 15 min) and low doses (0.01–0.02 mg/kg IV) are used.

In some instances, it may be challenging to determine if a patient is exhibiting excitement (dysphoria and emergency delirium), or if they are in respiratory distress due to airway obstruction and/or hypoxemia. If following sedation and oxygen supplementation, the patient's clinical signs to do not improve, anesthetic induction, tracheal intubation, and maintenance of anesthesia are likely required to permit reassessment of the airway.

The time that an orotracheal tube is maintained in place following reintubation will depend on the time required for airway swelling to subside and the availability of resources to manage an intubated patient. In some instances, prolonged intubation (e.g., 24 h) and ventilatory support are required.

Traditionally, if repeated attempts to extubate the patient are unsuccessful or the means to support a patient for a prolonged period with an orotracheal tube in place are unavailable, a temporary tracheotomy is recommended. Unfortunately, permanent or temporary tracheotomy is associated with high complication rates. To maximize the likelihood of success, the decision to perform a tracheostomy should be taken early and discussed with the owner before the procedure.

Several new approaches have been attempted to improve gas flow and gas exchange in brachycephalic patients recovering from anesthesia. Achieving positive pressure airway support using systems that include a helmet or high-flow nasal cannula has shown promise. A case series has also reported success of topical epinephrine, administered via nebulization, in reducing the severity of signs associated with BOAS as assessed by whole body barometric plethysmography (see Further Reading). Topical application of vasoconstrictor drugs, such as oxymetazoline or phenylephrine, is also used to reduce post-operative airway swelling.

Anesthesia of the Equine with Upper Airway Disease

In general, pre-anesthetic concerns for equine patients with upper airway disease are similar to those listed for small animal patients discussed in the preceding text. While equine patients do not regurgitate, patients with some upper airway conditions may have dysphagia that results in aspiration of food particles.

Pre-anesthesia Period

In general, horses with recurrent laryngeal neuropathy do not have other associated concurrent conditions. Standard pre-operative workup based on signalment and physical examination is appropriate. Patients with upper airway disease (for example, guttural pouch mycosis) that is associated with dysphagia may require further diagnostic workup, including thoracic radiography.

Anesthetic Period

Laryngoplasty is traditionally performed under general anesthesia with the horse placed in lateral recumbency. Standard anesthesia and monitoring protocols are appropriate for induction and maintenance of anesthesia. A partial-*mu* opioid agonist and an NSAID, most commonly butorphanol and phenylbutazone, respectively, are generally given before surgery. The latter is continued for several days post-operatively. As the surgical field is in the laryngeal region, the anesthetist needs to plan for the location of IV access ports and access to monitoring equipment. Direct arterial blood pressure measurement can be performed away from the head by using the lateral metatarsal artery. Endoscopy to assess the degree of arytenoid lateralization is generally performed after laryngoplasty with the patient spontaneously breathing before surgical wound closure. To reduce room contamination, inhalational anesthetics should be discontinued, and if necessary, anesthesia should be maintained with injectable anesthetics. During surgery, it is possible for the endotracheal tube cuff to be damaged during suturing. This should be considered if there is a reduction in breathing circuit pressure during the inspiratory phase of mechanical ventilation.

More recently, laryngoplasty has been performed in sedated standing horses in order to prevent the risks associated with general anesthesia, particularly in draft horses. Acepromazine at low doses is routinely administered 30–40 min before moving the horse into the surgical suite. Then, an alpha-2 adrenergic receptor agonist, detomidine or romifidine, combined with either butorphanol or morphine is given to provide a suitable level of sedation to permit surgery. Sedatives are generally administered immediately before or after moving into the surgical suite. Sedatives can be administered as either repeat boluses or as a continuous rate infusion (see Chapter 6 for CRI calculation). The opioid analgesic can be administered similarly. Earplugs and a hood with a blinker over the eye on the side of the surgery can minimize stimulation from the surgical team. The mucosal surface of the larynx can be desensitized with lidocaine delivered via an endoscope or by using a Chalmers catheter passed in the contralateral ventral nasal meatus with the location of the local anesthetic application facilitated by endoscopic visualization. Local infiltration of the tissues surrounding the surgical area with lidocaine or mepivacaine, or a unilateral ultrasound-guided cervical plexus block, can be performed to provide anesthesia.

Anesthetic Recovery and Post-anesthetic Period

For horses having undergone laryngoplasty under general anesthesia, the orotracheal or nasotracheal tube is maintained in place until the horse has recovered to standing.

Lower Airway Disease

Anesthesia may be required in patients with lower airway disease to permit collection of lower airway samples or for procedures unrelated to the respiratory system. The most frequently encountered lower airway diseases in companion animals presenting for anesthesia are feline asthma and canine chronic bronchiolitis. Inflammatory and allergic airway diseases are very common in mature horses of all ages and breeds.

Feline Asthma

Feline asthma is a disease of middle-aged cats, characterized by airway hyper-reactivity, airway inflammation, and airway gas flow limitation. Feline asthma is hard to differentiate from chronic bronchitis, pulmonary parasitic diseases, and heartworm associated respiratory disease. The unique characteristic of asthma is the fluctuation in severity of clinical signs, information that can be determined from the patient medical history.

The etiology of asthma is primarily allergic in origin. On physical examination, increased respiratory rate with increased respiratory effort characterized by activation of accessory muscles may be evident. A prolonged expiratory phase of respiration is typical, and wheezes may be heard on auscultation. Tracheal palpation may elicit a cough. Complete blood count may reveal an eosinophilia. Radiographic and CT imaging results can vary from normal findings to marked changes with a bronchial or bronchointerstitial lung pattern with lung collapse (Figure 18.15). Eosinophilic inflammation is characteristic of fluid obtained from airway samples using BAL.

Current treatment of feline asthma includes systemic or inhaled glucocorticoids and bronchodilators. The latter include short-acting and long-acting beta-2 adrenergic receptor agonists, methylxanthines and anticholinergics. The beta-2 adrenergic receptor agonists terbutaline and salbutamol, which can be administered systemically prior to anesthesia, are currently recommended due to the potential side effects of other bronchodilators. Inhaled salbutamol (albuterol) can also be used to treat acute bronchoconstriction.

Canine Chronic Bronchitis

Chronic bronchitis is an inflammatory lower airway disease of dogs that manifests clinically as reduced exercise tolerance and persistent cough. As many other conditions, such as mitral valve regurgitation or pneumonia, may present with similar presenting clinical signs, a thorough medical workup that includes diagnostic blood work and thoracic radiography is essential.

Glucocorticoids are the mainstay of therapy for patients with chronic bronchitis with bronchodilators, antimicrobials, and cough suppressants (butorphanol or hydrocodone), included as required.

Equine Inflammatory Airway and Obstructive Pulmonary Disease (Equine Asthma)

Lower airway conditions in the horse can range from airway hyper-reactivity and mild airway inflammation that only affects maximum athletic performance to marked airway inflammation with airway obstruction with mucus, airway remodeling, and breakdown of the alveolar structure such that horses that exhibit an increase in the work of breathing and experience impaired gas exchange at rest. There are likely many different etiologies contributing to equine lower airway disease including environmental allergens, genetics, viral disease, and bacterial infections. The more severe form of lower airway disease, which is of greatest concern as it relates to anesthesia, generally manifests in middle-aged to older horses of any breed.

Clinical signs of lower airway disease at rest include cough, nasal discharge, and an increase in expiratory effort. In severe cases, the horse's nostrils may be flared, and wheezes may be heard on thoracic auscultation.

Diagnostic investigation of horses presenting with lower airway disease includes a complete blood count, thoracic radiographs (in patients with severe disease), endoscopy, and BAL. In horses with performance limitation, pulmonary function testing may be required to detect airway hyper-reactivity and monitor the response to therapy.

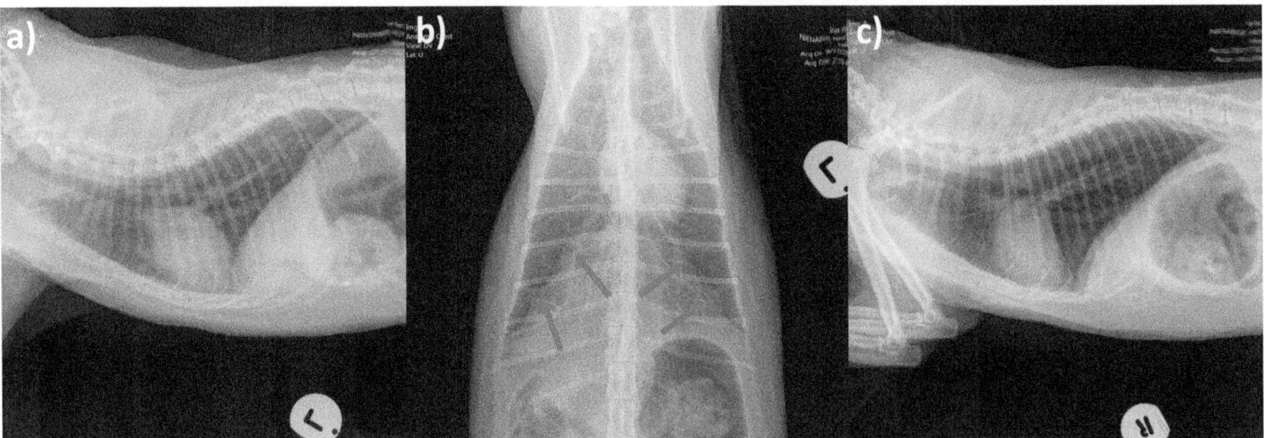

Figure 18.15 Series of left lateral (a), dorso-ventral (b), and right lateral thoracic radiographs in a cat with asthma. Note the hyperinflated lungs by identifying diaphragmatic tenting that is radiographically diagnosed by an undulating lung–diaphragm boarder (blue arrows) on the dorso-ventral view. (*Source:* Courtesy of Valley Farm Animal Hospital.)

Management of horses with lower airway disease includes reducing environmental exposure to allergens, in addition to treatment with inhaled or systemically administered glucocorticoids and bronchodilators. Unfortunately, glucocorticoid administration is associated with the development of laminitis, a factor to consider during the pre-operative examination of the horse.

Anesthetic Management of Dogs and Cats with Lower Airway Disease

Major concerns when anesthetizing companion animal patients with lower airway respiratory disease include the following:

- Potential for acute bronchospasm during anesthesia
- Potential need for shared airway during bronchoscopy
- Increased airway resistance requiring a prolonged expiratory time
- Risk of hypoxemia.

Pre-anesthesia Period

Before anesthesia, obtaining a thorough history regarding medications and thorough physical examination is essential. Depending on the underlying condition, animals may be receiving glucocorticoids, which will impact the ability to prescribe nonsteroidal anti-inflammatory drugs. Most nonsteroidal anti-inflammatory drugs inhibit the cyclo-oxygenase pathways of arachidonic acid metabolism for a lot longer than the lipoxygenase pathway. As a result, the production of leukotrienes may be increased. Leukotrienes trigger bronchoconstriction and can cause an acute asthmatic attack, and therefore the use of nonsteroidal anti-inflammatory drugs in cats is cautioned, with the possible exception of tepoxalin (10 mg/kg PO once daily for three days). CBC, biochemical profile, and thoracic radiographs are routinely recommended before anesthesia to characterize the severity of respiratory disease and screen for underlying disease. Medical management should be continued with the goal of optimizing the patient's condition before anesthesia. In cats with severe asthma, or cats undergoing airway procedures with a history of asthma, parenteral terbutaline (0.01 mg/kg SC) is recommended at least 30 min before anesthesia to reduce the risk of bronchospasm. Alternatively, salbutamol (100–200 micrograms) can be delivered via a mask and chamber (aids aerosolization) a few minutes before inducing general anesthesia.

As with patients with upper airway disease, the anesthesia workstation and supplies should be prepared before inducing anesthesia. For patients undergoing bronchoscopy, a bronchoscope adaptor, or means to insufflate oxygen during airway procedures, should be available. The anesthetist should also be prepared to assist with ventilation, either manually or with a ventilator, if available.

Anesthetic Period

Premedication is generally beneficial and can be tailored to the individual patient's behavior, coexisting disease, and the planned intervention. In mature patients, premedication with an opioid alone may be sufficient to provide a level of sedation and analgesia appropriate to permit IV catheter placement. Opioids possess antitussive properties that can reduce the response to tracheal intubation, bronchoscopy, and/or airway sample collection. Morphine and meperidine, when administered IV in particular, can induce systemic histamine release and subsequent bronchoconstriction. Therefore, they should not be administered via this route and alternative opioid analgesics are recommended if available. In hemodynamically stable patients with reactive airways, acepromazine may be beneficial due to its antihistamine effects. Anticholinergics block vagally mediated bronchoconstriction and reduce upper airway secretions that could trigger a lower airway response; therefore including glycopyrrolate or atropine as part of the premedication, along with an opioid and/or acepromazine, is recommended although they should be used with caution when included with alpha-2 adrenergic receptor agonists. However, if there is a suspicion of thicker respiratory secretions (e.g., infectious bronchitis), then including an anticholinergic is strongly cautioned because it can promote airway plugging with thick respiratory secretions.

Pre-oxygenation should be performed before inducing general anesthesia if it is well tolerated. The injectable anesthetics propofol and ketamine are associated with relaxation of airway musculature. Ketamine may induce upper airway secretions particularly when used at high doses, and therefore propofol may be the preferred agent. Although the effects of alfaxalone on airway tone are not as thoroughly studied, they are expected to be similar to those of propofol. Topical lidocaine, applied to the larynx in cats before intubation, is particularly important in cats with reactive airways. Intubation attempts at light planes of anesthesia should be avoided. In dogs, administering lidocaine (2 mg/kg IV) before intubation can be performed to reduce the risk of coughing and subsequent airway hyper-reactivity.

Like the injectable anesthetics, both sevoflurane and isoflurane result in relaxation of airway smooth muscle, resulting in bronchodilation. Injectable agents such as propofol or alfaxalone can also be administered as an IV infusion for maintaining anesthesia.

Monitoring should include SpO_2, $PE'CO_2$, ECG, and blood pressure in patients with lower airway disease, with blood gas analysis performed if concerns regarding oxygenation are present. Spirometry, specifically the measurement of airway gas flow and volume over time, is now included in some physiologic monitors and ventilators suitable for use in small animals. The information provided may be particularly useful in patients with lower airway disease as it can detect alterations to inspiratory and expiratory airway gas flow that may otherwise be challenging to detect until they are markedly impaired.

If positive pressure ventilation is required to maintain adequate ventilation, $PE'CO_2$ should be monitored, and the waveform should be observed to ensure complete exhalation between breaths. Using a lower respiratory rate will permit a longer inspiratory and expiratory time with an adequate expiratory pause.

Acute bronchoconstriction (bronchospasm) can occur during anesthesia in patients with asthma or bronchiolitis. The reduction in airway caliber results in increased airway resistance, which is most evident on expiration, manifesting as a prolonged expiratory time. Airway closure and air trapping in distal lung units can also occur. Patients can become hypoxemic even when receiving oxygen due to intrapulmonary shunting. Supporting patients using positive pressure ventilation and administering bronchodilators such as atropine (IV), terbutaline (IV), and/or salbutamol (albuterol) (nebulized) may reduce the severity of airway obstruction as evidenced by reduced peak airway pressures during positive pressure ventilation.

Anesthetic Recovery and Post-anesthetic Period

In canine patients that are not at risk of regurgitation and aspiration, extubation should be performed earlier than normal, once the patient is ventilating adequately but before return of a swallowing reflex to prevent triggering a cough response. Feline patients should also be extubated early, as routinely practiced, to prevent laryngospasm. Oxygen supplementation should be included as part of the post-anesthetic plan in patients with lower airway disease.

Anesthesia of the Equine Patient with Lower Airway Disease

Major concerns when anesthetizing equine patients with lower airway respiratory disease include the following:

- Risk of hypoxemia
- Increased airway resistance necessitating prolonged inspiration and expiratory phases of ventilation

Pre-anesthetic Period

Information regarding current medications and any adverse effects should be obtained. Based on physical examination, obtaining an arterial blood gas sample for analysis, if feasible, may be indicated to provide further information regarding the degree of gas exchange impairment before anesthesia.

Ideally, elective procedures are scheduled once the horse is stabilized with environmental and medical management. If interventions can be performed with the horse standing versus under general anesthesia, the former is highly recommended when respiratory compromise is evident at rest. In horses that require general anesthesia, dorsal recumbency will generally lead to the greatest impairment in gas exchange, and therefore maintaining the horse in lateral recumbency is preferred if possible.

Anesthetic Period

Typical anesthetic protocols are suitable (see Chapter 13); however, in cases with severe lower airway disease, means to provide oxygen and ventilatory support should be available. Fortunately, most sedative and anesthetic agents have minimal direct negative effects on lower airway tone. If hypoxemia occurs during anesthesia, it may be improved with ventilatory strategies that employ alveolar recruitment maneuvers and by applying a positive end expiratory pressure. Aerosolized salbutamol (albuterol, 100–200 mcg/100 kg) administered through the endotracheal tube has also been shown to be beneficial in some horses.

Anesthetic Recovery and Post-anesthesia Period

Oxygen supplementation should be provided in horses with lower airway disease during recovery from anesthesia.

Pleural Space Disease

Normally the pleural space is occupied by only a small volume of fluid (0.1–0.3 mL/kg) that acts as a lubricant between the visceral and parietal pleura. There is always a small amount of negative pressure within this potential space, which in most species keeps the lungs "sucked" up against the thoracic cage and pulls the diaphragm cranially. During spontaneous ventilation, higher negative intrapleural pressures during inspiration increases venous return resulting in an increase in cardiac output. The presence of air, fluid, soft tissue, or masses within the thorax can markedly increase the work of breathing, inhibit lung inflation, and impair gas exchange. As pleural pressures increase (even becoming positive), venous return and cardiac output fall. Concurrent conditions, including pulmonary atelectasis or contusions, are often present in patients with pleural space disease and sedation, and anesthesia may be required to permit adequate diagnostic investigation and permit appropriate management and/or treatment.

Pneumothorax

Air can enter the thoracic space, creating a pneumothorax, through the thoracic wall, esophagus, airways, or lung.

Traumatic pneumothorax resulting from penetrating injuries to the chest wall, or pulmonary contusions, is generally identified based on history and physical examination findings. Spontaneous pneumothorax, the accumulation of air in the pleural space in the absence of a traumatic or iatrogenic cause, can be primary or secondary to underlying lung disease. Primary spontaneous pneumothorax has been reported in dogs, with large-breed or deep-chested dogs being most represented. Histological findings in these patients include pulmonary bullae and blebs or occasionally general bullous emphysema. Secondary spontaneous pneumothorax occurs with lung disease that is inflammatory, infectious, or neoplastic in nature and is the most common form of spontaneous pneumothorax in other species. The differences in patients with pneumothorax versus a tension pneumothorax (a life-threatening emergency) are presented in Table 18.7.

Table 18.7 Observations and clinical signs of a dog or cat presenting with pneumothorax versus tension pneumothorax.

Observations and clinical signs	Pneumothorax		Tension pneumothorax	
	open	closed	open	closed
Common etiologies or mechanism of development	Trauma (large wound where lungs are visible) and elective surgery (thoracotomy)	Spontaneous (bullae disease and verminosis), trauma (esophageal tear, bruised or torn lung parenchyma, tracheal or bronchial rupture), and elective surgery (thoracoscopy)	Small penetrating wound with a one-way valve flap of tissue allows sucking in of air during inspiration but not expiration.	Dyspnea with an esophageal, tracheal or bronchial tear. Lung tears or bullae disease where intermittent positive pressure is applied
Level of consciousness	Awake	Awake	Awake but collapsed or could be comatose	
Posture	Abducted elbows, sternal recumbency	Abducted elbows and sternal recumbency	Panicked facial expression, staring into the distance, neck extended, and gasping for air (air hungry)	
Heart rate	Elevated due to other reasons such as pain	Elevated, especially if there is a concurrent pneumomediastinum	Progressive increase in heart rate to tachycardia then sudden bradycardia as myocardium becomes hypoxic	
Arterial blood pressure	Normal to decreased	Normal to decreased, especially if pneumomediastinum	Progressive decrease	
Pulse quality	Femoral: good Dorsal pedal: good or hard to feel	Femoral: good but hard to feel if pneumomediastinum Dorsal pedal: good or hard to feel	Femoral: hard to feel or absent Dorsal pedal: hard to feel or absent	
Venous return to the heart	Minimally decreased	Minimally decreased but can be greatly depressed if pneumomediastinum	Profoundly decreased	
Jugular veins	Normal on palpation	Normal to mildly distended on palpation	Very distended and often obvious to palpate as large distended tubes	
Cyanosis	Possible	More frequently than open pneumothorax	Common observation	
Breathing pattern	Costo-abdominal	Costo-abdominal to abdominal	Abdominal, the thoracic cavity is maximally distended and costal movement is usually not observed	
Respiratory rate	Normal or elevated if painful	Normal to elevated, especially if pneumomediastinum	Elevated	
Subjective assessment of flow of airway gases[a]	Easy to feel or appreciate flow of gases during exhalation	Easy to feel or appreciate flow of gases during exhalation	Open mouth gasping with no or very low flow of airway gases	
Immediate intervention	Routine stabilization	Routine stabilization and, if pneumomediastinum is present, then administer an isotonic fluid bolus (10–20 mL/kg) to improve cardiac return before inducing anesthesia.	Immediate thoracocentesis (even without radiograph evidence) using a large-bore intravenous catheter. Consider administering an isotonic fluid bolus (10–20 mL/kg) to improve cardiac return.	

a Animals < 5 kg hold a glass microscope slide by nares and see condensation of exhaled water vapor on slide.

Depending on the quantity of air within the pleural space, patients with a pneumothorax may be relatively asymptomatic or they may have severe respiratory and hemodynamic compromise. Reduced thoracic and pulmonary compliance, as a result of air accumulation, result in a rapid, shallow breathing pattern. Patients typically avoid recumbency and may stand with their elbows abducted. Auscultation reveals reduced lung sounds in the dorsal lung fields. Thoracic percussion in larger animals will help demarcate the extent of pneumothorax. Thoracic radiography is used to diagnose a pneumothorax although point-of-care thoracic ultrasonography is becoming more readily available and shows promise as a screening tool (Figure 18.16). In canine patients with suspected primary spontaneous pneumothorax, CT imaging, in multiple recumbencies, under general anesthesia, is recommended to determine the location(s) of lung bullae to assist with surgical planning.

Patients with traumatic wounds to the chest may require sedation and/or general anesthesia to repair a thoracic wound and/or address concurrent injuries. In dogs with primary spontaneous pneumothorax, lung lobectomy is generally performed via median sternotomy although the approach may also be via an intercostal thoracotomy or thoracoscopy.

Pleural Effusion, Chylothorax, Pyothorax, and Hemothorax

Several different medical conditions can lead to the accumulation of fluid within the intrapleural space. Unfortunately, congestive heart failure and neoplasia are common causes of fluid (transudates, exudates, or blood) accumulation in the thoracic space.

Clinical signs are highly variable depending on the underlying etiology; however, rapid shallow breathing with the muffling of heart and lung sounds on auscultation are consistent with the presence of fluid in the pleural space. Patients with hemothorax may also show signs related to loss of blood volume with pale mucus membranes, tachycardia, and poorly palpable peripheral pulses. In addition to the abnormalities detected in the respiratory

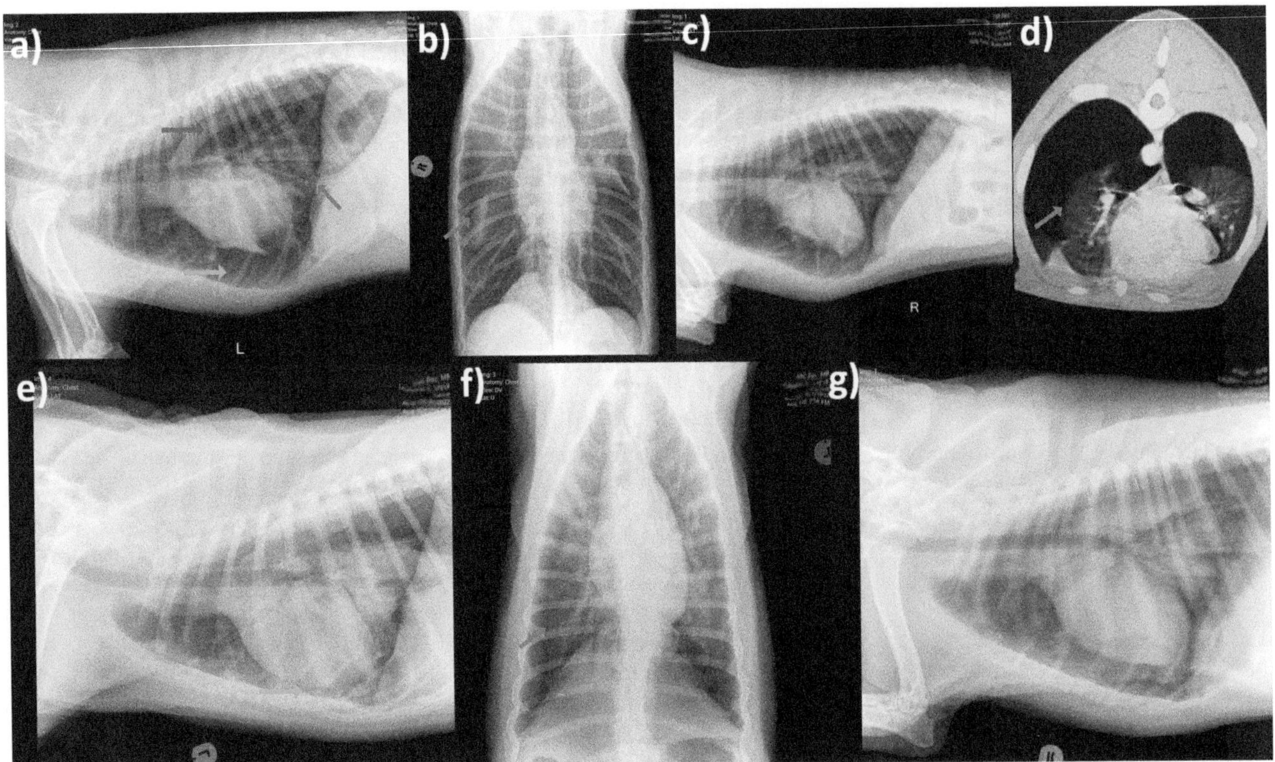

Figure 18.16 Left lateral (a), ventro-dorsal (b) and right lateral (c) thoracic radiographs, and (d) transverse image from a computed tomography scan in a dog with severe bilateral pneumothorax identified by the cardiac silhouette has no sternal or diaphragm contact (green arrow in (a)) and clearly defined aorta (red arrow in a) and caudal vena cava (blue arrow in (a)) on lateral views; and the large amount of gas in the pleural space with the lung parenchyma margin not clearly defined but clearly not making contact with the parietal pleura (blood arrow in (b) and (d)). Left lateral (e), dorso-ventral (f), and right lateral (g) thoracic radiographs of a dog with mild pneumothorax identified by a normal cardiac silhouette (green arrow in (e)) on the lateral views and a clearly defined lung parenchyma margin that is not making contact with the parietal pleura (blue arrow in (f)). (*Source:* Courtesy of Valley Farm Animal Hospital.)

system, pyothorax generally results in weight loss and anorexia. Diagnostic imaging including ultrasonography and radiographs are used to confirm the presence of fluid while collection of fluid via thoracocentesis confirms the nature of the fluid (Figure 18.17).

Patients with pleural fluid accumulation requiring anesthesia need a thorough diagnostic workup, including a cardiac evaluation in many instances to determine cardiac structure and performance, the presence of pericardial fluid, and characteristics of the pericardium.

The nature of the underlying disease will have a major impact on the pre-operative management of the patient and the choice of anesthetic protocol.

Diseases Affecting the Diaphragm

Abnormalities in the diaphragm most encountered in companion animals include diaphragmatic hernia and peritoneopericardial diaphragmatic hernia (PPDH). Diaphragmatic hernia is characterized by a lack of continuity in the diaphragmatic wall, while in animals with a PPDH, there is a communication between the abdomen and pericardial sac. In both instances, abdominal organs such as liver and intestines can migrate outside the confines of the abdominal space and become trapped, leading to organ dysfunction, abdominal pain, and anorexia and dyspnea.

Diaphragmatic Hernia

Diaphragmatic hernia can be congenital; however, in companion animals most are acquired secondary to trauma. Relatively high intrabdominal pressure relative to intrathoracic pressure associated with blunt trauma to the abdomen results in tears to the muscular component of the diaphragm.

Congenital or acquired diaphragmatic hernia may also occur in horses. Foals may present shortly after birth or following trauma. In adult horses, dystocia, strenuous exercise, or trauma may lead to the development of a diaphragmatic defect.

Clinical signs in patients with traumatic diaphragmatic hernia are highly variable and will depend on the viscera displaced into the thorax and its impingement on the lung and vascular system as well as current injuries. Some patients may present with only mild signs of respiratory compromise while others will present with signs of acute

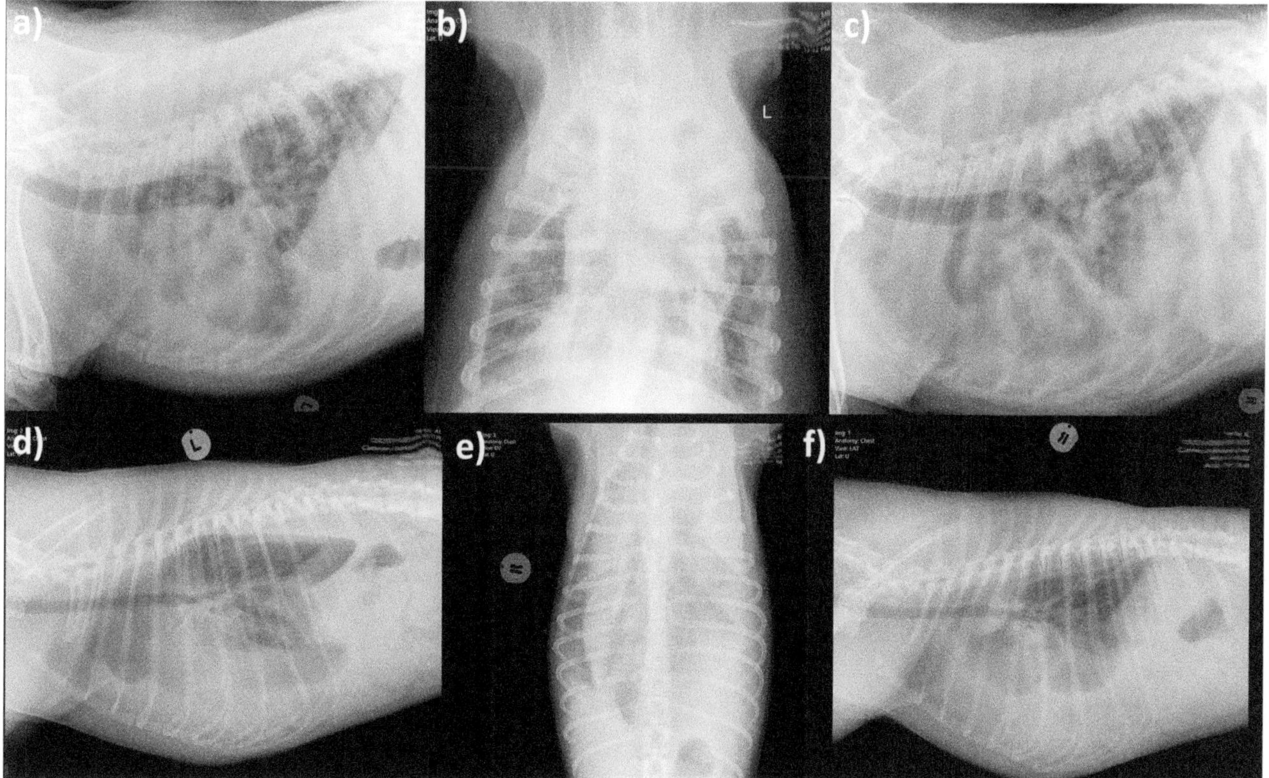

Figure 18.17 Left lateral (a), dorsal-ventral (b), and right lateral (c) thoracic radiographs of a dog with pleural effusions. Left lateral (d), dorso-ventral (e), and right lateral (f) thoracic radiographs of a cat with pleural effusions. In both series of lateral view radiographs, the air-filled lungs are displaced to the caudo-dorsal region of the thoracic cavity by the fluid in the pleural space and the fluid is radiopaque that makes defining the diaphragm margin challenging. (*Source:* Courtesy of Valley Farm Animal Hospital.)

respiratory distress including an increase in respiratory effort, tachypnea, and pale and/or cyanotic mucus membranes. Clinical signs consistent with a pneumothorax and/or hemothorax discussed in the preceding text may also be present. In horses, small intestinal migration into the thorax leads to signs of abdominal pain (colic).

Following trauma, comorbidities are extremely common, and animals should be examined carefully while receiving supportive therapy. Cardiac arrhythmias and hypovolemia secondary to internal or external blood loss are not uncommon along with fractures, soft-tissue wounds and neurological injuries.

Some patients may not exhibit clinical signs related to a diaphragmatic tear immediately after the traumatic incident but rather weeks to years after the trauma. Again, clinical signs can be highly variable, ranging from nonspecific weight loss to acute changes in respiratory or gastrointestinal function. In some cases, animals are asymptomatic and the defect is discovered incidentally during elective abdominal surgery or imaging studies.

Diagnosis of diaphragmatic hernia is generally performed with radiography and/or ultrasonography but contrast CT is required in some animals (Figure 18.18).

In cases presenting with respiratory compromise, surgery is generally recommended as soon as the patient is hemodynamically stable. Oxygen therapy can be initiated immediately and thoracocentesis performed if air or fluid is present in the pleural space while the patient is stabilized and prepared for surgery.

Peritoneopericardial Diaphragmatic Hernia

Peritoneopericardial diaphragmatic hernia is a congenital diaphragmatic malformation that can occur in both dogs and cats. Animals can present with signs of severe respiratory compromise at any age; however, they may also remain asymptomatic, with the defect only being discovered during diagnostic workup for other conditions or during elective abdominal surgery. Dogs with PPHD may have gastrointestinal signs such as anorexia, weight loss, or pain after eating. Patients may also have concurrent sternal or cardiac anomalies.

Physical examination finding typically include respiratory signs such as tachypnea and/or dyspnea with muffled heart sounds evident on auscultation. Abdominal pain may also be evident as organs can displace into the pericardial sac.

Diagnostic imaging used to confirm PPDH include radiographs, ultrasound, and CT (Figure 18.19).

Anesthetic Management of Patients with Pleural Space Disease

Major considerations when anesthetizing patients with intrapleural disease include the following:

- Risk of hypoxemia due to intrapulmonary shunting, ventilation/perfusion mismatching, and/or pulmonary parenchymal disease
- Risk of hemodynamic compromise secondary to an increase in intrapleural pressure

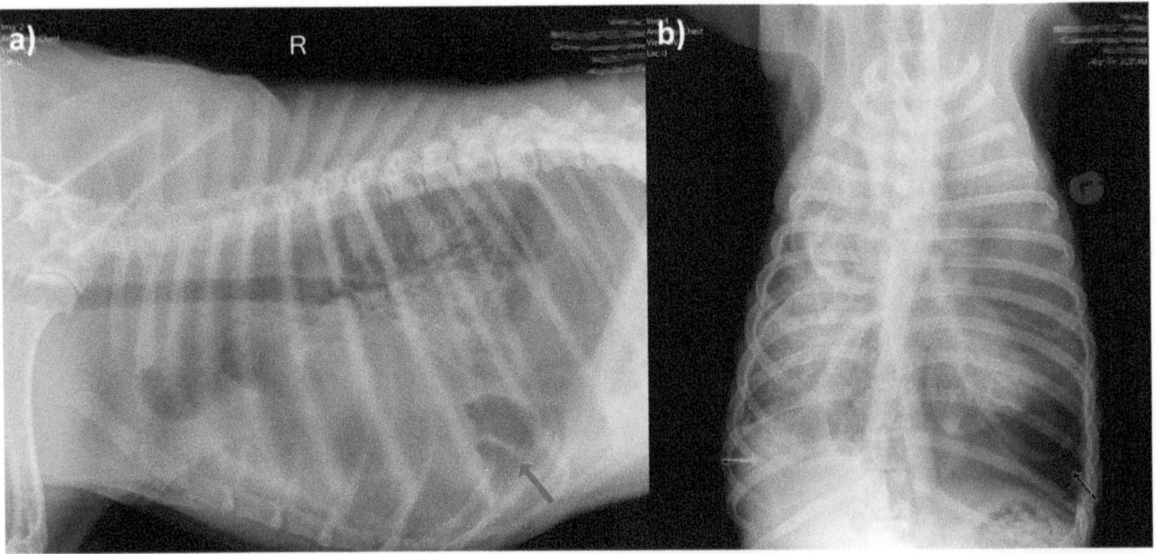

Figure 18.18 Right lateral (a) and dorso-ventral (b) thoracic radiographs of a dog with a diaphragmatic hernia. Note the gas-filled bowel loops (blue arrow) in the caudo-ventral region of the lateral thoracic radiograph and that the diaphragmatic boarder not clearly defined in both views, especially noticeable on the right-hand side (green arrow) of the dorso-ventral view and a pneumothorax on the left-hand side (red arrow). (*Source:* Courtesy of Valley Farm Animal Hospital.)

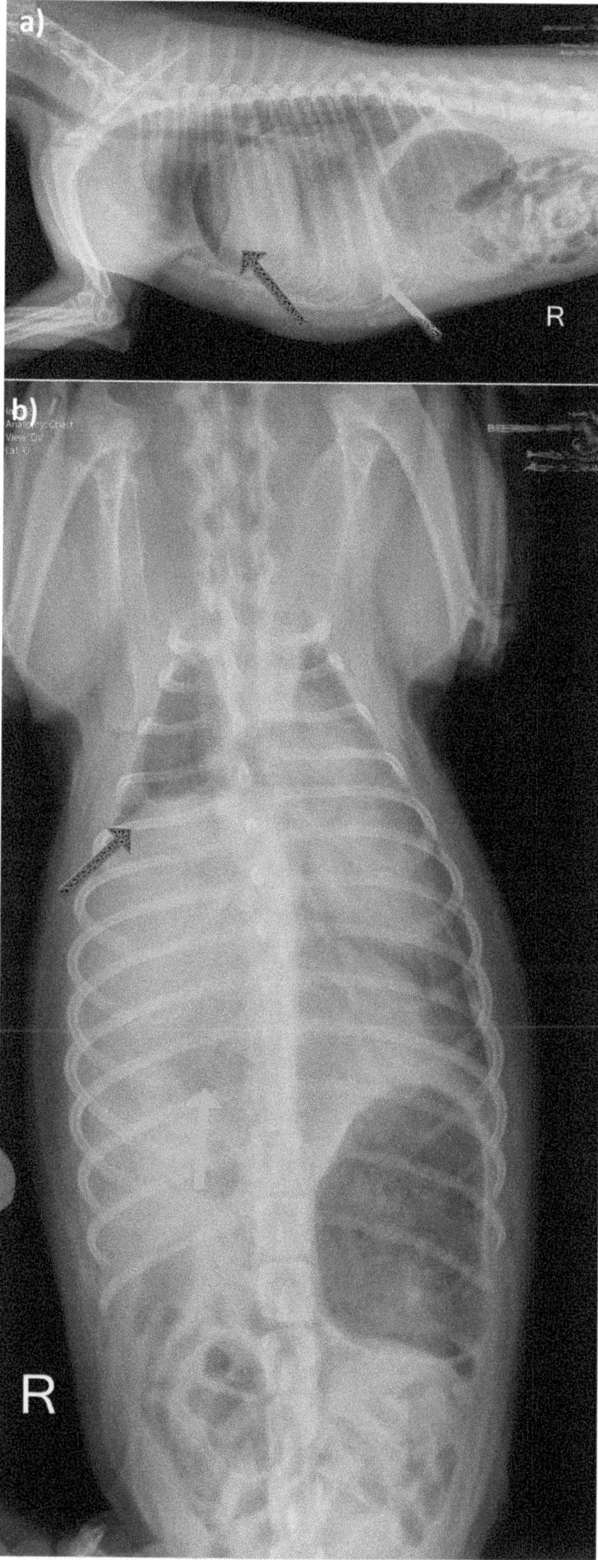

Figure 18.19 Right lateral (a) and dorso-vental thoracic radiographs of a cat with a peritoneopericardial diaphragmatic hernia. Note how well circumscribed the herniated organs are within pericardium inside the thoracic cavity (red arrows) and that the diaphragmatic border is not clearly defined (green arrows). (*Source:* Courtesy of Valley Farm Animal Hospital.)

- Increased work of breathing due to reduced thoracic and pulmonary compliance
- Potential for acute exacerbation of disease

Pre-anesthetic Period

In addition to a complete physical examination, the diagnostic workup of patients with pleural space disease before anesthesia should include the assessment of an ECG, arterial blood pressure and SpO_2, as well as a complete blood count and biochemical profile and thoracic radiography to screen for concurrent disease. In companion animals, images should be obtained in standing or sternal recumbency and/or in multiple positions to both screen for underlying pulmonary disease and to assess the severity of the patient's condition. As previously noted, thoracic ultrasound, if available, may also be used to confirm the presence of air in the pleural space, assess the continuity of the diaphragm, and screen for other abnormalities. Arterial blood gas analysis, if available, will also quantify the degree of gas exchange impairment.

Pre-operative stabilization, including O_2 supplementation and fluid therapy, should be administered based on individual patient needs. Patients with traumatic lesions or esophageal perforations can be extremely painful, and systemic analgesics can be used to improve patient comfort pre-operatively. Opioid analgesic administration should be titrated to effect to achieve analgesia while minimizing any negative impact on ventilation.

To minimize the patient's work of breathing and improve gas exchange, thoracocentesis should be performed if pneumothorax or abnormal pleural fluid is present. Placement of an indwelling thoracostomy tube or catheter using local anesthesia techniques to permit continuous or intermittent evacuation of air from the intrapleural space may be warranted if repeated thoracocentesis is required to maintain patient stability over time.

Anesthetic Period

Unless a thoracotomy is planned, means to ensure removal of air or fluid from the pleural space, either intermittently or continuously, should be in place throughout anesthesia. In large animal patients, repair of thoracic wounds may be performed under standing sedation using an alpha-2 adrenergic receptor agonist and an opioid analgesic in combination with local anesthesia. Sedative analgesic combinations can be administered as intermittent boluses or as a constant rate IV infusion. Intercostal nerve blocks, interpleural anesthesia, or infiltrative anesthesia can improve analgesia to the thoracic space and can be used in both conscious patients and patients undergoing general anesthesia. Gaseous or liquid pleural effusions increase the intrapleural space pressure (should be a negative pressure), and this can result in a decrease in venous blood return to the heart, decreased preload, and a decrease in cardiac output and blood pressure. When general anesthesia is required, ensuring access to the system used to evacuate the chest should be verified before the final preparation for surgery is performed.

The choice of anesthetic protocol is based on the individual patient condition and the planned procedure. In companion animals, general recommendations include pre-oxygenation before and during induction of anesthesia, using induction techniques that are tailored to the hemodynamic status of the patient and balanced anesthetic techniques to maintain anesthesia.

Strategies that result in the patient maintaining spontaneous ventilation are preferred when there is abnormal pulmonary parenchyma (i.e., pulmonary bullae leading to pneumothorax or evidence of pulmonary contusions).

In patients undergoing a thoracotomy (these procedures are generally restricted to specialist referral or academic hospital for appropriate anesthetic and post-operative care) under general anesthesia, including local anesthetic techniques before the start of surgery is recommended to reduce anesthetic requirements and provide pre-emptive analgesia. Positive pressure ventilation is required as the thorax is entered surgically. Use of a double lumen orotracheal tube with an endobronchial blocker can facilitate thorascopic lung lobectomy (see Further Reading). Before chest closure, the lung should be expanded slowly to a peak pressure of 15 cmH_2O while air is evacuated from the pleural space using an indwelling thoracostomy tube. In a patient with preexisting lung injury including chronic atelectasis, providing 2–3 large manual breaths to reinflate the lungs before surgical closure of a thoracotomy should not be performed as it will further lung injury.

In patients with a diaphragmatic hernia, ventilatory support will also be required. Manual ventilation to support breathing should be continued until the abdomen has been opened and the organs removed from the chest before intermittent positive pressure ventilation using a mechanical ventilator is started. This technique prevents cyclic high intrathoracic pressures that can decrease cardiovascular performance that may already be compromised because of poor venous return from the abdominal splenic organs.

Once the hernia is repaired, it is critical that air is removed from the pleural space. Generally, this is performed intra-operatively by the surgeon, who can place a catheter (such as an intravenous catheter with stylet removed immediately after entry into the thorax) through the diaphragm close to the thoracic wall (away from major vessels) after the diaphragm is closed. The catheter can be attached to extension tubing that facilitates aspirating air from the pleural space before closing the abdominal wall.

Monitoring airway pressures using in-circuit manometry, ventilation using capnography, and oxygenation using pulse oximetry and blood gas analysis, if available, and hemodynamic monitoring that includes an ECG and systemic blood pressure, ideally measured directly (arterial catheterization), are recommended.

Intra-operative complications that can occur in patients with pleural space disease include hypoxemia, arrhythmias, and continued air leakage into the pleural space. It is possible for the patient to develop a tension pneumothorax associated with positive pressure ventilation through continued air leakage from injured airways if the chest is not open or active evacuation of intrapleural air using a chest tube is not being performed. In patients undergoing a thoracotomy and lung lobectomy, iatrogenic laceration of the lung, hemorrhage due to laceration of the internal thoracic artery, and severe hypoxemia are possible.

Anesthetic Recovery and Post-anesthetic Period

All patients with pre-operative pleural space disease should be monitored intensively post-operatively due to the potential for air (recurrence of pneumothorax) or fluid accumulation within the chest. Following diaphragmatic hernia repair involving incarcerated organs, patients may develop pleural effusion, even if large quantities of pleural fluid were not evident pre-operatively.

Patients should receive O_2 supplementation post-operatively using previously described techniques until they can maintain normal hemoglobin oxygen saturation while breathing room air. An increase in respiratory rate and/or decrease in oxygenation should trigger an immediate assessment of the patient, focusing on the potential accumulation of intrapleural air or fluid. Chest radiographs or ultrasound can be repeated if clinical signs persist or worsen.

In companion animals, the administration of analgesic drugs including opioids, lidocaine, and/or ketamine by continuous infusion are recommended post thoracotomy. NSAIDs are suitable in hemodynamically stable patients but should be used cautiously in critically ill patients. Local anesthesia techniques can be repeated and opioid or lidocaine infusions can be used in large animal patients to improve patient comfort.

Patients with pleural space disease secondary to trauma (either thoracic or pulmonary parenchymal) are at increased risk of intrapleural infection or pneumonia post-operatively. Cardiac arrhythmias may also become evident in the post-operative period if myocardial contusions occurred, and therefore monitoring should include an ECG.

Complications reported following lung lobectomy include continued pneumothorax due to leakage at the site of lung lobectomy and wound complications.

Pulmonary Disease

Diffuse lung disease can result from a variety of causes including infectious pathogens, trauma, aspiration, sepsis, pancreatitis, and smoke inhalation. Pathological changes leading to impaired gas exchange include lung tissue consolidation with loss of functional alveolar space, thickened alveolar capillary membranes, and fluid accumulation in airways. To maintain adequate alveolar ventilation (and therefore normal arterial carbon dioxide levels) and oxygenation, an increase in respiratory rate and effort is observed on physical examination.

General anesthesia reduces normal mucociliary clearance, predisposes the lung to atelectasis, promotes hypoventilation (depressed response to carbon dioxide), reduces the pulmonary compensatory response to prevent hypoxemia (hypoxic pulmonary vasoconstriction), and in combination with surgery, and results in a neuroendocrine stress response that further suppresses the immune system. A combination of these factors can contribute to a worsening of pulmonary function following anesthesia in a patient with preexisting inflammatory and/or infectious lung disease.

While elective procedures requiring general anesthesia should not be performed in patients with pneumonia or pulmonary contusions, unfortunately some patients may require sedation or general anesthesia for emergency interventions, including ventilatory support.

Anesthetic Management of Patients with Pulmonary Parenchymal Disease

Major considerations when anesthetizing patients with lung disease include the following:

- Impaired gas exchange with impaired oxygen delivery to vital tissues in the peri-operative period
- Increased airway secretions that may create varying degrees of airway obstruction
- Increase in the work of breathing
- Change in respiratory pattern required to achieve gas exchange
- Potential for anesthesia to exacerbate preexisting lung disease
- Hemodynamic consequences of ventilatory support

Pre-anesthetic Period

As noted in the preceding text, patients are stabilized and elective procedures scheduled once normal pulmonary function is restored. Emergency procedures in patients that have pulmonary parenchymal disease but are maintaining adequate gas exchange while breathing room air may experience a deterioration in condition post-operatively. In general, anesthesia of patients with hypoxemia should be avoided. In emergency situations, companion animal patients are ideally stabilized on a ventilator that monitors patients' pulmonary mechanical properties and permits the application of positive end expiratory pressure to achieve gas exchange targets (PaO_2 over 80 mmHg and $PaCO_2$ below 55 mmHg). Most companion animal referral hospitals have the capacity to provide such support, and therefore referral to these centers is highly recommended.

Diagnostic investigation before anesthesia is based on the individual patient. In addition to a complete physical examination, thoracic radiographs, and assessment of gas exchange and metabolic status using arterial blood gases, are highly recommended. An ECG and blood pressure assessment are recommended as patients may have underlying cardiac disease, fluid deficits, and acid–base disturbances that impact cardiac rhythm, cardiac output, and vascular tone. In critically ill patients or in patients that have the potential to become further compromised following anesthesia, complete blood count and biochemistry profile should be performed before anesthesia.

Continuous O_2 supplementation should be maintained if there is evidence of hypoxemia or an increase in the work of breathing.

Medications including antimicrobials, bronchodilators, and anti-inflammatories should be continued in the perioperative period.

Anesthetic Period

In large animal patients with pulmonary parenchymal disease resulting in a change in respiratory function, local anesthesia and sedation should be used in place of general anesthesia to avoid recumbency and further impairment of pulmonary function when possible. Oxygen supplementation can be provided through the use of nasal cannulae during standing procedures if the animal has impaired gas exchange.

In small animal patients, local anesthesia and analgesic techniques should be included in the anesthetic protocol to assist with reducing the dose requirement for inhalant anesthetics. The anesthetist should be prepared to provide hemodynamic support measures including the use of inotropes and vasopressors.

For patients requiring general anesthesia, the protocol can be based on their hemodynamic stability and comorbidities. In patients achieving adequate gas exchange before anesthesia, it is preferrable to maintain spontaneous ventilation throughout anesthesia to minimize exposure of injured lungs to positive pressure. When ventilatory support is required (based on the assessment of oxygenation and ventilation), tidal volumes below 12 mL/kg should be used in combination with positive end expiratory pressure.

Due to the critical nature of patients with underlying pneumonia or pulmonary contusions, aggressive monitoring should be instituted including ECG, direct arterial blood pressure, PE′CO_2, SpO_2, and blood gas analysis. Monitoring should also include the observation of peak airway pressure on the anesthesia machine to prevent excessive airway pressures and assist with ventilatory management. Pneumothorax may develop during anesthesia, and increasing peak inspiratory pressures should trigger further investigation as to the etiology. Trending pulmonary mechanics using spirometry if available is ideal.

Anesthetic Recovery and Post-anesthetic Period

Oxygen supplementation and/or continued ventilatory support is likely to be required in the post-anesthesia period in patients with significant pulmonary compromise, even if it was not required before anesthesia. In companion animals and neonatal large animals in which recovery can be assisted, it is ideal if an arterial catheter can be maintained into the recovery period to permit continued monitoring of arterial blood gases and blood pressure.

Questions and Answers

There are more practice questions and answers available for this chapter on the website. Please visit http://www.wiley.com/go/VeterinaryAnesthesiaZeiler.

Questions

1) What is the fraction of inspired oxygen of room air?
   a) 0.12
   b) 0.21
   c) 0.28
   d) 0.31
   e) 0.32
2) A Husky dog presents collapsed, minimally conscious, gasping for air and has a cyanotic tongue. Answer the following questions:
   a) What is your immediate course of action?
   b) What oxygen support technique would you recommend?

Answers

1) b
   a) Perform an emergency thoracocentesis (it is diagnostic and therapeutic) by placing a large-bore intravenous cannula (catheter) into the thoracic cavity because a tension thorax is suspected. First, a quick thoracic auscultation can help confirm the suspicion of a tension thorax because there would be an absence of lung sounds during inspiration, and the thoracic cage will be distended with very little movement during inspiration and the jugular veins would be distended (very easy to palpate).
   b) Facemask (100 mL/kg/min) or via an endotracheal tube if tracheal intubation is possible if the dog loses consciousness, we can provide mechanical ventilation, if required.

Further Reading

Benatar S.R., Hewlett A.M., and Nunn J.F. (1973). The use of iso-shunt lines for control of oxygen therapy. *Br J Anaesth* 45: 711–718

Benumof J.L. (1994). Respiratory physiology and respiratory function during anesthesia. In: *Anesthesia*, 4e. (ed. R.D. Miller), Chapter 32. New York: Churchill Livingstone.

Couetil, L., Cardwell, J.M., Leguillette, R. et al. (2020). Equine asthma: current understanding and future directions. *Front Vet Sci* 7: 450.

Epstein, S.E. and Balso, I.M. (2020). Canine and feline exudative pleural diseases. *Vet Clin Small Anim* 50: 467–487.

Farnsworth, M.J., Chen, R., Packer, R.M.A. et al. (2016). Flat feline faces: is brachycephaly associated with respiratory abnormalities in the domestic cat (*Felis catus*)? *PLoS One* 11: e0161777.

Franklin, P.H., Liu, N.C., and Ladlow, J.F. (2021). Nebulization of epinephrine to reduce the severity of brachycephalic obstructive airway syndrome in dogs. *Vet Surg* 50: 62–70.

Freiche, V. and German, A.J. (2021). Digestive diseases in brachycephalic dogs. *Vet Clin Small Anim* 51: 61–78.

Gilday, C., Odunayo, A., and Hespel, A.M. (2021). Spontaneous pneumothorax: pathophysiology, clinical presentation and diagnosis. *Top Companion Anim Med* 45: 100563.

Jagodich, J.A., Bersenas, A.M.E., Bateman, S.W., and Kerr, C.L. (2020). Preliminary evaluation of the use of high-flow nasal cannula oxygen therapy during recovery from general anesthesia in dogs with obstructive upper airway breathing. *J Vet Emerg Crit Care (San Antonio)* 30: 487–492.

Kerr, C.L. and McDonell, W.N. (2009). Oxygen supplementation and ventilatory support. In: *Equine Anesthesia*, 2e (ed. W. Muir and J. Hubbell), Chapter 17, 332–352. Elsevier.

Krainer, D. and Dupre, G. (2022). Brachycephalic obstructive airway syndrome. *Vet Clin Small Anim* 52: 746–780.

Lumb, A.B. and Thomas, C.R. (2021). *Applied Respiratory Physiology*, 9e. London, UK: Elsevier.

MacPhail, C.M. (2020). Laryngeal disease in dogs and cats: an update. *Vet Clin Small Anim* 50: 295–310.

Maggiore, A.D. (2020). An update on tracheal and airway collapse in dogs. *Vet Clin Small Anim* 50: 419–430.

Marks, S.L., Kook, P.H., Papich, M.G. et al. (2018). ACVIM consensus statement: support for rational administration of gastrointestinal protectants to dogs and cats. *J Vet Intern Med* 32: 1823–1840.

McDonell, W.N. and Kerr, C.L. (2014). Physiology, pathophysiology, and anesthetic management of patients with respiratory disease. In: *Veterinary Anesthesia and Analgesia*, 5e (ed. K.A. Grimm, L.A. Lamont, W.J. Tranquilli et al.), 513–555. USA: Wiley-Blackwell.

Parente, E.J. (2018). Upper airway conditions affecting the equine athlete. *Vet Clin Equine* 34: 427–441.

Ranninger, E., Kantyka, M., and Bektas, R.N. (2020). The influence of anaesthetic drugs on the laryngeal motion in dogs: a systematic review. *Animals (Basel)* 10: 530.

Rossignol, F., Vitte, A., Boening, J. et al. (2015). Laryngoplasty in standing horses. *Vet Surg* 44: 341–347.

Rozanski, E. (2020). Canine chronic bronchitis. An update. *Vet Clin Small Anim* 50: 393–404.

Trzil, J.E. (2020). Feline asthma. Diagnostic and treatment update. *Vet Clin Small Anim* 50: 375–391.

Weisse, C., Berent, A., Violette, N. et al. (2019). Short-, intermediate-, and long-term results for endoluminal stent placement in dogs with tracheal collapse. *J Am Vet Med Assoc* 254: 380–392.

19

Approach to a Patient with Renal, Urinary, or Hepatobiliary Disease

Chantal McMillan and Gareth Zeiler

Introduction

The focus of this chapter is on dogs and cats with renal, urinary, or hepatobiliary disease; however, the overriding principles discussed here are transferrable to equine, cattle, and other mammalian species seen in veterinary practice.

Approach to a Patient with Renal or Urinary Disease

Overview of Pathology

The functional unit of the kidney is the nephron. The nephron's most important roles include urine production, removal of nitrogenous waste, and maintaining water and electrolyte balance. The nephron is composed of (1) the renal corpuscle that contains the glomerulus (unique arterial blood vessel capillary network with fenestrations that filter blood plasma) surrounded by the Bowman's capsule (cup-like structure that collects the filtrate) and (2) the renal tubules (processes the filtrate to form urine). If the glomerulus is irreversibly damaged, the associated tubule will degenerate. When disease is primary tubular in origin, the opposite occurs (e.g., tubular injury leads to eventual glomerular injury). As nephrons are lost, glomerular hypertension occurs in the remaining functional glomeruli leading to further injury and loss.

While the kidneys are responsible for the formation of urine, the bladder functions to store urine until micturition takes place. Micturition occurs through a complex reflex involving the neurological system and the urinary system. Normal micturition allows for ultimate excretion of metabolic by-products and toxins filtered by the kidneys. Of most significance for anesthetic management are urinary tract conditions that result in urinary tract obstruction as they can lead to metabolic disturbances.

Definitions

Azotemia

Glomerular filtration rate (GFR), despite being the most accurate assessment of renal function, is not commonly performed in clinical practice. Azotemia refers to increased concentrations of creatinine, blood urea nitrogen (BUN), and other nonprotein nitrogenous compounds in the blood. In small animal medicine, elevations in creatinine and/or BUN are used as markers of decreased renal function. Azotemia is not limited to primary renal disease and may also reflect pre-renal or post-renal etiologies, or a combination of these disorders. The urine specific gravity (USG; see later) is an important assessment to help differentiate whether azotemia is pre-renal, renal, or post-renal in origin.

- Pre-renal azotemia can occur with conditions leading to impaired renal perfusion and resultant decrease in GFR (e.g., dehydration, heart failure, and shock).
- Renal azotemia is the result of reduced GFR secondary to primary renal disease or injury. Azotemia arises with decreased GFR where there has been 75% or more loss of renal function. Therefore, creatinine and/or BUN is not a sensitive indicator of decreased function.
- Post-renal azotemia occurs with conditions leading to an obstruction or rupture of the urinary tract leading to an inability to excrete nitrogenous waste. With obstruction, there is also an increase in pressure in the renal tubular system, decreasing GFR. Azotemia typically resolves quickly after the obstruction is relieved and appropriate supportive therapy is provided, unless it is long-standing and has resulted in intrinsic renal damage.

It is important to note that azotemia can develop due to concurrent pre-renal, renal, or post-renal components, for example, a patient with chronic kidney disease (CKD; e.g., renal azotemia) that has decreased renal perfusion due to fluid deficits secondary to vomiting and inadequate water

Fundamental Principles of Veterinary Anesthesia, First Edition. Edited by Gareth E. Zeiler and Daniel S. J. Pang.

Companion Website: www.wiley.com/go/VeterinaryAnesthesiaZeiler

intake. In such a patient, the pre-renal component would be a correctable element of the azotemia. It is also possible that patients with a renal azotemia could have a concurrent post-renal component, for example, a ureterolith (calculi lodged in the ureter) in a patient with chronic kidney disease. This post-renal component would also represent a possible correctable component with appropriate diagnosis and therapy. Similarly, patients with post-renal azotemia can have a correctable pre-renal component (e.g., a dehydrated and hypovolemic obstructed cat). Correctable causes of azotemia are more likely to be pre-renal and post-renal compared to renal components.

Uremia

Uremia is a clinical syndrome comprising a myriad of symptoms that can result from decreased kidney function and can occur secondary to impaired glomerular, tubular, and endocrine functions. These impairments lead to accumulation of toxic metabolites, changes in composition of body fluids, and endocrine imbalances. The most common clinical signs recognized by pet owners will include weight loss, often with significant muscle wasting, gastrointestinal signs such as nausea and vomiting, lethargy, and decreased appetite. Uremia is not synonymous with azotemia. Azotemia refers to the accumulation of nitrogenous wastes secondary to a decrease in glomerular filtration rate. Not all animals with azotemia will have the clinical syndrome of uremia.

Renal Pathology

The most common renal conditions encountered include chronic kidney disease, primary glomerular disease, and acute kidney injury (AKI). Underlying pathologies affecting the renal system are diverse, as are the metabolic derangements that can arise secondary to a primary renal disease process.

Chronic Kidney Disease

CKD refers to structural and/or functional abnormalities of the kidneys that have been present for three months or longer. In reality, the practitioner will typically have no perspective on the chronicity of the condition at the time of presentation. CKD is one of the most common diseases veterinarians will diagnose with increasing frequency as cats age. It is less common in dogs but, when present, is also most common in the older population. There are a number of etiologies that result in CKD. These include, but are not limited to, congenital disease affecting function, neoplasia, infectious disease, sequelae to acute injury (e.g., toxic injury, ureteroliths, or nephroliths), immune, and inflammatory diseases. The specific cause underlying CKD is commonly undetermined.

Primary Glomerular Disease

This renal pathology is more commonly seen in dogs than cats. Primary glomerular disease can lead to similar complications as seen with CKD (e.g., azotemia and systemic hypertension). However, some unique manifestations, like hypoalbuminemia and hypercoagulability, can also occur. Primary disease of the glomerulus most commonly arises secondary to immune complexes, amyloidosis, or glomerulosclerosis. Hereditary glomerular diseases also exist.

Acute Kidney Injury

AKI occurs because the kidneys are at high risk of acute injury from ischemia and toxic insults. This predisposition is multifactorial and includes dependence on a large proportion of cardiac output, high metabolic activity, and concentration of nephrotoxins (e.g., ethylene glycol, nephrotoxic plants, and certain drugs) in tubular epithelial cells.

There are numerous etiologies of AKI including the following:

- Pre-renal causes occur secondary to decreases in renal perfusion. Some common risk factors include hypovolemia, hypotension, sepsis, anesthesia, nonsteroidal anti-inflammatory drugs (NSAIDs), and heart failure.
- Renal causes occur secondary to changes within the kidneys themselves (renal vasculature, glomeruli, tubules, or interstitium). Possible etiologies include pyelonephritis, infectious etiologies such as Leptosporosis, toxins (e.g., ethylene glycol, vitamin D), plants (e.g., grapes/raisins in dogs, lilies in cats such as *Lilium* sp. and *Hemerocallis* sp.), and drugs (e.g., aminoglycoside antimicrobials).
- Post-renal causes include disorders resulting in obstruction to urine flow such as would occur with ureteral or urethral obstruction. These can result in AKI if not identified and treated appropriately. Fortunately, most patients with urethral obstruction are easy to identify clinically due to their signs of lower urinary tract disease. Ureteral obstructions can be more subtle clinically as patients do not demonstrate obvious signs of urinary tract disease.

Even with appropriate diagnosis and therapy, AKI can result in patient morbidity and mortality. However, AKI does not always lead to long-term loss of function emphasizing the importance of identification of risks, early detection of injury, and appropriate therapy. With AKI, it must be understood that azotemia may not always be present following injury. Clinicians should be observant of increasing creatinine, even within the reference range in the euvolemic patient having risk factors for AKI. Whether azotemia is present or not, it is important to recognize potential for injury or early injury to make appropriate monitoring and therapeutic plans for the most positive patient outcome. If not recognized and left untreated, there can be increased risk of permanent damage resulting in CKD. Awareness of risk factors (e.g., nephrotoxin ingestion) and appropriate management is important to reduce the risk of AKI. One such risk factor for AKI is anesthesia, especially in patients that experience severe peri-anesthetic hypotension or have an ASA III or greater.

Urinary Pathologies

The most common urinary conditions encountered in which metabolic complications can arise are processes that have resulted in urinary tract obstruction (urethral calculi, obstructive feline lower urinary tract disease [FLUTD], and mass lesions) and bladder rupture. Underlying pathologies affecting the urinary system are diverse as are the metabolic derangements that can arise secondary to the primary disease process. Many of these derangements (azotemia and electrolyte abnormalities) are discussed elsewhere in this chapter.

Obstruction to Voiding Urine

Calculi

Calculi (stones) can form for several reasons including supersaturation of the urine with precursor constituents, combined with influences of urinary pH, the presence of certain microorganisms (e.g., Urease-positive bacteria), and even breed predispositions (e.g., Dalmatian dogs form urate calculi). If a calculus is passed into the urethra, this can result in an inability to void urine in both dogs and cats. Due to the smaller diameter of the male urethra in both species, obstruction is more common in males. With complete obstruction, patients will present with stranguria with a lack of urine production. Other signs can include licking the prepuce or vulva, pollakiuria, and, with incomplete obstructions, urine dribbling. Depending on duration, patients with complete obstruction may be systemically ill due to the development of metabolic disturbances such as hyperkalemia, azotemia, and acid–base abnormalities.

Treatment of a urethral obstruction requires sedation and, in some cases, anesthesia in order to pass a urinary catheter to relieve the obstruction, in addition to fluid therapy to correct electrolyte and acid–base disturbances, and often treat dehydration. Pending suspected stone composition, anesthesia is then also required in most cases on a less urgent basis to remove the cystic calculi via voiding urohydropropulsion or cystotomy and less commonly urethrotomy for urethral calculi (Figure 19.1). Calculi (also called "uroliths") can be sent for analysis to the University

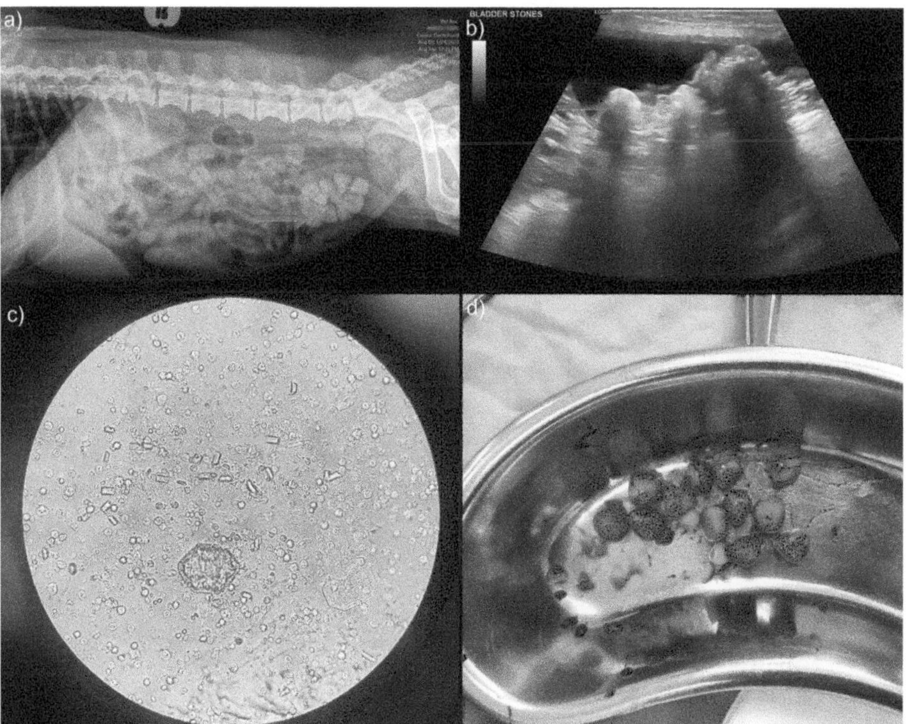

Figure 19.1 A right lateral radiograph (a) of an abdomen and an abdominal ultrasound of the urinary bladder (b) of a dog with cystic calculi (blue arrows; also called "bladder stones and uroliths"), and some smaller calculi (not shown in the radiograph) were intermittently obstructing the urethra prompting a cystotomy. These patients may have crystalluria (c) that is detected on urinalysis. The cystic calculi that were removed by cystotomy should be sent for urolith analysis (d).

of Minnesota, College of Veterinary Medicine, Minnesota Urolith Center (https://vetmed.umn.edu/urolith-center) at no cost (other than shipping).

Other etiologies of urethral obstruction resulting in the same metabolic disturbances can include neoplasia, strictures, and inflammatory disease.

Feline Lower Urinary Tract Disease "Feline lower urinary tract disease" is a common term referring to a number of disorders that can manifest in lower urinary tract signs in cats. Regardless of the cause, lower urinary tract disease typically results in a similar constellation of signs which can include hematuria, licking the penis/vulva, stranguria, dysuria, and pollakiuria. Some of the more common etiologies in cats include interstitial cystitis and urolithiasis, both of which can result in urethral obstruction. As noted in the preceding text, due to the narrow male urethra, it is far more common to see obstruction with these disorders in male cats. Acute management is aimed at correcting metabolic disturbances and relieving the obstruction. Fluid therapy plans should be individualized per case. Monitoring fluid balance is especially important once the obstruction is resolved because there can be a profound post-obstructive diuresis that increases the risk for dehydration, hypovolemia, and further AKI.

Urinary Bladder Rupture

Bladder rupture most commonly occurs following blunt trauma. Other etiologies include penetrating injuries, attempts to express the bladder manually in the presence of an obstructed devitalized bladder, and traumatic catheterization because of poor technique or rigid catheters. As urine will not be completely voided, patients will develop similar metabolic disturbances to those with obstruction including azotemia, acid–base disturbances, and hyperkalemia.

Often clinicians will have an index of suspicion of a ruptured bladder following trauma if their patient develops azotemia, hyperkalemia, lack of a palpable urinary bladder, and lack of an identifiable bladder on radiographs or ultrasound with the presence of free fluid in the abdomen. In the case of ureteral or renal injury, free fluid can be found in the retroperitoneal space.

Evaluation of fluid with creatinine concentrations (>2:1) and potassium (>1.9:1 cats or >1.4:1 dogs) when compared to serum helps confirm the diagnosis. Evaluation of urea is not helpful as it is a small molecule that readily diffuses across membranes. Peritonitis will typically develop within 12–18 h. Contrast studies (usually radiographs but also computed tomography) are commonly used to identify location of the injury. If the urine contains bacteria, urosepsis can occur and anesthetic principles for management of the septic patient would apply (see Chapter 16).

Management will involve stabilization with fluids to treat metabolic disturbances present and analgesia. Urinary diversion is also key in the acute stage and is typically used to help stabilize patients before surgical intervention for definitive repair. Urinary management will typically include a carefully placed urinary catheter to provide a conduit to empty the bladder of urine being produced. In some patients, depending on location of the trauma, a peritoneal catheter or cystostomy tube may be required. In some patients with small tears, the injury may heal spontaneously with placement of a urinary catheter. In cases where the urine is suspected to contain bacteria, antimicrobials will be part of the management plan.

Biochemical and Hematological Findings

Only the most common biochemical changes will be discussed in the following text.

Creatinine

Creatinine is a waste product arising from endogenous muscle tissue and protein metabolism of creatine phosphate. Muscle creatine is irreversibly converted to creatinine through nonenzymatic pathways at a constant rate of production. The greater the patients muscle mass the greater the production of creatinine. Creatinine is freely filtered by the glomeruli, not resorbed by renal tubules and ultimately excreted in the urine. Elevations of creatinine concentrations are seen with a decrease in GFR and are used in clinical practice to assess renal function. However, as mentioned previously, creatinine is insensitive as these elevations only occur with decreasing GFR that approximates a 75% or greater loss of function. Elevations in creatinine can be pre-renal, renal, or post-renal in origin. It is very important to note that creatinine arises primarily from endogenous muscle tissue and various conditions can lead to muscle wasting. Therefore, evaluating serum creatinine in the context of muscle condition is essential since patients with decreased muscle mass may have lower than expected serum creatinine concentrations that are not a reliable reflection of their GFR. For example, a thin hyperthyroid cat with concurrent CKD can have a creatinine within the reference range due to reduced muscle mass. This can lead to challenges when evaluating renal disease in patients with reduced muscle mass, in particular accurately staging patients with CKD.

Blood Urea Nitrogen

The majority of BUN measured arises from the hepatic urea cycle where circulating ammonia is converted to urea. BUN, like creatinine, is freely filtered by the renal glomeruli. Small amounts are resorbed by the renal tubules. Resorbed BUN is an important contributor to the medullary concentration gradient that allows for the formation of a concentrated urine. Like creatinine, BUN can be increased in the presence of decreased GFR due to pre-renal, renal, or post-renal etiologies. Other reasons for elevated BUN that must be taken into account when evaluating a patient include increased protein intake, gastrointestinal hemorrhage, and increased protein catabolism. Decreases in BUN can be seen with low protein diets, vascular shunting lesions of the liver (e.g., portosystemic shunt [PSS] without intrinsic liver disease), decreased liver function secondary to intrinsic liver disease, and in some cases in patients with severe polyuria/polydipsia (pu/pd). Because there are a number of factors that can result in elevated serum BUN (high-protein meal, gastrointestinal hemorrhage, and increased protein catabolism), creatinine is considered a more reliable surrogate for decreased GFR (renal function) in small animal patients.

Symmetric Dimethylarginine (SDMA)

SDMA is a methylated arginine residue of metabolism of intracellular proteins containing arginine. It is considered a specific biomarker of renal function as it is freely filtered by the glomerulus and is not reabsorbed by the renal tubules, thereby correlating well with GFR. SDMA is used clinically as an early marker of decreased GFR. It is assessed commonly in both dogs and cats when investigating for or monitoring progression of renal disease. Increases, on average, are reported to occur with a 25–40% decrease in renal function compared to the 75% that leads to increases in serum creatinine concentrations. Increases in SDMA may therefore be detected before elevations in serum creatinine. Persistent elevations suggest reduced renal function. SDMA increases alongside elevations in serum creatinine together with an inappropriately concentrated urine are consistent with renal disease.

Unlike creatinine, SDMA is not impacted by muscle mass and thus can be a useful marker when evaluating patients with muscle loss and concurrent renal disease (e.g., patients with hyperthyroidism or other illness's resulting in reduced muscle mass). As mentioned, patients with decreased muscle mass may have serum creatinine concentrations that do not correlate well with GFR, and clinicians can underestimate the severity of kidney dysfunction.

Albumin

Hypoalbuminemia is a common biochemical abnormality. This can occur secondary to decreased production from hepatic disease, increased loss, negative acute phase reaction, fluid overload, or sequestration (e.g., vasculitis). Increased loss often results in a more profound and clinically relevant hypoalbuminemia than what is associated with other etiologies listed in the preceding text. The most common causes of albumin loss in small animal patients are gastrointestinal (protein-losing enteropathy) and urinary (protein-losing nephropathy). With gastrointestinal disease, protein loss is most typically nonselective leading to a panhypoproteinemia (albumin and globulin loss). Albumin loss can also occur through the kidney. Due to its size and charge, albumin is normally only minimally filtered through the glomerulus, and the small amount that is filtered is reabsorbed by the proximal renal tubules. However, glomerular disease allows passage of albumin and can result in a profound hypoalbuminemia. Globulins are preserved as they are much larger than albumin, and as such the pattern of hypoproteinemia differs from that which is seen with gastrointestinal disease. One can confirm that hypoalbuminemia is secondary to renal loss through evaluation for proteinuria (described in the following text). With primary glomerular disease, the loss of albumin can be severe and have clinically relevant consequences.

Loss of albumin decreases intravascular oncotic pressure that may result in spontaneous cavitary effusions or interstitial edema formation, especially if albumin concentrations are less than 16 g/L. Higher albumin concentrations values can also lead to complications from decreased oncotic pressure if patients have concurrent inflammatory disease or conditions requiring fluid therapy. This predisposition to and the presence of effusions or edema are important considerations for anesthetic management.

Although patients with CKD can have proteinuria, it is typically lower grade and not correlated with hypoalbuminemia. Despite the lower-grade proteinuria, it is still of clinical significance in CKD as its presence is associated with an accelerated disease course.

Electrolytes

Phosphorous

Hyperphosphatemia is common in small animal patients with CKD. Its presence is associated with a more rapid disease progression and increased mortality in both dogs and cats. The physiology of this electrolyte disturbance is complex. In early stages of CKD, initial increases in phosphorous are counteracted by a reduction in calcitriol (1,25-dihydroxycholecalciferol; active vitamin D) concentration. In later stages, the increasing phosphorus is counteracted through increased parathyroid hormone (PTH) production. This compensation is eventually ineffective with further reductions in GFR and loss of functional nephrons decreasing phosphorous excretion by the kidneys. As phosphorous excretion is dependent on GFR, it should be noted that, like with azotemia, hyperphosphatemia can be pre-renal, renal, or post-renal in origin.

Renal diets are commonly prescribed as part of the standard of care when managing patients with CKD and are formulated with lower phosphorous concentrations. Other therapies to decreased serum phosphorous concentrations can include calcium or aluminum phosphorous binding agents for daily oral use.

Potassium

Hypokalemia is a common finding in cats with early stages of CKD (see International Renal Interest Society [IRIS] staging later). If hypokalemia is not recognized and managed, it can result in hypokalemic myopathy. The presence of hypokalemia is less common in cats with more advanced disease and is likely due to a marked reduction in GFR and resultant decrease in renal excretion. Canine patients with CKD are very commonly on angiotensin-converting enzyme (ACE) inhibitor drug therapy, and may be why hypokalemia is less commonly present in this species. To help prevent development of hypokalemia, renal diets often contain higher amounts of potassium. In some patients, oral supplementation is needed. In those that are receiving subcutaneous fluids on a consistent basis (every second or third day), potassium chloride can be added as a method of supplementation.

Hyperkalemia is commonly encountered in disorders resulting in post-renal azotemia (e.g., obstructive feline lower urinary tract disease and bladder rupture) and can also be encountered in some patients with AKI. The hyperkalemia that occurs secondary to these disorders can be severe and life-threatening, especially if there is a rapid increase in plasma concentration. Hyperkalemia causes an increase in the resting membrane potential of excitable tissues (notably cardiac muscle and nerves) and alters normal conduction of action potentials in these tissues. The result is usually a bradycardia with a decrease in cardiac output. Therapies to decrease potassium concentration (insulin, dextrose, IV fluids, and beta-2 adrenergic receptor agonists) and cardioprotective therapies to increase the threshold potential, which will normalize the gap between the resting and threshold potentials (calcium gluconate), are often used to stabilize patients with hyperkalemia before sedation and/or anesthesia to relieve urinary tract obstructions or repair the urinary tract.

Erythrogram (Red Blood Cell Count and Morphology)

Anemia of renal disease may be present in patients with CKD. With advanced disease, anemia can be of clinical significance and negatively impact the patient's quality of life. It can also contribute to further renal injury secondary to hypoxia. The main etiology of this anemia is a decreased production of erythropoietin, which is required for red cell production. Other factors include reduced red cell lifespan in the presence of azotemia, gastrointestinal loss, and poor nutrition. Anemia of CKD arising secondary to decreased erythropoietin production is typically characterized as a normocytic, normochromic, nonregenerative anemia. If the hematocrit is 20% (0.2 L/L) or less, and the loss was acute (within a few days) or if less than 15% (0.15 L/L) in chronic losses (>3 months), then it should generally be corrected before sedation and general anesthesia because the hematocrit decreases (by as much as 8%) in sedated and anesthetized animals. Either packed red blood cells or fresh whole blood could be considered as treatment in emergency or urgent situations. In elective procedures, treatment with drugs that stimulate erythrocyte production (e.g., darbepoetin with iron supplementation and vitamin B12) could be started before an elective surgery if time allows for appropriate response (2–3 months).

Patient Evaluation and *International Renal Interest Society Staging and Grading Systems*

All patients with renal or urinary disease that require sedation or general anesthesia should undergo a clinical examination and ASA physical status classification (see Chapter 2). This is in addition to renal-specific evaluations that include biochemical, hematological (as described in the preceding text), and urinalysis. Information gained from some of these renal-specific evaluations is used in the various renal disease scoring systems.

Urinalysis

A urinalysis is an essential part of the diagnostic evaluation of the renal and urinary systems. Only fundamental components of a complete urinalysis most pertinent to this chapter are discussed here. Information about the other components can be found elsewhere (see Further Reading).

Urine Specific Gravity

USG provides an estimate of the renal tubules ability to dilute or concentrate the glomerular filtrate. In patients with renal disease, decreased concentrating ability is not present until there has been approximately 70% loss of renal function.

Reagent urinalysis strips commonly used in small animal clinics for in-house assessments of urine often include an indicator for USG. However, these are not considered accurate. Rather, a standard refractometer with a refractive index for urine should be used.

Definitions such as hyposthenuria, isosthenuria, and adequately concentrated urine often help veterinarians organize their thought processes when interpreting USG in a clinical context and are discussed in the following text.

Hyposthenuria is defined as a USG < 1.008 (verbalized as "ten-o-eight"). A persistently hyposthenuric urine is supportive of an inability to concentrate urine; however, it also reflects the ability to produce dilute urine that requires functional renal tubules. Hyposthenuria can occur in disorders that can result in severe pu/pd such as hyperadrenocorticism, psychogenic polydipsia, and the uncommon conditions such as central and primary nephrogenic diabetes insipidus.

Isosthenuria refers to a USG between 1.008 and 1.012 ("ten-twelve"). Persistently isosthenuric urine can indicate an underlying disease resulting in pu/pd. If isosthenuria is present in a dehydrated animal (with or without azotemia) or in an adequately hydrated azotemic animal, then this is highly suggestive of renal disease.

Adequately concentrated urine requires a USG > 1.030 ("ten-thirty") in dogs and >1.035 ("ten-thirty-five") in cats. If these USGs are found in patients with azotemia, then these findings are consistent with a pre-renal azotemia and normal renal concentrating ability.

Values consistently less than adequately concentrated (typically <1.025) and greater than the isosthenuric range in patients with history of polydipsia fit with an underlying pu/pd disorder. Cats and dogs with renal disease will commonly have USGs that fall in this (>1.012 to <1.025) or the isosthenuric range.

The whole clinical picture must be taken into account when evaluating USG because many factors influence concentrating ability. Some examples of factors that must be considered when interpreting USG include hydration status, electrolyte concentrations (sodium, potassium, and calcium), the presence of glucosuria (causes an osmotic diuresis), BUN and creatinine concentrations, fluid therapy, and diet and any medications (e.g., corticosteroids and diuretics) that could be resulting in pu/pd from a variety of mechanisms. The veterinarian must also recognize that there can be tremendous daily variability in USG. Thus, veterinarians should not conclude that an inability to concentrate urine is present based on a single USG reading, especially in the absence of other signs associated with renal disease (e.g., azotemia and/or dehydration) or history fitting with pu/pd.

When interpreting the USG, veterinarians must consider exceptions to these guidelines of what is considered adequately and inadequately concentrated urine exist and relationship to renal disease. Disorders that can result in dehydration and azotemia can impact the kidneys' ability to adequately concentrate and are not due to primary renal disease. An example would be Addisonian (hypoadrenocorticism) patient presenting with dehydration and the frequent presence of azotemia. These patients often do not have an appropriately concentrated urine that may be due to hyponatremia.

Proteinuria

Proteinuria generally refers to the detection of excess protein in urine. In health, very little protein is present, if detected at all. The glomerulus is effective at minimizing the loss of serum proteins (albumin and larger proteins like globulins) while other substances such as water, small solutes, and waste products readily pass through for processing by the renal tubules (reabsorption or elimination). In addition, there is effective active tubular absorption of proteins that do reach the glomerular filtrate. As the renal tubular cells are responsible for processing proteins, increased amounts will not only exceed their capacity for reabsorption but increase their metabolic workload, leading to oxidative stress and tubular damage. Proteinuria can occur due to pre-renal, renal, or post-renal causes.

- Pre-renal proteinuria refers to clinical situations in which abnormally high levels of plasma proteins have traversed the glomerular capillary. Clinical examples include myoglobinuria secondary to muscle injury, hemoglobinuria secondary to intravascular hemolysis, and the presence of Bence Jones proteins secondary to multiple myeloma.
- Renal proteinuria refers to abnormal renal handling of normal levels of plasma proteins. This can occur due to transient functional reasons, such as fever or strenuous exercise. In these cases, proteinuria is typically mild and transient. Renal proteinuria can also occur secondary to structural or functional lesions within the glomerulus, renal tubules, or the renal interstitium. Proteinuria associated with glomerular lesions can be severe.
- Post-renal proteinuria refers to entry of protein into urine after it has entered the renal pelvis (hemorrhage or inflammation). This can occur secondary to disease of the renal pelvis, ureters, urinary bladder, and urethra (including prostatic urethra), which are termed "urinary etiologies." Extra-urinary etiologies are those that typically arise from the genital tract or external genitalia. In conditions arising from the genital tract or external genitalia, protein will be present in voided samples but should not be present in those attained via cystocentesis.

Urine Protein:Creatinine Ratio (UP:C or UPC)

In clinical practice, the UP:C is the most commonly used test to determine the magnitude of proteinuria and whether the protein present on routine urinalysis is in excess. Protein is measured in relation to creatinine concentration to account for the degree of concentration in the urine and to standardize the protein concentration. Creatinine is a good standard in most settings because it is freely filtered by the glomerulus but is not resorbed or secreted by the tubules (e.g., once filtered by the glomerulus, its concentration remains relatively constant).

In dogs, veterinarians can consider evaluating for proteinuria with a UP:C if 2+ or more protein is detected in a urine sample using a urine dipstick (Figure 19.2). However, if 1+ proteinuria is present and the urine has a USG of 1.025 or less, then the evaluation of UP:C is indicated as protein is more likely to be of significance when detected in dilute urine. In patients with CKD, if any amount of protein is detected, then a UP:C is recommended for accurate staging and therapeutic decision-making. A UP:C >0.5 in a dog or >0.4 in a cat is abnormal in a urine sample free of inflammation or discoloration from hematuria.

Elevations in UP:C can occur in patients with hematuria, bacteriuria, and pyuria. Clinicians should realize that corticosteroid therapy can also result elevations in UP:C which are typically mild. If proteinuria is significant and in the absence of hematuria, pyuria, or bacteriuria, then veterinarians should ensure it is persistent before therapy is instituted. There is no agreed upon number of UP:C measurements that is diagnostic for forms of renal disease but, in general, disorders that are primary glomerular in origin tend to have a more severe proteinuria (UP:C > 2). Detailed references are available with respect to diagnostic approach and therapeutic recommendations for proteinuria in patients with suspected glomerular disease and CKD. Determining the presence of proteinuria is an important part of the IRIS staging system (see later) in both cats and dogs with CKD as proteinuria is considered detrimental to renal health and is a therapeutic target to decrease its magnitude. Therapy typically involves the use of drugs such as ACE inhibitors and/or angiotensin receptor blockers.

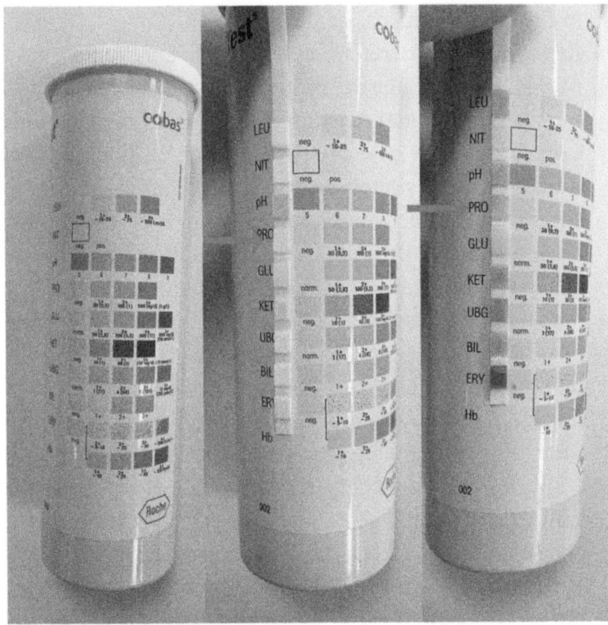

Figure 19.2 A human urine dip stick that is used during urinalysis in companion animal practice. From left to right: The container with all of the variables that can be analyzed, a clean dipstick before being dipped into the urine, a dipstick that has been dipped into urine, and the change in color of the various strips has occurred and can be read off the blocks on the right-hand side. Proteinuria has been detected (blue arrows).

Cytologic Examination of Urine

Cytologic examination is an important component of a complete urinalysis for assessing the clinical picture in both urinary and renal diseases. This can be used to evaluate cells (hematuria, pyuria, and atypical cells), casts (cellular or proteinaceous), or crystals (e.g., calcium oxalate monohydrate that occurs with ethylene glycol toxicity, evidence of urine supersaturation and possible increased risk of calculi formation, or hepatic disease [ammonium biurate with portosystemic shunts]).

International Renal Interest Society Staging and Grading Systems

IRIS Staging of CKD

The IRIS staging of CKD provides specific and standardized information with respect to the stage of disease present and therapeutic and monitoring recommendations. In both dogs and cats, IRIS staging stratifies patients into one of four stages based on their creatinine and/or SDMA concentrations. The use of both markers is preferred. Both dogs and cats are then sub-staged based on systemic blood pressure measurements and the presence or absence of proteinuria. The inclusion of determining the patient's SDMA is that it may allow for earlier detection of stage 1 disease where most clinical signs are not yet evident and may also be useful in patients with decreased muscle mass. The earlier detection may afford improved opportunities for early intervention and monitoring that can improve patient longevity and quality of life.

IRIS Grading of AKI

IRIS grading of AKI has been developed to facilitate standardized classification of patients. Unlike staging for CKD evaluation, in AKI patients grading does not imply a stable or steady state disease. Grading for AKI in dogs and cats is based on blood creatinine, urine formation, and the requirement for renal replacement therapy. Grading should be continually evaluated as part of routine assessments during therapy for AKI to assess response to therapy, guide therapeutic changes, and help determine prognosis.

Further information about the specifics of IRIS staging of CKD and grading of AKI can be found on the website www.iris-kidney.com.

Additional Complications of Renal Disease to Consider

Hypertension

Hypertension is common in both dogs and cats with CKD and patients with primary glomerular disease. Patients with persistent systolic arterial blood pressure >160 mmHg are typically classified as hypertensive. Severe hypertension is classified as systolic arterial blood pressure >180 mmHg. Hypertension can result in significant organ effects such as retinal hemorrhage and detachment which if left undetected can lead to permanent blindness. Other organs prone to hypertensive injury include the brain, kidneys (causing further damage), and the heart. The presence of hypertension can also worsen proteinuria. Patients with uncontrolled hypertension are more likely to have a more rapid progression of their renal disease.

Blood pressure should be assessed, as described elsewhere (see Chapter 4). If persistent hypertension is detected, treatment is strongly recommended, and therapy depends on severity. *Severe persistent hypertension* is defined as systolic arterial blood pressure measurement of >180 mmHg for 1–2 weeks, and >160 but <180 mmHg for 1–2 months of duration. If there is evidence of target organ damage consistent with hypertensive injury (e.g., retinal detachment), there is no need to evaluate for persistence of hypertension and therapy should be instituted immediately to prevent further damage. Therapies often include drugs that decrease systemic vascular resistance through calcium channel blockade (e.g., amlodipine) or decrease systemic vascular resistance by effects on the renin–angiotensin system. This includes ACE inhibitors (e.g., benazepril and enalapril) or angiotensin receptor antagonists (e.g., telmisartan). Recommendations for therapy in both dogs and cats with CKD are included in the IRIS guidelines (see Further Reading).

Hypercoagulability

Patients with proteinuria secondary to primary glomerular disease are often hypercoagulable predisposing them to thromboembolic disease. There are several proposed mechanisms of hypercoagulability including loss of antithrombin III, increased procoagulant factors, and increased platelet activity. However, it must be noted that the pathophysiology is not completely understood. Therapies commonly utilized in clinical practice for thromboprophylaxis make use of drugs decreasing platelet function and include low-dose aspirin and clopidogrel.

Anesthetic Management of Patients with Renal or Urinary Disease

Patients that have renal and/or urinary pathology may require sedation or general anesthesia to facilitate procedures (e.g., passing urinary catheters) or surgery (e.g., cystotomy and repair of ruptured bladder). Other patients may require anesthesia for diagnostic or therapeutic procedures related to renal system disease or to address comorbidities (e.g., dental assessments in patients with CKD). Potential complications of renal disease are important to recognize. The more common complications include hypertension, hypoalbuminemia, hypokalemia or hyperkalemia, and hypercoagulability. If present, they will influence the sedation and/or anesthetic and monitoring plan. In addition to recognition and management of complications of renal disease, adverse effects associated with anesthesia that can contribute to further renal damage (e.g., hypotension) should be monitored for and managed. Sedation (especially deep sedation) can carry a higher risk than general anesthesia because the frequency and complexity of peri-sedation monitoring, especially of arterial blood pressure, is often less compared to patients undergoing a general anesthetic.

Major Considerations for Sedation or Anesthesia

- Pain related to procedures (e.g., urinary catheterization and urohydropropulsion) can be experienced and requires providing analgesia.
- Systemic hypotension, with or without hypovolemia, or systemic hypertension.
- Assessment for electrolyte imbalances, especially potassium and phosphate.
- If there is severe hypoalbuminemia (<16 g/L), then the impact of any associated cavity effusions (e.g., ascites or pleural effusions) should be assessed (e.g., negative effects on venous return and/or ventilation) and corrected (i.e., drained by abdominocentesis or thoracocentesis) before general anesthesia.
- Determining urine output (or at least confirming urine production), especially if the patient has AKI.
- Anemia can be present in patients with renal disease and thus the hematocrit should be measured.
- Nausea and vomiting should be treated.
- In all cases, it is wise to prepare all that is required for the procedure or surgery prior to injecting drugs that cause sedation or general anesthesia in order to keep the anesthetic time as short as reasonably possible.
- In all cases, the intravascular volume should be resuscitated before inducing general anesthesia to minimize the occurrence of post-induction hypotension.

Sedation or Peri-anesthetic Management

Evaluation and, when necessary, stabilization and pre-anesthetic optimization of the patient's cardiovascular system (intravascular volume and functional performance) are critically important if there is concurrent/coexisting cardiac disease. Furthermore, a patient with renal disease can have a higher resting arterial blood pressure compared to healthy animals. This elevated arterial blood pressure is usually taken into account during anesthesia so that the minimal tolerated arterial blood pressure is often greater than that for healthy patients. A hematocrit of at least 20% (0.2 L/L) is suggested to minimize peri-anesthetic hypoxemia. Both hypotension and hypoxemia will worsen renal function or destabilize a patient by initiating an acute-on-chronic renal disease process, which can be life-threatening. This is especially true if anuric AKI develops. Patients with urinary tract pathology may have hyperkalemia, hypovolemia, and acid–base derangements, and these should be investigated and corrected (as much as possible) before general anesthesia is induced. Stratifying the patient into one of the ASA categories (see Chapter 2) will assist in drug and monitoring selection, and consideration of risk, while preparing the sedation or general anesthetic plan.

Most of the drugs used for sedation or general anesthesia require part or complete elimination of the active drug or its metabolites (active or inactive) via the renal system. Thus, drugs are selected to ensure optimal cardiovascular performance that provides adequate blood flow to the kidneys (and other vital organs). However, the use of thiopentone or ketamine is cautioned in most species because they can be associated with prolonged or stormy recoveries, respectively. If the patient is hypovolemic, hypotensive, has gastrointestinal hemorrhage, urinary pathology (obstruction to voiding urine and ruptured urinary bladder) or has AKI, then the administration of NSAIDs is not recommended. However, stable feline CKD patients can benefit from an NSAID (e.g., meloxicam or robenacoxib) for the treatment of inflammatory pain, if indicated. In dogs with CKD, NSAID use is currently not recommended. However, if an NSAID is required, then the lowest effective dose should be used initially and only in hydrated and euvolemic patients and titrated to effect with regular monitoring for adverse gastrointestinal or renal effects (see Further Reading). Drug protocols that can be considered in renal or urogenital diseased patients can be found in Table 19.1.

Table 19.1 Drugs commonly used in the immediate peri-anesthetic period in patients with renal or urinary disease.

Drug class	Drug	Dose (mg/kg)	Route	Comments
Premedication drugs				
ASA I–III				
Opioids	Butorphanol	0.1–0.4	IM, IV	Used for non- to minimally painful procedural sedation (i.e., radiographs and ultrasound). Only in patients that have not been given other opioids.
	Buprenorphine	0.015–0.03	IM, IV	Used in mild- to moderately painful dogs and in cats
	Methadone	0.2–0.3	IM, IV	Slow IV injection (over 2–3 min), used in moderate to severely painful patients
	Morphine	0.2–0.3	IM, IV	As for methadone
Alpha-2 adrenergic receptor agonists	Medetomidine	0.005–0.010	IM, IV	Cautioned use if there is an obstruction to urine outflow or cardiac disease. Contraindicated if hyperkalemia is present because a life-threatening bradycardia could occur.
	Dexmedetomidine	0.002–0.010	IM, IV	As for medetomidine
	Xylazine	N/A	N/A	More modern drugs in this class are preferred. Use only if other options are unavailable: 0.25 mg/kg (dogs) and 0.5 mg/kg (cats).
Phenothiazine derivatives	Acepromazine	0.01–0.03	IM, IV	Only used in normotensive and normovolemic patients
Benzodiazepines	Diazepam	0.2–0.3	IV only	Reserved for use as a co-induction drug
	Midazolam	0.2–0.3	IM, IV	Should be used in a drug combination to provide muscle relaxation

Table 19.1 (Continued)

Drug class	Drug	Dose (mg/kg)	Route	Comments
ASA IV and V				
Opioids	Butorphanol	0.1–0.2	IM, IV	As above
	Buprenorphine	0.02–0.03	IM, IV	As above
	Methadone	0.2–0.3	IM, IV	As above
	Morphine	0.2–0.3	IM, IV	As above
Alpha-2 adrenergic receptor agonists	Medetomidine	0.001–0.005	IV	Only to be used in noncompliant, fractious animals where the benefit of sedation outweighs the risk of cardiovascular compromise, self-inflicted trauma, distress, and injury to personnel. Contraindications are as described above.
	Dexmedetomidine	0.001–0.003	IV	As for medetomidine
	Xylazine	N/A	N/A	Not recommended
Induction drugs				
ASA I–III				
Benzodiazepines	Diazepam	0.2–0.3	IV only	Used as a co-induction drug with propofol or alfaxalone
	Midazolam	0.2–0.3	IM, IV	As for diazepam, with the advantage of IM administration route in fractious or noncompliant animals (in combination with alfaxalone or ketamine, and an opioid)
Phenol	Propofol	1–4	IV	Titrated in 1 mg/kg boluses every 15 s until tracheal intubation is possible. Heavily sedated or sick animals often do not require more than 2 mg/kg total dose to achieve tracheal intubation. High doses cause vasodilation, hypotension, hypoventilation, or apnea; these adverse effects are undesirable in this patient cohort.
Neurosteroids	Alfaxalone	0.5–2	IM, IV	As for propofol but to titrate in 0.5 mg/kg boluses IV over 15 s. Drug of choice for IM drug combinations (1–2 mg/kg, with midazolam and butorphanol [or other opioid]) in fractious or noncompliant patients. More reliable effects can be achieved with the addition of medetomidine (0.01 mg/kg)/dexmedetomidine (0.005 mg/kg) (adverse cardiovascular effects must be considered).
Cyclohexylamines	Ketamine	2–6	IM, IV	If alfaxalone and propofol are unavailable, then ketamine can be considered in fractious or noncompliant patients. However, recovery, especially in cats, can be prolonged. Cautioned used in obstructed cats, unless confident that obstruction will be relieved. IM drug combinations are similar to those used with alfaxalone.
ASA IV and V				
Benzodiazepines	Diazepam	0.2–0.3	IV only	Used as a co-induction drug usually with a full-*mu* opioid agonist
	Midazolam	0.2–0.3	IM, IV	As for diazepam
Opioids	Fentanyl	0.005–0.015 (i.e., 5–15 mcg/kg*)	IV	Used in critically ill or moribund dogs. Use in cats has been described but have an induction drug readily available in the rare event that excitement during induction occurs. Caution if hyperkalemia is present because a life-threatening bradycardia may occur. Other members of this group (sufentanil, alfentanil, and remifentanil) are suitable alternatives where available.
Phenol	Propofol	0.5–1	IV	As above, but titrated in 0.5 mg/kg boluses every 15 s until tracheal intubation is possible.
Neurosteroids	Alfaxalone	0.25–0.5	IV	As above but to titrate in 0.25 mg/kg boluses over 15 s.

(Continued)

Table 19.1 (Continued)

Drug class	Drug	Dose (mg/kg)	Route	Comments
Maintenance drugs (ASA I–V)				
Inhalational anesthetics	Isoflurane	1.0–1.3 × MAC	–	Preferred drug for maintaining anesthesia; however, hypotension and hypoventilation are common adverse effects. Therefore, providing good analgesia (i.e., local anesthetic blocks, opioids, etc.) helps reduce the MAC requirement (as well as providing analgesia).
	Sevoflurane	1.0–1.3 × MAC	–	As for isoflurane
Phenol	Propofol	0.1–0.5 mg/kg/min	IV	An infusion of propofol is preferred to administering intermittent boluses for maintaining anesthesia.
Neurosteroids	Alfaxalone	0.05–0.15 mg/kg/min	IV	As for propofol. Some animals appear "lightly anesthetized" despite being in an adequate surgical plane of anesthesia.
Ketamine	N/A	N/A	N/A	Contraindicated in this patient cohort
Analgesic drugs				
NSAIDs				
Oxicam derivative	Meloxicam	0.01–0.05 (cats)	SC, PO	As with all NSAIDs they must never be given to patients that have AKI, known sensitivity, gastrointestinal hemorrhage, or are hypotensive or hypovolemic. Low doses have been given once daily to cats with CKD with minimal adverse effects being reported. The listed dose is lower than labeled doses but are recommended for CKD cats (see Further Reading).
		0.05–0.1 (dogs)	SC, PO	Given once only. No guidelines have been established for dogs with CKD, and therefore caution is always advised and monitoring for gastrointestinal or renal adverse effects is recommended (see text for details). As above with regard to overriding warning of when never to use NSAIDs.
Coxib derivatives	Robenacoxib	1–2 (cats)	SC, PO	As for meloxicam. The dose is lower than labeled doses but are recommended for CKD cats.
Opioids				
Opioids	Butorphanol	0.1–0.3	IM, IV	Not a preferred analgesic drug, it has better sedative qualities.
	Buprenorphine	0.015–0.03	IM, IV	As above (see ASA I–III), but administered at 5–8 h intervals
	Methadone	0.2–0.3	IM, IV	As above (see ASA I–III), but administered at 4–5 h intervals
	Morphine	0.2–0.5	IM, IV	As above (see ASA I–III), but administered at 4–5 h intervals or as a constant rate infusion (0.05–0.1 mg/kg/h) in dogs. Some cats do not tolerate morphine (change in demeanor and anorexic) well and buprenorphine can be used instead.
	Hydromorphone	0.05–0.1 mg/kg	IM, IV	Administered at 4–6 h intervals or as CRI (0.02–0.04 mg/kg/h)
	Fentanyl	0.001–0.003 mg/kg/h (i.e., 1–3 mcg/kg/h) (cats)	IV	Recommended starting post-operative dose rates. The dose can be titrated upward to desired response. Very painful cats tolerate and respond well to a fentanyl infusion. If not tolerated (change in demeanor and anorexic), then buprenorphine can be given instead.
		0.003–0.005 mg/kg/h (i.e., 3–5 mcg/kg/h) (dogs)	IV	Well tolerated by dogs for the treatment of moderate-to-severe pain.
Others				
Drugs such as lidocaine (lignocaine) and ketamine infusions can be considered in very painful dogs. Usually given in conjunction with an opioid.				

Intravenous fluid administration during short periods (<30 min) of sedation is generally not required provided that arterial blood pressure is monitored and remains within an acceptable range, and the patient is classified as ASA I or II. However, if the patient has been given an intravenous contrast agent during a diagnostic imaging study then, to minimize the risk of contrast-induced AKI, a single bolus of an isotonic crystalloid (10 mL/kg over 60 min) has been anecdotally recommended to cause intravascular volume explanation. In stable normovolemic animals under anesthesia, a recommended 5 mL/kg/h for dogs and 3 mL/kg/h for cats of an isotonic crystalloid can be used. If urine output is monitored, then the rate of urine production can be added to the general recommended fluid rate. The administration of hydroxyethyl starch (HES) colloid solutions to patients with renal disease is generally not recommended. However, there is very limited evidence that AKI is caused by the tetrastarches (e.g., VetStarch, Voluven, and Venofundin) when used for volume expansion in animals. Blood products containing red blood cells (packed red blood cells or whole blood) can be used to increase the hematocrit before general anesthesia, if required.

Providing analgesia is important for anesthetic stability, patient well-being, and convalescence. See Table 19.1 for suggested analgesic drugs in these patients.

Physiologic monitoring during general anesthesia is essential, with a focus on regular measurements of systemic blood pressure and body temperature. Generally, if the patient maintains good cardiac output (hemodynamically stable) during anesthesia, then it is easier to maintain normothermia. Arterial blood pressure should be measured before premedication, before induction of anesthesia and at five-minute intervals (or less, in unstable patients) during anesthesia, and in the early recovery phase. Normotensive patients could be monitored using noninvasive blood pressure techniques (Doppler or oscillometric) that are practical, whereas hypertensive, hypotensive, or ASA IV or V patients should be stabilized first, if possible, and will benefit from invasive blood pressure measurement (see Chapter 16). Subjectively, renal perfusion and function can be assessed by measuring urine output though general anesthesia tends to greatly depress urine output even when arterial blood pressure is acceptable, rendering this approach insensitive and nonspecific. Capillary refill time and mucous membrane color serve a similar purpose in assessing perfusion of peripheral tissues but should not be used as substitute for arterial blood pressure monitoring. Efforts should be made to maintain normothermia, which usually requires active warming.

Approach to a Patient with Hepatobiliary Disease

Overview of Pathology

Patients with hepatobiliary disease often require anesthesia to collect diagnostic samples, correct underlying pathologies, or to provide means for enteral nutrition. Recognition of important hepatobiliary functions is essential for clinicians to help guide case management.

The liver plays a central role in numerous biological processes including metabolism of carbohydrates, lipids, proteins, and many hormones. Select vitamins and minerals, glycogen, blood, and triglycerides are stored in the liver.

The liver is also integrally involved in the detoxification and excretion of drugs and endogenous and exogenous toxins. The presence of hepatobiliary disease will therefore influence pharmacological choices. Additional peri-anesthetic considerations in patients with hepatobiliary disease can include the management of patients with hypoalbuminemia, the presence of ascites with some disorders (e.g., diseases resulting in portal hypertension and/or hypoalbuminemia, and bile peritonitis), predisposition to hypoglycemia, neurological symptoms, and bleeding tendencies due to the liver's central role in hemostasis.

There are a multitude of disorders that can affect the liver and can include infectious, metabolic, toxic, inflammatory, storage, neoplasia, and vascular anomalies. In this section, we review some key diagnostic principles and disorders. It is important to realize that the anesthetic and physiologic principles can be extrapolated to other patients requiring sedation and anesthesia with hepatobiliary diseases not covered here.

Liver Enzymes and Hepatic Injury

Due to the livers large reserve capacity, small animal patients often manifest clinical signs late in disease. Clinical signs of hepatic disease can also be vague or nonspecific such as decreased appetite and weight loss. In some cases, with more advanced disease, veterinarians may be able to identify clinical clues on their physical examinations directing them to consider disease of the hepatobiliary system. These clinical clues can include signs consistent with hepatic encephalopathy (HE) and examination findings such as icterus, microhepatica or hepatomegaly, or ascites.

Elevated liver enzymes can often be the first clue that a companion animal patient may have hepatic disease and can be considered sensitive indicators of liver disease or injury. However, it is essential that clinicians recognize that liver enzyme elevations are not specific to liver disease, are not indicators of liver function, sometimes arise secondary to extrahepatic disease, and the magnitude of increase does not indicate long-term prognosis. For example, some patients with dramatic changes in enzymes secondary to an acute insult can recover fully with timely recognition of their clinical condition and appropriate therapy. Another example is a patient with dramatic elevations of hepatic enzymes secondary to a mucocele causing extrahepatic biliary obstruction. These patients can have excellent long-term prognosis with appropriate diagnosis and therapy if they do not have concurrent intrinsic liver disease.

Disorders such as diabetes mellitus, congestive heart failure, and feline hyperthyroidism are common examples of diseases that do not have a primary hepatic etiology but can lead to elevated liver enzymes.

Enzymes are typically categorized as hepatocellular leakage or cholestatic enzymes. In some instances, critical evaluation of patterns of enzymatic changes may give clinical clues as to the underlying disease etiology.

Hepatocellular Leakage Enzymes

Alanine aminotransferase (ALT) and aspartate aminotransferase (AST) are hepatocellular enzymes released following damage to the hepatocyte membrane. The magnitude of increase is proportional to the number of hepatocytes affected with the most severe increases seen with hepatic inflammation and necrosis. However, the severity of elevation does not indicate decreased liver function or reflect irreversible injury. Additionally, declining values can occur with decreasing numbers of viable hepatocytes, for example in some cases of severe acute injury or end-stage chronic liver disease.

ALT and AST are not liver specific. ALT is present in highest concentrations in the liver with lower concentrations in the skeletal muscle. In addition to the liver, AST is found in skeletal muscle and red blood cells. Elevations in ALT are considered more specific to the liver than AST due to the lower concentrations of ALT in skeletal muscle when compared to AST. AST can be elevated in serum secondary to both hemolysis and skeletal muscle injury. Concurrent evaluation of AST and ALT together with creatinine kinase can help provide clues if elevations of these enzymes are secondary to hepatic or muscular sources.

Cholestatic Enzymes

Alkaline phosphatase (ALP) and gamma-glutamyl transferase (GGT) can both become elevated in diseases resulting in bile stasis. The mechanism for these increases is through increased synthesis and enhanced release from cell membranes. Of the hepatic enzymes, ALP has the lowest specificity for liver disease. Concurrent elevations in ALP and GGT will therefore increase the likelihood that ALP elevations are of hepatic etiology.

In dogs and cats there are two major isoforms of ALP: liver (L-ALP) and bone (B-ALP). The bone isoform may lead to mild increases in serum ALP most commonly in young growing animals. In dogs there is a third isoform: cortisol (C-ALP). C-ALP in this species can be induced by endogenous and exogenous steroids. ALP concentrations can also be induced resulting in increased serum concentrations with phenobarbital therapy. In cats, L-ALP is primarily responsible for serum concentrations. The absence of C-ALP, a shorter half-life, and less ALP in feline hepatic tissue make ALP increases more specific for hepatic disease in cats when compared to dogs.

Like ALP, GGT is also not exclusive to the liver; however, increased serum concentrations are most typically secondary to hepatobiliary disease. GGT may also be increased secondary to corticosteroid administration in dogs although to a lesser degree than what is seen in ALP concentrations.

Pathobiology of Decreased Liver Function

It is a common misconception that elevations in ALT, AST, ALP, and GGT indicate decreased liver function. These enzymatic changes are not indicators of function. There are other analytes on routine serum biochemistry profiling that can provide clues that decreased hepatic function is present. If decreased hepatic function is suspected, then specific hepatic function testing can be performed for confirmation if clinically indicated.

Routine Serum Biochemistry Profile of Decreased Liver Function

Glucose

Hypoglycemia can be an indicator of decreased liver function in patients with intrinsic liver disease and is estimated to occur with approximately 75% loss of function. Portosystemic shunts are another condition that often results in hypoglycemia on serum biochemical analysis. Hypoglycemia can arise in hepatobiliary disease due to the liver's central role in glucose homeostasis. This includes glycogen storage, gluconeogenesis, glycogenolysis, and insulin clearance.

Blood Urea Nitrogen

In healthy animals, ammonia from the splanchnic circulation is converted to BUN in the liver via the urea cycle. With significant reductions in liver function, or in cases of portosystemic shunts, there can be a decrease in

BUN production. Other etiologies of low BUN are noted in the preceding text, in the renal and urinary section.

Albumin

The liver is responsible for albumin synthesis. Hypoalbuminemia may be present when approximately 70% of liver function is lost and in cases of portosystemic shunt. The half-life of albumin in dogs (and likely in cats) is approximately eight days. Thus, hypoalbuminemia detected during acute liver injury might be because it is a negative acute phase protein in dogs and cats and not because of decreased production. However, in chronic hepatic failure, the hypoalbuminemia can be due to decreased production.

Hypoalbuminemia with hepatic disease is not typically as severe as with gastrointestinal or renal loss. In some forms of hepatic disease, ascites can occur (e.g., canine chronic hepatitis). While hypoalbuminemia may contribute to ascites in these patients, the pathophysiology of the ascites is most likely primarily due to the hepatic fibrosis and resultant portal hypertension.

Cholesterol

The liver is the primary site of cholesterol synthesis, excretion, and catabolism. In hepatobiliary disease, cholesterol concentrations can be increased, decreased, or normal. Hypocholesterolemia can be seen in end-stage liver disease where hepatic function is impaired and in portosystemic shunt patients because of the poorly developed liver and decreased functional hepatic mass. Hypercholesterolemia can develop in patients with cholestasis.

Bilirubin

Bilirubin is the major pigment in bile and is an end product of the metabolism of hemoproteins (hemoglobin, myoglobin, and cytochromes). Bilirubin is taken up by the liver where it then undergoes conjugation to a more soluble and less toxic form and is subsequently secreted in bile.

Hyperbilirubinemia results from disruption of the production and/or processing of bilirubin. Accumulation of bilirubin in tissues can cause visible icterus. Increased bilirubin and icterus are often categorized as pre-hepatic, hepatic, or post-hepatic in etiology (Figure 19.3).

Pre-hepatic hyperbilirubinemia occurs due to pathologically increased release of bilirubin as a consequence of hemolysis. With hemolysis, excess bilirubin overwhelms the liver's capacity to take up bilirubin, conjugate, and secrete it. Patients with a pre-hepatic etiology are not only icteric on physical examination, but astute veterinarians are also likely to appreciate pallor of the mucous membranes. Documenting an anemia with a complete blood count and/or hematocrit together with some characteristic red cell morphologic changes can provide support that the hyperbilirubinemia is pre-hepatic in origin.

Hepatic hyperbilirubinemia etiologies can occur secondary to decreased uptake, conjugation or secretion of bilirubin, and can occur as a consequence of severe, diffuse hepatic disease and thus often used as a marker of decreased liver function. Disorders resulting in disruption and disorganization of the hepatic parenchyma can also contribute to hepatic icterus due to physical disruption of intrahepatic bile flow. Cholestasis associated with sepsis can result in hyperbilirubinemia of hepatic etiology due to cytokine disruption of bilirubin transport pathways.

Post-hepatic hyperbilirubinemia etiologies arise secondary to disruption of bile outflow through the extrahepatic biliary system. Diagnostic imaging (e.g., ultrasound and computer tomography) is typically required to differentiate between hepatic and post-hepatic etiologies. Biochemically, these cases may have a disproportionate increase in cholestatic enzymes (ALP and GGT) and bilirubin when compared to hepatocellular enzymatic (AST and ALT) changes. In these cases, in the absence of concurrent intrinsic liver disease affecting liver function, elevated bilirubin and enzymatic changes commonly resolve if the obstruction can be corrected. Of note are the

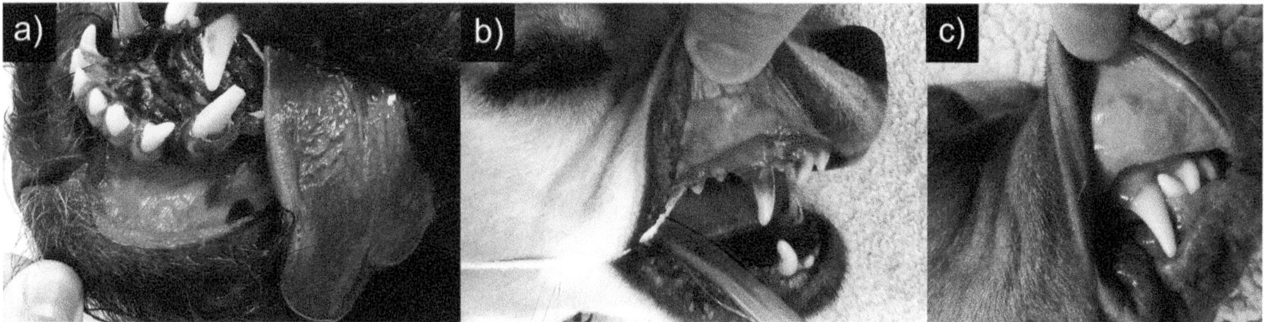

Figure 19.3 The mucous membrane color of a healthy dog (a) that is pink; (b) a dog with mild icterus, note the yellow color tinge to the pink mucous membranes; and (c) a dog with severe icterus (intravascular erythrolysis caused by Babesiosis).

differences between cats and dogs when bilirubin is evaluated on routine urinalysis. The renal tubular cells in dogs are capable of conjugating bilirubin during hemoglobin metabolism (males > females) and the renal tubules have a low threshold for reabsorption, meaning normal dogs may have small amounts of bilirubin in their urine in the absence of hyperbilirubinemia. Cats have a higher threshold for reabsorption, and the presence of bilirubinuria in a cat is significant and indicates that a hyperbilirubinemia will be present.

Testing Hemostasis

The liver plays a key role in hemostatic functions. Coagulopathies may arise in patients with hepatic disease due to decreased synthesis of coagulation factors and impaired activation of vitamin K–dependent factors. Impaired absorption of the fat-soluble vitamin K in cholestatic disorders could also contribute to impaired coagulation. Thrombocytopenia can occur in cases of hepatic disease or acute injury. Etiologies include disseminated intravascular coagulation (DIC), decreased production of thrombopoietin, activation of the endothelium, and primary hemostasis with hepatic injury. Spontaneous bleeding is uncommon in patients with hepatic disease. However, many patients will undergo therapeutic and diagnostic procedures, which may cause insidious, ongoing bleeding (e.g., liver biopsy). Patients with hepatic disease should have their platelet count evaluated and coagulation assessed through screening tests such as prothrombin time (PT) and activated partial thromboplastin time (aPTT) before interventional procedures so that appropriate precautions can be taken to avoid uncontrolled bleeding. Other tests to assess the coagulation system include viscoelastic analysis (thromboelastogram "TEG" or rotational thromboelastometry "ROTEM"). However, to gain the most information from these analyses, strict guidelines are to be followed from sample collection, transfer to the laboratory, and analytical procedures (see Further Reading), thus limiting viscoelastic analysis to major referral centers or academic hospitals with on-site clinical pathology laboratories.

Liver Function Testing

Beyond measuring the analytes that can be associated with decreased liver function, two additional tests can be performed that specifically focus on evaluating liver function: measurements of bile acids (BAs) and ammonia.

Bile Acids

Bile acids are synthesized in the liver from cholesterol and are stored in the gallbladder. The major functions of bile acids include cholesterol homeostasis, stimulation of bile flow, and absorption of fats and fat-soluble vitamins from the gastrointestinal tract. Shortly after a meal, the gallbladder contracts, releasing its contents into the duodenum. BAs undergo efficient enterohepatic recirculation with 95% being reabsorbed from the gastrointestinal tract and transported back to the liver via the portal vein. This efficient reuptake can be disrupted with decreased liver function and portosystemic shunts, leading to elevations in serum bile acid concentrations.

BAs are of limited value as an initial screening test for liver disease but are used to evaluate liver function and for the presence of portosystemic shunts. BAs will typically be elevated in both instances. The BAs test evaluates pre- and post-prandial serum concentrations (prandial means to eat food). Briefly, following a 12 hour withholding of food period, the pre-prandial blood sample is taken. This is followed by a small challenge meal, used to stimulate gallbladder contraction, releasing its contents into the gastrointestinal tract. In the healthy animal, BAs are taken up efficiently by the portal vein and taken back up by the liver. The post-prandial sample (taken two hours after a challenge meal) evaluates the efficiency of this reuptake. Clinicians should not evaluate BAs in patients that are suspected of having hepatic or post-hepatic etiologies of hyperbilirubinemia. The physiology of bile flow should make it intuitive that BAs would be increased and provides no additional clinical information.

Ammonia

Ammonia is primarily derived from colonic bacteria through digestion of dietary protein, gastrointestinal mucosal metabolism, and hemorrhage. It is subsequently transported to the liver through the portal vein and is converted to urea via the urea cycle. Ammonia concentrations are most commonly elevated in patients with decreased function and portosystemic shunts. However, despite being a test of liver function, ammonia concentration is infrequently assessed in general practice due to its labile nature and is therefore a less accessible test in facilities without an on-site machine to complete the analysis of ammonia expediently. By contrast, bile acid measurement is accessible to veterinarians and as such is the most used function test.

Selected Hepatobiliary Disorders

A summary of selected hepatobiliary disorders that can be diagnosed in cats and dogs is presented in Table 19.2. The selected hepatic disorders are those that are commonly seen in general practice.

Feline Hepatic Lipidosis

Hepatic lipidosis (HL) is a common hepatobiliary disease of cats. It can occur in cats of any age or sex, but there is

Table 19.2 A summary of selected hepatobiliary disorders in cats and dogs.

Disorder	Clinical and clinicopathologic signs	Management Considerations
Feline hepatic lipidosis	• GGT commonly normal or mildly increased despite moderate to marked increases in other cholestatic and hepatocellular enzymes (in the absence of concurrent hepatic condition) • Period of anorexia typically proceeds presentation • Hyperechoic liver on ultrasound	• Feline hepatic lipidosis is often a secondary disorder; therefore evaluate for underlying disease whenever possible • Electrolyte monitoring is essential as significant hypokalemia, and hypophosphatemia can develop with institution of nutritional support
Feline neutrophilic cholangitis	• May have fever and/or inflammatory leukogram • May have evidence of concurrent inflammatory bowel disease or pancreatitis (triaditis)	• If taking hepatic biopsies for histopathology-hepatic and bile culture, intestinal and pancreatic biopsies should also be considered • Consider feeding tube placement to support patients nutritionally to prevent hepatic lipidosis
Feline lymphocytic cholangitis	• Some patients may have hyperglobulinemia and/or abdominal effusion (ddx FIP) • May have evidence of concurrent inflammatory bowel disease or pancreatitis (triaditis)	• If taking hepatic biopsies for histopathology-hepatic and bile culture, intestinal and pancreatic biopsies should also be considered • Consider feeding tube placement to support patients nutritionally to prevent hepatic lipidosis
Portosystemic shunts	• Young patients developing neurological signs • Young patients presenting with lower urinary tract obstructions with radiolucent to semi-opaque calculi • Low BUN, albumin, and glucose may be present on serum biochemistry • Microcytosis may be present on CBC • Often dramatic elevations in pre- and post-prandial bile acids	• Management of HE before surgical correction • Consider pre- and peri-operative anti-epileptic medications
Canine portal vein hypoplasia	• Bile acids unlikely to be as high as seen in patients with PSS	• Rule out concurrent PSS • No corrective surgery or therapy, and management is supportive • Diagnosis requires biopsy and exclusion of congenital macroscopic vascular shunt
Canine chronic hepatitis	• Persistent elevations in ALT/AST can be early clues of underlying hepatitis	• The presence of acquired shunts and/or ascites typically indicates severe disease • Biopsies should be taken from multiple lobes for histopathology and copper quantification, and culture of hepatic tissue

Note: All cases of hepatic disease should have coagulation testing and appropriate treatment of existing clinically significant findings as part of their management prior to any surgical procedure.
ALT: alanine transaminase; AST: aspartate transaminase; BUN: blood urea nitrogen; ddx: differential diagnoses; GGT: gamma-glutamyl transferase; HE: hepatic encephalopathy; PSS: portosystemic shunt.

predisposition with increasing body weight. The disease is triggered when there is insufficient caloric consumption leading to release of fatty acids from peripheral adipose stores that exceed the liver's capacity for fat utilization and dispersal. The net result is lipid accumulation in the liver, liver dysfunction, and potential liver failure due to lipid accumulation overtaking the functional tissues of the liver.

Hepatic lipidosis may be primary (idiopathic) in which no underlying disease is recognized. This can occur during periods of forced rapid weight loss, unintentional food deprivation (e.g., change to an unacceptable food to the cat), or sudden change in lifestyle causing stress leading to inappetence. Hepatic lipidosis can also be secondary to concurrent disease such as pancreatitis or neoplasia. Underlying disease can act as the stimulus for anorexia, and therefore evaluation for underlying disease should be offered to owners as part of the diagnostic workup and to ensure appropriate management.

An abdominal ultrasound is recommended to rule out concurrent disease whenever possible as treatment is intensive and expensive and may not be pursued if significant underlying disease is identified early. Thoracic radiographs could also be considered to evaluate for concurrent disease. Ultrasound typically reveals an enlarged hyperechoic liver. It must be remembered that other disease processes can result in a similar appearance to the liver.

Diagnosis requires biopsy; however, this is not frequently performed if the clinical signs, physical examination, biochemical findings, and ultrasound are consistent with diagnosis. Biopsy carries significant risk in these patients as the liver is friable and patients are typically coagulopathic. An alternative to biopsy, with reduced risk of complications that is commonly performed, is fine needle aspirates to provide further support of the diagnosis.

Therapy is focused upon providing adequate nutrition so that lipid can be mobilized from the liver. This therapy is additional to suggested medical management of these patients (see Further Reading). These patients will commonly receive nutrition through nasoesophageal feeding tubes initially; however, once stabilized, they will require anesthesia so that a more permanent method of feeding can be instituted.

Feline Inflammatory Liver Diseases

In contrast to dogs, who commonly develop hepatitis, cats typically develop inflammatory disease affecting their biliary system and are grouped together as the cholangitis complex. Only the neutrophilic and lymphocytic forms are discussed here. Cholangitis can also occur secondary to liver flukes (e.g., *Opisthorchis felineus and Platynosomum fastosum*) in cats.

Neutrophilic Cholangitis

This disorder may result from translocation of bacteria through the biliary tree from the intestine. Enteric species such as *Escherichia coli*, *Enterococcus* sp., *Clostridium* sp., and *Salmonella* sp. are the most common organisms cultured from the bile and/or hepatic tissue.

Ultrasound is not diagnostic to determine the underlying etiology of disease; however, in some cases the liver can appear hyperechoic or heterogenous. There will commonly be changes observed with the gallbladder, which can include distention with the presence of echogenic material and wall thickening. The common bile duct often appears prominent. Changes consistent with pancreatitis and inflammatory bowel disease may be noted in some patients in a condition referred to as "triaditis."

Definitive diagnosis requires biopsy of the liver. Pancreatic and small intestinal biopsies are often pursued concurrently. Hepatic samples are taken for both culture and histopathology. Bile is cultured and cytology can be performed to evaluate for the presence of neutrophilic inflammation and bacteria to help support a diagnosis. At the time of surgery, the biliary system should be assessed to ensure patency. In such patients, esophageal or gastric feeding tubes are often placed to decrease the risk of developing HL (secondary to inappetence associated with systemic illness). Appropriate precautions should be taken beforehand to evaluate for and mitigate coagulopathies.

Histopathology reveals neutrophilic inflammation within the bile duct lumen, closely associated with the bile duct or between the biliary epithelial cells. With more chronic disease, there may be a mixed inflammation, fibrosis, and bile duct proliferation. If inflammation extends beyond the limiting plate and into the hepatic parenchyma, the diagnosis is termed "cholangiohepatitis."

Therapy centers on appropriate antimicrobial therapy based on culture and sensitivity testing. While awaiting results, antimicrobials that are secreted in the bile in the active form and target enteric aerobic and anaerobic bacteria are selected. A commonly used drug is amoxicillin with clavulanic acid. Cats should be provided appropriate analgesia as many are reportedly painful, which could reflect concurrent pancreatic pathology.

Lymphocytic Cholangitis

It is suspected that the lymphocytic form of cholangitis is immune in etiology. Some propose that this could be a more chronic form of neutrophilic cholangitis. Concurrent intestinal and pancreatic pathology occurs but less commonly than in cases of neutrophilic cholangitis.

Ultrasonographic findings are similar to cases of neutrophilic disease. Biopsies are required for definitive diagnosis, and sampling should be performed as suggested under the neutrophilic form of disease. Histopathology reveals a predominance of small lymphocytes in the bile duct lumen. Treatment with a corticosteroid (e.g., prednisolone) is instituted following attaining histopathology results and negative culture.

Vascular Liver Disease

The portal vein transports blood from the spleen, pancreas, and the gastrointestinal tract to the liver. The capillary system of the liver is where the smallest branches of the portal vein and the hepatic artery meet (hepatic sinusoids). The hepatic vein collects filtered blood from the hepatic sinusoids entering the caudal *vena cava* to return to the heart.

Congenital portosystemic shunts and portal vein hypoplasia (PVH; also termed "microvascular dysplasia") are vascular disorders the general practitioner will be presented with. Both result in a proportion of blood shunting directly from the portal to the systemic circulation.

Portosystemic Shunts

Portosystemic shunts can be classified as extrahepatic or intrahepatic, single or multiple, and congenital or acquired. Congenital disease will be focused on here.

Congenital PSS are more commonly encountered in dogs compared to cats. In both species, congenital PSS are most commonly extrahepatic. In dogs, extrahepatic PSS are most common in small breeds with predispositions in Miniature Schnauzers, Yorkshire Terriers, Maltese, Havanese, and Pugs. Intrahepatic PSS are more frequently seen in large-breed dogs, with Irish Wolfhounds, Labrador, and Golden Retrievers, Australian Cattle Dogs and Australian Shepherds having increased risk.

Acquired PSS are commonly seen in canine chronic hepatitis when fibrosis and cirrhosis develop resulting in portal hypertension or can be seen in other less common diseases resulting in portal hypertension. In these cases, increased hydrostatic pressure within the liver results in opening of fetal, vestigial blood vessels that provide an alternative route to transport blood from the splanchnic circulation. Unlike congenital PSS, these cannot be corrected surgically and are signs of end-stage liver disease.

With PSS, intestinal absorption of products that include endogenous and exogenous toxins, some of which lead to encephalopathy, is carried directly to the systemic circulation and can have detrimental effects. When blood bypasses the liver, trophic factors are not available to support hepatic growth resulting in poor hepatic development and resultant dysfunction. Consequently, the liver is unable to perform many of its metabolic functions. Some of these toxins result in hepatic encephalopathy that is a group of neuro-behavioral signs that most typically develop with a marked reduction in hepatic tissue mass with chronic disease, PSS, or acute fulminant hepatic necrosis. Ammonia is one of the most widely accepted toxins that cause HE, and most medical interventions in veterinary medicine are chosen to reduce ammonia production. Symptoms of hepatic encephalopathy can wax and wane and vary in severity. Most commonly, signs include lethargy, decreased alertness, ataxia, intermittent blindness, pacing, and head pressing. Signs of HE may appear within hours after ingesting a meal because of an increase in ammoniagenesis via urease producing bacteria in the colon. Seizures are uncommon.

Abdominal radiographs are commonly performed in small animal patients presenting to clinicians with a complaint of stranguria. Ammonium biurate calculi that can occur in some patients with PSS are radiolucent to semi-radio opaque. Microhepatica may also be noted and would help support the diagnosis (Figure 19.4).

Ultrasonography is often used for definitive diagnosis and requires documentation of the anomalous vessel(s). Other changes identified can include bladder calculi, renomegaly, and microhepatica. Ultrasound exam typically requires heavy sedation. Computer tomography scans using contrast are increasingly used and preferred by most radiologists as they have increased sensitivity for documenting the anomalous vessel(s).

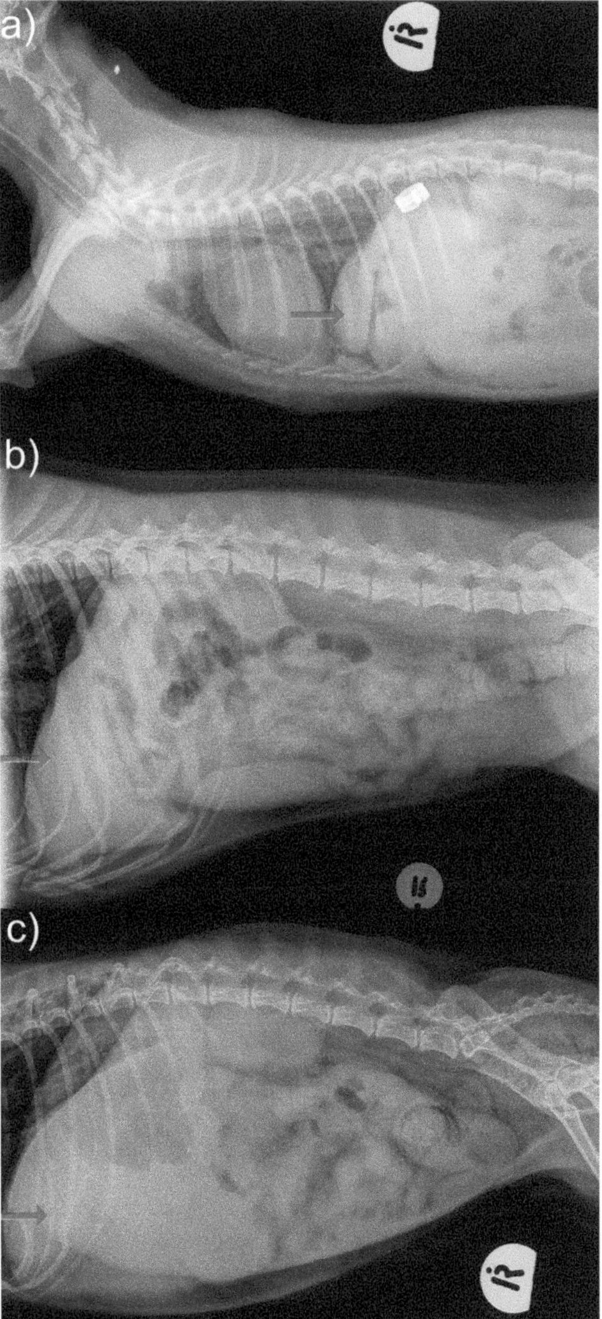

Figure 19.4 Right abdominal radiographs to show dogs with (a) microhepatica, (b) normal sized liver (within the costal arch), and (c) hepatomegaly. The blue arrows point to the liver in the radiographs.

In patients with HE, medical management is instituted pre-operatively to stabilize these patients, if residual shunting is present post-operatively and HE persists, or in cases where surgery is not feasible. Commonly used therapies for HE largely center around decreasing ammonia production. Lactulose, a nonabsorbable disaccharide, is used to acidify colonic contents decreasing ammonia absorption, may alter the bacterial population (decreases the population of urease producing bacteria), and enhances frequency of defecation (decreasing gastrointestinal contents exposure to bacteria and time for proliferation). Lactulose is usually given orally but in severely affected (stuporous to comatosed) patients, and it can be given per rectum. Cleansing enemas can be given to patients with severe manifestations to reduce nitrogenous waste and may also decrease bacterial content. Antibiotics are often used with the rational of altering the bacterial flora and decreasing ammonia production. Protein intake should be reduced from what patients are currently being fed and presented in a highly digestible form.

Definitive therapy for congenital PSS is closure of the anomalous vessel. These surgeries require referral; however, the general practitioner must be able to recognize this disease process, facilitate preliminary diagnostics, and be able to medically stabilize these patients until definitive therapy can occur.

Vascular occlusion encourages portal perfusion; however, the development of portal hypertension is a potential complication. If excessive portal hypertension occurs acutely, then these patients can develop ascites, intestinal congestion, diarrhea, hypoxia, and cell death in the gastrointestinal tract, resulting in a grave prognosis. If portal hypertension develops, secondary multiple acquired PSS may develop which are not amenable to surgical correction.

Following vascular closure, post-operative seizures unrelated to glucose levels, closure technique, or HE have been reported. This seems to be more common in cats. Prognosis is poor in animals with post-operative seizures. Seizure therapy can include phenobarbital, levetiracetam, or a constant rate infusion of propofol if status epilepticus cannot be controlled with traditional anti-seizure therapy. More recently, clinicians have been treating patients with levetiracetam (because it does not require liver metabolism) before surgery to decrease the incidence of post-operative seizures.

Portal Vein Hypoplasia

Portal vein hypoplasia is a congenital microscopic anomaly of the portal veins within the liver itself, resulting in abnormal communications between the portal and systemic system circulation. PVH can occur in isolation or with concurrent PSS. Breeds predisposed to PSS are also predisposed to PVH.

Serum biochemistry may demonstrate mild elevations in liver enzymes. Although BAs are commonly elevated unless a concurrent macroscopic shunt is present, they are typically less severe than seen with PSS. Biopsy is required for diagnosis. For symptomatic cases, one should treat as per PSS to control HE if present because no surgical treatment is available.

Canine Chronic Hepatitis

Hepatitis refers to the inflammation of the hepatic parenchyma. Chronic hepatitis is uncommon in cats but is a common diagnosis in canine patients. Various etiologies are responsible, including immune, copper storage, drugs, toxic insults, and infectious agents. Etiologic agents can initiate changes resulting in chronic hepatitis; however, the initial insult is often undetermined due to the late onset of clinical signs and diagnosis so that the disease is often termed "idiopathic."

Any breed can be affected by chronic hepatitis. Certain breeds have a strong association with hepatic copper accumulation, a common etiology of chronic hepatitis. These include Bedlington Terriers, West Highland White Terriers, and Labrador Retrievers.

Long-standing inflammation can result in hepatic fibrosis and cirrhosis which is irreversible. With fibrosis and cirrhosis, patients can develop acquired PSS due to portal hypertension. These patients may also develop ascites secondary to portal hypertension with possible contributions from hypoalbuminemia if present. This will indicate advanced disease.

Definitive diagnosis and important prognostic information (degree of fibrosis) are achieved with biopsy. Evaluation for the presence of coagulopathy should be performed beforehand. When performing hepatic tissue sampling in dogs, samples should be submitted for culture (bile and liver), histopathology (liver), and copper quantification (liver). Copper is the most frequently identified underlying cause of hepatitis in some parts of the world.

Early identification and treatment of this disease is key. Often early clues will be an increase in hepatocellular enzymes ALT and/or AST. If persistent, even if mild and especially in predisposed breeds for hepatitis or copper storage disease, biopsies should be considered.

Anesthetic Management of Patients with Hepatobiliary Disease

Major Considerations for Sedation or Anesthesia

- Pain is often experienced with these conditions and analgesia should be provided.
- Raised liver enzymes do not necessarily indicate the liver's ability to metabolize drugs used for sedation or general anesthesia is compromised, but it is wise to use drugs that have multiple routes of metabolism (not exclusively hepatic metabolism).
- Hypoglycemia can occur with decreased liver function, young animals, and those with PSS, and should be measured and corrected before general anesthesia, with monitoring continuing intra- and post-operatively.
- Coagulopathies are common in patients with liver disease, and thus the assessment of hemostasis is prudent.
- Surgery on the liver, especially when inflamed, can result in rapid and severe hemorrhage
- Decreased liver function can result in difficulty managing peri-operative normothermia because metabolism within the liver is a major contributor to maintaining core body temperature.
- General anesthesia can result in a temporary worsening of hepatic encephalopathy during recovery (typically for several hours).
- Gastrointestinal hemorrhage can worsen after sedation or general anesthesia.
- Nausea and vomiting should be treated.
- In all cases, it is wise to prepare all necessary material before beginning sedation/anesthesia in order to keep the anesthetic time as short as possible.

Sedation or Peri-anesthetic Management

Patients that require sedation or general anesthesia to perform procedures such as placement of a nasogastric tube or esophagostomy tube for feeding are not always fully stabilized. This is because the placement of these tubes may be part of the patient treatment plan. However, at minimum, intravascular volume, systemic arterial blood pressure, and glucose should be stabilized before any sedation or anesthetic event. If surgery is required, especially within a body cavity, then the assessment of hemostasis should be performed (thrombocyte count, hematocrit, PT, and aPTT), and plasma (or fresh whole blood if thrombocytopenia and/or anemia is present) should be given before surgery. Stratifying the patient into one of the ASA categories (see Chapter 2) will assist in drug and monitoring selection.

Most drugs that are used for sedation and general anesthesia undergo hepatic metabolism. If hepatic function is adequate, then it can be assumed that metabolism of these drugs should be minimally affected. Using drugs that have additional sites of metabolism are preferred to promote a rapid recovery from drug effect. Furthermore, drugs that have antagonists are useful to include because if an emergency event arises, their effects can be rapidly reversed. Generally, drugs with minimal cardiovascular depressive effects are preferred choices to include in the anesthetic plan in an effort to support arterial blood pressure and hepatic perfusion. Drug protocols that can be considered in patients with hepatobiliary disease can be found in Table 19.3.

Intravascular isotonic fluid in normovolemic patients is administered at 3 mL/kg/h (cats) to 5 mL/kg/h (dogs). Patients that are hypoglycemic may require the addition of dextrose to the isotonic fluid to make a 5% dextrose solution (e.g., 100 mL of 50% dextrose to 1 L isotonic fluid bag infused at intra-operative rates). Blood glucose should be monitored at induction, midway through the anesthetic, and in recovery in stable patients and more frequently (every 30 min) in unstable patients. Fresh whole blood should be available in the event of acute hemorrhage that is difficult to control, but stored whole blood is acceptable in an emergency. However, administering stored whole blood to a patient with HE might worsen their state because of an increased concentration of ammonia. If there are no coagulation concerns, then administering packed red blood cells is a preferred treatment in these cases. Hemorrhage can be difficult to quantify, especially if it is insidious (e.g., continuous oozing during a surgical procedure). Quantifying hemorrhage is useful as blood loss >15 mL/kg requires some form of intervention (isotonic crystalloids or synthetic colloids or blood products) and >30 mL/kg often requires a fresh whole blood transfusion. Fluid administration can be titrated to ongoing losses and as an initial treatment for hypotension.

Providing analgesia is important for anesthetic stability, patient well-being, and convalescence. See Table 19.3 for

Table 19.3 Drugs commonly used in the immediate peri-anesthetic period in patients with hepatobiliary disease.

Drug class	Drug	Dose (mg/kg)	Route	Comments
Premedication drugs				
ASA I–III				
Opioids	Butorphanol	0.1–0.4	IM, IV	Used for nonpainful or minimally painful procedural sedation (i.e., radiographs, ultrasound, and fine needle aspirates). Only in patients that have not been given other opioids.
	Buprenorphine	0.015–0.03	IM, IV	Used in mildly to moderately painful dogs and in cats
	Methadone	0.2–0.3	IM, IV	Slow IV injection (over 2–3 min), used in moderately to severely painful patients
	Morphine	0.2–0.5	IM, IV	As for methadone, but it has been the prototypical opioid that is cautioned in dogs that have a sphincter of Oddi, and it is best to time its administration 2 h before or after a meal.
	Hydromorphone	0.05–0.1 mg/kg	IM, IV	Used in moderately to severely painful patients
Alpha-2 adrenergic receptor agonists	Medetomidine	0.005–0.010	IM, IV	Contraindicated if hyperkalemia is present because a life-threatening bradycardia could occur.
	Dexmedetomidine	0.002–0.007	IM, IV	As for medetomidine
	Xylazine	N/A	N/A	Use is mostly contraindicated, but if it is the only sedative available, use at 0.25 mg/kg (dogs) and 0.5 mg/kg (cats)
Phenothiazine derivatives	Acepromazine	0.01–0.03	IM, IV	Only used in normotensive and normovolemic patients
Benzodiazepines	Diazepam	0.2–0.3	IV only	Benzodiazepines, especially diazepam, are generally not recommended in animals with decreased liver function because it can have a prolonged duration of effect. Controversial in dogs with hepatic encephalopathy.
	Midazolam	0.2–0.3	IM, IV	Can be used in a drug combination to provide muscle relaxation.
ASA IV and V				
Opioids	Butorphanol	0.1–0.4	IM, IV	As above
	Buprenorphine	0.015–0.03	IM, IV	As above
	Methadone	0.2–0.3	IM, IV	As above
	Hydromorphone	0.05–0.1	IM, IV	As above
	Morphine	0.2–0.3	IM, IV	As above
Alpha-2 adrenergic receptor agonists	Medetomidine	0.001–0.005	IM, IV	Only to be used in noncompliant, fractious animals where the benefit of sedation outweighs the risk of cardiovascular compromise, self-inflicted trauma, distress, and injury to personnel. Contraindications are as described above.
	Dexmedetomidine	0.001–0.003	IM, IV	As for medetomidine
	Xylazine	N/A	N/A	Not recommended
Induction drugs				
ASA I–III				
Benzodiazepines	Diazepam	0.2–0.3	IV only	Used as a co-induction drug with propofol or alfaxalone, but generally this class of drug should be avoided if there is any indication of decreased liver function.
	Midazolam	0.2–0.3	IM, IV	As for diazepam. In fractious or noncompliant animals, it is used in IM drug combination with alfaxalone or ketamine, and an opioid.

Table 19.3 (Continued)

Drug class	Drug	Dose (mg/kg)	Route	Comments
Phenol	Propofol	1–4	IV	Titrated in 1 mg/kg boluses every 15 s until tracheal intubation is possible. Heavily sedated animals often do not require more than 2 mg/kg total dose to achieve tracheal intubation. High doses cause vasodilation, hypotension, hypoventilation, or apnea; all adverse effects are undesirable in this patient cohort.
Neurosteroids	Alfaxalone	0.5–2	IM, IV	As for propofol but to titrate in 0.5 mg/kg boluses over 15 s. Drug of choice for IM drug combinations (1–2 mg/kg, with midazolam and butorphanol [or other opioid]) in fractious or noncompliant patients. Deeper sedation can be achieved, if needed, with the addition of medetomidine (0.01 mg/kg)/demedetomidine (0.005 mg/kg). Consider cardiovascular adverse effects of medetomidine/dexmedetomidine.
Cyclohexylamines	Ketamine	2–6	IM, IV	If alfaxalone/propofol are not available, then ketamine can be considered in fractious or noncompliant patients. However, recovery can be prolonged if hepatic function is decreased. IM drug combinations are similar to those used with alfaxalone.
ASA IV and V				
Benzodiazepines	Diazepam	0.2–0.3	IV only	Used as a co-induction drug, usually with a full-*mu* opioid agonist if midazolam is not available and if hepatic function is not decreased.
	Midazolam	0.2–0.3	IM, IV	As for diazepam
Opioids	Fentanyl	0.005–0.015 (i.e., 5–15 mcg/kg[a])	IV	Used in critically ill or moribund dogs (administered with a benzodiazepine). Use in cats has been described but have an induction drug readily available in the rare event that excitement during induction occurs. Caution if hyperkalemia is present because a life-threatening bradycardia could occur. Other members of this group (sufentanil, alfentanil, and remifentanil) are suitable alternatives where available.
Phenol	Propofol	0.5–1	IV	As above, but titrated in 0.5 mg/kg boluses every 15 s until tracheal intubation is possible.
Neurosteroids	Alfaxalone	0.25–0.5	IV	As above but to titrate in 0.25 mg/kg boluses over 15 s.
Maintenance drugs (ASA I–V)				
Inhalational anesthetics	Isoflurane	1.0–1.3 × MAC	–	Preferred drug for maintaining anesthesia; however, hypotension and hypoventilation are common side effects. Therefore, providing good analgesia (i.e., local anesthetic blocks, opioids etc.) often decreases the MAC requirement.
	Sevoflurane	1.0–1.3 × MAC	–	As for isoflurane
Phenol	Propofol	0.1–0.5 mg/kg/min	IV	An infusion of propofol is preferred to administering intermittent boluses for maintaining anesthesia.
Neurosteroids	Alfaxalone	0.05–0.15 mg/kg/min	IV	As for propofol. However, infusions in patients with decreased liver function have not been investigated yet.
Ketamine	N/A	N/A	N/A	Contraindicated in this patient cohort.
Analgesic drugs				
NSAIDs				
Oxicam derivative	Meloxicam	0.01–0.05 (cats)	SC, PO	As with all NSAIDs, they must never be given to patients that are in shock, hypotensive, hypovolemic, have known sensitivity, or gastrointestinal hemorrhage. Conservative doses are proposed for cast with decreased liver function but see labeled dose for country of practice.

(Continued)

Table 19.3 (Continued)

Drug class	Drug	Dose (mg/kg)	Route	Comments
		0.05–0.1 (dogs)	SC, PO	Given once daily. No guidelines have been established for dogs with decreased liver function. Therefore, monitoring for adverse effects is recommended. As above with regard to overriding warning of when never to use NSAIDs. Conservative doses are proposed but see labeled dose for country of practice.
Coxib derivatives	Robenacoxib	1–2 (cats)	SC, PO	As for meloxicam. Conservative doses are proposed but see labeled dose for country of practice.
Propionic acids	Carprofen	4.4 (dogs)	SC/ PO	Generally, not recommended in dogs with anorexia and decreased liver function.
Opioids				
Opioids	Butorphanol	0.2–0.4	IM, IV	Not a preferred analgesic drug, and it has better sedative qualities.
	Buprenorphine	0.015–0.03	IM, IV	As above, for ASA I–III but administered at 5–8 h intervals
	Methadone	0.2–0.3	IM, IV	As above, for ASA I–III but administered at 4–5 h intervals
	Hydromorphone	0.05–0.1	IM, IV	Administered at 4–6 h intervals or as CRI (0.02–0.04 mg/kg/h)
	Morphine	0.2–0.5	IM, IV	As above, for ASA I–III but administered at 4–5 h intervals or as a constant rate infusion (0.05–0.1 mg/kg/h) in dogs. Some cats do not tolerate morphine well (change in demeanor and anorexic), and buprenorphine can be used instead. Historically, use is cautioned in dogs as they have a sphincter of Oddi (morphine may cause sphincter contraction and pain). Recommended administration 2 h before or after a meal.
	Fentanyl	0.001–0.003 mg/kg/h (i.e., 1–3 mcg/kg/h) (cats)	IV	Very painful cats tolerate and respond well to a fentanyl infusion. If not tolerated (change in demeanor and anorexic), then buprenorphine can be given instead.
		0.003–0.005 mg/kg/h (i.e., 3–5 mcg/kg/h) (dogs)	IV	Well tolerated by dogs for the treatment of moderate-to-severe pain.
Others				
Drugs such as lidocaine (lignocaine) and ketamine infusions can be considered in very painful dogs. Usually given in conjunction with an opioid.				

suggested analgesics drugs in these patients. Physiologic monitoring during general anesthesia is essential and similar to the recommendation made for patients with renal or urogenital diseases (see the preceding text).

Questions and Answers

There are more practice questions and answers available for this chapter on the website. Please visit http://www.wiley.com/go/VeterinaryAnesthesiaZeiler.

Questions

Renal and Urinary Disease Questions

1) In patients with reduced muscle mass why can SDMA assist with the assessment of renal health?
2) In what form of renal disease are patients at increased risk of developing a severe hypoalbuminemia? What are some complications of severe hypoalbuminemia (i.e., <16 g/L) and why can these be important to recognize in the anesthetized patient?

3) What parameters are used to assess stage and substage chronic kidney disease in dogs and cats with the IRIS staging system? Why is staging important?

Hepatobiliary Questions

1) How can the following be used to assess liver disease?
   a) Serum albumin
   b) Serum BUN
   c) Serum bilirubin
   d) Serum cholesterol
   e) Serum glucose concentration
   f) Bile acids

Answers

Renal and Urinary Disease Answers

1) SDMA is a specific biomarker of renal function as it is freely filtered by the glomerulus and is not reabsorbed by the renal tubules; therefore, it correlates well with GFR. Increases in SDMA are generally associated with a 25–40% decrease in renal function. This contrasts with the 75% decrease in renal function that leads to increases in serum creatinine concentrations. Increases in SDMA may therefore be detected before elevations in serum creatinine.

   Unlike creatinine, SDMA is not impacted by muscle mass and thus can be a useful marker when evaluating patients with reduced muscle mass and concurrent renal disease.
2) Patients with glomerular disease are at risk of developing a severe hypoalbuminemia that can result in spontaneous effusions or interstitial edema formation due to decreased intravascular oncotic pressure. The predisposition and the presence of effusions or edema are important considerations for anesthetic management. If pleural effusion is present and interferes with respiration, thoracocentesis should be performed before anesthesia. Large abdominal effusions may also interfere with ventilation and should be drained before anesthesia to a volume that will not interfere with respiration. Assessment of draining effect can be made based on improvements in respiratory rate and effort.
3) Staging is completed with creatinine and/or SDMA concentrations (preferably both) with substages defined based on proteinuria and blood pressure as per IRIS staging of CKD. Staging is important as this will guide therapeutic and monitoring recommendations, and help track disease progression.

Hepatobiliary Disease

1)
   a) The liver is responsible for albumin synthesis. Hypoalbuminemia may be present when approximately 70% of liver function is lost, resulting in decreased production. Hypoalbuminemia also occurs in cases of portosystemic shunt.
   b) In healthy animals, ammonia from the splanchnic circulation is converted to BUN in the liver via the urea cycle. With significant reductions in liver function, or in cases of portosystemic shunt, there can be a decrease in BUN production.
   c) Hyperbilirubinemia results from disruption of the production and/or processing of bilirubin. In cases of primary hepatic disease, increased serum bilirubin indicates decreased ability to produce/process bilirubin.
   d) The liver is the primary site of cholesterol synthesis, excretion, and catabolism. In hepatobiliary disease, cholesterol concentrations can be increased, decreased, or normal. Hypocholesterolemia can be seen in end-stage liver disease where hepatic function is impaired and in portosystemic shunt patients because of the poorly developed liver and decreased functional hepatic mass. Hypercholesterolemia can also develop in patients with cholestasis.
   e) Hypoglycemia can be an indicator of decreased liver function in patients with intrinsic liver disease and is estimated to occur with approximately 75% loss of function. Portosystemic shunts are another condition that often results in hypoglycemia. Hypoglycemia can arise in hepatobiliary disease due to the liver's central role in glucose homeostasis through glycogen storage, gluconeogenesis, glycogenolysis, and insulin clearance.
   f) Bile acids (BAs) are synthesized in the liver from cholesterol and are stored in the gallbladder. Shortly after a meal, the gallbladder contracts, releasing its contents into the duodenum. BAs undergo efficient enterohepatic recirculation with 95% reabsorbed from the gastrointestinal tract and transported back to the liver via the portal vein. This efficient reuptake can be disrupted with decreased liver function and portosystemic shunts, leading to elevations in serum bile acid concentrations.

Further Reading

Renal and Urinary Disease Section

Information about IRIS grading and staging. Please Visit: http://www.iris-kidney.com.

Acierno, M.J., Brown, S., Coleman, A.E. et al. (2018). ACVIM consensus statement: guidelines for the identification, evaluation, and management of systemic hypertension in dogs and cats. *J Vet Intern Med* 32: 1803–1822.

Brown, S., Atkins, A., Bagley, R. et al. (2007). Guidelines for the identification, evaluation, and management of systemic hypertension in dogs and cats. *J Vet Intern Med* 21: 542–558.

De Santis, F., Boari, A., Dondi, F. et al. (2022). Drug-dosing adjustment in dogs and cats with chronic kidney disease. *Anim* 12 (262): 1–26.

Littman, M.P., Daminet, S., Grauer, G.E. et al. (2013). Consensus recommendations for the diagnostic investigation of dogs with suspected glomerular disease. *J Vet Intern Med* 27: S19–S26.

Lees, G.E., Brown, S.A., Elliot, J. et al. (2005). Assessment and management of proteinuria in dogs and cats: 2004 AACVIM forum consensus statement (small animal). *J Vet Intern Med* 19: 377–385.

Monteiro, B., Steagall, P.V.M., Lascelles, B.D.X. et al. (2019). Long-term use of non-steroidal anti-inflammatory drugs in cats with chronic kidney disease: from controversy to optimism. *J Sm Anim Prac* 60: 459–462.

Mugford, A., Li, R., and Humm, K. (2013). Acute kidney injury in dogs and cats 1: pathogenesis and diagnosis. *In Pract* 35: 253–264.

Oiech, T.L. and Wycislo, K.L. (2019). Importance of urinalysis. *Vet Clin Small Anim* 49: 233–245.

Quimby, J. (2016). Update on medical management of clinical manifestations of chronic kidney disease. *Vet Clin Small Anim* 46: 1163–1181.

Relford, R., Robertson, J., and Clements, C. (2016). Symmetric dimethylarginine improving the diagnosis and staging of chronic kidney disease in small animals. *Vet Clin Small Anim* 46: 941–960.

Stafford, J.R. and Bartges, J.W. (2013). A clinical review of pathophysiology, diagnosis, and treatment of uroabdomen in the dog and cat. *J Vet Emerg Critic Care* 23: 216–229.

Vaden, S. and Elliot, J. (2016). Management of proteinuria in dogs and cats with chronic kidney disease. *Vet Clin Small Anim* 46: 1115–1130.

Hepatobillary Disease Section

Boland, L. and Beatty, J. (2017). Feline cholangitis. *Vet Clin Small Anim* 47: 703–724.

Goggs, R., Brainard, B., deLaforcade, A.M. et al. (2014). Partnership on rotational viscoelastic test standardization (PROVETS): evidence-based guidelines on rotational viscoelastic assays in veterinary medicine. *J Vet Emerg Critic Care* 24: 1–22.

Gow, A. (2017). Hepatic encephalopathy. *Vet Clin Small Anim* 47: 585–599.

Lawrence, Y. and Steiner, J. (2017). Laboratory evaluation of the liver. *Vet Clin Small Anim* 47: 539–553.

Valtolina, C. and Favier, R. (2017). Feline hepatic lipidosis. *Vet Clin Small Anim* 47: 683–702.

Webster, C. (2017). Hemostatic disorders associated with hepatobiliary disease. *Vet Clin Small Anim* 47: 601–615.

Webster, C., Center, S., Cullen, J. et al. (2019). ACVIM Consensus statement on the diagnosis and treatment of Chronic Hepatitis in Dogs. *J Vet Intern Med* 33: 1173–1200.

20

Anesthetic Complications and Cardiopulmonary Resuscitation

Tamara Grubb, Daniel Pang, and Gareth Zeiler

Anesthetic Incidents and Accidents

The field of patient safety in veterinary medicine is relatively new though awareness has rapidly increased in the past few years. What follows is a very basic introduction, and in-depth descriptions are available for interested readers. *Patient safety* has been defined as "the reduction of risk of unnecessary harm associated with health care to an acceptable minimum." Most of what we know about errors, accidents, and their prevention and investigation originally emerged from aviation. In turn, lessons learned from aviation have been adopted into human medicine, which provides a useful clinical correlate to veterinary medicine. Helpfully, while areas of practice may differ (e.g., small versus large animals), the concepts in this section apply to all types of clinical veterinary practice.

When considering preventable negative outcomes that cause harm to patients, there are several key concepts to consider.

First, humans make mistakes, and this can be viewed as inherent to human nature irrespective of levels of training or experience, or motivation to do the right thing. Second, the likelihood of mistakes occurring is affected by our personal performance at a given time as well the system in which we work. While mistakes are common everyday occurrences, patient harm is less common. Third, by reflecting upon the potential factors that contribute to patient harm, we can better understand contributing factors in a given situation and hopefully reduce the risk of a similar future event.

Before discussing these three concepts, there are a few definitions to present. For each of the following terms, numerous definitions exist, with none universally accepted. Those presented here have been selected by the authors based on widespread use, personal preference, and ease of understanding:

1) *Error* (mistake): The mental, or physical, activities of individuals that fail to achieve an intended outcome.
2) *Adverse event* (accident): An incident that resulted in harm to a patient. (Where incident is "an event or circumstance that could have resulted, or did result, in unnecessary harm to a patient.")
3) *Near miss* (close call): An incident that did not reach a patient, either through chance or intervention.

Errors (Mistakes)

Errors occur daily in veterinary medicine and can be further classified as skill-based, decision-based, or perceptual. Skill-based errors represent those common everyday tasks with which we are familiar and able to perform "without thinking." Examples could include locking a car after parking it, performing a simple drug calculation, and turning the oxygen on when a patient is connected to the anesthetic machine. Nevertheless, these apparently simple tasks can and do go wrong (forgetting to lock the car, making a drug miscalculation, and distracted from turning on the oxygen). Skill-based errors are implicated in over half of adverse events in human health care. Medication errors are a particularly common example of skill-based errors (see the following text). Decision-based errors reflect a plan that goes as intended, but the plan itself is flawed. It may be inadequate or inappropriate for the situation. Examples could include a new veterinary graduate planning a drug sedation protocol for an aggressive dog and the dog being inadequately sedated despite all drugs being given as intended. Or, an experienced practitioner anesthetizing a species with which they are unfamiliar and encountering problems inducing and maintaining anesthesia. Decision-based errors generally improve with training and experience. Perceptual errors result from an altered perception of the environment. This might include attempting to

Fundamental Principles of Veterinary Anesthesia, First Edition. Edited by Gareth E. Zeiler and Daniel S. J. Pang.

Companion Website: www.wiley.com/go/VeterinaryAnesthesiaZeiler

perform anesthesia in a darkened environment, such as during ophthalmic or arthroscopic procedures when room lighting is reduced. Perceptual errors are generally the least common of these error types.

Medication Errors

Medication errors are often considered as a separate case as they are so commonly encountered, with the vast majority being a form of skill-based error. Medication errors can affect any part of the medication pathway, including prescribing, manufacturing/compounding, dispensing, and administration. Medication errors are commonly described as the "5Ws": Wrong drug, Wrong patient, Wrong time, Wrong route, and Wrong dose. Of these, wrong dose and wrong drug are more common, with typical examples including decimal point errors (calculating a 0.1 mg/kg dose instead of the intended 0.01 mg/kg dose) and syringe swaps (picking up and administering the contents of the wrong syringe).

Adverse Events (Accidents)

When accidents occur, they typically represent multiple failures within different layers of the system in which we work. The best known model in use for understanding adverse events is the "Swiss Cheese Model," based on the work of James Reason (Reason 2008). This model uses layers of Swiss cheese to represent defensive layers within a system (Figure 20.1). The holes in each layer represent weaknesses. These weaknesses are not fixed, but rather move, open, and close depending on current events, reflecting the often dynamic nature of the system. Layers can be identified as representing different parts of a system, such as "unsafe acts," "preconditions for unsafe acts," "supervision," and "organizational influences." Unsafe acts include errors (as described in the preceding text) and is the layer closest to the patient, reflecting that errors are usually the last line of defense. Behind this, preconditions are closely associated with unsafe acts as these are the local factors that can increase or decrease the likelihood of a mistake being made. Such factors include being distracted, fatigued, or sick. Importantly, team performance is a precondition. That is, when a team is functioning well together, there is a greater likelihood of things going well, with the inverse being true that a team functioning suboptimally will have a greater risk of errors and adverse events. Factors influencing team performance include communication, coordination, interaction with the physical environment, and the use of cognitive aids (e.g., checklists). Supervision factors can play an important role, with the quality of supervision positively and negatively affecting performance. Poor supervision could involve requests to perform tasks without necessary training or being asked to exceed a reasonable workload, among others. Organizational factors often exert an influence through workplace culture, and policies and procedures. For instance, there is still a tendency in some, perhaps many, clinics to hide adverse events and not benefit from learning from them through discussion (morbidity and mortality rounds; see Further Reading). This outdated approach fails to recognize the "systems approach" reflected by considering the layers of a system and, in doing so, tends to fall back on "blaming and shaming" of individuals.

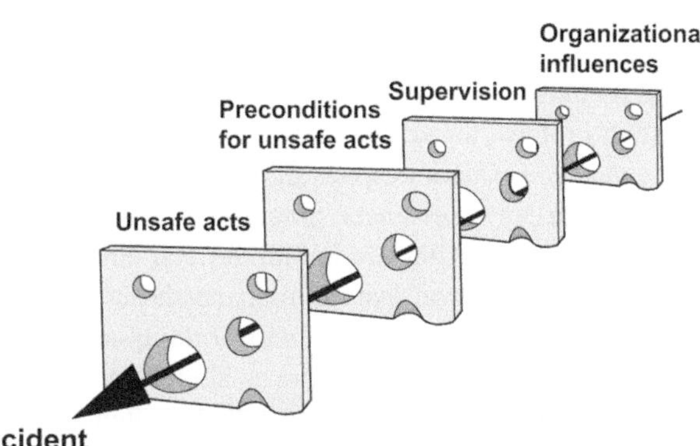

Figure 20.1 Reason's Swiss Cheese Model. (*Source:* Adapted from Pang (2022).)

Near Miss (Close Call)

Near misses are fairly common but often go unrecognized. Discussing and analyzing near misses can be instructive as we can learn what triggered avoidance of an adverse event in the hope of preventing a similar future scenario. Often, adverse events are avoided through the good performance of team members and individual resilience to errors; however, these are not finite resources. As errors mount, the likelihood of one continuing on its course to cause an adverse event increases.

Error Prevention

Error prevention can take many forms. Ultimately, engineering solutions that minimize reliance on human behavior to avoid errors are ideal; however, these may not be applicable in all cases. An engineering solution in use in human medicine is to have different syringe tips for different routes of injection (e.g., a drug intended for intrathecal administration will be placed in a syringe that cannot be connected to an IV line). Other approaches use knowledge of the Swiss Cheese Model to make different layers more resistant to error. These could include a culture of self-reporting when unfit for work (e.g., sick), clear policies and procedures for performing tasks (e.g., always labeling syringes), the use of cognitive aids (see the following text), structured training, etc. At the level of caregivers, self-awareness and situational awareness play important roles. Early recognition of limitations in individual performance and situations getting out of hand can help prevent errors occur.

Cognitive Aids

Cognitive aids are prompts (usually physical) to help users complete a task. The best known and most widely used example is the safe surgery checklist (Haynes et al. 2009). It is currently unknown to what extent checklists are used in veterinary anesthesia. An example used at one of the author's institutions is applied immediately before induction (Figure 20.2). This checklist serves two purposes: (1) as a checklist to ensure all items are confirmed/completed and (2) as a teaching aid, to help students work efficiently and reduce the stress of managing anesthesia. Checklists are ideally suited for tasks that have multiple steps; steps that must be performed in a certain order and tasks that may need to be performed in difficult/stressful conditions. Relying on memory in any of these situations is particularly error-prone. Checklists are applicable in many areas of anesthesia and surgery, including pre-induction, pre-incision, patient transfer, and anesthetic machine check. A less known benefit of using checklists is that, when used correctly, they promote communication between team members and break down hierarchies that serve as barriers to communication (e.g., a junior team member reticent to raise a concern with a senior team member).

Understanding Accidents

The approach to understanding factors contributing to an accident and learning from what went wrong is based on the Swiss Cheese Model. A structured approach can be taken, prompting users to consider key factors. One such approach is a fishbone (Ishikawa) diagram (Figure 20.3). Here, the "head" of the fish is the accident (or near miss) and the spines represent potential contributing factors. In most adverse events, there are multiple contributing factors (see Further Reading), with some being more important than others. Reviewing and discussing adverse events can be difficult, particularly for those proximal to the event (directly involved with the error(s)), and it is important that this is performed in a supportive environment where the goal is to *reflect and learn* rather than to *blame and shame*. Many clinics hold morbidity and mortality rounds but little is described in the veterinary literature regarding their format and structure (see Further Reading).

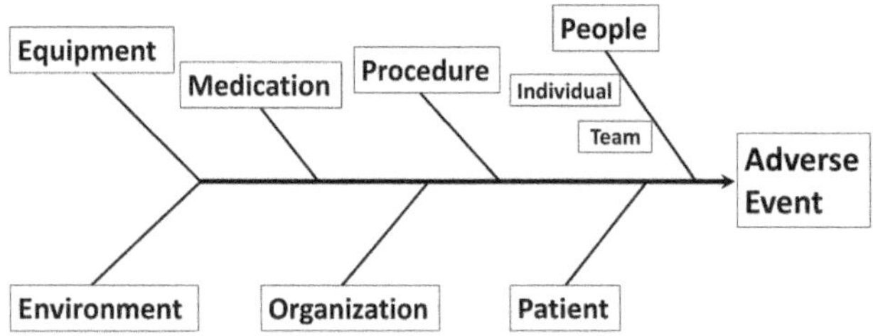

Figure 20.3 Fishbone (Ishikawa) diagram for investigating and understanding adverse events and near misses.

Figure 20.2 Pre-induction checklist. (*Source:* Daniel Pang, with permission.)

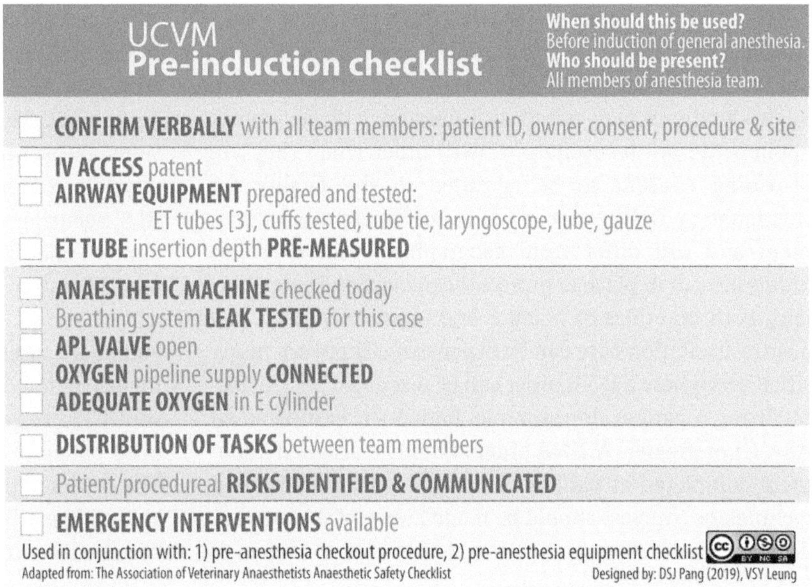

UCVM
Pre-induction checklist

When should this be used?
Before induction of general anesthesia.
Who should be present?
All members of anesthesia team.

- [ ] **CONFIRM VERBALLY** with all team members: patient ID, owner consent, procedure & site
- [ ] **IV ACCESS** patent
- [ ] **AIRWAY EQUIPMENT** prepared and tested:
  ET tubes [3], cuffs tested, tube tie, laryngoscope, lube, gauze
- [ ] **ET TUBE** insertion depth **PRE-MEASURED**
- [ ] **ANAESTHETIC MACHINE** checked today
- [ ] Breathing system **LEAK TESTED** for this case
- [ ] **APL VALVE** open
- [ ] **OXYGEN** pipeline supply **CONNECTED**
- [ ] **ADEQUATE OXYGEN** in E cylinder
- [ ] **DISTRIBUTION OF TASKS** between team members
- [ ] Patient/procedureal **RISKS IDENTIFIED & COMMUNICATED**
- [ ] **EMERGENCY INTERVENTIONS** available

Used in conjunction with: 1) pre-anesthesia checkout procedure, 2) pre-anesthesia equipment checklist

Adapted from: The Association of Veterinary Anaesthetists Anaesthetic Safety Checklist
Designed by: DSJ Pang (2019), VSY Leung

RECOVER Initiative and Cardiopulmonary Resuscitation

The RECOVER (Reassessment Campaign of Veterinary Resuscitation) initiative started in 2010 by a team of veterinarians who are specialists in veterinary emergency and critical care. Their goal is to develop and disseminate evidence-based veterinary cardiopulmonary resuscitation (CPR) guidelines for dogs and cats. Furthermore, this non-profit, volunteer-based program within the American College of Veterinary Emergency and Critical Care (ACVECC; www.acvecc.org) and Veterinary Emergency and Critical Care Society (VECCS; www.veccs.org) is dedicated to provide high-quality education and training of CPR to veterinarians and animal care givers, to continue conducting research and evidence searchers about veterinary CPR, and to continue updating CPR guidelines. The current RECOVER guidelines identify and provide information on five critical areas of CPR: preparedness and prevention, basic life support (BLS), advanced life support (ALS), monitoring, and post-cardiac arrest care. This chapter includes information from those reviews, particularly from the clinical guidelines published in RECOVER part 7. For training opportunities and more information about the RECOVER initiative, please visit a definitive and detailed resource at www.recoverinitiative.org. Successful CPR in foals and adult horses (and other species of animals) are sporadically reported on with an overall better survival rate in foals compared to adult horses. Comparative CPR techniques are described at the end of the chapter.

Do-Not-Resuscitate Orders

Each veterinary practice requires their own plan for a patient's unplanned response to treatment (including an anesthetic event) which could result in cardiac arrest. Such situations may entail a discussion with an owner about a "do-not-resuscitate" (DNR) order when they are providing consent to be admitted to the facility for treatment. A DNR order is not a universally used document and can differ from geographical region. These orders are put in place to protect the owners and veterinarians, both on ethics of practice and financially (CPR and post-resuscitation care can be expensive). There are many situations where a DNR order can be discussed before hospitalizing a patient, for example, patients classified as an ASA III or greater. A DNR order should be a signed document completed at patient admission. Veterinarians and technicians (nurses) should be made aware of the owner's decision.

Overview of Cardiopulmonary Arrest and Cardiopulmonary Resuscitation

Cardiopulmonary arrest (CPA) can be described as the cessation of flow of blood and gases within the cardiac and respiratory systems, respectively. As a consequence, there is failure of tissue oxygen delivery and carbon dioxide elimination. The result is hypoxemia and acidosis, which cause cell death and organ damage/death if not immediately corrected. The only "treatment" for CPA is cardiopulmonary resuscitation (also known as "cardiopulmonary cerebral resuscitation" [CPCR]). During CPR, the goal is to restore oxygen delivery to the tissues by supporting/restoring function of both the cardiovascular and respiratory systems. *Initial success of CPR* is defined as return of spontaneous circulation (ROSC) with the further goal of a return to normal physiologic function and discharge from the hospital. CPR in anesthetized patients is generally more successful than CPR in nonanesthetized patients. This is likely due to a number of reasons, including cause of CPA (i.e., drug overdose versus end-stage systemic disease), that the patient is already intubated and receiving supplemental oxygen, physiologic monitoring is already being performed, and multiple team members are likely to be present/nearby to assist with CPR, all of which minimize any delay to beginning resuscitation.

CPR success is also improved with a patient care team that is knowledgeable of CPR concepts and is trained in its delivery (with regular re-training). A stocked, maintained (regularly checked for expired drugs), and conveniently located "crash cart," along with drug-dosing charts, and a CPR algorithm (Figure 20.4) are important. Successful CPR is highly correlated with team training. The team should read the documents and carry out mock trials to practice CPR, even if the actual compressions cannot be practiced.

There are two levels of CPR: basic life support and advanced life support. The complete CPR algorithm can be found in Appendix 1. All veterinary clinics are capable of BLS, but ALS requires a greater skill set and additional equipment. The BLS phase is focused on chest compressions and ventilation, whereas the ALS phase focuses on physiologic monitoring of the patient and its response to BLS, securing an intravenous access point (if not already done), and administering advanced therapies (drug administration and electrical defibrillation).

Potential Causes/Predictors of CPA

Identification of patients at high risk for CPA can help prevent CPA or guide treatment if CPA occurs. For anesthetized patients, risk for CPA generally parallel ASA status. The causes of pulseless electrical activity (PEA) are invaluable to learn because treating the Hs and Ts before they become life-threatening can prevent a CPA (Table 20.1).

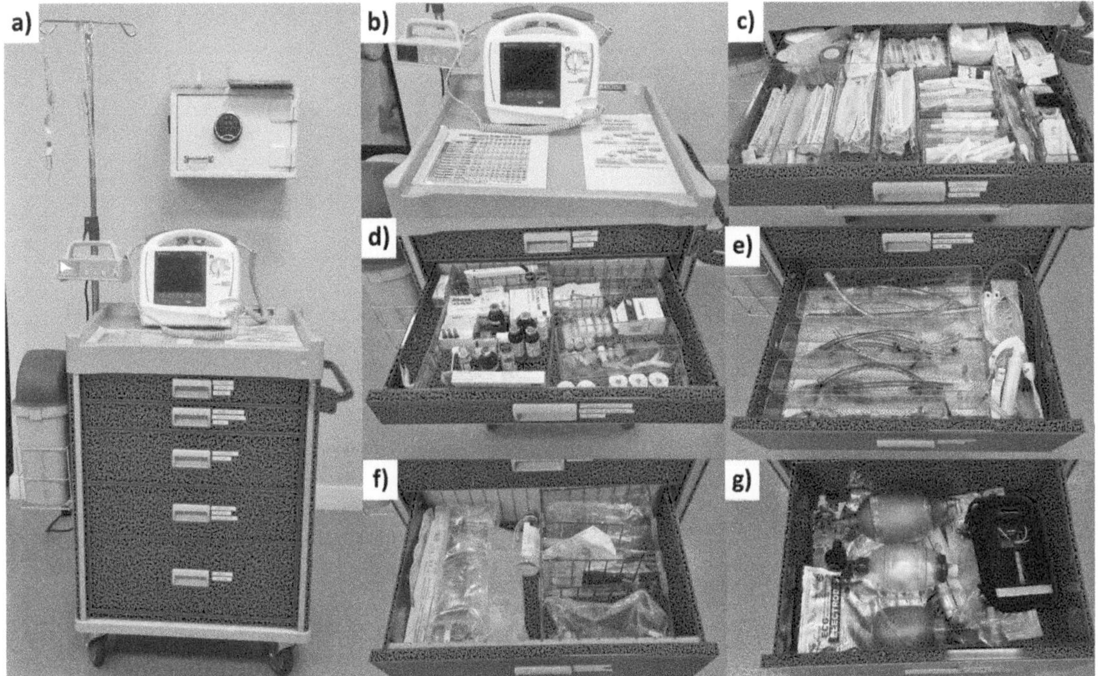

Figure 20.4 An emergency crash cart (a) placed in close proximity to a triage area or operating room. Each area of the crash cart serves a purpose. On top (b) rests the defibrillator, RECOVER CPR flow diagram, and emergency drug-dosing chart; needles, syringes, and over-the-needle intravenous catheters in the top drawer (c); emergency drugs in the second drawer (d); airway equipment for dogs and cats in the third drawer (e); various intravenous fluids in the fourth drawer (f); and AMBU bags and some monitoring equipment in the bottom drawer (g).

Table 20.1 The causes of cardiopulmonary arrest (CPA) are grouped into the Hs and Ts. Treating these causes early in their progression can help prevent CPA.

Causes of CPA	Potential lifesaving treatment
The Hs	
Hypotension	Fluid bolus, administering a catecholamine, and treating heart failure and cardiac arrhythmias.
Hypovolemia	Fluid bolus: administering fresh whole blood if exsanguinating, administering a vasopressor in the presence of relative hypovolemia.
Hypothermia	Actively warming patient using forced-air warming device, heated blankets, heating lamps (with caution).
Hyperthermia	Actively cooling patient by running cold tap water over coat (if no external injuries to skin), and placing insulated ice packs to neck, and between thoracic limbs against chest, and between the pelvic limbs.
Hypoventilation (and apnea)	Secure the airway (might require general anesthesia) and provide manual breaths.
Hypoxemia	Provide supplemental oxygen via a face mask, nasal prongs, or if very severe, consider securing the airway and providing oxygen via an endotracheal tube.
Hyperkalemia	Consider a fluid bolus to dilute excess potassium. Measure glucose, and if normal or low, provide a glucose bolus (0.5–1 mL/kg of dextrose 50% diluted to 1:4 with isotonic crystalloid fluid). If glucose is high, provide rapid acting short-lasting insulin (0.1 IU/kg); if acidotic and heart rate within normal reference intervals or elevated, treatment may not be required. If bradycardic (typical of a "blocked" cat that presents collapsed), administer a bolus of 10% calcium gluconate at 0.5–1 mL/kg over 10 min. The calcium restores the difference between the threshold and resting membrane potentials but does not treat hyperkalemia.
Hypocalcemia	Administer an intravenous bolus of 10% calcium gluconate (0.5–1.0 mL/kg) slowly, ideally while monitoring the ECG or heart rate. If given too fast, you could induce bradycardia.

(Continued)

Table 20.1 (Continued)

Causes of CPA	Potential lifesaving treatment
The Ts	
Tension thorax	Could be any fluid or air accumulating in the thorax (pneumothorax, pyothorax, hemothorax, chylothorax, etc.), and if the volume is large enough, it decreases venous return of blood to the heart and causes a decrease in cardiac output. The lifesaving intervention is a thoracentesis, and if fluid returns, placement of a thoracic drain can be considered.
Tamponade	Cardiac tamponade is treated by pericardiocentesis, and the tamponade is usually caused by an accumulation of fluid (blood, transudate, exudate, modified transudate, etc.). Low-volume rapidly developing effusions usually result in a sudden life-threatening tamponade, whereas slowly developing effusions accumulate to a large volume. If a pericardiocentesis needs to be performed regularly and if the fluid is not whole blood, then a pericardiectomy could be considered.
Tympani	Usually referred to as a "gastric dilatation" with or without a volvulus and can occur because of aerophagia often seen in patients with respiratory distress. Generally, a light plane of general anesthesia to secure the airway before passing a gastric tube down the esophagus is the most effective method of rapidly deflating the stomach. Alternatively, in sedated, moribund or anesthetized animals, a nasogastric tube can also be passed into the stomach to evacuate the gas, or a transabdominal needle (large-bore 12–18 gauge IV catheter) trocar can be considered.
Thromboembolism	Poorly recognized and diagnosed in dogs and cats. Generally, supportive treatment, ensuring optimal cardiovascular function and preventing further clot formation (aspirin and clopidogrel), is performed.

Identification of CPA

A rapid decrease in blood pressure and/or end-tidal carbon dioxide (PE′CO_2) concentrations (Figure 20.5) with weak pulses can indicate impending CPA. As CPA occurs, there will be no peripheral pulse, no audible heart beat on auscultation, apnea (occasionally "gasping" efforts), and fixed and dilated pupils. Identification of CPA is easier and quicker in patients connected to a physiological monitor (such as during general anesthesia) where ECG, capnography, pulse oximetry, and indirect or invasive blood pressure are monitored. There are four cardiac arrhythmias of cardiac arrest that can be recognized: (1) pulseless electrical activity (PEA, the most sinister of them all because the ECG tracing appears normal), (2) asystole, (3) ventricular fibrillation, and (4) pulseless ventricular tachycardia (Figure 20.6).

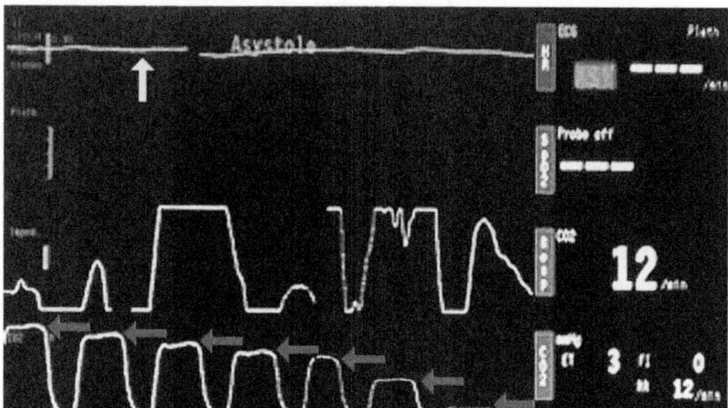

Figure 20.5 Photograph of a multiparameter monitoring screen in a mechanically ventilated dog that was euthanized while under general anesthesia. The electrocardiogram (yellow arrow) indicates asystole, and the height of the capnograph waveform is decreasing (indicating a decrease in end-tidal carbon dioxide; red arrows) with each mechanical breath. Patients in asystole and not mechanically ventilated will be apneic. This figure shows the value of capnography in resuscitation, in that end-tidal carbon dioxide will only be above 15 mmHg if there is sufficient cardiac output. The white tracing above the capnograph is measuring the respiratory rate by electrical impedance measured from the electrocardiogram leads. This tracing should not be confused with the capnograph.

Nonanesthetized patients can have a witnessed (caregiver sees the animal "faint") or unwitnessed (animal found collapsed and unresponsive) rapid loss of consciousness (faint; collapsed and unresponsive) and are apneic. Therefore, all unconscious/unresponsive animals that are apneic should be assumed to have CPA and treated immediately with BLS. With this presentation, it is critically important to minimize time wasted trying to listen for a heartbeat or palpate a peripheral pulse. Every minute that BLS is delayed reduces the chance of recovery. Starting BLS will not harm your patient. If you discover that the animal is not in CPA, then this patient should be investigated to identify why CPA was suspected. The person identifying CPA should begin chest compressions and call for help. A properly managed CPR effort requires four people, if possible. One person performs chest compressions, one person secures an airway and provides intermittent positive pressure ventilation (IPPV) and oxygen support, one person obtains intravenous access and administers resuscitation drugs and reversal agents (pharmaceutical antagonists), and the fourth person records treatments and timings, and attaches monitoring equipment to the patient.

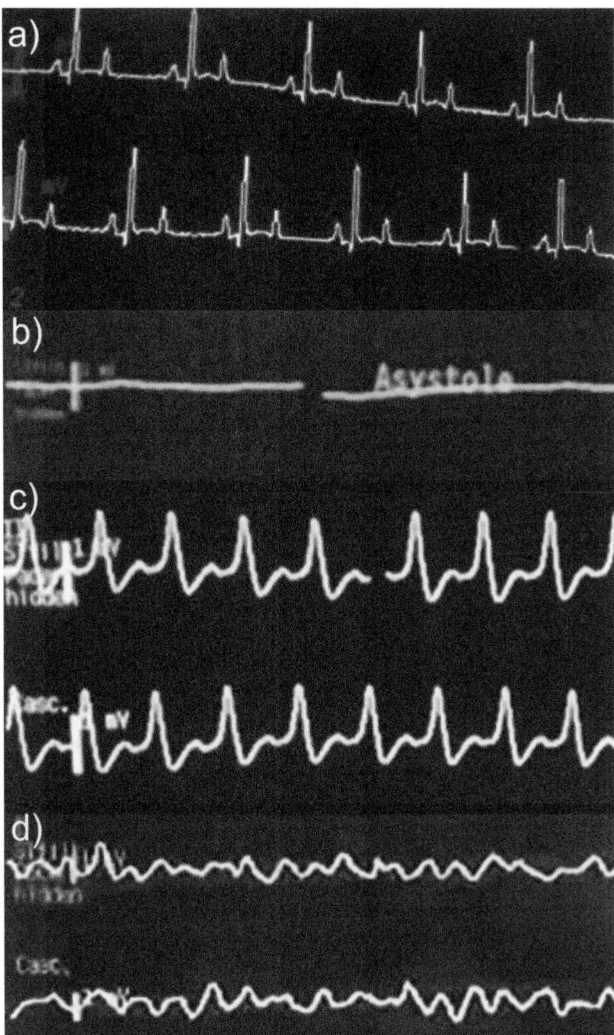

Figure 20.6 The four important electrocardiograph tracings of patients in cardiopulmonary arrest. (a) Pulseless electrical activity (formerly electromechanical dissociation) is a normal sinus tracing but with no associated pulses and apnea. The rate can change as hypoxemia develops (initially an increase and then a decrease to severe bradycardia of <30 beats per minute). Tracing (b) is asystole, where no electrical activity is identifiable. The trace is an iso-electric line. Tracing (c) is ventricular tachycardia. To be confirmed as pulseless ventricular tachycardia, there must be no pulse. If a pulse is present, this rhythm could be a ventricular tachycardia or accelerated idioventricular arrythmia (these latter rhythms do not require electrical defibrillation). Tracing (d) is ventricular fibrillation. Tracings (c) and (d) require electrical defibrillation.

Performing Effective Cardiopulmonary Resuscitation

Basic Life Support

The sooner BLS starts after identifying CPA the greater the chance of ROSC occurring. Chest compressions should start immediately (Figure 20.7). As stated in RECOVER part 7, "the evidence strongly reinforced the importance of early delivery of high-quality chest compressions with minimal interruption." Compressions are so crucial to the likelihood of success that the old moniker for CPR, "ABC" (airway, breathing, and compressions) has more appropriately become "CAB" (compressions, airway, and breathing). If the patient is under general anesthesia, then all anesthetic drugs must be stopped immediately. If intravenous drugs have been used to maintain anesthesia, then the duration (at least 30 min) of resuscitation should be longer to allow enough time for drug redistribution. If inhalational anesthesia was used for maintenance, then the vaporizer should be turned off and the breathing system flushed of anesthetic gases (temporarily disconnect the breathing system from the patient, occlude the patient end of the breathing hose, and activate the oxygen flush valve for 5–10 s; see Chapter 5).

Chest Compressions

Effectiveness of compressions depends, in part, on the position of the patient (based on body type) and the location of the resuscitator's hands on the patient's thorax. Blood flow is optimized by direct cardiac compression (i.e., "cardiac pump" theory) in small dogs, cats, and narrow-chested medium–large dogs (e.g., sighthounds). In small dogs (<5 kg) and cats, the fingers of one hand should be placed directly over the heart on one side of the chest and the thumb on the other side of the chest, and compressions performed by squeezing the fingers and thumb together. Narrow-chested, medium–large-breed dogs should be placed in lateral recumbency (either right or left, and right may be preferred if open chest cardiac massage is expected), and the resuscitator's hands should be placed one over the other (palm of top hand on back of lower hand with fingers intertwined) and then placed on the thorax directly over the heart. For medium–large-breed dogs with round chests (e.g., Rottweilers and Labradors), blood flow is optimized using the movement of the thorax (i.e., "thoracic pump" theory) by placing both hands together on the widest part of the thorax in the laterally recumbent patient. In barrel-chested dogs (e.g., Bulldogs and other brachycephalic breeds), blood flow is optimized by placing the patient in dorsal recovery with the resuscitator's hands placed on the sternum. In patients where compressions are performed in lateral recumbency and where the resuscitator applies pressure to one side of the thorax during compressions, then ensuring that the patient is on a firm surface is important. Removing patient cushioning ensures good chest wall movements during compression. In deep-chested animals, placing a sandbag (or 1 L fluid bag) between the ventral chest and surface they are lying on will help balance the patient and prevent them from sliding away from the resuscitator and improve the quality of the compressions.

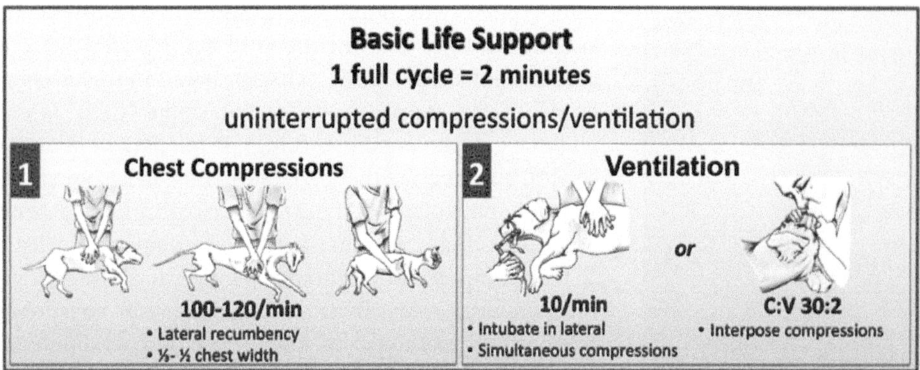

Figure 20.7 Basic life support steps during cardiopulmonary resuscitation. (*Source:* Reproduced with permission from Fletcher et al. (2012).)

Also, to prevent pushing the patient away from the resuscitator, it is best for the resuscitator to stand at the dorsal side of the animal during chest compressions (Figure 20.8).

Compressions should be delivered at a rate of 100–120 per minute with a 1:1 compression time to relaxation time ratio. To maintain this rate (and to relax and focus the team on the job at hand), some people hum or sing certain songs, such as "Stayin Alive" (Bee Gees; released 1977 by RSO records [UK]) for optimistic teams and "Another One Bites the Dust" (Queen; released 1980 by EMI [UK] and Elektra [USA]) for less optimistic teams. Compressions, regardless of hand position, should compress the chest by approximately 1/3 of its width (or depth, in dorsal recumbency), and the chest should be allowed to completely recoil (i.e., return to resting position) during relaxation. Chest recoil is important for promoting flow of blood and is just as important as compression. Perform chest compressions for a *full two minutes* without stopping. Compressions should continue at all costs because any pause results in a dramatic decrease in blood flow and myocardial perfusion, decreasing the chance of ROSC. Even with optimal chest compressions, cardiac output is only a fraction of normal levels (around 15%), meaning that pauses in compressions cause a precipitous drop in cardiac output. The resuscitator has the most important initial role during the CPR effort and must be open to constructive criticism from the team on technique to ensure that effective chest compressions are delivered. Common pitfalls are leaning on the patient (preventing complete recoil), failing to maintain an adequate compression rate, failure to achieve adequate compression depth, and overzealous compressions that cause excessive injury (bruising of myocardium and lungs or rib fractures). When done properly, performing chest compressions is tiring, and it is expected that the person performing compressions will change regularly (often every 2 min). Switching resuscitators should be rapid, taking no longer *than 10 s*. Resume compressions immediately if no cardiac activity is detected (i.e., confirmed by the assessment of electrocardiogram (ECG) tracing and the absence of a peripheral pulse).

Airway/Breathing

Every patient experiencing CPA should be intubated if at all possible but not at the expense of thoracic compressions. While preparing for intubation, oxygen should be delivered via facemask. The patient should be intubated in the 10 s pause between switching the person performing compressions or during compressions (without changing patient body position). Team members should practice intubation in patients, in these recumbencies, in nonurgent situations. Placement of the endotracheal tube in the trachea, rather than the esophagus, is critical, and the visualization of the tube passing through the arytenoids is the best way to determine correct placement. A laryngoscope will aid visualization. If saliva or other fluids are obscuring the view, they should be suctioned or swabbed (e.g., with gauze). If intubation is not possible, then another device (e.g., supraglottic airway device [SGAD] in cats/rabbits) can be used. With SGADs, there is always a risk of dislodgement of the device or accidental (partial or complete) obstruction of the airways during CPR because of head and neck movement during chest compressions. Therefore, observing thoracic excursion when delivering a breath is critically important. In some cases, if chest compressions are good, the presence of a capnograph trace will confirm adequate placement of these devices. If there is upper airway obstruction (tumors, trauma, swelling, etc.) preventing orotracheal intubation, a tracheotomy will be necessary to secure an airway. During CPR, often a large-bore (20–16 gauge) over-the-needle intravenous catheter can be inserted into the trachea (needle tracheostomy) distal to the cricoid cartilage. Connecting the catheter to a

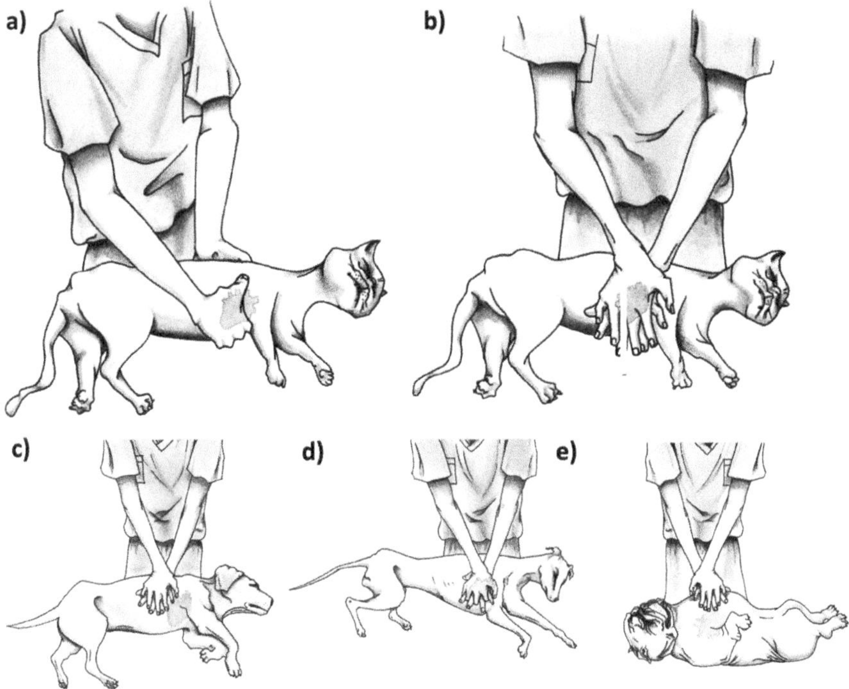

Figure 20.8 Techniques of performing external compressions in animals: under 10 kg using a single-handed technique (a) and a two-handed technique (b); heavier than 10 kg (c), deep-chested (keel-chested) dogs (d), and barrel-chested (e) dogs. (*Source:* Reproduced with permission from Fletcher et al. (2012).)

supplemental oxygen source at a flow rate of 1–2 L/min can be lifesaving.

Once an airway has been secured, the patient should receive supplemental oxygen and intermittent positive pressure ventilation (i.e., providing manual breaths) at 10 breaths per minute. These breaths can be delivered using an AMBU bag or an anesthetic machine. The inspiratory phase should be completed within 1–2 s and the chest observed to confirm inflation. When a chest rise is seen, then this generally translates into a tidal volume of 10 mL/kg with a peak airway pressure of <20 cmH_2O. If a ventilator is available, this can be used to provide IPPV. Do not stop chest compressions to ventilate the patient. If an airway cannot be secured (via intubation, SGAD, or tracheotomy), ventilation can be attempted by closing the mouth and performing mouth-to-nose ventilations. Make sure the head and neck are in a straight line to promote gas flow through the upper airway and into the lungs. If this method of providing a breath is used, then chest compressions should be stopped, two breaths given rapidly, and then chest compressions resumed. A 30:2 sequence is recommended (cycles of 30 chest compressions followed by 2 breaths).

Single Rescuer Administering CPR

If a single rescuer is performing CPR, anesthesia should be discontinued (if anesthetized), all reversal drugs should be administered intravenously with flush between drugs, and continuous (uninterrupted) compressions should be initiated at the ratio of 30 chest compressions to 2 breaths.

Advanced Life Support

ALS is the second phase of CPR and, if the team is large enough, should begin during the first two-minute cycle of BLS. The focus of ALS is to begin physiologic monitoring, obtain intravenous access, and administer advanced therapies (Figure 20.9).

Physiologic Monitoring

There are two desirable variables to monitor during CPR, the electrocardiogram and end-tidal carbon dioxide. Other monitoring techniques like auscultation of the heart, feeling for peripheral pulses, and using pulse oximetry or

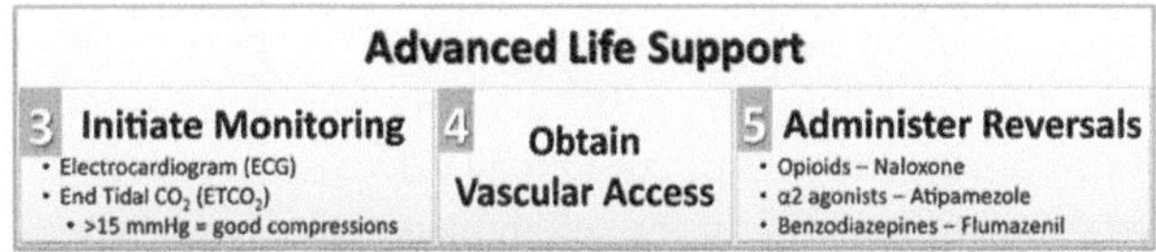

Figure 20.9 Advanced life support steps during cardiopulmonary resuscitation. (*Source:* Reproduced with permission from Fletcher et al. (2012).)

Doppler probes are not recommended because they are not reliable or informative under CPR conditions.

The ECG is used to determine the electrical actively of the heart and is interpreted during the 10 s switching period where a new chest compressor is taking over compressions. There are four common waveforms, see Figure 20.6, and two require commencement of chest compressions (PEA and asystole) and two require electrical defibrillation (ventricular fibrillation and pulseless ventricular tachycardia). Ventricular fibrillation and ventricular tachycardia are easy waveforms to identify. Determining if the ventricular tachycardia is pulseless, it is somewhat harder to confirm, and capnography will assist in interpretation.

The capnograph allows waveform visualization of the exhaled CO_2 during a breath (unlike a capnometer that only displays a number or an indicator of a range). For this to occur, there needs to be blood flowing through the alveolar capillaries of the lungs. A $PE'CO_2$ > 15 mmHg is a good indicator that chest compressions are effective and that there is flow of blood through the lungs, and it is assumed there is systemic blood flow, and most importantly, myocardial blood flow. If the $PE'CO_2$ is less than 15 mmHg, then the quality of chest compressions is inadequate or there is another cause such as pericardial effusions, plural effusions, pneumothorax, distended abdominal organs (gastric dilatation because of aerophagia commonly seen during respiratory failure or gastric dilatation and volvulus), or large abdominal organ hemorrhage, for example, hindering good blood flow despite "effective" external chest compressions. Therefore, if changing the chest compression technique (or swapping out a tired chest compressor) does not improve the $PE'CO_2$, then consideration for open chest CPR needs to be discussed (see Further Reading).

If ROSC occurs, this will be identified, most often, as a rapid rise in the $PE'CO_2$ to >45 mmHg, and the chest compressor might even be able to feel the heart beating in the chest. This indicates that the heart is able to generate a pulse wave of blood that can also be felt by palpating a peripheral (dorsal pedal) or central (femoral) artery. Thus, the capnograph is used to help differentiate between pulseless ventricular tachycardia ($PE'CO_2$ < 25 mmHg) and ventricular tachycardia ($PE'CO_2$ > 40 mmHg).

Obtaining Intravenous Access

Intravenous access is essential for any CPR effort because this is the most effective route of administering drugs and fluids during the ALS phase. Often IV access is already present; however, catheters are often placed into a peripheral vein (cephalic or saphenous) and could become dislodged if inadequately secured because of limb movement during chest compressions. Chest compressions should not be stopped when investigating catheter placement and patency. If IV access has been lost or if IV access needs to be established, this should be done while performing good-quality chest compressions. If there is excessive limb movement and no help to try to stabilize the limb during chest compressions, then at least one minute of good-quality compressions should be performed before the briefest of pauses to allow catheter placement by the most skilled member of the team. The catheter placer must be fully prepared to attempt catheter placement in the shortest period (site should be shaved and prepared before the pause) of time to allow the recommencement of chest compressions. If the patient does not have IV access, then the placement of a catheter into a jugular vein is often easiest and, with experience, can be placed during chest compressions. Attaching an extension set to the catheter helps prevent potential dislodgment while injecting drugs via a "moving target." If it is impossible to obtain IV access, then a large-bore (14–18 gauge 1.5–2.0 inch long) hypodermic needle should be placed into a bone marrow cavity (usually the femur or tibia). Direct intra-cardiac injections, especially if repeated, and if injecting drugs like adrenaline, injures the already hypoxic myocardium even more and could result in post-ROSC arrhythmias that are difficult to control. Furthermore, accidently tearing a myocardial blood vessel, such as a coronary artery, diminishes a occurrence of ROSC and could cause a rapid developing pericardial tamponade. Preparing for and attempting an intra-cardiac injection also wastes valuable BLS time and is thus not recommended. Injecting drugs into the lower airways via a tube (eight French gauge nasogastric feeding tube) placed past the carina (tracheal bifurcation into the main stem bronchi) is not recommended because it is mostly ineffective and large volumes of fluids and drugs need to be used compared to intravenous administration. Once intravenous (or intraosseous) access has been established, advanced therapies can be initiated, including administering drugs.

If the animal has a low intravascular volume because of an absolute (hemorrhage, history of ongoing severe vomiting and diarrhea, etc.) or relative (hypersensitivity reaction) hypovolemia, then an intravenous bolus (20–30 mL/kg) of isotonic fluids should be initiated immediately at a rapid rate of administration (>1000 mL/h). If the arrest was because of congestive heart failure, acute kidney injury with anuria, etc., then these patients might be hypervolemic, and fluid bolusing during CPR is not recommended because it worsens the outcome and lowers the probability of achieving ROSC. Regardless of the fluid therapy plan during CPR, there must be fluids made available in order to "flush" all of the drugs that are given during the ALS phase. Recommended intravenous (or intraosseous) "flush" volumes are 10 mL for animals under 5 kg, 20 mL for animals between 5 and 15 kg, and 40 mL for animals >15 kg. This fluid "flush" bolus ensures adequate movement of the given drug to the desired effect site.

Advanced Therapies

Drugs that are given during ALS have three major functions: to reverse the effects of anesthetic or analgesic drugs (if the patient is anesthetized or been given these types of drugs recently, within the last two hours), to facilitate the flow of blood toward the heart, and to cause parasympatholysis (high vagal nerve tone decreases the effectiveness of the CPR effort to result in ROSC).

Anesthetic and analgesics drugs that can be reversed belong to the opioid, alpha-2 adrenergic receptor agonist, and benzodiazepine agonist groups of drugs and can be antagonized using naloxone, atipamezole, and flumazenil, respectively (see Chapter 7). The doses for these drugs can be found on the CPR emergency drugs and doses chart (Appendix 2). The reversal drugs should be given as quickly as possible, soon after starting BLS. If the patient is under general anesthesia, then all anesthetic drugs used during maintenance should be stopped immediately if not already done so. Drugs that have vasopressor effects are used to facilitate the flow of blood toward the heart, specifically drugs that increase vasoconstriction of peripheral (and central) veins will help recruit a pool of blood from these capacitance vessels. The most frequently used drug is epinephrine (adrenaline), and it should be administered early on at an initial low dose of 0.01 mg/kg. Patients undergoing CPR become progressively acidotic, and after 10 min, a higher dose of epinephrine is recommended (0.1 mg/kg) because there is downregulation of the alpha-adrenergic receptors that occur during acidosis, making its vasopressor effect less potent. Using high doses of epinephrine early on during the CPR is discouraged because if ROSC does occur it is associated with tachyarrythmias and a decrease in myocardial perfusion (perfusion is greatest during diastole). Furthermore, epinephrine causes vasoconstriction of the coronary blood vessels which also results in a decreased perfusion. The hypoxic myocardium requires the best perfusion to rapidly reoxygenate the muscle tissue. If available, vasopressin (0.8 U/kg) could be used instead of epinephrine to cause vasoconstriction and facilitate blood flow to the heart. This drug will have a clinical effect regardless of the patient's blood acid–base status. The most commonly used drug to cause parasympatholysis is atropine (0.04 mg/kg). Processes that increase vagal tone in an arresting animal could include pulmonary edema, laryngeal injury, traumatic brain injury (increased intracranial pressure), and distention of any part of the gastrointestinal tract (gastric dilatation is common). A routine single dose of atropine should be considered in every CPR effort to standardize the approach and make team training easier. Atropine is often given at the same time as the first dose of epinephrine.

Advanced therapies, other than administering emergency drugs, include defibrillation and treating the common causes of PEA. A description of these advanced therapies is outside the scope of this chapter, and information can be found in Further Reading.

Concluding CPR

The BLS and ALS cycles of CPR should be started as soon as possible and continued for a "long enough" period of time before stopping if ROSC is not achieved. The recommended or ideal duration of a CPR effort is not established for veterinary medicine, but the sentiment of "you are not dead until you are warm and dead" holds true. Thus, if the patient is <34 °C, it should be actively warmed to 36 °C before pronouncing death. If CPA is related to anesthetic or analgesic drugs, then a 15–20 minute CPR effort could be considered adequate. If the arrest was because of other non-drug-related reasons, then rapidly identifying the cause while a CPR effort is underway is important. If pericardial or any other effusions are detected, or a pneumothorax or profound gastric distention is identified, then they must be corrected while the CPR effort is underway. Usually arrest from unknown causes warrants a 30–40 minute CPR effort. Another general remark is that if the BLS effort produces a $PE'CO_2 > 20$ mmHg, this is an incentive to continue CPR efforts as a chance of ROSC remains. The longer it takes for ROSC to occur the greater the risk of rearrest (within the first four hours) and brain injury. In practices where there is not advanced support and expertise, if ROSC is not achieved within 15–20 min, then it is perhaps best to pronounce the animal dead. Once ROSC occurs, then the patient moves into the post-CPA period and the team must orientate their attention to prevent a rearrest and minimize brain injury. Achieving ROSC is a great feeling of accomplishment for the CPR team, but it must be realized that the patient requires a lot of monitoring and intensive care and at least 75% of the "job" still remains to try and get the patient home.

Post-CPA Care (Post-ROSC Care)

A post-CPA algorithm has been described based on the best level of current evidence (Figure 20.10). It is important to appreciate that the proportion of animals that leave the clinic following CPA is low, approximately 2–10%. This is despite ROSC occurring in 35–45% of CPA cases. This difference reflects several, potentially overlapping, factors: ongoing disease, organ damage secondary to CPA, insufficient post-ROSC monitoring, and supportive care.

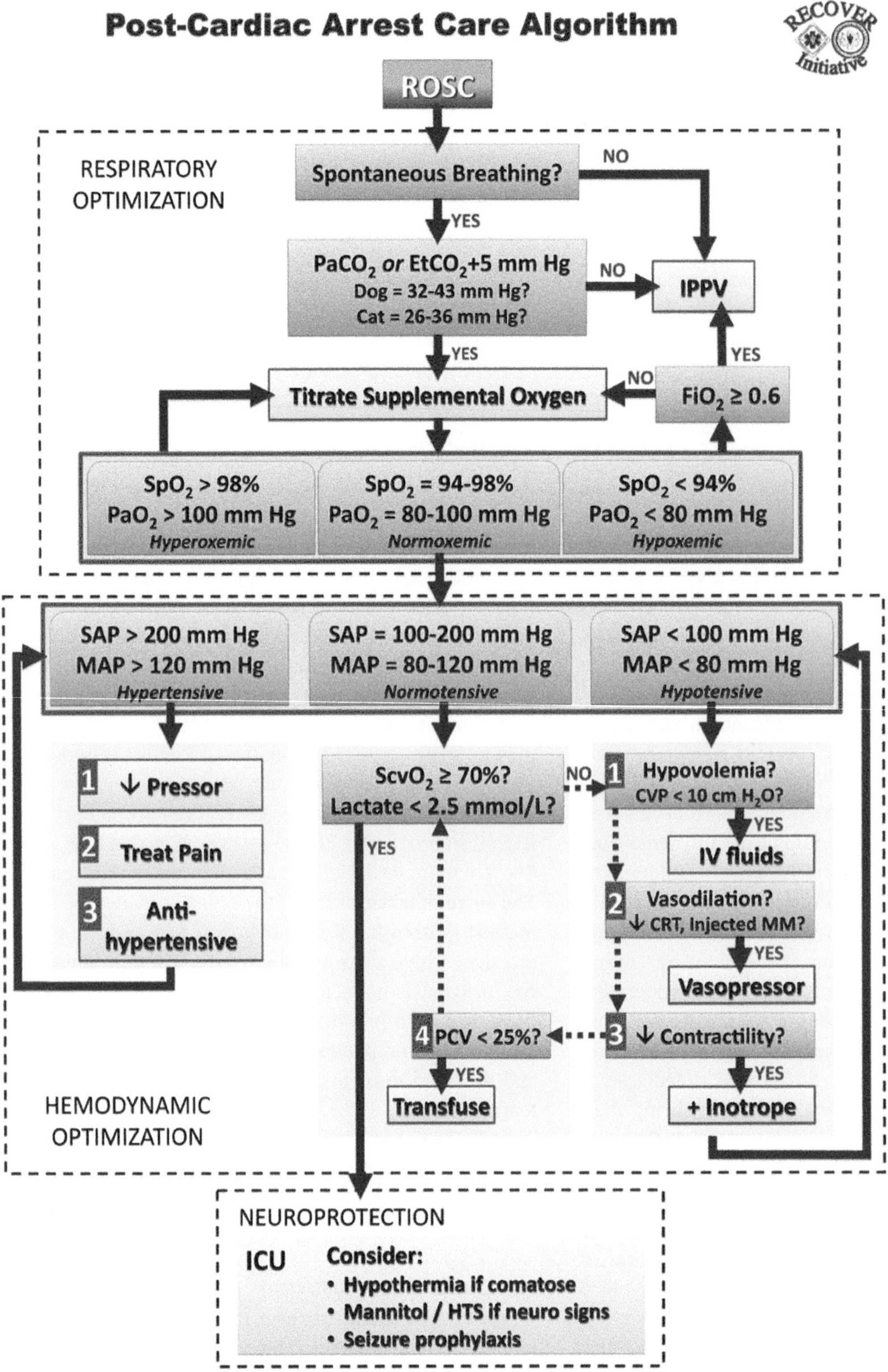

Figure 20.10 Post-cardiac arrest algorithm of the RECOVER initiative. (*Source:* Reproduced with permission from Fletcher et al. (2012).)

Good post-CPA care requires a very close monitoring of the patient for the first 24 h. Ideally, the cause of the CPA should be identified or understood so that is can be treated, if possible, to prevent a re-arrest. The two main goals of post-CPA care are to resolve the acidosis (because this will often result in a re-arrest) and to prevent or minimize the development of brain edema. The RECOVER guidelines propose a post-CPA arrest algorithm where the goal is to optimize respiratory and cardiovascular functions and to provide neuroprotection. Patients that achieve ROSC have a very high circulating CO_2 load that should be removed as soon as possible, and this can be achieved by providing IPPV for 2–6 h (sometimes longer). This treatment resolves a large contribution toward the post-CPA acidosis that almost always develops. The acidosis decreases cardiovascular function through a decrease in inotropy and an increase in vasodilation. Thus, treating the acidosis with effective ventilation will assist in improving cardiovascular function. The next goal is to achieve adequate cardiovascular function by trying to achieve a normal blood pressure and circulating volume. This optimization will help organ reperfusion and a quick return of organ function. Often, all electrolyte, lactate, and glucose derangements will self-correct once the optimization of the respiratory and cardiovascular system function has been achieved. However, regular (initially every 15–30 min post-CPA) monitoring of electrolytes, glucose, and lactate can help guide additional therapies during the post-CPA period. Providing neuroprotective care and prophylactic treatment is recommended if the CPR lasted longer than 15 min. Post-ROSC blindness commonly occurs, and generally this blindness is temporary, lasting for a few days and in worse cases up to 6 months. Often in these cases, return to consciousness could take a few hours. Neuroprotective care includes elevating the cranial half of the body higher than the caudal part (reverse Trendelenburg position), extending the neck to a natural position to optimize jugular venous draining of the head, avoiding use of the jugular as a venipuncture site (or catheter site), and optimizing cardiovascular function to ensure good cerebral blood flow and prefusion pressures. The authors' regularly give mannitol (0.5–1.0 g/kg) or 7.5% hypertonic saline (4 mL/kg) once to all post-CPA patients that achieved ROSC after 15 min of CPR.

CPR in Horses

The causes of CPA (and indicators of impending arrest) and the approach to performing CPR and goals for ROSC in horses are similar to those described for the dog and cat.

CPR in adult horses should always be attempted. Despite being generally ineffective, there are sporadic reports of successes. For BLS, the provision of chest compression and ventilation needs to be started as soon as CPA is identified. Chest compressions are potentially effective if performed by a person (resuscitator, greater than 70 kg) bouncing on, or jumping on, the widest part of the thorax, in an effort to apply a "thoracic pump" (Figure 20.11). Another technique described is where the resuscitator stands caudal to the thoracic limbs and repetitively kneels on the thorax over the region of the heart (Figure 20.12). The recommended compression rate is at least 80 compressions per minute, but a rate of 40–60 compressions per minute may be more realistic. For ventilation, endotracheal intubation (via nasal or oral route, or tracheostomy) is critical because mouth-to-nose ventilation from a human cannot provide adequate respiratory tidal volumes for an adult horse. Rather, a large animal anesthetic machine (see Chapter 5) or a demand valve can be used to provide ventilation (Figure 20.13). The recommended ventilation rate is 10 breaths per minute. If the horse was anesthetized, then all anesthetic drugs should be discontinued and antagonists administered

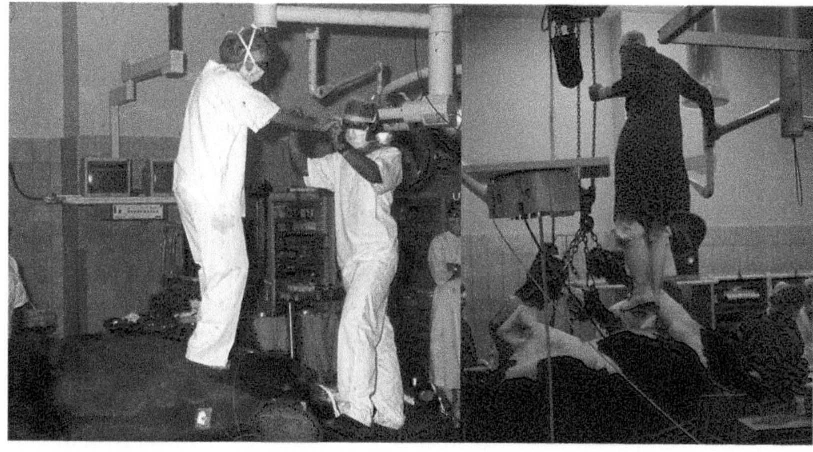

Figure 20.11 External chest compressions in a horse (left) and a cow (right). Cardiopulmonary efforts in large animals (>100 kg) are generally ineffective, with occasional reports of success. (*Source:* Courtesy of Prof. George F. Stegmann, University of Pretoria.)

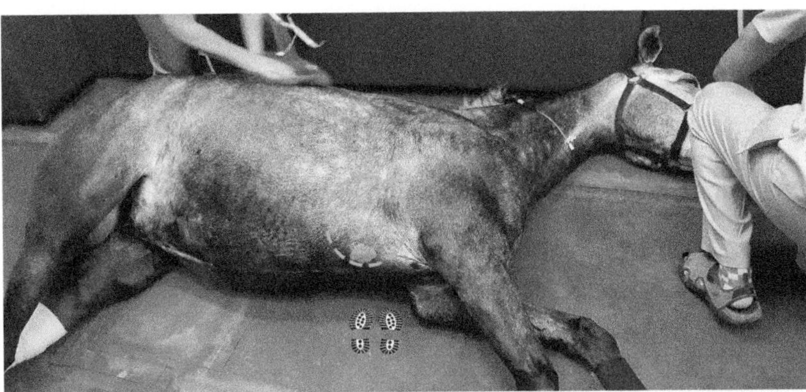

Figure 20.12 The resuscitator can perform chest compression by standing caudal to the thoracic limbs (boot prints) and repetitively kneel on the thorax over the area of the heart (green circle).

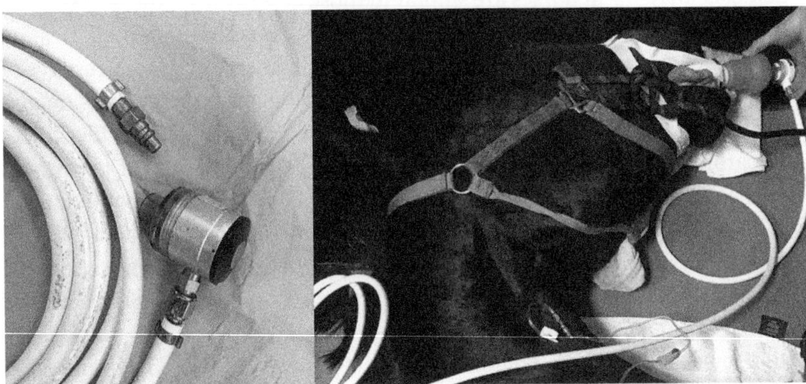

Figure 20.13 A demand valve (left) can be used to provide oxygen support and deliver a manual breath to the horse (right). To deliver a manual breath, the demand valve is connected to an oxygen supply and attached to the breathing circuit end of the endotracheal tube. The activation button is pressed and held to inflate the lungs with oxygen. The activation button should be held until a chest rise is seen. Care should be exercised in small horses and foals as the lungs will inflate quickly, with a risk of barotrauma if the inflation time is excessive.

(e.g., naloxone, atipamezole, etc.). Physiologic monitoring and intravenous access are discussed in the following text.

Resuscitation of foals is more likely to be successful than in adult horses, primarily because their small body size permits more effective chest compressions. Depending on size, compressions can either be performed directly over the heart (foals < 50 kg) or over the widest part of the thorax (foals > 50 kg), as described in the section for small animals. The recommended compression rate is 100–120 compressions per minute. As in smaller species, there should be adequate time for thoracic recoil between compressions, and compressions should continue for minimum periods of 2 min, minimizing the duration and frequency of any pauses (e.g., to assess the ECG or change the person performing compressions). For ventilation, endotracheal intubation (via nasal or oral route, or tracheostomy) is recommended but mouth-to-nostril ventilation can be successful. For mouth-to-nostril ventilation, one nostril should be occluded as air is blown into the other. The recommended ventilation rate is 10 breaths per minute.

For both adult horses and foals, physiologic monitoring should be used to monitor ROSC. Capnography and ECG are the key physiologic variables to be monitored as these will also guide CPR efforts. As with small animals, epinephrine (and/or vasopressin) should be administered IV every 3–5 min early in CPR. Atropine use in alive anesthetized horses is controversial since the drug is highly likely to cause ileus in horses. However, horses have a high vagal tone; therefore, at least a single dose of atropine (IV) during CPR is warranted. Furthermore, animals in CPA have an absence of circulation and organ perfusion (i.e., death). This situation does not promote gastrointestinal function, rendering a decision to avoid administering atropine questionable. Intestinal motility can be addressed if the horse survives. Drug doses in horses are the same as those listed for small animals.

As with other species, early identification of pending arrest and vigorous post-CPA care are imperative to raise the likelihood of a successful outcome. More information on CPR in horses can be found in Further Reading.

Questions and Answers

There are more practice questions and answers available for this chapter on the website. Please visit http://www.wiley.com/go/VeterinaryAnesthesiaZeiler.

Questions

1) What are the core components of basic life support when performing cardiopulmonary resuscitation?
2) What are the recommended physiologic variables that should be monitored to guide a cardiopulmonary resuscitation?
3) At what time interval should epinephrine be administered during cardiopulmonary resuscitation?
4) What are the target organ systems to monitor and support once return of spontaneous circulation is achieved and during the post-CPA period?

Answers

1) Chest compressions and ventilation
2) Electrocardiogram (ECG) and capnography (end-tidal carbon dioxide)
3) Every 3–5 min
4) Brain (neuroprotection) and cardiovascular (hemodynamic optimization) and respiratory (respiratory optimization) systems

Further Reading

Boller, M. and Fletcher, D.J. (2012). RECOVER evidence and knowledge gap analysis on veterinary CPR. Part 1: evidence analysis and consensus process: collaborative path toward small animal CPR guidelines. *J Vet Emerg Crit Care* 22 (Suppl 1): S4–S12.

Brainard, B.M., Boller, M., and Fletcher, D.J. (2012). RECOVER monitoring domain worksheet authors. RECOVER evidence and knowledge gap analysis on veterinary CPR. Part 5: monitoring. *J Vet Emerg Crit Care* 22 (Suppl 1): S65–S84.

Bussières, G. (2022). Equine cardiopulmonary resuscitation. In: *Manual of Equine Anesthesia and Analgesia*, 2e (eds.: T. Doherty, A. Valverde, R.A. Reed). USA: Wiley-Blackwell.

Fletcher, D.J., Boller, M., Brainard, B.M. et al. (2012). RECOVER evidence and knowledge gap analysis on veterinary CPR. Part 7: clinical guidelines. *J Vet Emerg Crit Care* 22 (Suppl 1): S102–S131.

Haynes, A., Weiser, T., Berry, W. et al. (2009). A surgical safety checklist to reduce morbidity and mortality in a global population. *N Engl J Med* 360: 491–499.

Hopper, K., Epstein, S.E., Fletcher, D.J., and Boller, M. (2012). RECOVER basic life support domain worksheet authors. RECOVER evidence and knowledge gap analysis on veterinary CPR. Part 3: basic life support. *J Vet Emerg Crit Care* 22 (Suppl 1): S26–S43.

Ludders, J.W. and McMillan, M. (2016). *Errors in Veterinary Anesthesia*, 1e. USA: Wiley-Blackwell.

McMichael, M., Herring, J., Fletcher, D.J., and Boller, M. (2012). RECOVER preparedness and prevention domain worksheet authors. RECOVER evidence and knowledge gap analysis on veterinary CPR. Part 2: preparedness and prevention. *J Vet Emerg Crit Care* 22 (Suppl 1): S13–S25.

McMillan, M. and Pang, D. (2023). An Introduction to patient safety. In: *Veterinary Anesthesia and Analgesia*, 6e (eds.: K. Grimm, L. Lamont, W. Tranquilli et al.). USA: Wiley-Blackwell.

Pang, D., Rousseau-Blass, F., and Pang, J. (2018) Morbidity and mortality conferences: a mini review and illustrated application in veterinary medicine. *Front Vet Sci* 5:43.

Pang, J., Yates, E., and Pang, D. (2021). A closed "pop-off" valve and patient safety incident: a human factors approach to understanding error. *Vet Rec Case Rep* 9: e189.

Pang, D. (2022). Accident and error management. In: *Equine Anesthesia and Co-Existing Disease* (ed. S. Clark-Price, K. Mama), 352–384. Hoboken, NJ: Wiley-Blackwell.

Reason, J. (2008). *The Human Contribution*. Hampshire: Ashgate Publishing Limited.

Rozanski, E.A., Rush, J.E., Buckley, G.J. et al. (2012). RECOVER advanced life support domain worksheet authors. RECOVER evidence and knowledge gap analysis on veterinary CPR. Part 4: advanced life support. *J Vet Emerg Crit Care* 22 (Suppl 1): S44–S64.

Runciman, W., Hibbert, P., Thomson, R. et al. (2009). Towards an international classification for patient safety: key concepts and terms. *Int J Qual Health Care* 21: 18–26.

Smarick, S.D., Haskins, S.C., Boller, M., and Fletcher, D.J. (2012). RECOVER post-cardiac arrest care domain worksheet authors. RECOVER evidence and knowledge gap analysis on veterinary CPR. Part 6: post-cardiac arrest care. *J Vet Emerg Crit Care* 22 (Suppl 1): S85–S101.

Appendix 1

RECOVER CPR Algorithms

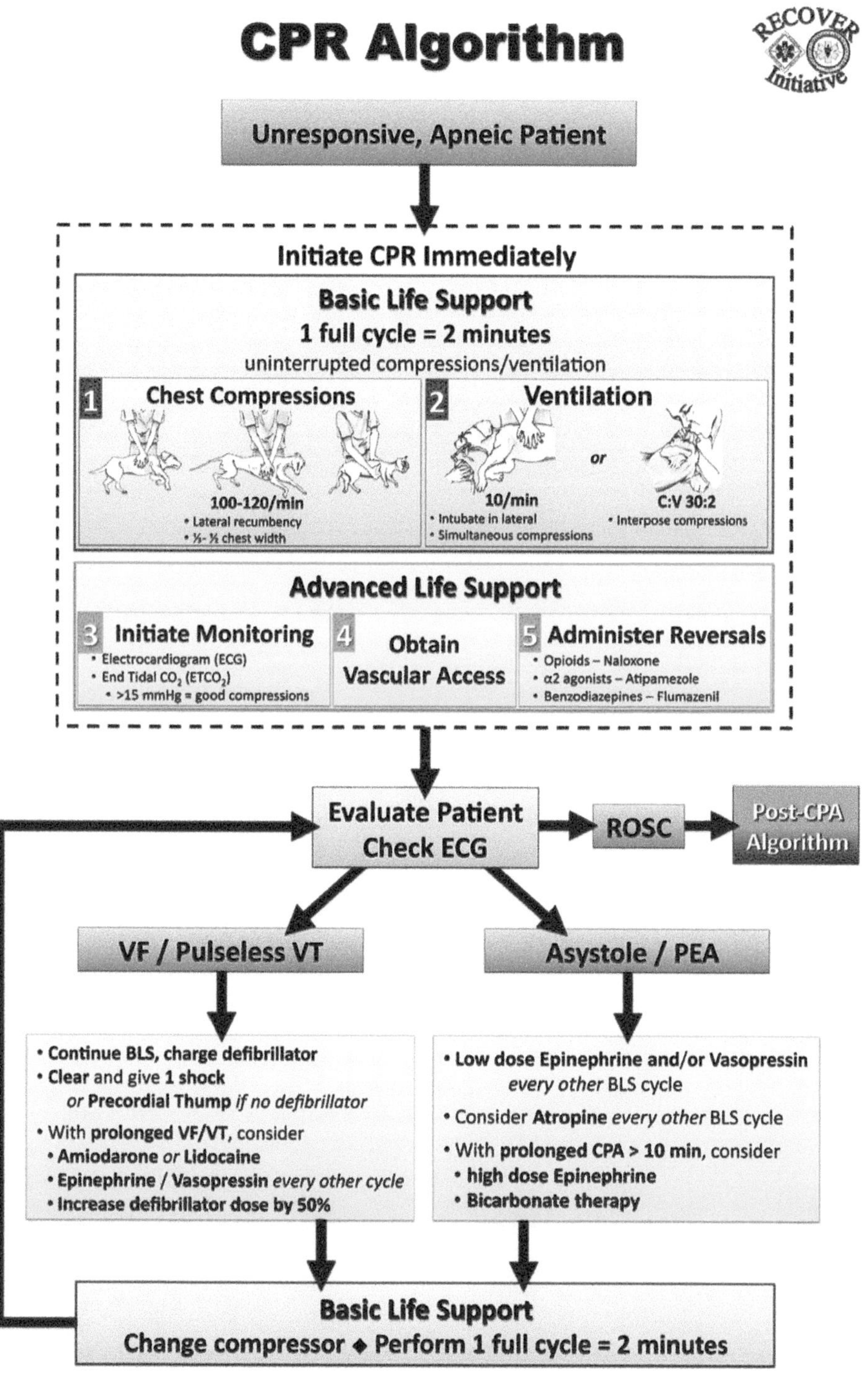

Fundamental Principles of Veterinary Anesthesia, First Edition. Edited by Gareth E. Zeiler and Daniel S. J. Pang.

Companion Website: www.wiley.com/go/VeterinaryAnesthesiaZeiler

Appendix 2

RECOVER CPR Emergency Drug Dose Charts

CPR Emergency Drugs and Doses

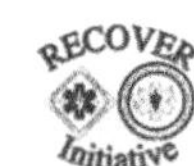

		Weight (kg)	2.5	5	10	15	20	25	30	35	40	45	50
		Weight (lb)	5	10	20	30	40	50	60	70	80	90	100
	DRUG	DOSE	ml	ml	ml	ml	ml	ml	ml	ml	ml	ml	ml
Arrest	Epi Low (1:1000; 1mg/ml) every other BLS cycle x3	0.01 mg/kg	0.03	0.05	0.1	0.15	0.2	0.25	0.3	0.35	0.4	0.45	0.5
Arrest	Epi High (1:1000; 1 mg/ml) for prolonged CPR	0.1 mg/kg	0.25	0.5	1	1.5	2	2.5	3	3.5	4	4.5	5
Arrest	Vasopressin (20 U/ml)	0.8 U/kg	0.1	0.2	0.4	0.6	0.8	1	1.2	1.4	1.6	1.8	2
Arrest	Atropine (0.54 mg/ml)	0.04 mg/kg	0.2	0.4	0.8	1.1	1.5	1.9	2.2	2.6	3	3.3	3.7
Anti-Arrhyth	Amiodarone (50 mg/ml)	5 mg/kg	0.25	0.5	1	1.5	2	2.5	3	3.5	4	4.5	5
Anti-Arrhyth	Lidocaine (20 mg/ml)	2 mg/kg	0.25	0.5	1	1.5	2	2.5	3	3.5	4	4.5	5
Reversal	Naloxone (0.4 mg/ml)	0.04 mg/kg	0.25	0.5	1	1.5	2	2.5	3	3.5	4	4.5	5
Reversal	Flumazenil (0.1 mg/ml)	0.01 mg/kg	0.25	0.5	1	1.5	2	2.5	3	3.5	4	4.5	5
Reversal	Atipamezole (5 mg/ml)	100 µg/kg	0.06	0.1	0.2	0.3	0.4	0.5	0.6	0.7	0.8	0.9	1
Defib Monophasic	External Defib (J)	4-6 J/kg	10	20	40	60	80	100	120	140	160	180	200
Defib Monophasic	Internal Defib (J)	0.5-1 J/kg	2	3	5	8	10	15	15	20	20	20	25

Fundamental Principles of Veterinary Anesthesia, First Edition. Edited by Gareth E. Zeiler and Daniel S. J. Pang.

Companion Website: www.wiley.com/go/VeterinaryAnesthesiaZeiler

Appendix 3

Checklists

Anaesthetic Safety Checklist

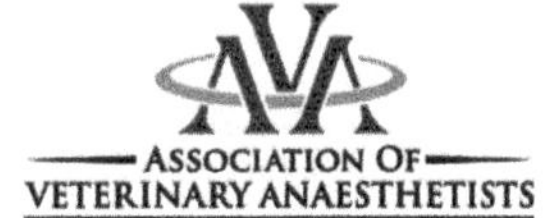

Pre-Induction

- ☐ Patient NAME, owner CONSENT & PROCEDURE confirmed
- ☐ IV CANNULA placed & patent
- ☐ AIRWAY EQUIPMENT available & functioning
- ☐ Endotracheal tube CUFFS checked
- ☐ ANAESTHETIC MACHINE checked today
- ☐ Adequate OXYGEN for proposed procedure
- ☐ BREATHING SYSTEM connected, leak free & APL VALVE OPEN
- ☐ Person assigned to MONITOR patient
- ☐ RISKS identified & COMMUNICATED
- ☐ EMERGENCY INTERVENTIONS available

Pre-Procedure — Time Out

- ☐ Patient NAME & PROCEDURE confirmed
- ☐ DEPTH of anaesthesia appropriate
- ☐ SAFETY CONCERNS COMMUNICATED

Recovery

- ☐ SAFETY CONCERNS COMMUNICATED
  Airway, Breathing, Circulation (fluid balance), Body Temperature, Pain
- ☐ ASSESSMENT & INTERVENTION PLAN confirmed
- ☐ ANALGESIC PLAN confirmed
- ☐ Person assigned to MONITOR patient

This checklist was written by the AVA with design and distribution support from 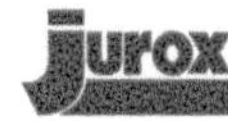

Fundamental Principles of Veterinary Anesthesia, First Edition. Edited by Gareth E. Zeiler and Daniel S. J. Pang.

Companion Website: www.wiley.com/go/VeterinaryAnesthesiaZeiler

Recommended Procedures

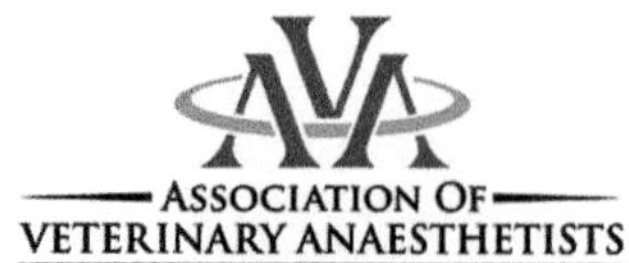

Pre-Anaesthesia

★ Has anything significant been identified in the history and/or clinical examination?

★ Do any abnormalities warrant further investigation?

★ Can any abnormalities be stabilised prior to anaesthesia?

★ What complications are anticipated during anaesthesia?

★ How can these complications be managed?

★ Would the patient benefit from premedication?

★ How will any pain associated with the procedure be managed?

★ How will anaesthesia be induced & maintained?

★ How will the patient be monitored?

★ How will the patient's body temperature be maintained?

★ How will the patient be managed in the post-anaesthetic period?

★ Are the required facilities, personnel & drugs available?

Anaesthetic Machine

- ☐ PRIMARY OXYGEN source checked
- ☐ BACK-UP OXYGEN available
- ☐ OXYGEN ALARM working (if present)
- ☐ FLOWMETERS working
- ☐ VAPORISER attached and full
- ☐ Anaesthetic machine passes LEAK TEST
- ☐ SCAVENGING checked
- ☐ Available MONITORING equipment functioning
- ☐ EMERGENCY equipment and drugs checked

Drugs / Equipment

- Endotracheal tubes (cuffs checked)
- Airway aids (e.g. laryngoscope, urinary catheter, lidocaine spray, suction, guide-wire/stylet)
- Self-inflating bag (or demand valve for equine anaesthetics)
- Epinephrine/adrenaline
- Atropine
- Antagonists (e.g. atipamezole, naloxone/butorphanol)
- Intravenous cannulae
- Isotonic crystalloid solution
- Fluid administration set

Drug charts & CPR algorithm (http://www.acvecc-recover.org/)

This checklist was written by the AVA with design and distribution support from 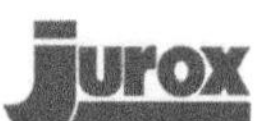

Pre-anesthesia checkout procedure (including machine leak test)

A pre-anesthesia checkout procedure is considered an important step in the safe provision of anesthesia. Failure to properly check anesthesia equipment is associated with patient morbidity and mortality.[1,2]

^before the first case of the day
*before each use

1. ^Electrical supply: check anesthetic machine is connected to the electrical supply (if applicable) and switched on.
2. Oxygen
   a. ^Confirm secondary oxygen source (oxygen cylinder) is available and functioning
      i. Open cylinder valve, check adequate contents (usually at least 50% full, or 1000 psig) and close cylinder valve (unless cylinder will be primary oxygen source).
   b. ^Pipeline gas: confirm gas pressure is ≥ 50 psig (400 kPa)
      i. perform "tug test" - ensure correct and secure connection between pipeline (gas hose) and supply terminal (socket).
3. Vaporizer(s)
   a. *Check vaporizers are adequately filled and filling ports are closed.
   b. ^Check that vaporizers are properly seated on back bar and secured.
   c. ^Check vaporizer dial turns smoothly throughout range.
   d. *Turn off at end of testing and ensure off before use.
4. *Carbon dioxide absorbent
   a. Check absorbent is not exhausted (colour change may be lost if absorbent has not been used for some time - capnography during anesthesia recommended).
5. ^Flowmeter
   a. Confirm flow valve operates and that bobbin moves smoothly throughout full range.
6. Confirm function of emergency oxygen flush valve: gas flow is present when activated, without a decrease in pipeline pressure, and flow stops when control released.
7. Leak test
   a. ^Vaporizer leak test
      i. Turn on oxygen (approx. 3 l/min) and occlude common gas outlet with vaporizer dial in on and off position. Flowmeter bobbin should dip.
   b. *Breathing system leak testing
      i. Visually inspect system components to confirm correct assembly and free of obstruction.
      ii. Connect system securely to common gas outlet.
      iii. Circle leak test: occlude patient end (hand or plug), close APL valve and pressurize system via oxygen flowmeter to approx. 30 cmH_2O. Turn off oxygen flow and observe pressure gauge. Pressure should be maintained for 10 seconds. Open APL valve and confirm that reservoir bag deflates (pressure gauge should return to zero). Uncover/unplug patient end. A leak rate of ≤ 200 ml/min is considered acceptable.

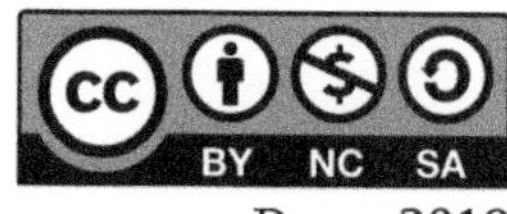

(1) Check unidirectional valve function (see "Two-bag test", below).
(2) If a co-axial Circle system is in use, confirm inner limb connection as described below for Bain system.

iv. Bain leak test: occlude patient end (hand or plug), close APL valve and pressurize system via oxygen flowmeter to approx. 30 cmH_2O. Turn off oxygen flow and observe pressure gauge. Pressure should be maintained for 10 seconds. Open APL valve and confirm that reservoir bag deflates (pressure gauge should return to zero). Uncover/unplug patient end. A leak rate of ≤ 200 ml/min is considered acceptable.
(1) Test inner limb of system: with oxygen flowing at approx. 3 L/min, occlude inner limb (plunger from 3 ml syringe) - flowmeter bobbin should dip.

v. Two-bag test: perform after checking vaporizer(s) and breathing system. Attach reservoir bag to patient end of breathing system, turn on oxygen (3 l/min) and manually ventilate.
(1) Confirm whole breathing system is patent.
(2) Circle system: observe unidirectional valve function during manual ventilation.
(3) APL valve: squeeze both reservoir bags to check APL valve.

8. ^Anesthetic gas scavenging system
   a. Check that active scavenging system is correctly connected to machine and breathing system.
   b. Confirm that reservoir bag deflates at conclusion of leak test.
   c. Occlude patient end of breathing system and activate emergency oxygen flush valve with APL valve open. Confirm that breathing system pressure gauge reading is below 10 cmH_2O.
   d. If using a charcoal cannister passive scavenging system, ensure that bottom holes are not occluded and confirm in records that charcoal is not exhausted (if in doubt, weigh and refer to manufacturer guidelines).
9. *Ensure required monitors are available, connected to the electrical supply and switched on.
   a. Confirm gas sampling lines are unobstructed and connected.
   b. Check appropriate frequency of NIBP measurement is selected.
   c. Check alarm limits are appropriate (where available).
10. *Check that ancillary equipment is available and working: this includes laryngoscope, ET tubes, tube tie, gauze.
11. *Log: document completion of checkout procedure (date, time, initial) in patient record.

NB: this checkout procedure was developed for the machines in current use at the UCVM (2019) and is not exhaustive. Users should be familiar with the specific requirements of their equipment.

Adapted from: AAGBI Safety Guideline (Anaesthesia 2012 67:660-668), Recommendations for Pre-Anesthesia Checkout Procedures (2008) Sub-Committee of ASA Committee on Equipment and Facilities, the BSAVA Manual of Small Animal Anaesthesia and Analgesia (chapters 4 and 5) and Ward's Anaesthetic Equipment (5th edition).

[1]Cooper JB, Newbower RS, Kitz RJ. An Analysis of Major Errors and Equipment Failures in

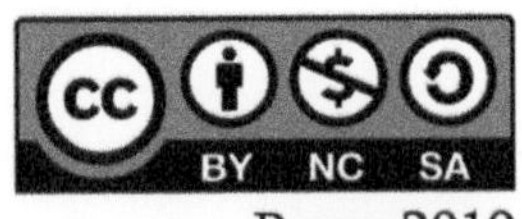

Anesthesia Management: Considerations for Prevention and Detection. Anesthesiology 1984;60:34-42.

[2]Arbous MS, Meursing AE, van Kleef JW, de Lange JJ. Impact of Anesthesia Management Characteristics on Severe Morbidity and Mortality. Anesthesiology 2005; 102:257–68

ANESTHETIC EQUIPMENT CHECKLIST

Carbon Dioxide Absorbent

- ☐ Change the CO_2 absorbent regularly based on individual anesthesia machine manufacturer recommendations.
- ☐ The useful lifespan of absorbent varies with the patient size and fresh gas flow rate.
- ☐ Color change is not an accurate indicator of remaining absorption capacity.

Oxygen

- ☐ Ensure supply lines are attached.
- ☐ Ensure the flowmeter is functioning.
- ☐ Ensure the supply tank and at least one spare tank are sufficiently full.
    - To calculate the estimated remaining tank volume, follow this example: *An E-cylinder contains 660 L, and has a full pressure of 2,200 psi. Pressure drop is proportional to remaining O_2 volume. A tank with 500 psi has 150 L. When used at a flow rate of 1 L/min, it will last approximately 2.5 hours.*

Endotracheal Tubes and Masks

- ☐ Have access to various sizes of masks and endotracheal tubes.
- ☐ Provide a light source such as a laryngoscope.
- ☐ Check cuff integrity and amount of air needed to properly inflate the cuff.

Breathing System

- ☐ Refer to anesthesia machine's documentation for proper leak-checking procedures.
- ☐ Conduct a check before every procedure.
- ☐ Select the appropriate size and type of reservoir bag and breathing circuit.
- ☐ Non-rebreathing systems are generally used in patients weighing less than 5–7 kg or when the work of breathing associated with the circle system might not be easily sustainable by an individual patient.

Inhalant

- ☐ Ensure the vaporizer is sufficiently full.

Waste-Scavenging Equipment

- ☐ Verify a functioning scavenging system.
- ☐ If using a charcoal absorbent canister, ensure there is sufficient capacity remaining for the duration of the procedure.
- ☐ Observe all regulations concerning the dispersion of waste anesthesia gases.

Electronic Monitoring Equipment

- ☐ Ensure devices are operational and either are connected to a power source or have adequate battery reserve.
- ☐ Check alarms for limits and activation.

Bednarski, Richard, Kurt Grimm, Ralph Harvey, et al. "AAHA Anesthesia Guidelines for Dogs and Cats," *Journal of the American Animal Hospital Association* 47, no. 6 (Nov/Dec 2011): 381, https://doi.org/10.5326/JAAHA-MS-5846.

UCVM
Pre-induction checklist

When should this be used?
Before induction of general anesthesia.
Who should be present?
All members of anesthesia team.

- ☐ **CONFIRM VERBALLY** with all team members: patient ID, owner consent, procedure & site

- ☐ **IV ACCESS** patent
- ☐ **AIRWAY EQUIPMENT** prepared and tested:
  ET tubes [3], cuffs tested, tube tie, laryngoscope, lube, gauze
- ☐ **ET TUBE** insertion depth **PRE-MEASURED**

- ☐ **ANAESTHETIC MACHINE** checked today
- ☐ Breathing system **LEAK TESTED** for this case
- ☐ **APL VALVE** open
- ☐ **OXYGEN** pipeline supply **CONNECTED**
- ☐ **ADEQUATE OXYGEN** in E cylinder

- ☐ **DISTRIBUTION OF TASKS** between team members

- ☐ Patient/procedureal **RISKS IDENTIFIED & COMMUNICATED**

- ☐ **EMERGENCY INTERVENTIONS** available

Used in conjunction with: 1) pre-anesthesia checkout procedure, 2) pre-anesthesia equipment checklist

Adapted from: The Association of Veterinary Anaesthetists Anaesthetic Safety Checklist

Designed by: DSJ Pang (2019), VSY Leung

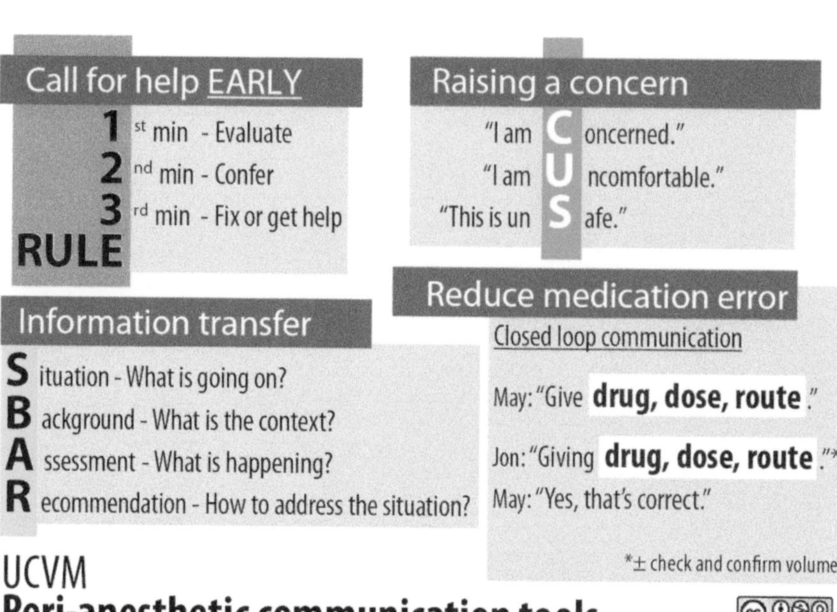

UCVM
Peri-anesthetic communication tools

Designed by: VSY Leung

Appendix 4

Peri-anesthetic Monitoring Sheets

Click here to add logo

Anaesthesia record

Date:

ASSOCIATION OF VETERINARY ANAESTHETISTS

Name:
Owner:
Breed:
Age: Sex:
Weight:
Anaesthetist:
Clinician:

History:

Clinical findings/results/medications:

Temperament:
HR: RR:
Pulse quality:
MM: CRT:
Thoracic auscultation:
Temperature: °C

ASA classification
- I No organic disease
- II Mild systemic disease
- III Severe systemic disease (not incapacitating)
- IV Severe disease (constant threat to life)
- V Moribund (life expectancy < 24 h)

Add 'E' for emergencies

ASA Grade:

Procedure(s):

Anticipated problems:

Pre-GA medication	Dose	Route	Time
....	....	....	....
....	....	....	....
....	....	....	....

Anaesthetic Safety Checklist completed ☐ (see overleaf)

Induction agent(s)	Dose	Route	Time
....	....	....	....
....	....	....	....

☐ IV catheter Position: Size:

ET tube / LMA / Mask | Cuffed / Uncuffed | Size:

Breathing system: ☐ Eye(s) lubricated

Fluids/Drugs/Monitoring Time

Patient position

Patient warming

Throat pack: Placed ☐ Removed ☐

Swabs: In: Out:

Sharps: In: Out:

Notes

220 210 200 190 180 170 160 150 140 130 120 110 100 90 80 70 60 50 40 30 20 10

Iso / Sevo %

O_2 / N_2O / Air L/min

SpO_2 %

Jaw tone -/+/++

Palpebral -/+

Eye position ↓ / →

Symbols
- ● HR
- o RR ø IPPV
- v SAP – MAP ^ DAP
- ⊗ Doppler

RECOVERY instructions:

	T+0	T+15	T+30	T+45
Time				
Heart rate				
Resp. rate				
MM & CRT				
Temp.				
Pain score				

IV catheter care: ☐ Remove once recovered ☐ Maintain & flush

Fundamental Principles of Veterinary Anesthesia, First Edition. Edited by Gareth E. Zeiler and Daniel S. J. Pang.

Companion Website: www.wiley.com/go/VeterinaryAnesthesiaZeiler

Index

Note: Page numbers in *italics* refer to figures; those in **bold** to tables.

Fundamental Principles of Veterinary Anesthesia, First Edition. Edited by Gareth E. Zeiler and Daniel S. J. Pang.

Companion Website: www.wiley.com/go/VeterinaryAnesthesiaZeiler

b

d